Current and Emerging Therapies in Pancreatic Cancer

Contents

1 **Pancreatic Cancer Epidemiology and Environmental Risk Factors** 1
Mahender Yellu, Chandana Kamireddy, and Olugbenga O. Olowokure

2 **Anatomy of the Pancreas and Biliary Tree** 23
Constantinos P. Zambirinis and Peter J. Allen

3 **Pathology: Premalignant and Malignant Diseases and Molecular Genetics** 49
Wei Chen, Ming Jin, and Wendy L. Frankel

4 **Screening for Pancreatic Cancer: Who to Screen and How to Follow-Up?** 97
Phil A. Hart, Peter P. Stanich, and Heather Hampel

5 **Staging and Prognostic Implications** 109
Amit Mahipal and Richard Kim

6 **Current and Emerging Therapies in Pancreatic Cancer** 119
Maria Diab and Philip A. Philip

7 **Imaging of Pancreatic Malignancies** 135
Ferenc Czeyda-Pommersheim, Bobby Kalb, and Diego Martin

8 **Advanced Endoscopic Procedures** 151
James J. Farrell

9 **How to Treat Resectable Disease** 171
Mary Dillhoff and Mark Bloomston

10 **The Management of Locally Advanced Nonmetastatic Pancreas Cancer** 183
Brent T. Xia, Young Kim, and Syed A. Ahmad

11 Cytotoxic Therapy in Advanced Pancreatic Cancer: Where We Are and Where We Are Headed 205
Namrata Vijayvergia and Steven J. Cohen

12 Molecularly Targeted Therapies in Pancreatic Cancer 219
Walid L. Shaib and Bassel F. El-Rayes

13 Targeting the Tumor Microenvironment 235
Julia Carnevale and Andrew H. Ko

14 Synthetic Lethality: Achilles Heel in Select Patient Subpopulations 257
Min Yuen Teo and Eileen M. O'Reilly

15 Immunotherapies in Pancreatic Cancer 271
Mohamad Bassam Sonbol and Mitesh J. Borad

16 Vaccine Therapy in Pancreatic Cancer 281
Benjamin A. Weinberg and Michael J. Pishvaian

17 Virotherapies in Pancreatic Cancer 309
Daniel H. Ahn and Ramesh Ramanathan

18 Novel Radiotherapy Modalities 323
Lauren M. Rosati, Shalini Moningi, Lauren Colbert, Sweet Ping Ng, and Joseph M. Herman

19 The Role for Palliative Surgical Interventions in Pancreatic Cancer 349
Alexandra G. Lopez-Aguiar and Shishir K. Maithel

20 Current and Emerging Therapies in Pancreatic Cancer: Do They Provide Value? 361
Astrid Belalcazar and Olatunji B. Alese

Index 369

Contributors

Syed A. Ahmad, M.D. Division of Surgical Oncology, Department of Surgery, The University of Cincinnati Medical Center, Cincinnati, OH, USA

Daniel H. Ahn, D.O. Mayo Clinic, Department of Hematology/Medical Oncology, Phoenix, AZ, USA

Olatunji B. Alese Winship Cancer Institute, Emory University, Atlanta, GA, USA

Peter J. Allen, M.D. Hepatopancreatobiliary Service, Department of Surgery, Memorial Sloan Kettering Cancer Center, New York, NY, USA

Astrid Belalcazar Winship Cancer Institute, Emory University, Atlanta, GA, USA

Mark Bloomston, M.D. 21st Century Oncology, Fort Myers, FL, USA

Mitesh J. Borad, M.D. Department of Hematology/Medical Oncology, Mayo Clinic, Phoenix, AZ, USA

Julia Carnevale, M.D. Helen Diller Family Comprehensive Cancer Center, University of California San Francisco, San Francisco, CA, USA

Wei Chen, M.D., Ph.D. Department of Pathology, The Ohio State University Wexner Medical Center, Columbus, OH, USA

Steven J. Cohen, M.D. Abington Hospital-Jefferson Health, Abington, PA, USA

Lauren Colbert, M.D., M.S. Department of Radiation Oncology, MD Anderson Cancer Center, University of Texas, Houston, TX, USA

Ferenc Czeyda-Pommersheim, M.D. Department of Medical Imaging, Banner-University, Tucson, AZ, USA

Maria Diab Wayne State University, Detroit, MI, USA

Mary Dillhoff, M.D., M.S. James Cancer Center and Solove Research Institute, Ohio State University, Columbus, OH, USA

Bassel El-Rayes, M.D. Department of Hematology and Oncology, Winship Cancer Institute, Emory University, Atlanta, GA, USA

James J. Farrell, M.D. Yale Pancreatic Disease Program, Interventional Endoscopy, Yale University School of Medicine, New Haven, CT, USA

Wendy L. Frankel, M.D. Department of Pathology, The Ohio State University Wexner Medical Center, Columbus, OH, USA

Heather Hampel, M.S., C.G.C. Division of Human Genetics, The Ohio State University Wexner Medical Center, Columbus, OH, USA

Phil A. Hart, M.D. Division of Gastroenterology, Hepatology, and Nutrition, The Ohio State University Wexner Medical Center, Columbus, OH, USA

Joseph M. Herman, M.D., M.Sc. Department of Radiation Oncology and Molecular Radiation Sciences, The Johns Hopkins University School of Medicine, Baltimore, MD, USA

Department of Radiation Oncology, MD Anderson Cancer Center, University of Texas, Houston, TX, USA

Ming Jin, M.D., Ph.D. Department of Pathology, The Ohio State University Wexner Medical Center, Columbus, OH, USA

Bobby Kalb, M.D. Department of Medical Imaging, Banner University Medical center, Tucson, AZ, USA

Chandana Kamireddy, M.D. Department of Internal Medicine, University of Cincinnati, Cincinnati, OH, USA

Young Kim, M.D. Division of Surgical Oncology, Department of Surgery, The University of Cincinnati Medical Center, Cincinnati, OH, USA

Richard Kim, M.D. Department of Gastrointestinal Oncology, Moffitt Cancer Center, Tampa, FL, USA

Andrew H. Ko, M.D. Helen Diller Family Comprehensive Cancer Center, University of California San Francisco, San Francisco, CA, USA

Alexandra G. Lopez-Aguiar, M.D. Winship Cancer Institute, Division of Surgical Oncology, Department of Surgery, Atlanta, GA, USA

Amit Mahipal, M.B.B.S., M.P.H. Department of Oncology, Mayo Clinic, Rochester, MN, USA

Shishir K. Maithel, M.D. Winship Cancer Institute, Division of Surgical Oncology, Department of Surgery, Atlanta, GA, USA

Diego Martin, M.D., Ph.D. Department of Medical Imaging, Banner University Medical Center, Tucson, AZ, USA

Shalini Moningi, M.D. Department of Radiation Oncology, MD Anderson Cancer Center, University of Texas, Houston, TX, USA

Sweet Ping Ng, M.B.B.S., B.Med.Sci. Department of Radiation Oncology, MD Anderson Cancer Center, University of Texas, Houston, TX, USA

Eileen M. O'Reilly Department of Medicine, Memorial Sloan Kettering Cancer Center, New York, NY, USA

Weill Cornell Medical College, New York, NY, USA

Olugbenga O. Olowokure, M.D. Division of Hematology and Oncology, University of Cincinnati, Cincinnati, OH, USA

Philip A. Philip, M.D. Karmanos Cancer Institute, Wayne State University, Detroit, MI, USA

Michael J. Pishvaian, M.D., Ph.D. Division of Hematology and Oncology, Lombardi Comprehensive Cancer Center, Georgetown University, Washington, DC, USA

Ramesh Ramanathan, M.D. Mayo Clinic, Department of Hematology/Medical Oncology, Phoenix, AZ, USA

Lauren M. Rosati, B.S. Department of Radiation Oncology and Molecular Radiation Sciences, The Johns Hopkins University School of Medicine, Baltimore, MD, USA

Sidney Kimmel Comprehensive Cancer Center, The Johns Hopkins University School of Medicine, Baltimore, MD, USA

Walid Shaib, M.D. Department of Hematology and Oncology, Winship Cancer Institute, Emory University, Atlanta, GA, USA

Mohamad Bassam Sonbol, M.D. Department of Hematology/Medical Oncology, Mayo Clinic, Phoenix, AZ, USA

Peter P. Stanich, M.D. Division of Gastroenterology, Hepatology, and Nutrition, The Ohio State University Wexner Medical Center, Columbus, OH, USA

Min Yuen Teo Department of Medicine, Memorial Sloan Kettering Cancer Center, New York, NY, USA

Namrata Vijayvergia, M.D. Fox Chase Cancer Center, Philadelphia, PA, USA

Benjamin A. Weinberg, M.D. Division of Hematology and Oncology, Lombardi Comprehensive Cancer Center, Georgetown University, Washington, DC, USA

Brent T. Xia, M.D. Division of Surgical Oncology, Department of Surgery, The University of Cincinnati Medical Center, Cincinnati, OH, USA

Mahender Yellu, M.D. Division of Hematology and Oncology, University of Cincinnati, Cincinnati, OH, USA

Constantinos P. Zambirinis, M.D., M.Res. Hepatopancreatobiliary Service, Department of Surgery, Memorial Sloan Kettering Cancer Center, New York, NY, USA

Chapter 1
Pancreatic Cancer Epidemiology and Environmental Risk Factors

Mahender Yellu, Chandana Kamireddy, and Olugbenga O. Olowokure

Pancreatic cancer (PC) is one of the leading causes of cancer deaths worldwide. It is the fourth leading cause of cancer-related death in both men and women in the United States and has <10% 5-year overall survival rate for all stages [1]. Worldwide, PC is the eighth leading cause of cancer death in men (about 138,100 deaths annually) and the ninth in women (about 127,900 deaths annually). In general it affects more individuals residing in the Western and industrialized parts of the world with the highest incidence reported in New Zealand, Black American and Hawaiians and the lowest incidence reported among people living in Nigeria and India [2, 3]. Based on data obtained from the surveillance epidemiology and end results (SEER) database, the incidence and death rate of PC is 12.4 and 10.9 per 100,000 men and women per year, respectively. In the United States, an estimated 53,070 people will be diagnosed with PC in the year 2016, and 41,780 people will die secondary to it [1]. PC occurs less commonly before age 45, but its incidence rises sharply thereafter with more than half of the patients over 70 years at diagnosis. As the average lifespan is expected to increase in the future, it is likely that PC would become more prevalent.

Over 85% of exocrine PCs are adenocarcinomas with other variants making up the rest [4]. Majority of PCs are idiopathic in nature with exception of few cases where an actual risk factor could be identified. Some of the nonfamilial risk factors that have been identified which may contribute to the development of PC include smoking, alcohol, diabetes, impaired glucose metabolism, insulin resistance, obesity, infections, coffee and non-blood group 'O'. Age is considered one of the most common risk factors with an obvious dramatic increase in incidence of PC as one gets older. Racial factor may play a role in development and outcome of PC.

M. Yellu, M.D. • O.O. Olowokure, M.D. (✉)
Division of Hematology and Oncology, University of Cincinnati,
3125 Eden Ave, Cincinnati, OH 45219, USA
e-mail: olowokoo@ucmail.uc.edu

C. Kamireddy, M.D.
Department of Internal Medicine, University of Cincinnati, Cincinnati, OH, USA

T. Bekaii-Saab, B. El-Rayes (eds.), *Current and Emerging Therapies in Pancreatic Cancer*, DOI 10.1007/978-3-319-58256-6_1

Analysis based from the SEER database in the United States reveals African Americans having the highest incidence of PC and American Indian/Alaska natives are at lowest risk (Fig. 1.1) [1]. These are closely mirrored by the death rates with blacks having the highest (Fig. 1.2). Asians are found to have better survival which may be attributed to the aggressiveness of the disease, timing of diagnosis and operative approaches. Blacks appear to have more frequent Kras mutations as opposed to other races [5].

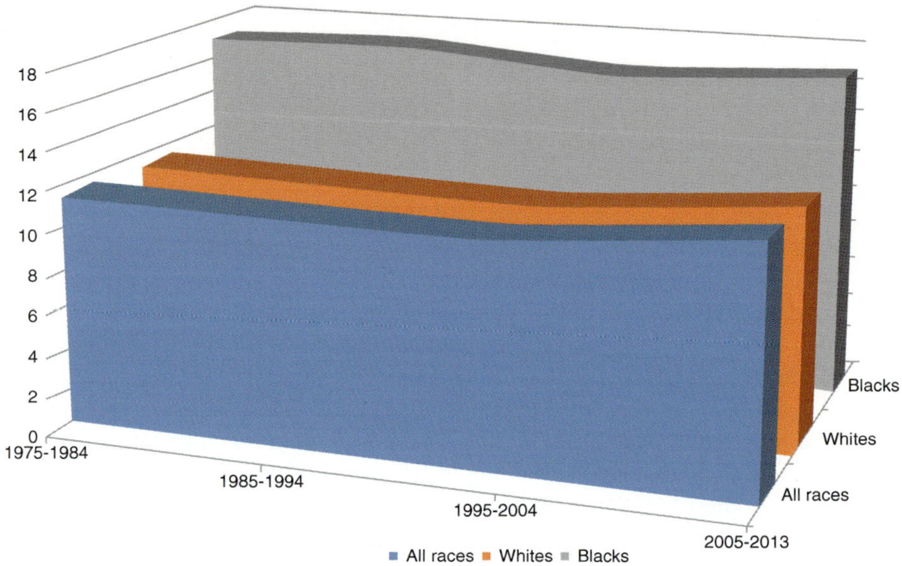

Fig. 1.1 US average age-adjusted incidence rates (per 100,000) by all races, whites and blacks

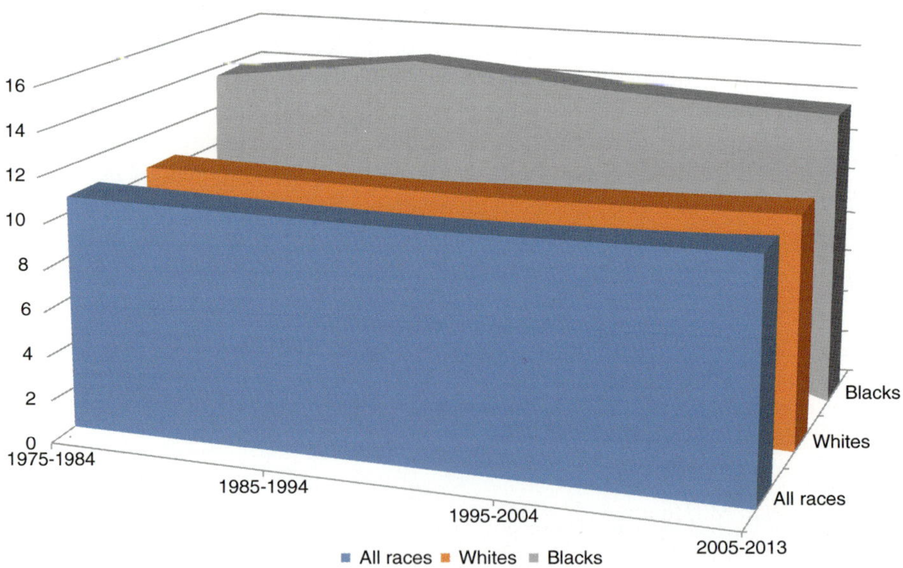

Fig. 1.2 US average age-adjusted death rates (per 100,000) by all races, whites and blacks

Inherited Risk Factors

Familial Pancreatic Cancer

Approximately 5–10% of patients have a family history of PC, and it is estimated that 10–15% of patients will have a genetic cause specific for PC [6]. Risk appears to be particularly high for individuals from families with a case of PC diagnosed under the age of 50. Patients from affected families tend to present at an earlier age than those with non-inherited disease [7]. Patients with family history of PCs may present at a later stage similar to sporadic PC [8]. Inherited PC is broadly divided into two categories, familial PC in which a specific genetic abnormality has not been identified and defined syndromes in which patients are at increased risk for PC and various other malignancies. Familial pancreatic cancer (FPC) is generally defined as a patient who does not meet the criteria for a known genetic predisposition syndrome but has an inherited predisposition based upon family clustering in families with multiple first and second degree relatives with adenocarcinoma of the pancreas.

Inherited genes alone may be inadequate to cause PC, but it is suspected that a complex interaction of many factors leads to the development of PC. Some of them include variable gene penetrance, environmental factors, family size and chance.

The risk of developing PC in FPC depends on the number of affected blood relatives. For example, first-degree relatives of patients with PC are at highest risk, and this is supported by two prospective studies. Families enrolled in National Familial Pancreas Tumor Registry were followed to estimate the risk and incidence of PC in first-degree relatives of patients with PC. This was compared with the SEER database [8] and revealed an 18-fold increase in PC in patients with first-degree relatives having PC and 57-fold increase in patients with three or more family members affected with PC [8]. This study concluded that the risk was largely confined to relatives over age 60 years and recommended screening high-risk patients. An extension of this study was performed with an increased study population of 5179 individuals of whom 3957 individuals had at least one first-degree relative with PC from 839 kindreds (370 familial PC kindreds, 468 sporadic PC kindreds). The study revealed that the expected rate of PC was significantly elevated in members of familial PC kindreds [9.0; 95% confidence interval (CI), 4.5–16.1] but not in the SPC kindreds (1.8; 95% CI, 0.22–6.4). In individuals with three, two or one first-degree relatives, the risk was (32.0; 95% CI, 10.2–74.7), (6.4; CI, 1.8–16.4) and (4.6; CI, 0.5–16.4), respectively [6].

In a Canadian population-based study, an attempt to analyse germline mutations was made using next-generation sequencing and a custom multiple gene panel [9]. Probands were selected from Ontario Pancreas Cancer Study (OPCS) and included a sample size of 290 patients. Eleven pathogenic mutations were identified in this study including three in ATM, one in BRCA1, two in BRCA2, one in MLH1, two in MSH2, one in MSH6 and one in TP53. The prevalence of mutations in all 13 genes was 3.8% (95% confidence interval, 2.1–5.6%). Carrier status was associated significantly with breast cancer in the proband or first-degree relative ($p < 0.01$), colorectal cancer in the proband or first-degree relative (<0.01) but not family history of PC, age at diagnosis or stage at diagnosis. This study concluded that in known predisposition genes, a small but clinically important proportion of PC is associated with mutations. It also demonstrated the value of using a multiple-gene panel in PC due to the heterogeneity of mutations identified [9].

A susceptibility locus was mapped to chromosome 4q32–34 in a large kindred with family history of PC in an autosomal dominant inheritance pattern [10]. Studying all detoxifying genes, CYP1B1-4390-GG and uridine 5-diphosphoglucur onosyltransferase were found to reduce the risk of PC, whereas variants in others, such as GSTM1, increased the risk. The exact mechanism through which these genes might contribute to the development of PC is still unknown [11]. Autosomal dominant penetrance was noted in a small study of 47 patients from 18 nuclear families (defined as a family group consisting of a pair of adults and their children); two or more cases of PC was observed in the first-degree relatives [12].

Genetic Predisposition Syndromes

Hereditary Pancreatitis

Hereditary pancreatitis accounts for 3–6% of all pancreatitis. These patients have an increased risk of PC with a lifetime risk of about 40–55% [13]. There are at least three different inherited patterns, autosomal dominant hereditary pancreatitis (most common), autosomal recessive hereditary pancreatitis associated with cystic fibrosis and mutations in the serine protease inhibitor Kazal type 1 gene (SPINK-1) and complex genetics. Autosomal dominant hereditary pancreatitis is most often caused by a mutation in serine protease 1 gene (PRSS1) located on chromosome 7q35, which encodes cationic trypsinogen with variable expressivity and penetrance of about 80%. The cumulative risk of PC in a French study of 78 families with 200 patients was 10, 19 and 54 percent at 50, 60 and 75 years, respectively [13]. The same study reported that at ages 50 and 75 years, the cumulated risk of PC was 11% and 49% for men and 8% and 55% for women.

Breast Cancer-Associated Gene Mutations

Mutations in BRCA1 and BRCA2 genes have been studied, although the percentage of their association with PC has been varied. PC is considered an integral part of hereditary breast-ovarian syndrome (HBOC). BRCA2 was found to be more commonly associated with PC compared to BRCA1 [12]. Thompson et al. studied the risk of BRCA1 mutation in a population-based study of over 11,000 individuals and found a significant association with PC (RR 2.26, p 0.004) [14]. However, in a study involving 66 patients with PC from National Familial Pancreas Tumour Registry who had at least two additional relatives with PC, it was noted that none of these patients harboured BRCA1 gene mutations [15]. In another study, PC approximately doubled in female BRCA carriers [16]. In addition to several other cancers, BRCA2 was associated with PC with a relative risk of 5.9 [17]. A study with 187 Jewish patients with PC, of whom tissue was available for 145 patients. Eight subjects (5.5%) had a BRCA founder mutation (two with BRCA1 [1.3%], six with BRCA2 [4.1%]). As many mutation carriers in this series did not have a family history of typical BRCA-associated cancers, the authors suggested clinicians may wish to consider the diagnosis of pancreatic cancer in an Ashkenazi individual an independent reason to consider BRCA founder mutation testing [18].

Partner and localizer of breast cancer 2 (PALB2) gene mutations have been found to be associated with familial breast cancer in 1–2% and PC up to1–4%. BRCA2 (FANCD1) and PALB2 (FANCN) are Fanconi anaemia genes that function in a FA-breast cancer (BRCA) DNA repair pathway. Slater et al. identified three truncating mutations (3.7%) in PALB2 gene each producing different stop codons after direct sequencing of 13 exons that affected index patients of 81 FPC families [19].

Familial Atypical Multiple Mole Melanoma

Familial atypical multiple mole melanoma (FAMMM) syndrome is an autosomal dominant disorder and is associated with PC which is the second most common cancer associated with this syndrome. In this syndrome FAMMM phenotype with both malignant melanoma and PC, CDKN2A (p16) mutation was found to be significant. The affected family members could have incidence of PC over 20 times compared to the general population [20].

Peutz-Jeghers Syndrome

Peutz-Jeghers (PJ) syndrome is an autosomal dominant disorder characterized by hamartomatous gastrointestinal polyps and mucocutaneous pigmentation [21]. Germline mutations in SKT11 gene are associated with PJ syndrome and both somatic and germline mutations have been identified in patients with PC [22]. A 100-fold increase in PC was noted compared to general population in 13 unrelated kindreds with PJ syndrome [21]. In a systematic review of 1 meta-analysis and 20 cohort studies, a significant increase in PC was noted in patients with PJ syndrome [23].

Ataxia Telangiectasia

Ataxia telangiectasia (AT) is an autosomal recessive disorder, characterized by progressive cerebellar ataxia, oculocutaneous telangiectasia and cellular and humoral immune deficiency; a twofold increase in PC was observed in blood relatives of patients with AT [24]. However, the risk of PC in patients with ATM mutations is still being studied actively. In a study using next-generation sequencing, only severely affected families with three or more PC cases were studied, and this revealed four deleterious ATM mutations among 87 families ($p = 0.009$) [25].

Lynch Syndrome

Hereditary nonpolyposis colorectal cancer (HNPCC) also called Lynch syndrome is an autosomal dominant disease caused by germline mutations in mismatch repair genes (MMR), MLH1, MSH2, MSH6 and PMS2. MSH2 is the most common mutation making up to 60%, followed by MLH1 approximately 30%. The association between Lynch syndrome and PC was studied, with an increased risk identified [26]. Data analysis of over 6, 000 individuals from 147 families with MMR gene mutations revealed 21.1% of families (47 PCs) having at least one case of PC with a cumulative risk of about 1.31% up to age 50 years and 3.68% up to age 70 years representing an 8.6-fold increase in risk of PC compared to the general population [27]. Medullary phenotype and wild type Kras gene status were associated with poor differentiation; therefore, evaluation of these patients for Lynch syndrome may be useful [28].

Other Risk Factors

Chronic Pancreatitis

Chronic pancreatitis although rare, regardless of its etiology (alcoholic, non-alcoholic, hereditary, tropical), is associated with PC [29]. The risk of developing PC in chronic pancreatitis is about 5% but can be several fold higher for someone with chronic pancreatitis secondary to hereditary and tropical causes. It is believed that PC can occur after one to two decades of repeated episodes of pancreatitis; however, if it occurs 1–2 years after the initial episode of pancreatitis, it is possibly due to tumour-related ductal obstruction [30]. Multiple case-control and cohort studies have found similar increase in risk of PC in patients with chronic pancreatitis [31, 32].

Cystic Fibrosis

Cystic fibrosis (CF) has been associated with PC although the data is not as strong as for chronic pancreatitis. CF is an autosomal recessive condition caused by a defect in protein cystic fibrosis transmembrane conductance regulator (CFTR) which regulates mucus in lung and gastrointestinal tract. The risk of PC in patients with cystic fibrosis is relatively low, approximately 1/100,000/year (nine PCs in 1.2 million person-years) [33]. Since the average lifespan of cystic fibrosis is increasing, it is felt that the incidence of PC in these patients will rise in the future. Two studies analysed the risk of PC in patients with cystic fibrosis, the first one included 712 patients and found no significant excess risk, but the second study with 412 patients noted a significantly increased risk of pancreatic and small intestine cancers [34–36].

Diabetes and Glucose Metabolism

Diabetes has been linked to PC; however, conflicting reports have been published. The relationship is bidirectional, and new onset of diabetes in a middle-aged, lower BMI individual that has no family history of diabetes could increase one suspicion for an association with PC. One must however remember that until features are identified that differentiate PC-associated diabetes from other causes of new-onset diabetes, CT screening in order to discover a small number of PCs is not feasible. In some patients PC could unmask the diabetes. The incidence of PC in diabetics was found to be 2.2-fold higher than the normal population in one study, but the calculated absolute risk was much lower at 0.5% [36]. Diagnosis of diabetes within 3 years of diagnosis of PC is much more common compared to the diagnosis of other types of cancer [37]. Gestational diabetes may also increase the risk of PC [38].

In a meta-analysis of 11 case-control and 9 cohort studies of having at least 1 year elapsed between diagnosis of diabetes and PC, the relative risk of PC was 2.1 with 95% CI 1.6–2.8. The relative risk in cohort studies (RR = 2.6; 95% CI: 1.6–4.1) was found to be higher compared to case-control studies (RR = 1.8; 95% CI: 1.1–2.7). The meta-analysis concluded that patients with long standing history of diabetes may have increased risk for developing PC [39].

Abnormal glucose metabolism has been implicated in developing PC. Post-load plasma glucose concentration and risk of PC mortality were evaluated in a prospective study in the absence of self-reported diabetes [40]. This association was noted to be independent of other risk factors including age, race, cigarette smoking and BMI and was found to be unchanged within the first 5 years of follow-up even after exclusion of subjects who died due to this malignancy. The Chicago Heart Association (CHA) Detection Project in Industry cohort project with 12 years of follow-up found that the baseline glucose load was higher in patients who died of PC compared to those who have normal glucose load; however, the effect was found only in men [41]. Men who had normal glycaemic index, PC mortality and post-load plasma glucose concentration were inversely associated according to another study [42].

Pernicious Anemia and ABO Blood Group

The occurrence of atrophic gastritis with hypergastrinaemia was thought to be associated with both gastric and PC in patients with pernicious anaemia. In a 7-year follow-up of a Swedish cohort study of over 300 participants, the association between pernicious anemia and PC was found to be significant ($p < 0.02$, Poisson analysis). Pancreatic malignancy was the primary cause of death in 4% of 134 patients who died during follow-up. Among 127 unselected patients with PC, the prevalence of pernicious anemia was found to be 3% [43]. In another population-based study of patients with pernicious anemia, younger age at diagnosis was noted to be associated with PC [44]. Compared to blood group 'O' individuals, individuals with non-blood group 'O' appear to have a higher incidence of PC. An increased risk of PC in subjects with non-blood group 'O' as compared to blood group 'O' was demonstrated in one study, with two large independent prospective cohorts. The Nurses' Health Study and the Health Professionals Follow-Up Study reported incidence rates of pancreatic cancer per 100,000 person-years for blood group O, A, AB and B were 28.9, 39.9, 41.8 and 44.5, respectively [45].

Environmental Risk Factors

PC is distributed unequally throughout the world; in some countries, the incidence is as high as five to seven times compared to low-risk countries [46]. Environmental factors likely contribute to this unequal distribution. These factors among others likely include smoking, occupational exposure, alcohol, dietary habits and medications.

Smoking

An association of smoking and PC has been well known for decades, and this was particularly evident when smoking increased in Japan between 1950s and 1990s which has now plateaued due to decreased smoking. It is estimated that about 15% decrease in PC would occur if all patients who smoke suddenly stop smoking [47]. Therefore quitting smoking would reduce the incidence of a sizeable number of PC cases [47].

Smoking tobacco has been consistently associated with PC, and there are multiple articles published in various journals that are related to smoking and PC. It is thought that carcinogens from smoking reach the pancreas via the blood stream, although direct exposure to pancreatic ductal system from ingested tobacco is also a possibility [48]. A pooled analysis of 12 case-controlled studies demonstrated increased risk of PC in smokers with an odds ratio of 1.2 in former smokers and 2.2 in current smokers. The risk increased proportionally with amount and duration of smoking [48]. Exposure to second-hand smoke may also result in increased risk of PC [49].

In a large cohort study conducted in the Netherlands, an increased risk of PC per increment of 10 years of smoking (HR, 1.15; 95% CI, 1.08–1.22) and per increment of 10 cigarettes/day (HR of 1.08, 95% CI, 0.98–1.19) was observed. No association was noted with PC risk and passive smoking exposure in women. The risk of PC in smokers has been reduced to that in non-smokers after quitting smoking for more than 20 years [50]. Historically epidemiological data showed that implementation of smoking reduction programs showed a decline in the PC mortality [51].

Effect of cigar and pipe smoking and smokeless tobacco use on risk of PC was analysed in a large pooled analysis of case-control studies. Results showed that cigar smoking alone or the combination of cigarette with cigar or pipe smoking has been associated with increased PC similar to that of cigarette smoking [52]. The increased risk was thought to be due to similar composition of cigars and cigarettes. No significant association for pipe smoking on excess risk of PC was found in a meta-analysis [52].

Effect of smokeless tobacco on PC has been controversial. A systematic review of the effect of smokeless tobacco in Europe and North America showed no increased risk, whereas cohort studies conducted in Norway and Sweden suggested increased risk. The difference in the effects may be due to the differences in the smokeless tobacco products between the populations considered [52, 53]. The tobacco-specific nitrosamines with the greatest proportions in snuff (4-(nitrosomethylamino)-1-(3-pyridyl)-1-butanone [NNK] and N′-nitrosonornicotine [NNN]) have been implicated to be carcinogenic to the pancreas, and these tobacco-specific nitrosamines have been found in the pancreatic juice of smokers compared to non-smokers [54].

Smoking has a late-stage effect on pancreatic carcinogenesis suggested by the greater risk for total exposure delivered at lower intensity for longer duration than for higher intensity for shorter duration [55]. A nested case-control study of 272 members of 28 familial PC kindreds found smoking to increase the risk of PC in kindred especially in males under the age of 50 years. It was also found to hasten the onset of the disease by approximately one decade in the subjects who smoke. A similar effect of smoking hastening the onset of PC was found in individuals with hereditary pancreatitis. This further highlights the importance of the need for behavioural modification in individuals who have a high familial risk [56, 57]. Table 1.1 highlights some of the important studies and meta-analysis demonstrating the association of smoking and PC.

Table 1.1 Studies (including meta-analysis) pertinent to smoking and PC

Author	Aim of study	Study design	No. of participants	Results	Conclusion	Comments
Bosetti C et al.	Dose-response relationship between cigarette smoking and PC	Pooled analysis	6507 cases of adenocarcinoma of pancreas and 12,890 controls, within the International PC Case-Control Consortium (PanC4)	Odds ratio was 1.2 (95% confidence interval [CI] 1.0–1.3) for former smokers and 2.2 (95% CI 1.7–2.8) for current cigarette smokers OR = 3.4 for ≥35 cigarettes per day, *P* for trend <0.0001)	Current smokers with twofold increased risk of PC, risk increases with increasing number of cigarettes smoked and duration of smoking	A 20% excess risk of PC in former smokers declines with time since quitting and reached the level of never cigarette smokers ~20 years after quitting
Vrieling A et al.	Cigarette smoking and exposure to ETS with PC risk	Prospective cohort study in ten European countries	465,910 participants including 524 first incident PC cases diagnosed, median follow-up time of 8.9 years	Risk of PC for current cigarette smokers (HR = 1.71, 95% CI = 1.36–2.15)	71% increased risk of PC in current smokers Statistically non-significant 19% increased risk in former cigarette smokers compared to never smokers	PC risk among never smokers daily exposed to ETS during childhood (HR = 2.61, 95% CI = 0.96–7.10) and exposed to ETS at home and/or work (HR = 1.54, 95% CI = 1.00–2.39) Exposure to ETS at home and/or work was borderline statistically significant, with increased PC risk among never smokers

Iodice S, Gandini S, Maisonneuve P, Lowenfels AB	Association between smoking and PC, the risk of pipe and cigar smoking	Meta-analysis	Analysis of 82 published case-control and cohort studies between 1950 and 2007 about smoking and PC	Risk of PC for current and former smokers was 1.74 (95% CI 1.61–1.87) and 1.2 (95% CI 1.11–1.29)		Risk of PC for current and former pipe and/or cigar smokers was, respectively, 1.47 (95% CI 1.17–1.83) and 1.29 (95% CI 0.68–2.45) For former smokers, the risk remains elevated for 10 years after cessation
Lynch SM, Vrieling A, Lubin JH, et al.	Pooled analysis of cigarette smoking and PC	Meta-analysis	1481 cases, 1539 controls	Current smokers had elevated risk (OR) = 1.77, 95% (CI): 1.38, 2.26) Risk increased with (≥30 cigs/day: OR = 1.75, 95% CI: 1.27, 2.42), duration (≥50 years: OR = 2.13, 95% CI: 1.25, 3.62) and cumulative smoking dose (≥40 pack-years: OR = 1.78, 95% CI: 1.35, 2.34)		Risk more than 15 years after smoking cessation was similar to that for never smokers, suggesting smoking has a late-stage effect on pancreatic carcinogenesis

(continued)

Table 1.1 (continued)

Author	Aim of study	Study design	No. of participants	Results	Conclusion	Comments
The Netherlands Cohort study, Mirjam M Heinen et al.	The role of active cigarette smoking, smoking cessation and passive smoking as determinants for PC	Cohort study	120,852 men and women who completed a baseline questionnaire in 1986, with 16.3 years of median follow-up	Increased risk per increment of 10 years of smoking (HR, 1.15; 95% CI, 1.08–1.22) and an HR of 1.08 per increment of 10 cigs/d (95% CI, 0.98–1.19)		No association for passive smoking exposure and PC risk in women
Zhou J et al.	Exposure to ETS and risk of PC	Meta-analysis	Analysis of literature search using MEDLINE and EMBASE published in October 2011	Exposure to ETS during childhood was not associated with risk of PC-RR 1.12; 95% CI 0.89 to 1.43. No association with exposure to ETS during adulthood at home-RR 1.23; 95% CI 0.86–1.77 or at work RR 0.94; 95% CI 0.67–1.33	No evidence between exposure to ETS and risk of PC	

OR odds ratio, *CI* confidence interval, *HR* hazard ratio, *ETS* environmental tobacco smoke

Alcohol

The direct effect of alcohol on the incidence of PC is difficult to ascertain due to the concomitant use of tobacco in many instances, but direct insult from heavy alcohol consumption and indirect effect through development of chronic pancreatitis are felt to be some of the reasons. Several mechanisms have been proposed to explain the effect of alcohol on pancreas. Oxidative and non-oxidative damage from the metabolites of alcohol can initiate inflammatory and fibrotic cascades resulting in subsequent carcinogenesis. Molecular and genetic characteristics in individuals such as specific mutations in the Kras oncogene were found to be more common in alcohol consumers with PC. A molecular study was done in genetically engineered mouse models where oncogenic Kras mutation is activated in pancreatic cell types. It demonstrated that insults to the pancreas, in the form of acute and chronic pancreatitis, in the context of oncogenic Kras mutation can dramatically increase the risk of malignant transformation [58, 59].

PC-related deaths identified from cancer prevention study II in non-smokers found that consuming three or more drinks of liquor per day can increase the risk of pancreatic cancer independent of smoking [60]. However, pooled analysis of ten case-control studies with over 5000 subjects found insignificant association of alcohol and PC with ≤4 drinks per day but noted increased risk with ≥9 drinks per day [61]. Similar conclusion was made in another meta-analysis in which low to moderate alcohol intake was found to have no significant effect on PC risk, but high alcohol intake especially high liquor intake was associated with increased risk. This could be explained by the association of the high alcohol intake with chronic pancreatitis [62]. Also acetaldehyde, the main metabolite of alcohol, is considered carcinogenic by several studies. The increased risk associated with high liquor intake compared to other alcoholic beverages like beer and wine could be explained by the substantially higher concentration of alcohol in liquor compared to others [62].

A multicentric cohort study showed alcohol and tobacco use to be associated with earlier onset of PC. Patients who drink excess alcohol were found to have a median of 5.3 years earlier age of presentation compared to non-alcoholics [63].

Occupational Exposure

Occupational exposure is largely preventable, and one meta-analysis estimated that 12% of all PCs may be attributable to this [64]. A statistically significant association was found in a meta-analysis conducted by Ojajarvi et al. for chlorinated hydrocarbon compounds and nickel compounds [64]. Chlorinated hydrocarbons are used in variety of applications and products such as solvents, pesticides and plastics. Although there are different types of hydrocarbons, only metal degreasers and dry cleaners were found to be significantly associated with risk of PC, whereas others have increased risk but were non-statistically significant [65]. Chlorinated hydrocarbon pesticides include insecticides and organochlorines (dichlorodiphenyltrichloroethane, DDT), and the latter was restricted due to reported health concerns. In a case-control study, exposure to DDT was found to have increased risk of PC by

4.8-fold with mean duration of exposure of 47 months; a 7.4-fold increase in risk was noted [66]. Other pesticides such as fungicides and herbicides such as pendimethalin and S-ethyl dipropyl carbamothioate (EPTC) were found to have a significant increased risk of PC [67, 68]. Polycyclic aromatic hydrocarbons (PAH) include hundreds of compounds and are used in manufacturing various products. In a meta-analysis, the use of PAH was noted to be associated with a non-statistically significant increased risk of PC [64]. N,N-Diethyl-meta-toluamide (DEET) was shown to have some neurological effects, but it has not been linked to an increased risk in PCs [69].

Dietary Habits

The association of dietary habits and PC has been studied in large prospective trials. One prospective study evaluated five healthy lifestyle patterns assigning a score of one point for each category consisting of strict Mediterranean diet, non-smoking, limited alcohol, BMI of 18–25 kg/m^2 and regular exercise. This study reported a 58% reduction in PC for patients who scored all five points [70]. Another prospective study found that eating red meat especially when cooked at very high temperatures is associated with increased risk of PC but only in men [71]. Conflicting results have been published regarding the relationship between eating vegetables and fruits and their association with PC. For example, a population-based study included over half a million participants and found that there is no significant association between consuming vegetables, fruits and PC [72]. The relationship between total or available carbohydrate intake, glycaemic index, glycaemic load and PC was also studied with no association found except increased risk with high fructose intake [73]. These findings need to be confirmed by other studies. It is suspected that high fat content is a risk factor for PC; however, the evidence has been conflicting [74, 75].

The data regarding the association of coffee and pancreatic cancer is conflicting. A study aimed at evaluating the association of coffee with PC was conducted by MacMohan et al. in the 1980s. This study found a significant dose-response relationship with a relative risk of 1.8 for drinking up to two cups per day and 2.7 with three or more cups per day. This significance persisted even after adjusting it for cigarette smoking [76]. A large meta-analysis of 14 prospective studies concluded a decreased risk of PC (4% reduction with one cup per day) in subjects drinking coffee, with a pooled relative risk of 0.82 for regular coffee drinkers, 0.86 for low to moderate coffee drinkers and 0.68 for high coffee drinkers [77].

Medications

Human PC harbours renin-angiotensin system (RAS) and expresses angiotensin II and angiotensin II type 1 receptor. The role of local RAS in multiple pathways of carcinogenesis is well known, and in pancreatic cancer it appears to interfere with cell proliferation, apoptosis and angiogenesis [78, 79]. Research studying the impact of angiotensin converting enzyme inhibitors (ACEI) and angiotensin receptor blockers (ARB) on PC has also been conducted. ACEI and ARBs have showed protective effect against PC, according to one study reported by Khurana et al. [80]. They reported similar outcome in patients at Veteran Affairs (VA) after controlling for common variables [81]. One Taiwan-based case-control study examined about 12,000 participants taking either ACEI or ARBs and found reduced risk of PC even after adjusting for other variables [80]. On the other hand, some studies reveal increased risk of cancer incidence with ARBs (Sipahi et al., 2010) [82]. A retrospective study evaluated the effect of ACEI and ARBs on PC patients receiving gemcitabine therapy showed improved prognosis of the disease in advanced stages [83].

Dipeptidyl peptidase-4 (DPP-4) inhibitors (sitagliptin, saxagliptin and alogliptin) and glucagon-like peptide-1 (GLP-1) receptor agonists (exanetide and liraglutide) are incretin-based drugs and a relatively new group of drugs being used in the management of diabetes. An analysis of the FDA adverse event reporting database suggests that the sitagliptin and exanetide could have some unintended side effects. It showed the rate of PC reported was 2.7 and 2.9 times higher with sitagliptin and exanetide, respectively, compared to other oral antidiabetic drugs. In a rat model, sitagliptin caused increased pancreatic ductal turnover and acinar to ductal metaplasia. Similar characteristics of ductal proliferation and metaplasia have been seen with chronic pancreatitis in humans. This could explain the increased concern as chronic pancreatitis increases risk of PC [84].

A large international multicentre cohort study reported that the use of incretin-based drugs in diabetic patients followed for up to 8 years was not associated with an overall increased risk of PC compared with the use of sulfonylureas. The risk did not vary by class and evidence of a duration-response relation was lacking. However, additional prospective studies are required in this regard with long-term surveillance owing to the latency of this cancer [85].

Two other large multicentre cardiovascular outcome trials in patients with type 2 diabetes treated with incretin-based drugs—the Saxagliptin Assessment of Vascular Outcomes Recorded (SAVOR study) and the Examination of Cardiovascular Outcomes with Alogliptin versus Standard of Care (EXAMINE study) were conducted. Both trials found no increase in the rate of acute or chronic pancreatitis in the patients on DPP-4 inhibitor treatment [86–88]. The FDA and European Medicine Agency (EMA) conducted an extended review of more than 200 trials, preclinical and epidemiological studies, and reported that there is no causal relationship between DPP-4 inhibitors and either pancreatitis or PC [89]. Onitilo et al. reviewed the association of diabetic medications with pancreatic cancer and found that hyperinsulinemia and drugs that increase circulating insulin such as exogenous insulin, insulin analogues and insulin secretagogues have been associated with increased PC risk with a hazard ratio of 4.63 [90].

Statins have been considered to have antineoplastic properties. They were shown to inhibit the signalling pathways involved in pancreatic tumorigenesis. Secondly, they are anti-angiogenic and anti-inflammatory and have pro-apoptotic effects. A meta-analysis of 16 studies with over 7000 PC patients showed a non-significant decreased risk of PC in all statin users (RR 0.89) [91]. The use of fish oil is routinely recommended due to their cardioprotective nature, but its effect on cancer is less well understood. Based on a mouse model, eicosapentaenoic acid, a component of fish oil was noted to decrease the risk of PC [92]. However no human studies have confirmed this finding.

NSAIDs

NSAIDs including aspirin have been explored as emerging agents for chemoprevention for different cancers, including PC. The major mechanism by which aspirin is thought to have antineoplastic effect is via the inhibition of COX-1/COX-2 and modulation of NFkB or STAT3 pathway [93–95]. The effect of aspirin on PC reveals conflicting results with some studies showing a protective effect, while others found no association [96–99]. A large pooled analysis of 25,570 patients in eight randomized trials showed survival benefit with daily aspirin use (at a dose of 75 mg). The benefit was also shown to increase with the duration of treatment [93, 100].

The UK General Practice Research Database studied the effect of NSAIDs on PC and found reduced risk if consumed for over 5 years [101]. A randomized controlled study using aspirin for cardiovascular risk reduction found significant reduction in PC if used for over 5 years; however, this was not as strong in a follow-up study in the US Cancer Prevention Study II Nutrition Cohort [102–104]. Naproxen can induce cell apoptosis by downregulating bcl-2 and upregulating Bax [104].

Selenium, an antioxidant was found to be inversely associated with the risk of PC, but the observed association was attenuated by selenium supplementation [105]. Vitamin D has demonstrated reduced risk of PC and other cancers; therefore, its use in cancer prevention is currently being evaluated [106]. Possible mechanisms include 1,25-dihydroxyvitamin D3 receptor expression in pancreatic cell lines or calcitriol, and its analogues inhibit PC cell proliferation, induce differentiation and promote apoptosis [106, 107]. In one study, no association was found between the use of retinol and calcium intake and PC [108].

Obesity

Obesity defined as a body mass index greater than 30 kg/m^2 has been linked to an increased risk of many cancer types with PC also noted to have an increased incidence in obese individuals. A meta-analysis involving six case-control and eight cohort studies aimed at assessing the risk of obesity in PC found an increased risk of PC per unit increase in body mass index. The estimated risk in obese (30 kg/m^2) patients was 19% higher as compared with normal individuals [109]. Another meta-analysis analysing 21 prospective studies noted an increased relative risk of 1.12 with every 5 kg/m^2 increase in body mass index [110]. A subsequent meta-analysis showed a non-statistically significant increased risk of PC with every 5 kg/m^2 increase in body mass index. According to this study the calculated relative risk for men was 1.07 and that for women was 1.12 [111].

Infections

Infections such as *Helicobacter pylori* and hepatitis B virus in one study each were shown to increase the risk of PC [112, 113]. In another study, hepatitis C viral infection was noted to increase the risk of PC slightly, but the effect was found to be non-significant when adjusted to common variables [114].

Screening and Surveillance

There is currently no consensus on screening individuals for PC. Patients with high risk based on inherited cancer susceptibility syndromes and hereditary pancreatitis have severalfold increased risk of PC. In 2007, Brand RE et al. published suggestions of the expert consensus group on inherited diseases of the pancreas; however, they could not reach a consensus on the specific approaches to screening in high-risk individuals and recommended that surveillance be performed only as part of a peer-reviewed screening protocol. Even though there are no consensus on when to start or stop screening or how often to perform screening, the consensus group recommended that familial PC screening be considered at age 40–45 or 10–15 years younger than the youngest relative with PC, and one should tailor individual recommendations taking into account additional factors such as the patient's level of concern, study protocols and clinical history.

Current arguments against screening for PC are mainly threefold, with no study ever showing that screening improves survival till date. The yield of screening has not been uniformly high, and although intraductal papillary mucinous neoplasms (IPMNs) and pancreatic intraepithelial neoplasia (PanIN) act as precursor lesions to invasive PC, only a small fraction of such patients progress to PC.

Tumour markers are not always reliable, and CT imaging is unable to assess non-dilated pancreatic ducts in addition to radiation exposure. Invasive approaches such as endoscopic retrograde cholangiopancreatography (ERCP) may not be appropriate due to high cost, risk of morbidity and mortality with such procedures, while endoscopic ultrasound (EUS) is highly operator dependent. A very small study combining both EUS and ERCP tested 35 members of 13 FPC families and found abnormal findings in 15 individuals. Those with abnormal findings had a surgical resection done, either total (12 individuals) or partial pancreatectomy (3 individuals). The study concluded that PC screening is cost-effective with increased patient life expectancy in selected members of familial pancreatic cancer kindreds; however, the cost-effectiveness of repeated screening remains to be determined [115].

A multicenter study evaluated asymptomatic individuals with increased risk of PC at Johns Hopkins Institute and Mayo Clinic. Patients in this study were screened with EUS, and abnormal tissue was aspirated using fine-needle aspiration. Out of 38 patients, six were found to have abnormal tissue of which only two had clinically significant neoplasia. The study concluded that screening individuals with EUS is feasible [116]. Although based on these small studies EUS appears to be feasible for screening for PC, these are not powered to make definite conclusions.

References

1. Siegel RL, Miller KD, Jemal A. Cancer statistics, 2016. CA Cancer J Clin. 2016;66(1):7–30.
2. Boyle P, et al. Epidemiology of pancreas cancer (1988). Int J Pancreatol. 1989;5(4):327–46.
3. Hariharan D, Saied A, Kocher HM. Analysis of mortality rates for pancreatic cancer across the world. HPB (Oxford). 2008;10(1):58–62.
4. Horner MJ, et al. SEER cancer statistics review, 1975–2006. Bethesda: National Cancer Institute; 2009.
5. Pernick NL, et al. Clinicopathologic analysis of pancreatic adenocarcinoma in African Americans and Caucasians. Pancreas. 2003;26(1):28–32.
6. Klein AP, et al. Prospective risk of pancreatic cancer in familial pancreatic cancer kindreds. Cancer Res. 2004;64(7):2634–8.
7. Brune KA, et al. Importance of age of onset in pancreatic cancer kindreds. J Natl Cancer Inst. 2010;102(2):119–26.
8. Tersmette AC, et al. Increased risk of incident pancreatic cancer among first-degree relatives of patients with familial pancreatic cancer. Clin Cancer Res. 2001;7(3):738–44.
9. Grant RC, et al. Prevalence of germline mutations in cancer predisposition genes in patients with pancreatic cancer. Gastroenterology. 2015;148(3):556–64.
10. Eberle MA, et al. A new susceptibility locus for autosomal dominant pancreatic cancer maps to chromosome 4q32-34. Am J Hum Genet. 2002;70(4):1044–8.
11. Jang JH, et al. Genetic variants in carcinogen-metabolizing enzymes, cigarette smoking and pancreatic cancer risk. Carcinogenesis. 2012;33(4):818–27.
12. Lynch HT, et al. Familial pancreatic cancer: clinicopathologic study of 18 nuclear families. Am J Gastroenterol. 1990;85(1):54–60.
13. Rebours V, et al. Risk of pancreatic adenocarcinoma in patients with hereditary pancreatitis: a national exhaustive series. Am J Gastroenterol. 2008;103(1):111–9.
14. Thompson D, Easton DF. Cancer incidence in BRCA1 mutation carriers. J Natl Cancer Inst. 2002;94(18):1358–65.
15. Axilbund JE, et al. Absence of germline BRCA1 mutations in familial pancreatic cancer patients. Cancer Biol Ther. 2009;8(2):131–5.
16. Iqbal J, et al. The incidence of pancreatic cancer in BRCA1 and BRCA2 mutation carriers. Br J Cancer. 2012;107(12):2005–9.
17. van Asperen CJ, et al. Cancer risks in BRCA2 families: estimates for sites other than breast and ovary. J Med Genet. 2005;42(9):711–9.
18. Ferrone CR, et al. BRCA germline mutations in Jewish patients with pancreatic adenocarcinoma. J Clin Oncol. 2009;27(3):433–8.
19. Slater EP, et al. PALB2 mutations in European familial pancreatic cancer families. Clin Genet. 2010;78(5):490–4.
20. Bergman W, et al. Systemic cancer and the FAMMM syndrome. Br J Cancer. 1990;61(6):932–6.
21. Giardiello FM, et al. Increased risk of cancer in the Peutz-Jeghers syndrome. N Engl J Med. 1987;316(24):1511–4.

22. Su GH, et al. Germline and somatic mutations of the STK11/LKB1 Peutz-Jeghers gene in pancreatic and biliary cancers. Am J Pathol. 1999;154(6):1835–40.
23. van Lier MG, et al. High cancer risk in Peutz-Jeghers syndrome: a systematic review and surveillance recommendations. Am J Gastroenterol. 2010;105(6):1258–64. author reply 1265
24. Swift M, Chase CL, Morrell D. Cancer predisposition of ataxia-telangiectasia heterozygotes. Cancer Genet Cytogenet. 1990;46(1):21–7.
25. Roberts NJ, et al. ATM mutations in patients with hereditary pancreatic cancer. Cancer Discov. 2012;2(1):41–6.
26. Win AK, et al. Colorectal and other cancer risks for carriers and noncarriers from families with a DNA mismatch repair gene mutation: a prospective cohort study. J Clin Oncol. 2012;30(9):958–64.
27. Kastrinos F, et al. Risk of pancreatic cancer in families with Lynch syndrome. JAMA. 2009;302(16):1790–5.
28. Goggins M, et al. Pancreatic adenocarcinomas with DNA replication errors (RER+) are associated with wild-type K-ras and characteristic histopathology. Poor differentiation, a syncytial growth pattern, and pushing borders suggest RER+. Am J Pathol. 1998;152(6):1501–7.
29. Lowenfels AB, et al. Pancreatitis and the risk of pancreatic cancer. N Engl J Med. 1993;328(20):1433–7.
30. Raimondi S, et al. Pancreatic cancer in chronic pancreatitis; aetiology, incidence, and early detection. Best Pract Res Clin Gastroenterol. 2010;24(3):349–58.
31. Bansal P, Sonnenberg A. Pancreatitis is a risk factor for pancreatic cancer. Gastroenterology. 1995;109(1):247–51.
32. Bracci PM, et al. Pancreatitis and pancreatic cancer in two large pooled case-control studies. Cancer Causes Control. 2009;20(9):1723–31.
33. Maisonneuve P, Marshall BC, Lowenfels AB. Risk of pancreatic cancer in patients with cystic fibrosis. Gut. 2007;56(9):1327–8.
34. Sheldon CD, et al. A cohort study of cystic fibrosis and malignancy. Br J Cancer. 1993;68(5):1025–8.
35. Neglia JP, Wielinski CL, Warwick WJ. Cancer risk among patients with cystic fibrosis. J Pediatr. 1991;119(5):764–6.
36. Gupta S, et al. New-onset diabetes and pancreatic cancer. Clin Gastroenterol Hepatol. 2006;4(11):1366–72. quiz 1301
37. Aggarwal G, Kamada P, Chari ST. Prevalence of diabetes mellitus in pancreatic cancer compared to common cancers. Pancreas. 2013;42(2):198–201.
38. Sella T, et al. Gestational diabetes and risk of incident primary cancer: a large historical cohort study in Israel. Cancer Causes Control. 2011;22(11):1513–20.
39. Everhart J, Wright D. Diabetes mellitus as a risk factor for pancreatic cancer. A meta-analysis. JAMA. 1995;273(20):1605–9.
40. Gapstur SM, et al. Abnormal glucose metabolism and pancreatic cancer mortality. JAMA. 2000;283(19):2552–8.
41. Levine W, et al. Post-load plasma glucose and cancer mortality in middle-aged men and women. 12-year follow-up findings of the Chicago Heart Association Detection Project in Industry. Am J Epidemiol. 1990;131(2):254–62.
42. Smith GD, et al. Post-challenge glucose concentration, impaired glucose tolerance, diabetes, and cancer mortality in men. Am J Epidemiol. 1992;136(9):1110–4.
43. Borch K, et al. Increased incidence of pancreatic neoplasia in pernicious anemia. World J Surg. 1988;12(6):866–70.
44. Karlson BM, et al. Cancer of the upper gastrointestinal tract among patients with pernicious anemia: a case-cohort study. Scand J Gastroenterol. 2000;35(8):847–51.
45. Wolpin BM, et al. Pancreatic cancer risk and ABO blood group alleles: results from the pancreatic cancer cohort consortium. Cancer Res. 2010;70(3):1015–23.
46. Parkin DM, Muir CS. Cancer incidence in five continents. Comparability and quality of data. IARC Sci Publ. 1992;120:45–173.

47. Mulder I, et al. Smoking cessation would substantially reduce the future incidence of pancreatic cancer in the European Union. Eur J Gastroenterol Hepatol. 2002;14(12):1343–53.
48. Bosetti C, et al. Cigarette smoking and pancreatic cancer: an analysis from the International Pancreatic Cancer Case-Control Consortium (Panc4). Ann Oncol. 2012;23(7):1880–8.
49. Vrieling A, et al. Cigarette smoking, environmental tobacco smoke exposure and pancreatic cancer risk in the European Prospective Investigation into Cancer and Nutrition. Int J Cancer. 2010;126(10):2394–403.
50. Heinen MM, et al. Active and passive smoking and the risk of pancreatic cancer in the Netherlands Cohort Study. Cancer Epidemiol Biomark Prev. 2010;19(6):1612–22.
51. Adair T, et al. Tobacco consumption and pancreatic cancer mortality: what can we conclude from historical data in Australia? Eur J Pub Health. 2012;22(2):243–7.
52. Bertuccio P, et al. Cigar and pipe smoking, smokeless tobacco use and pancreatic cancer: an analysis from the International Pancreatic Cancer Case-Control Consortium (PanC4). Ann Oncol. 2011;22(6):1420–6.
53. Sponsiello-Wang Z, Weitkunat R, Lee PN. Systematic review of the relation between smokeless tobacco and cancer of the pancreas in Europe and North America. BMC Cancer. 2008;8:356.
54. Luo J, et al. Oral use of Swedish moist snuff (snus) and risk for cancer of the mouth, lung, and pancreas in male construction workers: a retrospective cohort study. Lancet. 2007;369(9578):2015–20.
55. Lynch SM, et al. Cigarette smoking and pancreatic cancer: a pooled analysis from the pancreatic cancer cohort consortium. Am J Epidemiol. 2009;170(4):403–13.
56. Rulyak SJ, et al. Risk factors for the development of pancreatic cancer in familial pancreatic cancer kindreds. Gastroenterology. 2003;124(5):1292–9.
57. Lowenfels AB, et al. Cigarette smoking as a risk factor for pancreatic cancer in patients with hereditary pancreatitis. JAMA. 2001;286(2):169–70.
58. Gupta S, et al. Risk of pancreatic cancer by alcohol dose, duration, and pattern of consumption, including binge drinking: a population-based study. Cancer Causes Control. 2010;21(7):1047–59.
59. Carriere C, et al. Acute pancreatitis markedly accelerates pancreatic cancer progression in mice expressing oncogenic Kras. Biochem Biophys Res Commun. 2009;382(3):561–5.
60. Gapstur SM, et al. Association of alcohol intake with pancreatic cancer mortality in never smokers. Arch Intern Med. 2011;171(5):444–51.
61. Lucenteforte E, et al. Alcohol consumption and pancreatic cancer: a pooled analysis in the International Pancreatic Cancer Case-Control Consortium (PanC4). Ann Oncol. 2012;23(2):374–82.
62. Wang Y-T, et al. Association between alcohol intake and the risk of pancreatic cancer: a dose-response meta-analysis of cohort studies. BMC Cancer. 2016;16:212.
63. Anderson MA, et al. Alcohol and tobacco lower the age of presentation in sporadic pancreatic cancer in a dose-dependent manner: a multicenter study. Am J Gastroenterol. 2012;107(11):1730–9.
64. Ojajarvi IA, et al. Occupational exposures and pancreatic cancer: a meta-analysis. Occup Environ Med. 2000;57(5):316–24.
65. Ojajarvi A, et al. Risk of pancreatic cancer in workers exposed to chlorinated hydrocarbon solvents and related compounds: a meta-analysis. Am J Epidemiol. 2001;153(9):841–50.
66. Garabrant DH, et al. DDT and related compounds and risk of pancreatic cancer. J Natl Cancer Inst. 1992;84(10):764–71.
67. Andreotti G, et al. Agricultural pesticide use and pancreatic cancer risk in the Agricultural Health Study Cohort. Int J Cancer. 2009;124(10):2495–500.
68. Ji BT, et al. Occupational exposure to pesticides and pancreatic cancer. Am J Ind Med. 2001;39(1):92–9.
69. Koren G, Matsui D, Bailey B. DEET-based insect repellents: safety implications for children and pregnant and lactating women. Can Med Assoc J. 2003;169(3):209–12.

70. Jiao L, et al. A combined healthy lifestyle score and risk of pancreatic cancer in a large cohort study. Arch Intern Med. 2009;169(8):764–70.
71. Stolzenberg-Solomon RZ, et al. Meat and meat-mutagen intake and pancreatic cancer risk in the NIH-AARP cohort. Cancer Epidemiol Biomark Prev. 2007;16(12):2664–75.
72. Vrieling A, et al. Fruit and vegetable consumption and pancreatic cancer risk in the European Prospective Investigation into Cancer and Nutrition. Int J Cancer. 2009;124(8):1926–34.
73. Jiao L, et al. Glycemic index, carbohydrates, glycemic load, and the risk of pancreatic cancer in a prospective cohort study. Cancer Epidemiol Biomark Prev. 2009;18(4):1144–51.
74. Dawson DW, et al. High-fat, high-calorie diet promotes early pancreatic neoplasia in the conditional KrasG12D mouse model. Cancer Prev Res (Phila). 2013;6(10):1064–73.
75. Nöthlings U, et al. Meat and fat intake as risk factors for pancreatic cancer: the multiethnic cohort study. J Natl Cancer Inst. 2005;97(19):1458–65.
76. MacMahon B, et al. Coffee and cancer of the pancreas. N Engl J Med. 1981;304(11):630–3.
77. Dong J, Zou J, Yu X-F. Coffee drinking and pancreatic cancer risk: a meta-analysis of cohort studies. World J Gastroenterol. 2011;17(9):1204–10.
78. Amaya K, et al. Angiotensin II activates MAP kinase and NF-kappaB through angiotensin II type I receptor in human pancreatic cancer cells. Int J Oncol. 2004;25(4):849–56.
79. Fujimoto Y, et al. Angiotensin II type 1 receptor expression in human pancreatic cancer and growth inhibition by angiotensin II type 1 receptor antagonist. FEBS Lett. 2001;495(3):197–200.
80. Chiang Y-Y, et al. Lowered cancer risk with ACE inhibitors/ARBs: a population-based cohort study. J Clin Hypertens. 2014;16(1):27–33.
81. Khurana V, Sheth A, Caldito G, Barkin JS. Angiotensin converting enzyme inhibitors reduce the incidence of pancreatic cancer: a study of half a million US veterans. Gastroenterology 2006;130(4), Suppl. 2, M 2163 A-425–426.
82. Sipahi I, et al. Angiotensin-receptor blockade and risk of cancer: meta-analysis of randomised controlled trials. Lancet Oncol. 2010;11(7):627–36.
83. Nakai Y, et al. Inhibition of renin-angiotensin system affects prognosis of advanced pancreatic cancer receiving gemcitabine. Br J Cancer. 2010;103(11):1644–8.
84. Elashoff M, et al. Pancreatitis, pancreatic, and thyroid cancer with glucagon-like peptide-1-based therapies. Gastroenterology. 2011;141(1):150–6.
85. Azoulay L, et al. Incretin based drugs and the risk of pancreatic cancer: international multicentre cohort study. BMJ. 2016;352:i581.
86. Scirica BM, et al. Saxagliptin and cardiovascular outcomes in patients with type 2 diabetes mellitus. N Engl J Med. 2013;369(14):1317–26.
87. White WB, et al. Alogliptin after acute coronary syndrome in patients with type 2 diabetes. N Engl J Med. 2013;369(14):1327–35.
88. Monami M, Dicembrini I, Mannucci E. Dipeptidyl peptidase-4 inhibitors and pancreatitis risk: a meta-analysis of randomized clinical trials. Diabetes Obes Metab. 2014;16(1):48–56.
89. Egan AG, et al. Pancreatic safety of incretin-based drugs--FDA and EMA assessment. N Engl J Med. 2014;370(9):794–7.
90. Onitilo AA, et al. Diabetes and cancer II: role of diabetes medications and influence of shared risk factors. Cancer Causes Control. 2012;23(7):991–1008.
91. Cui X, et al. Statin use and risk of pancreatic cancer: a meta-analysis. Cancer Causes Control. 2012;23(7):1099–111.
92. Fukui M, et al. EPA, an omega-3 fatty acid, induces apoptosis in human pancreatic cancer cells: role of ROS accumulation, caspase-8 activation, and autophagy induction. J Cell Biochem. 2013;114(1):192–203.
93. Amin S, Boffetta P, Lucas AL. The role of common pharmaceutical agents on the prevention and treatment of pancreatic cancer. Gut Liver. 2016;10(5):665–71.
94. Ulrich CM, Bigler J, Potter JD. Non-steroidal anti-inflammatory drugs for cancer prevention: promise, perils and pharmacogenetics. Nat Rev Cancer. 2006;6(2):130–40.
95. Yue W, et al. Repurposing of metformin and aspirin by targeting AMPK-mTOR and inflammation for pancreatic cancer prevention and treatment. Cancer Prev Res (Phila). 2014;7(4):388–97.

96. Bonifazi M, et al. Aspirin use and pancreatic cancer risk. Eur J Cancer Prev. 2010;19(5):352–4.
97. Tan XL, et al. Aspirin, nonsteroidal anti-inflammatory drugs, acetaminophen, and pancreatic cancer risk: a clinic-based case-control study. Cancer Prev Res (Phila). 2011;4(11):1835–41.
98. Capurso G, et al. Meta-analysis: the use of non-steroidal anti-inflammatory drugs and pancreatic cancer risk for different exposure categories. Aliment Pharmacol Ther. 2007;26(8):1089–99.
99. Larsson SC, et al. Aspirin and nonsteroidal anti-inflammatory drug use and risk of pancreatic cancer: a meta-analysis. Cancer Epidemiol Biomark Prev. 2006;15(12):2561–4.
100. Cui XJ, et al. High-dose aspirin consumption contributes to decreased risk for pancreatic cancer in a systematic review and meta-analysis. Pancreas. 2014;43(1):135–40.
101. Bradley MC, et al. Non-steroidal anti-inflammatory drugs and pancreatic cancer risk: a nested case–control study. Br J Cancer. 2010;102(9):1415–21.
102. Rothwell PM, et al. Effect of daily aspirin on long-term risk of death due to cancer: analysis of individual patient data from randomised trials. Lancet. 2011;377(9759):31–41.
103. Jacobs EJ, et al. Daily aspirin use and cancer mortality in a large US cohort. J Natl Cancer Inst. 2012;104(16):1208–17.
104. Kim MS, et al. Naproxen induces cell-cycle arrest and apoptosis in human urinary bladder cancer cell lines and chemically induced cancers by targeting PI3K. Cancer Prev Res (Phila). 2014;7(2):236–45.
105. Han X, et al. Antioxidant intake and pancreatic cancer risk: the Vitamins and Lifestyle (VITAL) Study. Cancer. 2013;119(7):1314–20.
106. Kawa S, et al. Vitamin D analogues up-regulate p21 and p27 during growth inhibition of pancreatic cancer cell lines. Br J Cancer. 1997;76(7):884–9.
107. Zugmaier G, et al. Growth-inhibitory effects of vitamin D analogues and retinoids on human pancreatic cancer cells. Br J Cancer. 1996;73(11):1341–6.
108. Skinner HG, et al. Vitamin D intake and the risk for pancreatic cancer in two cohort studies. Cancer Epidemiol Biomark Prev. 2006;15(9):1688–95.
109. de Gonzalez AB, Sweetland S, Spencer E. A meta-analysis of obesity and the risk of pancreatic cancer. Br J Cancer. 2003;89(3):519–23.
110. Larsson SC, Orsini N, Wolk A. Body mass index and pancreatic cancer risk: a meta-analysis of prospective studies. Int J Cancer. 2007;120(9):1993–8.
111. Renehan AG, et al. Body-mass index and incidence of cancer: a systematic review and meta-analysis of prospective observational studies. Lancet. 2008;371(9612):569–78.
112. Trikudanathan G, et al. Association between Helicobacter pylori infection and pancreatic cancer. A cumulative meta-analysis. JOP. 2011;12(1):26–31.
113. Hassan MM, et al. Association between hepatitis B virus and pancreatic cancer. J Clin Oncol. 2008;26(28):4557–62.
114. El-Serag HB, et al. Risk of hepatobiliary and pancreatic cancers after hepatitis C virus infection: a population-based study of U.S. veterans. Hepatology. 2009;49(1):116–23.
115. Rulyak SJ, et al. Cost-effectiveness of pancreatic cancer screening in familial pancreatic cancer kindreds. Gastrointest Endosc. 2003;57(1):23–9.
116. Canto MI, et al. Screening for pancreatic neoplasia in high-risk individuals: an EUS-based approach. Clin Gastroenterol Hepatol. 2004;2(7):606–21.

Chapter 2
Anatomy of the Pancreas and Biliary Tree

Constantinos P. Zambirinis and Peter J. Allen

Pancreas

The pancreas derives its name from the Greek words "*παν*" (*whole*) and "*κρέας*" (*flesh*), due to its fleshy consistency as well as the absence of bones or ligaments [1]. The pancreas has a complex microscopic structure and functions as both an exocrine and an endocrine organ. The exocrine component, which is responsible for the digestive functions of the pancreas, represents the bulk of the organ's mass (approximately 98%). The exocrine component is composed of an intricate network of blind sacs (acini) that produce an array of digestive enzymes and form small ductules that interconnect to form larger ducts of progressively increasing caliber, ultimately leading to the main pancreatic duct. This acinar network is supported by loose connective tissue that contains blood vessels, nerves, and pancreatic stellate cells. Interspersed within the exocrine gland are the pancreatic islets of Langerhans, which constitute the endocrine component of the pancreas. The islets of Langerhans are clusters of β, α, δ, PP, and ε cells (in decreasing order of abundance), which are responsible for the production of the hormones insulin, glucagon, somatostatin, pancreatic polypeptide, and ghrelin, respectively.

Embryology

The developmental biology of the pancreas has attracted the interest of the scientific community not only because of the complexity of the pancreatic structure but also because of the multiple diseases that result from developmental aberrations of this organ. Although significant progress has been made with the recent advances of

C.P. Zambirinis, M.D., M.Res. • P.J. Allen, M.D. (✉)
Hepatopancreatobiliary Service, Department of Surgery, Memorial Sloan Kettering Cancer Center, New York, NY 10065, USA
e-mail: allenp@mskcc.org

T. Bekaii-Saab, B. El-Rayes (eds.), *Current and Emerging Therapies in Pancreatic Cancer*, DOI 10.1007/978-3-319-58256-6_2

molecular biology that enable lineage tracing of the different cell types, many aspects of pancreatic development remain unclear.

The pancreas originates from the foregut as two separate primordia suspended in the mesentery. These separate components fuse to form the final organ that rests in the retroperitoneum (Fig. 2.1). Near the end of the fourth week of gestation, a mesenchymal condensation is formed dorsal to the primitive foregut, at the level of the future duodenum. This in turn induces the underlying foregut endodermal lining to form the dorsal pancreatic bud (Fig. 2.2). Specifically, mesenchymal fibroblast growth factor 2 (*FGF2*) and activin relieve the inhibition imposed on the foregut endoderm by Sonic Hedgehog (*SHH*) signaling, therefore enabling differentiation

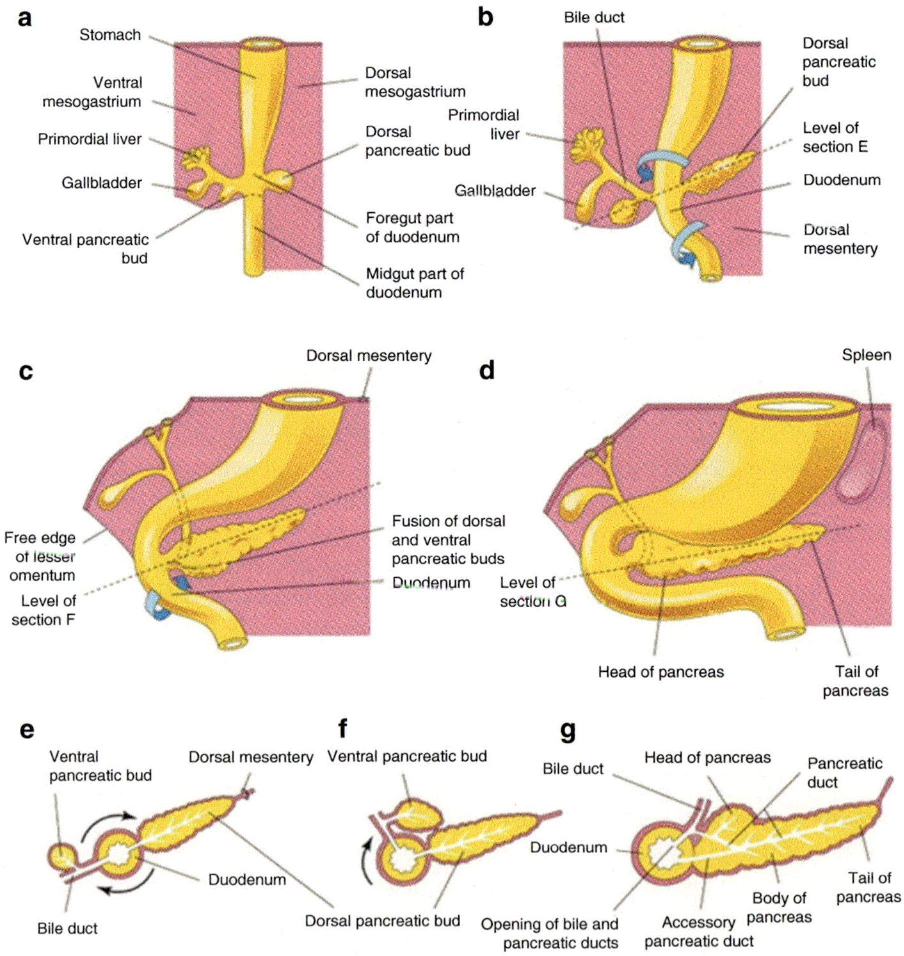

Fig. 2.1 Embryologic development of the pancreas. (**a–d**) Successive stages in the development of the pancreas from the fifth to eighth weeks. (**e–g**) Diagrammatic transverse sections through the duodenum and developing pancreas. Growth and rotation *(arrows)* of the duodenum bring the ventral pancreatic bud toward the dorsal bud, and the two buds subsequently fuse. Reproduced with permission from [2]

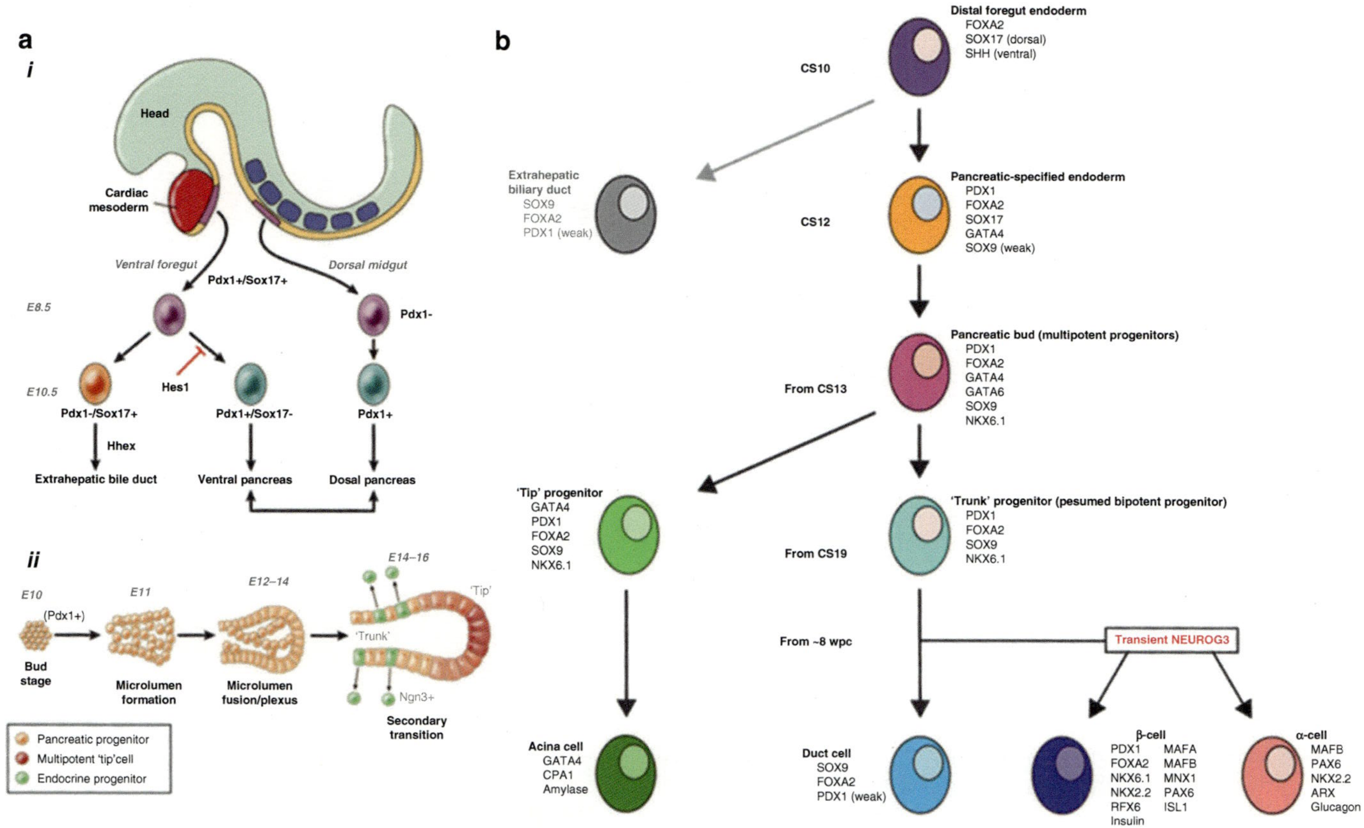

Fig. 2.2 Cellular and molecular interactions defining mammalian pancreas development. (**a**) Regulation of pancreas development in the mouse. Pancreatic specification begins with signals derived from the mesenchyme, with serial expression of different transcription factors (***i***). The "tip-trunk" model explains the intricate microarchitecture of the pancreas (***ii***). From [3]. (**b**) Transcription factors and other key markers that identify different cell types and stages during early pancreas specification and subsequent lineage commitment in humans (based on immunohistochemical studies). Only dorsal pancreas specification is shown for simplicity (markers for the extrahepatic biliary duct are in gray). CS, Carnegie stage; wpc, weeks postconception. Reproduced with permission from [4]

into the pancreatic primordium. The latter results from epithelial expression of the transcription factors pancreatic and duodenal homeobox 1 (*PDX1*) immediately followed by pancreas-specific transcription factor 1a (*PTF1A*) [3]. The importance of these transcription factors in pancreatic development is underscored by the fact that mutations in either gene lead to *pancreatic agenesis*. Both PDX1 and PTF1A have been exploited in various genetically engineered mouse models of pancreatic diseases, especially in mouse models of pancreatic cancer [5]. Furthermore, uncoordinated expression of pancreas-licensing signals can facilitate the development of *ectopic pancreatic tissue*—most commonly found in the mucosa of the stomach, duodenum, jejunum, or the ileal diverticulum (of Meckel)—that may lead to atypical gastrointestinal symptoms (e.g., bleeding or even cancer).

At the microscopic level, pancreatic development follows a process of branching morphogenesis. The inner cells of the growing pancreatic buds that lack contact with the surrounding tissues form microlumens (Fig. 2.2a). Adjacent microlumens subsequently fuse to form duct-like structures, while the epithelial lining is separated into proximal "trunk" and distal "tip" regions. The cells at the trunk regions will develop into cells with ductal and endocrine function. The cells of the tip region initially remain multipotent, but after progressive branching and elongation, the distal tip cells commit to the acinar lineage and will have exocrine function. Complex expression patterns of multiple transcription factors regulate the fate of each cell to give rise to the different lineages found in the adult pancreas (Fig. 2.2b).

Pancreatic parenchymal cells proliferate early in gestation resulting in an increase in the volume of the developing gland. The dorsal bud grows earlier than the ventral bud, taking a progressively oblong shape. The rotation of the stomach and duodenum influences the anatomy and orientation of the pancreatic primordia (Fig. 2.1). The ventral pancreatic bud follows the rotation of the duodenum, moving first to the right and then to its final dorsal position (Fig. 2.1). The two buds fuse in the retroperitoneum to form a single organ. The ventral bud eventually lies posterior to the superior mesenteric vessels and posterior and inferior to the dorsal pancreatic bud, giving rise to the bulk of the uncinate process and the inferior portion of the head of the pancreas. The rest of the head of the pancreas, the neck, body, and tail are all derived from the dorsal bud.

Each of the two pancreatic buds has its own separate main duct (Fig. 2.1). The duct of the ventral bud lies in continuity with the main bile duct. The two ductal systems join into one during the rotation of the duodenum and the pancreas (Figs. 2.1 and 2.3a). The ventral bud forms the proximal main pancreatic duct (of Wirsung), while the duct of the dorsal bud forms the rest of the main pancreatic duct spanning the majority of the gland. The proximal part of the duct of the dorsal bud persists as an accessory pancreatic duct (of Santorini) that opens in the minor duodenal papilla (Fig. 2.3a).

Abnormalities in the rotation and/or fusion of the two pancreatic buds may result in pathologic entities. The most common congenital anomaly of the pancreas is *pancreas divisum*. It is a consequence of failure of fusion of the ventral and dorsal duct system and can be subclassified depending on the extent of communication and the location of the two duct systems (Fig. 2.3a). It is found in approximately 10% of

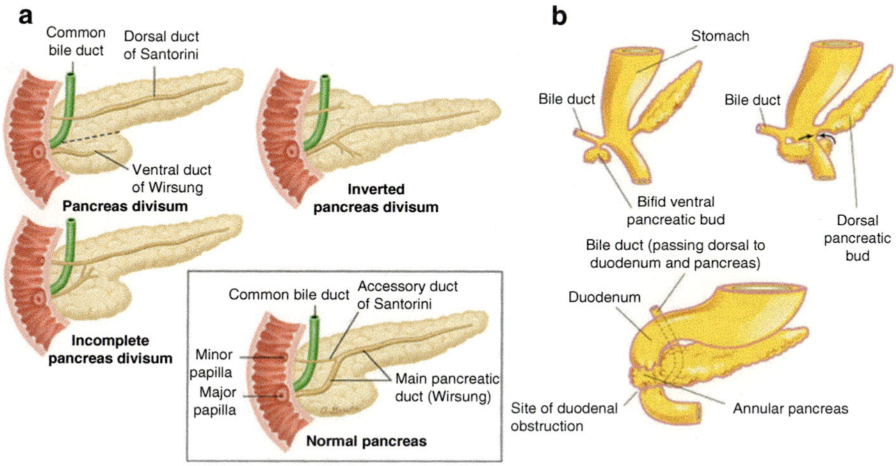

Fig. 2.3 Rotation of the pancreas primordia and its ductal system and related anomalies. (**a**) The rotation of the duodenum brings the two pancreatic buds together. Their ducts, initially separate, usually fuse to form the adult main pancreatic duct that drains into the duodenum. Failure of fusion results in pancreas divisum, whereby the two parts of the pancreas remain distinct to variable extent, each with its own duct [Source: UpToDate.com; Graphic 78,995 Version 3.0]. (**b**) Improper rotation of the pancreatic buds may lead to annular pancreas, in which the gland encircles the duodenum. This birth defect produces complete obstruction (atresia) or partial obstruction (stenosis) of the duodenum. Reproduced with permission from [2]

Box 2.1 Anatomic categorization of congenital pancreatic anomalies and variants

Ventral/dorsal ductal malfusion
1. Pancreas divisum
2. Incomplete pancreas divisum
3. Isolated dorsal segment
Rotation or migration problems
1. Annular pancreas
2. Ectopic pancreas
3. Ectopic papillae
Agenesis or hypoplasia
Ductal duplication
Atypical ductal configuration
Anomalous pancreatobiliary ductal junction
Cystic malformations

individuals, and although it is generally asymptomatic (in over 95% of individuals), it may manifest as recurrent abdominal pain with or without acute pancreatitis. Another notable, albeit rare, developmental anomaly is termed *annular pancreas*. In this case the ventral pancreatic bud has a bifid configuration, which leads to the encirclement and risk of potential strangulation of the duodenum during the rotation and fusion sequence (Fig. 2.3b). Approximately half of patients with annular pancreas also have pancreas divisum [6, 7]. A list of congenital pancreatic anomalies is shown in Box 2.1.

Surgical Anatomy

In the healthy adult, the pancreas is a soft, glandular organ, situated in a transverse to slightly oblique retroperitoneal position, immediately anterior to the spine at the level of L1–L2 vertebrae (Fig. 2.4). Its volume varies significantly among individuals (mean 70–80 mL) and is greater in males. It increases with age, peaking in the fourth decade, while the organ progressively atrophies after 60 and is replaced with fat.

The pancreas is divided into five parts: the head, neck, body, tail, and uncinate process (Fig. 2.4). The neck, head, and uncinate process form a C-loop to the anatomic right of the midline that follows the natural curvature of the duodenum and is in intimate relationship with the superior mesenteric vessels. The body extends laterally to the anatomic left, posterior to the stomach, with the tail terminating in the splenic hilum. The organ is surrounded by a thin capsule that is loosely attached to its surface. Most of the anterior surface of the pancreas is coated with peritoneum, except where it is crossed by the transverse mesocolon and the root of the mesentery, as well as at its contact areas with the first part of the duodenum and the splenic hilum (Fig. 2.4).

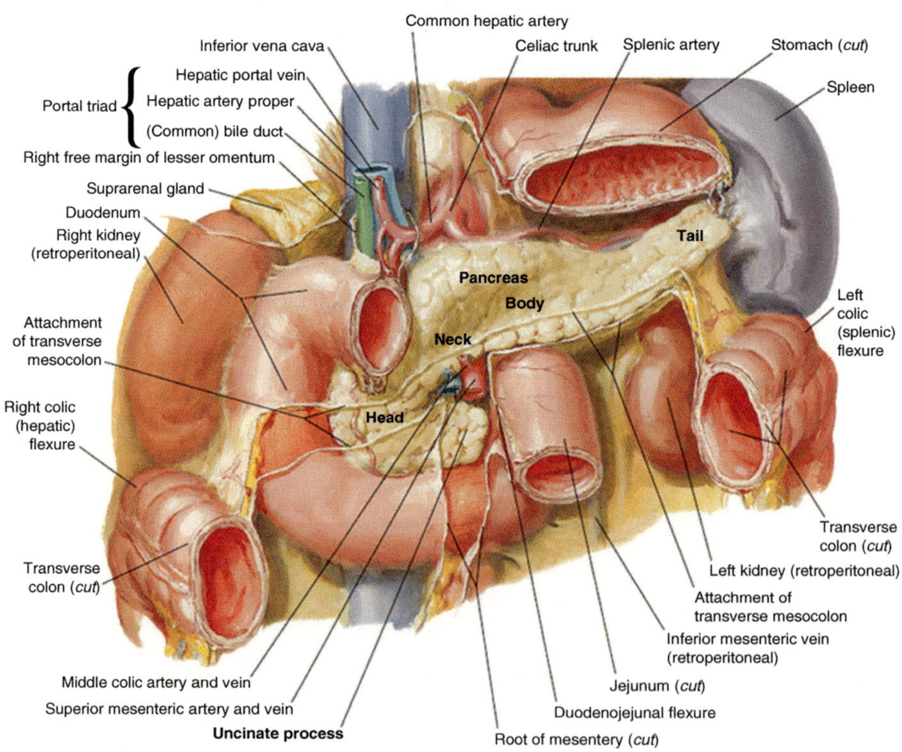

Fig. 2.4 The pancreas in situ. Reproduced with permission from [8]

The head of the pancreas is the thickest part of the gland. Anteriorly, it is related to the origin of the transverse mesocolon. Posteriorly, the head is related to the inferior vena cava (IVC), the right gonadal vein near its entrance into the vena cava, and the right crus of the diaphragm. The common bile duct runs either on the posterior surface of the pancreatic head or is embedded within the parenchyma of the gland.

The transitional zone between the head and the body of the pancreas is termed the neck. It is defined by its anatomic location anterior to the formation of the portal vein (usually by the confluence of the superior mesenteric and splenic veins). It is approximately 2 cm wide, and it is usually the most anteriorly located portion of the pancreas. Anteriorly the neck is covered by peritoneum and is related to the pylorus. Its posterior aspect is grooved by the superior mesenteric vein (SMV) and the portal vein (PV).

The body of the pancreas is anatomically the largest region. Its anterior surface is covered by the peritoneal layer that constitutes the posterior wall of the lesser sac (Fig. 2.5a). Toward the inferior border of the pancreas, the peritoneal layer is reflected anteroinferiorly to form the transverse mesocolon (Fig. 2.5). The posterior surface of the body lies on the fusion fascia of Toldt in the retroperitoneum and is related to the abdominal aorta and the origin of the superior mesenteric artery (SMA), the left crus of the diaphragm, the left renal vein, the left kidney, and the left adrenal gland, from right to left (Figs. 2.4 and 2.5a). The pancreas is surrounded by multiple blood vessels. The splenic vein runs on the posterior surface of the gland in a groove of variable depth, sometimes almost entirely embedded within the pancreatic parenchyma (Fig. 2.5). The celiac trunk and its branches emanate along the superior border of the body, with the common hepatic artery running to the right and the splenic artery to the left (Figs. 2.4 and 2.5b). The inferior border of the pancreas is crossed posteriorly by the inferior mesenteric vein (IMV), typically at its confluence with the splenic vein, and it serves as a useful landmark for identification of the former vessel on cross-sectional imaging (Fig. 2.5b).

The tail of the pancreas is the relatively mobile, leftmost part of the pancreas that is confined between the layers of the splenorenal ligament together with the splenic artery and the origin of the splenic vein (Figs. 2.4 and 2.5a). It is 1.5–3.5 cm long in adults and may extend up to the hilum of the spleen in 50% of cases. The tail of the pancreas is at risk of injury during splenectomy at the time of ligation of the splenic vessels.

The uncinate process is generally considered as a separate part of the pancreas due to its distinct embryologic origin and its location posterior to the superior mesenteric vessels (Figs. 2.4 and 2.5). It is wedged between the superior mesenteric vein and artery anteriorly and the aorta posteriorly (Fig. 2.5b). Superiorly, it relates to the left renal vein. It lies immediately superior to the third part of the duodenum, such that uncinate process tumors may compress the former leading to gastroduodenal obstruction symptoms (Figs. 2.4 and 2.5b).

The main pancreatic duct of Wirsung begins at the tail of the pancreas and runs through the body roughly halfway between the superior and inferior border (Fig. 2.3a). It receives multiple small ductules throughout its course that drain the pancreatic parenchyma, thus increasing progressively in diameter from 1 mm in the

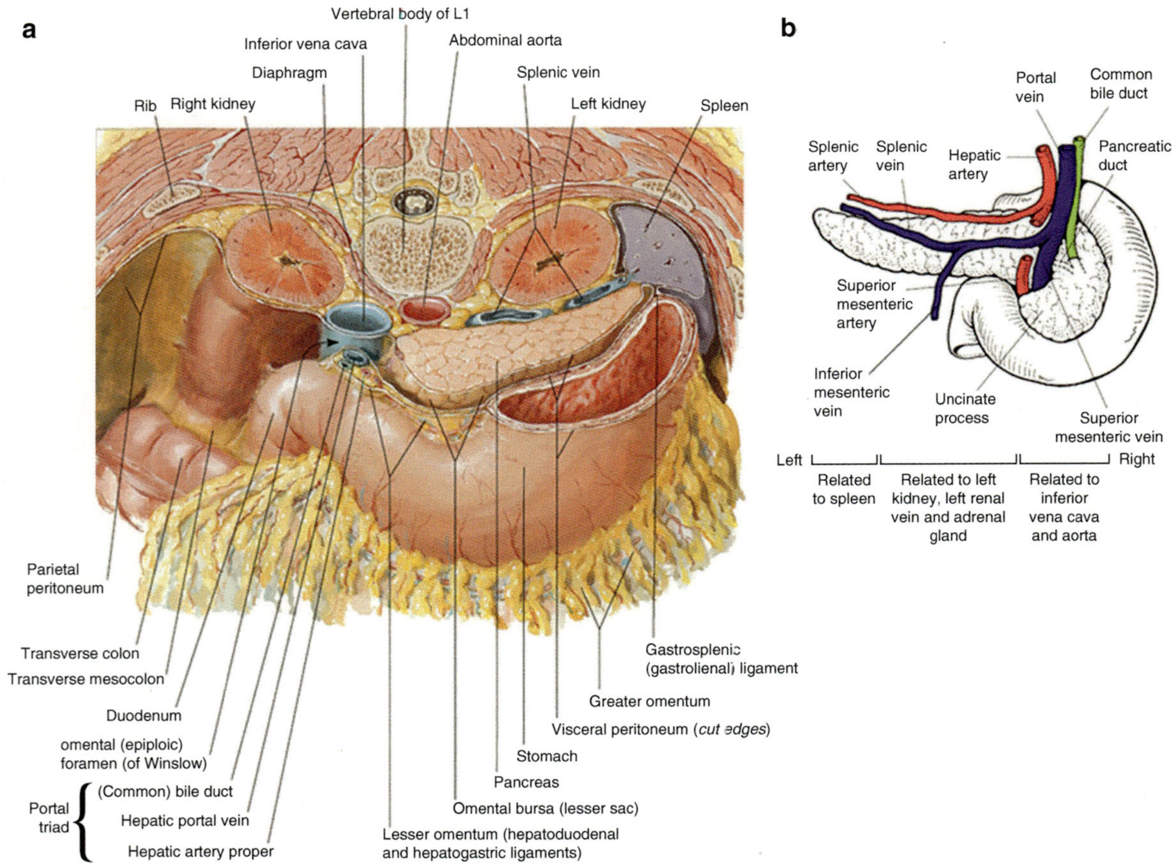

Fig. 2.5 Descriptive anatomy of the pancreas and its relationships to surrounding organs and vascular structures. (**a**) Axial cross section at the level of L1 vertebral body. The omental bursa or lesser peritoneal sac is evident. Peripancreatic inflammation can lead to obliteration of this potential space by adhesions and complicate pancreatic dissection. (**b**) The posterior relationships of the duodenum and pancreas. Reproduced with permission from [8] (**a**); [9] (**b**)

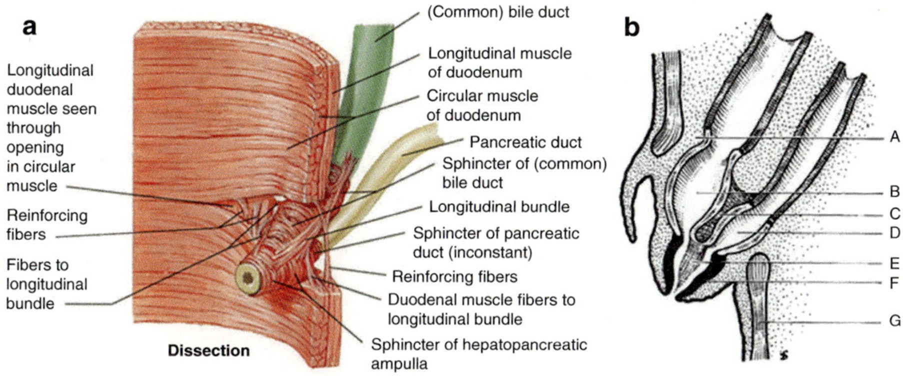

Fig. 2.6 Pancreatic duct and sphincter of Oddi. (**a**) Anatomy of the pancreatic duct at its junction with bile duct within the duodenal wall. (**b**) Schematic representation of the sphincter of Oddi: notch (**A**), biliary sphincter (**B**), transampullary septum (**C**), pancreatic sphincter (**D**), membranous septum of Boyden (**E**), common sphincter (**F**), smooth muscle of duodenal wall (**G**). Reproduced with permission from [8] (**a**); [9] (**b**)

tail to 3 mm in the head. It deviates inferiorly and posteriorly at the head. The pancreatic duct and bile duct are separated by the transampullary septum before joining in a "Y" configuration within the duodenal wall (Fig. 2.6). The terminal part of the two ducts is surrounded by a complex circular arrangement of smooth muscle fibers known as the sphincter of Oddi (Fig. 2.6). The sphincter of Oddi is anatomically distinct from the muscular layers of the duodenum, and it has a dual function: (a) to regulate flow of biliary and pancreatic secretions into the duodenal lumen and (b) to impede reflux of intestinal content into the pancreatobiliary ductal system.

The accessory duct of Santorini runs superior and parallel to the duct of Wirsung. It drains part of the head of the pancreas into the minor duodenal papilla, roughly 2 cm proximal to the papilla of Vater. The main and accessory ducts communicate to a variable extent or may be completely separate. Multiple anatomic variations have been described, some of which might predispose to pancreatitis. Pancreas divisum is the most common and has been described above.

Regional Blood Supply and Lymphatic Drainage

The celiac trunk emerges from the aorta upon its passage through the aortic hiatus of the diaphragm, just superior to the border of the pancreas (Fig. 2.4). It runs anteriorly for a very short distance and then typically trifurcates into the left gastric artery (LGA), the splenic artery, and the common hepatic artery (CHA) (Figs. 2.4 and 2.7a). The LGA may occasionally arise directly off of the aorta as a separate branch (Fig. 2.4). The splenic artery, the largest of the three celiac branches, runs a tortuous course posterior to the superior border of the pancreas toward the splenic hilum (Fig. 2.4). The splenic artery provides blood supply to the stomach via multiple short gastric arteries as well as the left gastroepiploic artery, the pancreas, and the spleen.

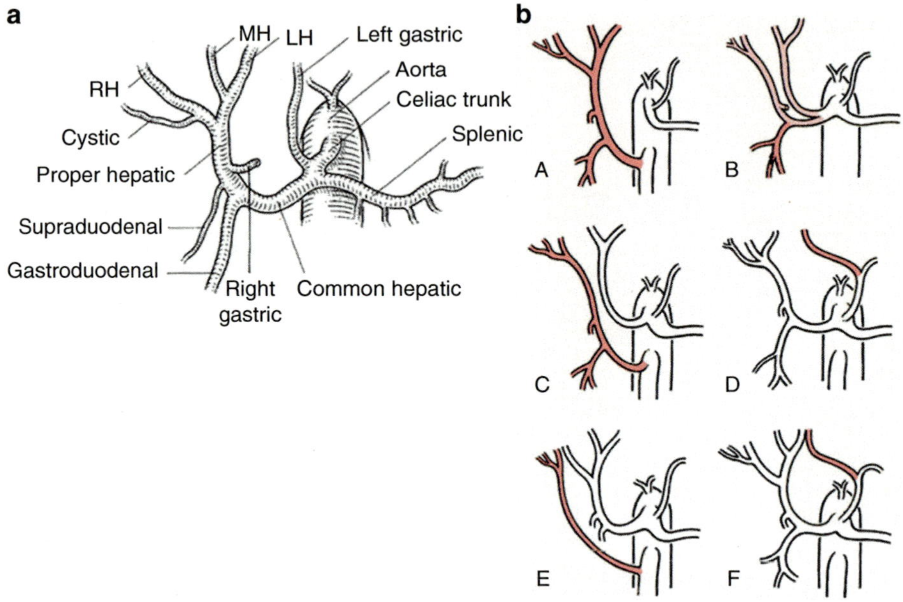

Fig. 2.7 Arterial inflow to the liver, biliary tree, and pancreas. (**a**) Usual anatomy of the celiac trunk. *LH* left hepatic artery; *MH* middle hepatic artery; *RH* right hepatic artery. Reproduced with permission from: [9]. (**b**) Common anatomic variations of the branches of the celiac trunk

The CHA initially travels forward into the retroperitoneum and then curves to the right just above the pancreas. It gives rise to the gastroduodenal artery (GDA) and the right gastric artery, after which it becomes the proper hepatic artery. The proper hepatic artery ascends in the hepatoduodenal ligament to the left of the CBD and anterior to the portal vein for a short distance (Fig. 2.5a) and divides into left hepatic (LH) and right hepatic (RH) arteries (Fig. 2.7a). The LH artery extends vertically toward the base of the umbilical fissure of the liver, giving off one or more branches to the caudate lobe as well as a branch to the quadrate lobe (segment IV) known as the middle hepatic artery. The RH artery usually passes behind the common hepatic duct and enters the hepatocystic triangle on its way to the right liver. It gives off the cystic artery that supplies the gallbladder, as well as branches to the caudate lobe.

The SMA arises from the aorta in an acute angle at the level of L1, about 1 cm distal to the origin of the celiac trunk (Fig. 2.5b). It runs inferiorly, posterior to the neck of the pancreas, the PV and SMV, and anterior to the left renal vein, the uncinate process, and the third part of the duodenum, eventually continuing into the small bowel mesentery to branch off into colic, ileal, and jejunal arteries (Fig. 2.5b). Near its origin it is surrounded by fatty tissue containing lymphatics and nerves which is frequently violated by pancreatic tumors. Preservation of this fatty plane is a critical determinant of resectability of pancreatic cancer.

The classic anatomy of the arterial blood supply to the liver, biliary tree, and pancreas is found in only approximately 60% of cases. A great degree of variability exists, and knowledge of these variations is critical for liver and pancreatic surgery (Fig. 2.7b). The CHA may arise from the SMA instead of the celiac trunk (Fig. 2.7b-A), coursing to the left of the portal vein and posterolateral to the CBD. This variation is important because it places the CHA at risk of operative injury should it go unrecognized. The GDA may originate from the right hepatic artery (Fig. 2.7b-B) and may be duplicated. The RH artery arises from the SMA in up to 25% of cases (Fig. 2.7b-C, E) and may, or may not, anastomose with the LH artery. In a similar proportion of cases, the LH artery may be replaced by a branch arising from the left gastric artery (Fig. 2.7b-D) or duplicated (Fig. 2.7b-F). In rare occasions, either of the two hepatic arteries may be derived independently from the celiac trunk.

The pancreas is a richly vascularized organ. Consistent with its embryologic origin from the foregut-midgut junction, the pancreas receives its arterial inflow from branches of the celiac trunk as well as the SMA, which form multiple arcades within and around the gland (Fig. 2.8). The head and uncinate process along with the adjacent duodenum are supplied by two main arterial vessels: the superior pancreaticoduodenal artery (SPDA), a branch of the gastroduodenal artery, and the inferior pancreaticoduodenal artery (IPDA), a branch of the SMA (Fig. 2.8). Each of these arteries divides into anterior and posterior branches. The anterior arteries unite to form the anterior (or ventral) pancreaticoduodenal arcade, and the posterior branches may unite in a posterior (dorsal) arcade (Fig. 2.8). The two arcades are connected by multiple small arteries that either run in the pancreaticoduodenal groove or traverse the pancreatic parenchyma. Usually a large branch known as the communicating artery (or middle pancreaticoduodenal arcade) runs between the main and accessory pancreatic ducts to connect the anterior arcade with the SPDA.

The body and tail of the pancreas are supplied by branches of the splenic artery (Fig. 2.8). These arteries enter the substance of the gland at its superior and inferior borders. During pancreatectomy, they should be ligated at the borders of the pancreas prior to transection, to prevent bleeding. Three large branches deserve special attention. The most prominent is the dorsal pancreatic artery, usually originating from the initial 2 cm of the splenic artery (Fig. 2.8). It supplies multiple small

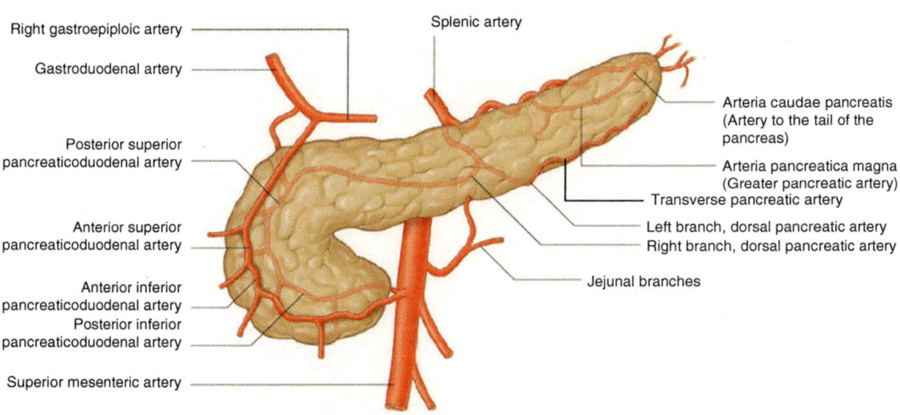

Fig. 2.8 The arteries supplying the pancreas form a rich anastomotic network around and within the gland. Reproduced with permission from [10]

branches and divides into right and left terminal branches. The right runs toward the head to unite with the pancreaticoduodenal arcades, while the left branch courses toward the tail, eventually uniting with the transverse pancreatic artery. The other two large named branches are the great pancreatic (arteria pancreatica magna) and the artery to the tail of the pancreas (arteria caudae pancreatis), both of which may join the transverse pancreatic artery running along the inferior border of the gland.

The pancreas drains into multiple peripancreatic lymph node stations via an extensive lymphatic network. Lymphatic vessels lying within the connective tissue septa of the gland unite to form larger branches that travel along the regional arteries. The lymphatic drainage of the body and tail of the pancreas occurs into the nodes of the splenic artery, the inferior pancreatic, and the splenic hilar and from there to the celiac and preaortic nodes. The neck and head of the pancreas have a much wider drainage to the nodal stations of the supplying arteries. Lymph node status is one of the most important prognostic factors of pancreatic cancer; therefore, adequate resection and appropriate staging (including number of involved lymph nodes and presence of lymphatic invasion) are paramount for appropriate management of these patients.

Innervation

The pancreas has a rich autonomic innervation that contributes to the regulation of both the exocrine and the endocrine functions of the gland. Parasympathetic nerve fibers distributed throughout the gland within the interlobular connective tissue transmit impulses to and from the vagus via its hepatic, gastric, and celiac branches. This is integrated with additional feedback from enteric neurons of the stomach and duodenum as well as sympathetic efferent neurons. In addition, sympathetic nerves innervate the intrapancreatic blood vessels and ducts, causing vasoconstriction and inhibiting exocrine secretion. Pain associated with pancreatic diseases is conveyed via visceral afferents of the celiac plexus and thoracic splanchnic nerves to the T6–T12 dorsal root ganglia, thus explaining its poor localization and ill-defined nature. However, in cases of extensive inflammatory or infiltrative processes involving the retroperitoneum, the regional somatic nerves may be involved leading to pain localized to the lower thoracic spine.

Biliary Tree

The biliary tree comprises a series of epithelium-lined ductal structures which function as a reservoir for the bile produced by the liver as well as a conduit for its delivery into the intestine. The biliary tree is divided into intrahepatic and extrahepatic portions, with the latter being further subdivided into the extrahepatic bile ducts and the accessory biliary apparatus (gallbladder and cystic duct). An in-depth understanding of the anatomy of the biliary tree and its associated vasculature constitutes essential knowledge that must be possessed by every upper abdominal surgeon and general surgeon. Cholecystectomy is the most common abdominal procedure performed in developed countries, and biliary injury during this procedure continues to occur.

Embryology

The events leading to the embryologic development of the liver and biliary tree have some similarity to the ones described above for the pancreas. The liver primordium appears in the middle of the third week of gestation as an outgrowth of the endodermal lining at the ventral aspect of the distal foregut. The hepatic progenitor cells, or hepatoblasts, proliferate rapidly and penetrate the basal lamina to expand into the septum transversum—a mesodermal plate separating the pericardial cavity and the future abdominal cavity. As this outgrowth (termed hepatic diverticulum or liver bud) continues to grow into the septum transversum, the connection to the distal foregut becomes progressively narrower leading to the formation of the bile duct (Fig. 2.1). The part of the septum transversum lying between the liver and the ventral abdominal wall eventually transforms into the falciform ligament, while the part of it between the liver primordium and the foregut forms the lesser omentum. An evagination at the ventral aspect of the developing bile duct gives rise to the gallbladder and cystic duct. Bile formation commences around the 12th week of gestation.

Bidirectional communication of the endodermal liver primordium with the septum transversum mesenchyme and the overlying cardiac mesoderm is critical for liver specification. The entire gut endoderm has the potential to form liver tissue, but this is suppressed by the action of surrounding tissues, particularly the notochord. Bone morphogenetic proteins (BMPs) originating from the septum transversum enable the endoderm to respond to liver-inducing signals [11]—a phenomenon termed hepatic competence and mediated by expression of forkhead box protein A (*FOXA*) transcription factors. Next, fibroblast growth factors (FGF) from the cardiac mesoderm disinhibit the liver specification program, which is tonically repressed, leading to liver induction. Vessel-forming endothelial cells also contribute to this process.

The proliferating hepatoblasts give rise to both mature hepatocytes and biliary epithelial cells, while the surrounding mesoderm of the septum transversum forms the stromal cells of the liver (primarily liver sinusoidal endothelial cells, hepatic stellate cells, and Kupffer cells) and its vasculature. Notably, at this stage of embryogenesis, the liver is an important site for hematopoiesis. Portal and hepatic vein radicals begin to form derived from the vitelline veins. The bipotential hepatoblasts initially express genes for adult hepatocytes (*ALB*, *HNF4A*) and biliary epithelial cells (*KRT19*). Subsequently, they downregulate either of the two and commit to the opposite lineage (Fig. 2.9a). This event appears to depend on the proximity of the cells to portal vein tributaries, possibly under the control of

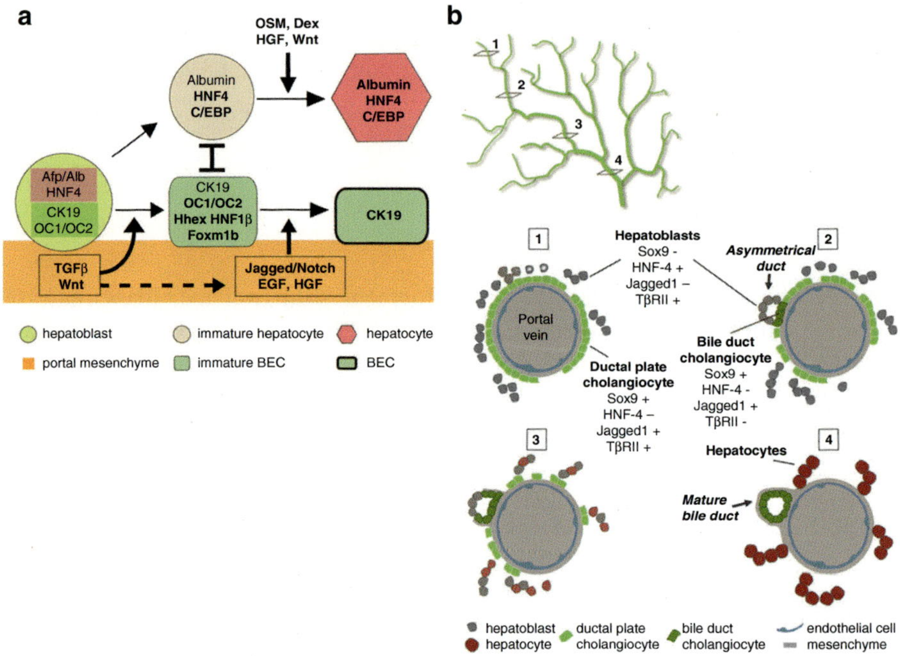

Fig. 2.9 Embryologic development of the liver and biliary tree. (**a**) Model of hepatoblast differentiation into hepatocytes or biliary epithelial cells (BEC). Hepatoblasts are bipotential, which is reflected in expression of both hepatocytes (albumin) and BECs (CK19). Interaction with the periportal mesenchyme promotes differentiation to BECs by expression of BEC promoting (OC1, OC2, HNF1β) and repression of mature hepatocyte (HNF4 and C/EBP) transcription factors. On the contrary, hepatoblasts not influenced by periportal mesenchyme signals (such as Wnt and TGF-β) undergo differentiation toward mature hepatocytes. Additional signals from the periportal mesenchyme (Notch, EGF, and HGF) facilitate ductal plate remodeling, while other factors (OSM, Dex, HGF, and Wnt) promote hepatocyte maturation. Reproduced with permission from Zorn, A.M., Liver development (October 31, 2008), StemBook, ed. The Stem Cell Research Community, StemBook, doi/10.3824/stembook.1.25.1, http://www.stembook.org. Copyright 2008 Aaron M. Zorn. (**b**) Formation of bile duct progresses from the hilum to the periphery of the liver. Sections at different stages of maturation are shown, with the least mature at the periphery (ductal plate; Sect. 1) and mature bile ducts near the hilum (Sect. 4). Part of the ductal plate cells form asymmetrical ducts that result in mature bile ducts, while the rest regress. Reproduced with permission from [12]

signals such as transforming growth factor-β (TGF-β) and Wnt originating in the periportal mesenchyme (Fig. 2.9).

A subpopulation of hepatoblasts encircles the portal veins to form a band of potential biliary epithelial cells. This band is termed the "ductal plate," and its constituent cells are called cholangiocytes (Fig. 2.9b). Soon this transforms into a bilayer with focal dilations. The latter give rise to the intrahepatic bile ducts in the portal triads. Remodeling of the ductal plates begins at the oldest ductal plates surrounding the larger portal veins near the hilum and progresses toward the periphery of the liver, following the portal vein system. The remaining ductal plate cells that were not incorporated into bile ducts then involute via apoptosis. The ductal plate is an important source of vascular endothelial growth factor (VEGF) that drives hepatic artery development [12]. The significance of the developmental relationship between the bile ducts, the portal vessels (hepatic artery, portal vein), and the portal mesenchyme is highlighted by *ductal plate malformations* that result from inappropriate interactions and ductal plate remodeling [13]. For example, *Alagille syndrome* is an autosomal dominant disease associated with mutations in *JAG1* and *NOTCH2* in which the bile ducts are absent from the portal tract, whereas there are increased numbers of hepatic arteries and fibrosis.

It is worth mentioning that ductal plate malformations are fundamentally different from biliary atresia. Biliary atresia begins with a normally developed biliary tree that is subsequently obliterated by inflammation and fibrosis due to perinatal environmental insults to the fetus (infectious and/or noninfectious). It involves predominantly the extrahepatic biliary tree and manifests as progressive neonatal jaundice that culminates in cirrhosis at a very young age, if left untreated. Although rare, it is critical that it is recognized as early as possible since portoenterostomy (Kasai operation and its variants) can have dramatically better outcomes if performed prior to 3 months of age and possibly spare the infant from a liver transplantation procedure.

Surgical Anatomy

The surgical anatomy of the biliary tree is intertwined with the hepatic anatomy due to their common embryologic origin and their integrated physiologic role. Although multiple classifications of the hepatic structural anatomy have been proposed, the most surgically relevant is the one described by Couinaud [14]. The liver is subdivided into eight distinct segments—each with its own discrete biliary drainage, vascular inflow that enters the segment as a pedicle, and vascular outflow (Fig. 2.10a). The functional unit of the liver is the hepatic lobule, which consists of sheets of hepatocytes radiating outward from a central vein (Fig. 2.11). At the periphery of these polygonal units are multiple portal triads—each composed of a branch of the hepatic artery, a branch of the portal vein and a bile duct, encased within trabeculae of connective tissue termed portal tracts. The hepatic artery and portal vein branches represent the vascular inflow to the hepatic lobule. The blood then circulates between the hepatocytes in spaces termed sinusoids in a centripetal manner, subsequently draining into the central vein (Fig. 2.11). The latter are tributaries of the hepatic veins and constitute the vascular outflow of the hepatic lobule, ultimately draining into the IVC. As the hepatocytes carry out their metabolic functions, they secrete bile into canaliculi that terminate at the bile duct tributaries found within the portal triads. Bile duct tributaries from adjacent lobules merge to form bile ductules of progressively larger caliber, which eventually lead to the segmental bile ducts, each draining one of the eight liver segments (Fig. 2.10).

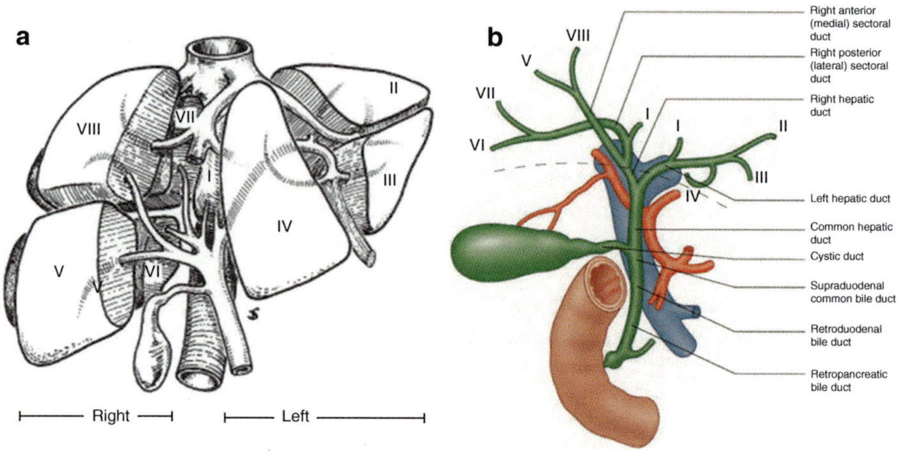

Fig. 2.10 Biliary drainage of the liver. (**a**) The functional division of the liver and its segments according to Couinaud's nomenclature, along with the biliary drainage of the two functional hemilivers is shown. Reproduced with permission from [9]. (**b**) The overall arrangement of the intrahepatic and extrahepatic biliary tree. Note that segment I (caudate lobe) often drains via both right and left hepatic ducts. The dashed line represents the level of the liver parenchyma at the porta hepatis. Reproduced with permission from [10]

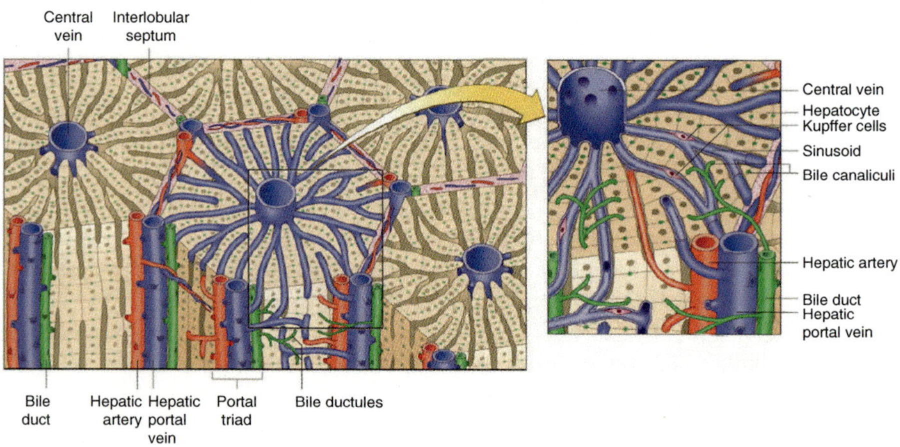

Fig. 2.11 Microarchitecture of the liver. Reproduced with permission from [10]

Intrahepatic Bile Duct Anatomy

The left liver (segments II, III, and IV) drains its bile into the left hepatic duct, and the right liver (segments V, VI, VII, and VIII) drains into the right hepatic duct (Fig. 2.10). Bile ducts generally course above the corresponding portal venous branches. Segmental branches join to form sectoral ducts, which derive their names from their location within the liver parenchyma (Fig. 2.10b). Thus, the bile ducts of segments II and III merge to form the left lateral sectoral duct, which is subsequently joined by the duct of segment IV to form the left hepatic duct. Similarly, the ducts of segments VI and VII form the right posterior (or lateral) sectoral duct, and the ducts of segments V and VIII form the right anterior (medial) sectoral duct. The right posterior sectoral duct runs a horizontal course and turns inferiorly to join the vertically coursing right anterior sectoral branch to form the right hepatic duct. The smaller caudate lobe (segment I) has a more pervasive biliary drainage such that in 78% of cases, it drains into both the right and left hepatic ducts, while in 15 and 7% of cases, it drains exclusively into the left or right hepatic duct system, respectively (Fig. 2.10b).

The biliary anatomy is subject to significant variation (Fig. 2.12) [9, 14, 15]. Such anatomic variations are more common in women [16]. Up to 15% of individuals lack a defined right hepatic duct; instead a "trifurcation pattern" is encountered, whereby the common hepatic duct (CHD) is formed by the union of the right posterior and right anterior sectoral ducts with the left hepatic duct (Fig. 2.12). An equally common variant involves a right sectoral duct (more often the anterior) with low insertion directly into the CHD. Less frequently a right sectoral duct (usually the posterior) may drain into the left hepatic duct. Variations involving ectopic drainage of individual segmental ducts may also occur [17]. Notably, a subvesical duct has been reported in 20–50% of cases, joining either the CHD or the right hepatic duct. It does not drain any specific liver territory and never communicates with the gallbladder, unlike the true ducts of Luschka [18]; however, it is at risk of injury and postoperative biliary leak during cholecystectomy if appropriate dissection with preservation of the cystic plate is not performed. Anatomic variations of the left-sided ductal system are less common and usually involve either variations of the site of drainage of segment IV duct (most commonly joining the duct of segment III) or multiple segmental branches emerging from segment IV.

Extrahepatic Bile Duct Anatomy

The extrahepatic biliary tree can be divided into the extrahepatic bile ducts and the accessory biliary apparatus (Fig. 2.10b). The former comprises the extrahepatic segments of the right and left hepatic ducts, joining to form a single main bile duct that drains into the duodenum. The right hepatic duct is nearly vertical with a short extrahepatic course (0.5–2.0 cm). The extrahepatic portion of the left hepatic duct runs a more horizontal course, posterior to the inferior border of the quadrate lobe (segment IV), and is longer (1.5–3.5 cm in adults). It is worth noting that ligation of an extrahepatic duct results in atrophy of the corresponding hepatic lobe with a high probability of subsequent cholangitis and even abscess formation. Therefore, any bile duct injury should be repaired when recognized and whenever feasible.

The right and left hepatic ducts unite anterior to the portal venous bifurcation and the origin of the right branch of the portal vein (Fig. 2.10b). This confluence is situated to the right of the hepatic hilar fissure, immediately posterior to the quadrate lobe of the liver. The hepatic plate/sheath system is a fusion of the Glisson capsule and the connective tissue enclosing the biliary and vascular elements

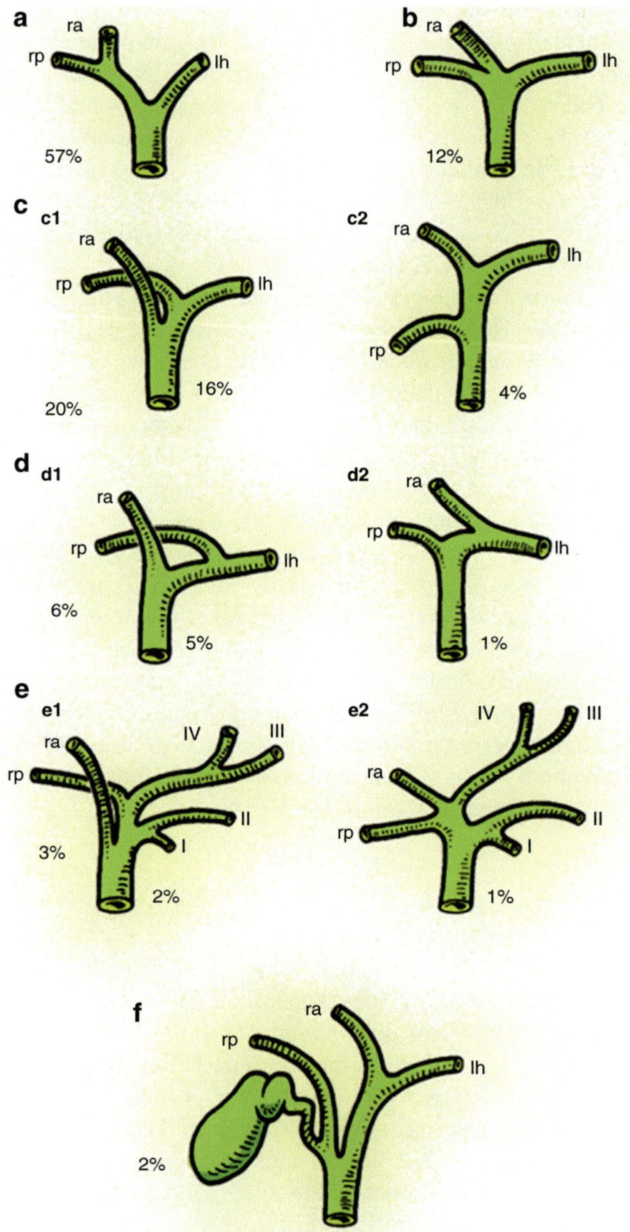

Fig. 2.12 Anatomic variations of the bile ducts. Main variations of the hepatic duct confluence [14]. (**a**) Typical anatomy of the confluence. (**b**) Triple confluence. (**c**) Ectopic drainage of a right sectoral duct into the common hepatic duct (C1, right anterior [ra] duct draining into the common hepatic duct; C2, right posterior [rp] duct draining into the common hepatic duct). (**d**) Ectopic drainage of a right sectoral duct into the left hepatic ductal system (D1, right posterior sectoral duct draining into the left hepatic [lh] ductal system; D2, right anterior sectoral duct draining into the left hepatic ductal system). (**e**) Absence of the hepatic duct confluence. (**f**) Absence of right hepatic duct and ectopic drainage of the right posterior duct into the cystic duct

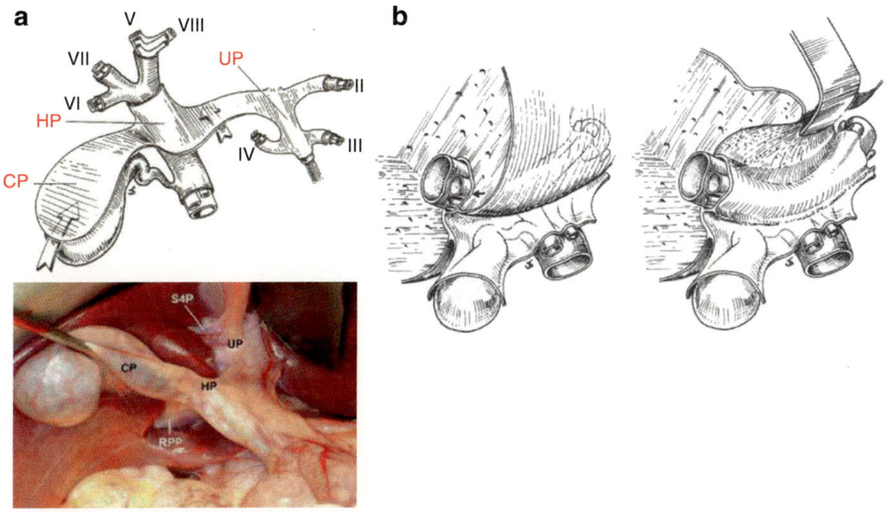

Fig. 2.13 The hepatic plate/sheath system. (**a**) Schematic representation (top) and in situ appearance (bottom) of the plate/sheath system, showing the cystic plate (CP) covered by the gallbladder, the hilar plate (HP), and the umbilical plate (UP). The large, curving arrows indicate the plane of dissection of the cystic plate during cholecystectomy and of the hilar plate during approaches to the left hepatic duct. S4P, segment 4 pedicle; RPP, right posterior pedicle. (**b**) The biliary confluence and left hepatic duct can be exposed by lifting the quadrate lobe upward after incision of the Glisson capsule at its base. This technique, "lowering of the hilar plate" [19], generally is used to display a dilated bile duct above an iatrogenic stricture or hilar cholangiocarcinoma. Reproduced with permission from [20] (photograph), and [9] (schematics)

(Fig. 2.13). It consists of flat fibrous planes on the undersurface of the liver termed "plates," and tubular extensions termed "sheaths" that radiate into the liver parenchyma to transmit the portal bilio-vascular structures. Familiarity with the anatomy of the plate system is very important as it is ideal for dissection of perihepatic structures due to its avascular nature. Thus, the hilar plate can be divided at the inferior border of the quadrate lobe, and the latter elevated to facilitate access to the biliary confluence and left hepatic duct—a maneuver termed *lowering of the hilar plate* (Fig. 2.13) [19].

The main bile duct is divided in two portions by the entry of the cystic duct (CD) (Fig. 2.10b). The upper portion, the CHD, is approximately 2–3 cm long and has an average diameter less than 6 mm in adults. It descends in the free edge of the lesser omentum, situated anterior to the portal vein and to the left of the hepatic artery proper. The lower portion is the common bile duct (CBD). The CBD has a luminal diameter of less than 8 mm (based on radiological measurements) that may increase in people older than 60 years (Box 2.2). It is 6–8 cm long and can be subdivided in three parts according to its relations to the duodenum and pancreas (Fig. 2.10b). The supraduodenal part (3–4 cm long) descends posteroinferiorly anterior to the IVC, situated within the hepatoduodenal ligament anterolaterally to the PV and to the right of the hepatic artery (Fig. 2.5a). The retroduodenal part crosses behind the first part of the duodenum, to the right of the GDA. The retropancreatic part runs through the parenchyma of the head of the pancreas (or occasionally behind it), anterior to

Box 2.2 Size of common pancreatobiliary structures

Structure	Diameter (luminal)
Cystic duct	1–3 mm
Common hepatic duct	≤6 mm
Common bile duct	≤8 mm
Main pancreatic duct	≤3 mm

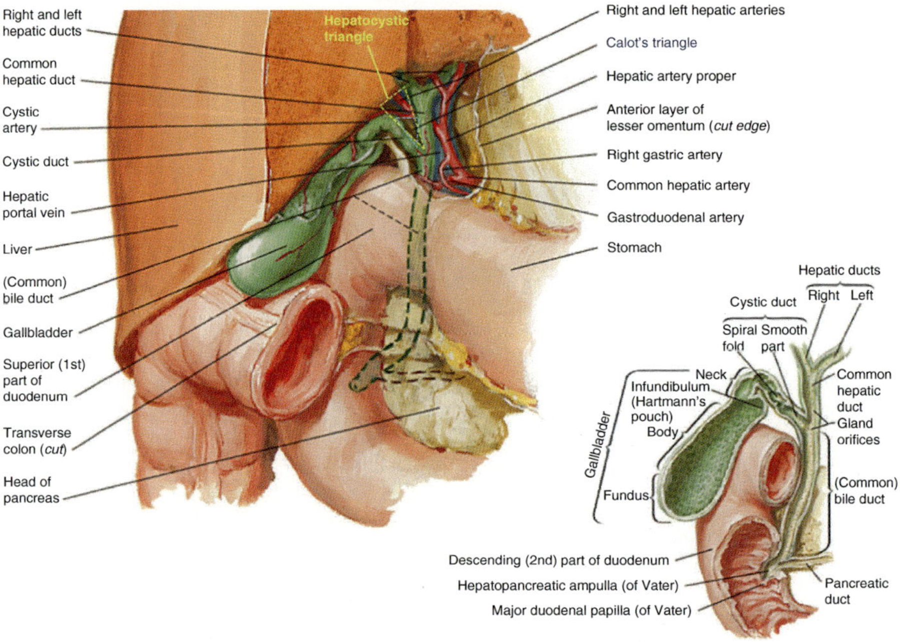

Fig. 2.14 Anatomy of the gallbladder and cystic duct. Note the *hepatocystic triangle*, limited by the common hepatic duct, right hepatic duct, cystic duct, and inferior liver edge. The *triangle of Calot* is limited by the common hepatic duct, the cystic duct, and the cystic artery. Reproduced with permission from [8]

the right renal vein and posterior to the SPDA. Its caudal end enters into the wall of the second portion of the duodenum together with the main pancreatic duct of Wirsung in a Y configuration. The two ducts unite within the duodenal wall forming a common channel, 2–10 mm long, that is focally dilated, and hence it is called the hepatopancreatic ampulla of Vater (Figs. 2.6 and 2.14).

Gallbladder and Cystic Duct

The accessory biliary apparatus is comprised of the gallbladder and CD (Fig. 2.14) and functions as a reservoir for bile during periods of fasting as well as a modifier of bile composition, mainly by concentrating it. The gallbladder is classically described as flask shaped. It varies in size and its volume can reach up to 50 mL. It consists of a fundus, a body, and a neck. The neck lies close to the porta hepatis. It transitions into the body at an angle, forming the infundibulum (or Hartmann's pouch) which is more prominent in the presence of gallstone disease. The neck and body lie anterior to the second part of the duodenum (Fig. 2.14). The fundus is located more anterolaterally and may project beyond the liver edge in close proximity to the anterior abdominal wall at the level of the ninth costal cartilage. If elongated, the fundus may be highly mobile, and, in rare occasions, it can result in folding back on the body. This variant, termed "Phrygian cap," can be identified radiologically and may be misinterpreted as an apparent septum in an otherwise normal gallbladder or at times be confused for a malignancy. Various rare anomalies of the gallbladder anatomy have been described [15].

The gallbladder is situated within the cystic fossa on the undersurface of the liver and serves as the external sign of the division between the right and left liver (Cantlie's line) (Fig. 2.14). Its surface is covered by peritoneum except at the cystic fossa, where it is intimately associated with the liver. The neck almost always has a short peritoneal attachment to the liver (mesentery) that usually contains the cystic artery. Occasionally, the gallbladder may be completely surrounded by peritoneum and be suspended from the liver in its own mesentery, rendering the gallbladder susceptible to torsion. On the other hand, less frequently it might be situated deep into the hepatic parenchyma or even be completely buried within the liver (intrahepatic gallbladder). The latter case may be misinterpreted as gallbladder agenesis. Even more uncommon is the scenario where the gallbladder lies to the left of the round ligament.

The connective tissue between the gallbladder and the liver comprises the cystic plate (Fig. 2.13a). It is ovoid anteriorly and narrows posteriorly to join the sheath of the right portal pedicle and the hepatic plate. During cholecystectomy, the dissection of the gallbladder off the liver proceeds along the avascular plane between the cystic plate and the gallbladder, which is filled with areolar tissue. Caution should be exercised in cases of chronic inflammation in which the cystic plate might be scarred and contracted, bringing the bilio-vascular structures of the right pedicle in close proximity to the gallbladder. In such cases, dissection of the gallbladder can be performed in a "top-down" or retrograde fashion to minimize the risk of injury to the right pedicle structures. Occasionally, the cystic plate may be penetrated by submillimeter accessory bile ducts that drain directly into the gallbladder. These are termed "ducts of Luschka" and are important because if severed during cholecystectomy, they can result in clinically significant bilomas postoperatively. Further, a subvesical duct from the right hemiliver may be deeply embedded in the cystic plate on its way to joining the right hepatic duct or the CHD, and it is at risk of injury if the cystic plate is not recognized and preserved at the time of cholecystectomy.

The CD arises from the neck of the gallbladder and descends in a posteromedial direction to join the CHD, marking the beginning of the CBD. It is lined by mucosa that has multiple crescentic intraluminal projections arranged in a spiral configuration, which are termed the "valves of Heister" (Fig. 2.14). The CD has a luminal diameter of 1–3 mm and is usually 2–4 cm long. Its length varies depending on the type of union with the extrahepatic bile duct system. In 75–80% of cases, the CD enters the main bile duct in a supraduodenal location; however, this union may occur more caudally at the retroduodenal or even retropancreatic part of the

CBD. Conversely, the CD may occasionally join the right hepatic duct or even a right hepatic sectoral duct. The orientation and mode of union may also vary. Most commonly, the CD joins the CHD from the right side in an angular fashion. However, the CD may merge in a parallel or even spiral fashion, at the anterior, posterior, or medial aspect of the main bile duct. Rarely, the gallbladder or cystic duct may receive aberrant drainage directly from intrahepatic ducts.

Regional Blood Supply and Lymphatic Drainage

The main regional arteries supplying the hepatobiliary structures (celiac trunk, hepatic artery, SMA) and their variations have been described above. The right and left hepatic arteries branch off the hepatic artery proper and enter the liver enclosed in sheaths of connective tissue that are part of the plate/sheath system, forming the right and left portal triads. They bifurcate into smaller branches along with the portal vein and bile duct branches to form pedicles corresponding to individual segments. The right hepatic (RH) artery usually passes behind the CHD and enters the hepatocystic triangle of Calot (Fig. 2.14). However, in some cases it courses anterior to the bile duct, which is important in surgical exposure of the latter. The hepatocystic triangle is defined as the triangular space bordered by the common hepatic duct, the cystic duct, and the inferior surface of the right lobe of the liver (Fig. 2.14). It is of critical importance during cholecystectomy, as it has to be dissected in order to identify and ligate the cystic artery en route to the gallbladder. The term "hepatocystic triangle" is nowadays used interchangeably with "Calot's triangle," although the original definition of the latter included the cystic artery instead of the inferior surface of the liver as the superior border. Notably, if there is a replaced or accessory common or right hepatic artery, it usually runs behind the cystic duct to enter the triangle of Calot.

The cystic artery usually arises from the RH artery and may cross the common hepatic duct anteriorly or posteriorly. It divides into anterior and posterior branches upon contact with the gallbladder. This division, however, may occur before the artery reaches the gallbladder wall, in which case one of the two branches may be unrecognized and divided without proper ligation during cholecystectomy, leading to hemorrhage. Multiple variations of the anatomy of the cystic artery exist; hence, the surgeon should be vigilant and prepared to recognize them in order to avoid inadvertent hemorrhage or injury to biliary structures in an attempt to control the bleeding. The venous drainage of the gallbladder occurs via multiple small cystic veins that traverse the cystic plate to join segmental portal veins. Uncommonly, distinct cystic veins run parallel to the cystic artery to empty into the main portal vein.

The blood supply of the main bile duct can be considered by dividing the latter in three parts: hilar, supraduodenal, and retropancreatic. The supraduodenal duct is supplied by branches of the GDA, the superior pancreaticoduodenal artery, the retroduodenal artery, the RH, and the cystic artery (Fig. 2.15). These branches run in an axial fashion at the 3 and 9 o'clock positions of the duct (Fig. 2.15a). They form a rich anastomotic network on the surface as well as within the wall of the duct (Fig. 2.15b). The hilar ducts receive ample blood supply from the neighboring arteries, in continuity with the epicholedochal plexus of the supraduodenal part

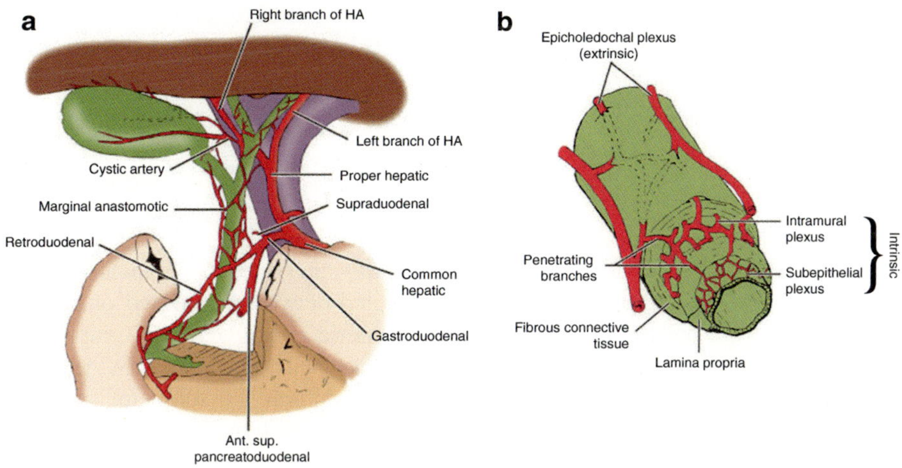

Fig. 2.15 (**a**, **b**) Arterial blood supply to the extrahepatic bile ducts showing the epicholedochal arterial plexus. HA, hepatic artery. Reproduced with permission from [15]

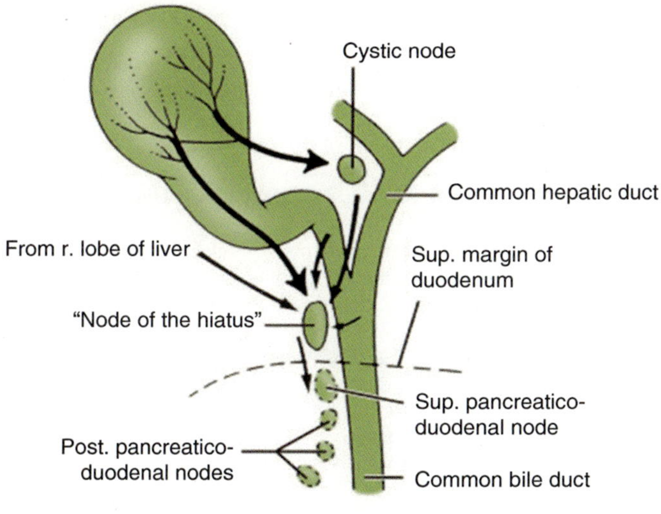

Fig. 2.16 Lymphatic drainage of gallbladder and biliary tract. Reproduced with permission from [15]

(Fig. 2.15a). The retropancreatic part of the duct is mainly supplied by branches of the retroduodenal artery that run around the duct to contribute to its arterial plexus (Fig. 2.15a). The veins of the extrahepatic bile ducts follow the same course as the corresponding arteries coursing mainly at the 3 and 9 o'clock positions. They communicate with the venous outflow of the gallbladder and drain into the portal venous system indirectly, via the liver.

The lymphatic drainage of the gallbladder is mainly to the hepatoduodenal ligament lymph nodes (Fig. 2.16). This can occur via the cystic node, which lies in the hepatocystic triangle, via lymphatics that descend along the CBD, or via lymphatics of the hepatic aspect of the gallbladder that drain into intrahepatic lymph vessels first. Subsequently the lymph can drain into multiple peripancreatic nodal stations, ultimately reaching the celiac, superior mesenteric, and preaortic lymph nodes.

Innervation

The extrahepatic biliary tree and gallbladder are innervated by branches of the hepatic plexus. The hepatic plexus is an integrated network composed of sympathetic fibers from the celiac and superior mesenteric plexus and parasympathetic fibers derived mainly from the anterior branch of the vagus. The latter provide motor stimulation to the bile ducts and gallbladder and inhibit the sphincter of Oddi. Sympathetic afferent fibers are the primary source of pain sensation, via the greater and lesser splanchnic nerves.

References

1. Tsuchiya R, Fujisawa N. On the etymology of "pancreas". Int J Pancreatol. 1997;21(3):269–72.
2. Moore KL, et al. The developing human: clinically oriented embryology. 10th ed. Philadelphia: Saunders; 2015.
3. Stanger BZ, Hebrok M. Control of cell identity in pancreas development and regeneration. Gastroenterology. 2013;144(6):1170–9.
4. Jennings RE, Berry AA, Strutt JP, Gerrard DT, Hanley NA. Human pancreas development. Development. 2015;142(18):3126–37.
5. Mazur PK, Siveke JT. Genetically engineered mouse models of pancreatic cancer: unravelling tumour biology and progressing translational oncology. Gut. 2012;61(10):1488–500.
6. Sandrasegaran K, Patel A, Fogel EL, Zyromski NJ, Pitt HA. Annular pancreas in adults. Am J Roentgenol. 2009;193(2):455–60.
7. Zyromski NJ, Sandoval JA, Pitt HA, Ladd AP, Fogel EL, Mattar WE, et al. Annular pancreas: dramatic differences between children and adults. J Am Coll Surg. 2008;206(5):1019–25. discussion 25-7
8. Netter FH. Atlas of human anatomy. 6th ed. Philadelphia: Saunders; 2014.
9. Jarnagin WR, Blumgart LH, Jarnagin WR, Brody LA, Brown KT, Covey AM, et al. Blumgart's surgery of the liver, biliary tract and pancreas. 5th ed. Philadelphia: Elsevier Saunders; 2012.
10. Standring S. Gray's Anatomy: the anatomical basis of clinical practice. 41st ed; 2016.
11. Rossi JM, Dunn NR, Hogan BL, Zaret KS. Distinct mesodermal signals, including BMPs from the septum transversum mesenchyme, are required in combination for hepatogenesis from the endoderm. Genes Dev. 2001;15(15):1998–2009.
12. Si-Tayeb K, Lemaigre FP, Duncan SA. Organogenesis and development of the liver. Dev Cell. 2010;18(2):175–89.
13. Raynaud P, Tate J, Callens C, Cordi S, Vandersmissen P, Carpentier R, et al. A classification of ductal plate malformations based on distinct pathogenic mechanisms of biliary dysmorphogenesis. Hepatology. 2011;53(6):1959–66.
14. Couinaud C. Le foie; études anatomiques et chirurgicales. Paris: Masson; 1957.
15. Skandalakis JE, Colborn GL. Skandalakis' surgical anatomy the embryologic and anatomic basis of modern surgery. Athens: Paschalidis Medical Publications, Ltd.; McGraw-Hill (distributor); 2004.

16. Cucchetti A, Peri E, Cescon M, Zanello M, Ercolani G, Zanfi C, et al. Anatomic variations of intrahepatic bile ducts in a European series and meta-analysis of the literature. J Gastrointest Surg. 2011;15(4):623–30.
17. Healey JE Jr, Schroy PC. Anatomy of the biliary ducts within the human liver; analysis of the prevailing pattern of branchings and the major variations of the biliary ducts. AMA Arch Surg. 1953;66(5):599–616.
18. Schnelldorfer T, Sarr MG, Adams DB. What is the duct of Luschka?--a systematic review. J Gastrointest Surg. 2012;16(3):656–62.
19. Hepp J, Couinaud C. Approach to and use of the left hepatic duct in reparation of the common bile duct. La Presse medicale. 1956;64(41):947–8.
20. Fischer JE, et al. Fischer's mastery of surgery. 6th ed. Philadelphia: Wolters Kluwer Health/ Lippincott Williams & Wilkins; 2012.

Chapter 3
Pathology: Premalignant and Malignant Diseases and Molecular Genetics

Wei Chen, Ming Jin, and Wendy L. Frankel

Introduction

Epidemiology

Although pancreatic cancer barely makes the top ten most common cancers in the USA, it is the fourth leading cause of cancer death according to Cancer Statistics 2016 [1]. The incidence and death rates of pancreatic cancer continue to increase. Total deaths due to pancreatic cancers are projected to increase dramatically, and pancreatic cancer will become the second leading cause of cancer-related deaths (after lung cancer) by 2020 [2].

Most pancreatic cancers are already advanced in stage at the time of diagnosis. The nonspecific presenting symptoms and the retroperitoneal location of the pancreas make it challenging for early detection of pancreatic cancer. The most common clinical presentation of pancreatic cancer includes back pain, unexpected weight loss, jaundice, pruritus, diabetes mellitus, depression, acute pancreatitis, and migratory thrombophlebitis. Imaging studies, pancreatic cyst fluid analysis, serology, fine needle aspiration cytology, and core needle biopsy are the major diagnostic modalities.

W. Chen, M.D., Ph.D. • M. Jin, M.D., Ph.D. • W.L. Frankel, M.D. (✉)
Department of Pathology, The Ohio State University Wexner Medical Center,
1645 Neil Ave, 129 Hamilton Hall, Columbus, OH 43210, USA
e-mail: Wendy.Frankel@osumc.edu

T. Bekaii-Saab, B. El-Rayes (eds.), *Current and Emerging Therapies in Pancreatic Cancer*, DOI 10.1007/978-3-319-58256-6_3

With a 5-year relative survival rate of only 6%, pancreatic cancer is listed as one of the deadliest cancers in the *Recalcitrant Cancer Research Act* (2013) [3]. It should also be noted that the survival rate for pancreatic cancer has not improved substantially for the last 40 years, and research efforts are essential for improving prevention, detection, and treatment of pancreatic cancer.

Histology of the Normal Pancreas

The pancreas is composed of exocrine (85%) and endocrine (15%) tissue. Microscopically, the pancreas is organized into lobules (Fig. 3.1a). The cellularity in each lobule is composed predominantly of exocrine acini, which secrete pancreatic enzymes that drain into the ductal system (Fig. 3.1b). Scattered within the lobules are the islets of Langerhans where 90% of endocrine cells in the pancreas reside (Fig. 3.1b). The remainder of the endocrine cells distributes among the acini and larger ducts. While the ductal system represents only a small portion of the pancreatic tissue, over 90% of pancreatic neoplasms originate from the ducts.

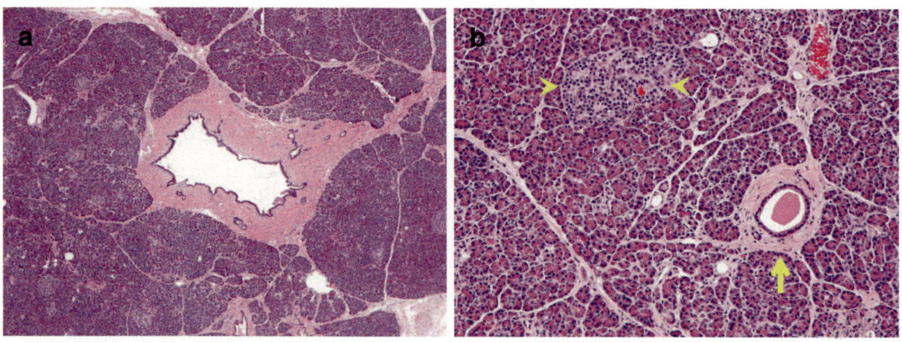

Fig. 3.1 Normal pancreas. Lobules of exocrine acini surround a central pancreatic duct (**a**, 20×). Intermediate power (**b**, 200×) demonstrates an islet of Langerhans (*arrowheads*) and an interlobular pancreatic duct (*arrow*) in a background of normally crowded pancreatic acini [**a** and **b**: Hematoxylin & eosin (H&E) stain]

Classification of Pancreatic Neoplasms

According to WHO 2010 classification [4], primary tumors in the pancreas are divided into four major categories: epithelial tumors (benign and malignant), mature teratoma, mesenchymal tumors, and lymphomas (see Table 3.1). Among these, epithelial tumors are the predominant tumor type in the pancreas.

Secondary tumors refer to neoplasms that have spread to the pancreas from an extrapancreatic primary. They account for 4–15% of all malignancies in the pancreas found at autopsy [5, 6]. The most common secondary tumors of the pancreas include (1) by direct extension (cancers of the ampulla of Vater, duodenum, and distal common bile duct) and (2) by lymphohematogenous spread (renal cell carcinomas, melanomas, colorectal carcinomas, breast carcinomas, and sarcomas).

Table 3.1 WHO 2010 classification of tumors of the pancreas

Epithelial tumors
Benign
• Acinar cell cystadenoma
• Serous cystadenoma
Premalignant lesions
• Pancreatic intraepithelial neoplasia with high-grade dysplasia
• Intraductal papillary mucinous neoplasm (IPMN)
• Intraductal tubulopapillary neoplasm (ITPN)
• Mucinous cystic neoplasm (MCN)
Malignant
• Ductal adenocarcinoma
– Adenosquamous carcinoma
– Colloid carcinoma (mucinous noncystic carcinoma)
– Hepatoid carcinoma
– Medullary carcinoma
– Signet ring cell carcinoma
– Undifferentiated carcinoma with and without osteoclast-like giant cells
• Acinar cell carcinoma
• Acinar cell cystadenocarcinoma
• IPMN and MCN with an associated invasive carcinoma

(continued)

Table 3.1 (continued)

• Mixed carcinomas (mixed acinar-ductal carcinoma, mixed acinar-neuroendocrine carcinoma, mixed acinar-neuroendocrine-ductal carcinoma, and mixed ductal-neuroendocrine carcinoma)
• Pancreatoblastoma
• Serous cystadenocarcinoma
• Solid pseudopapillary neoplasm
Neuroendocrine neoplasms
• Pancreatic neuroendocrine microadenoma
• Neuroendocrine tumor (NET)
– Nonfunctional pancreatic NET, G1, G2
– NET G1
– NET G2
• Neuroendocrine carcinoma (NEC)
– Large cell NEC
– Small cell NEC
• EC cell, serotonin-producing NET (carcinoid)
• Gastrinoma
• Glucagonoma
• Insulinoma
• Somatostatinoma
• VIPoma
Mature teratoma
Mesenchymal tumors
Extrapancreatic mesenchymal tumors
• Gastrointestinal stromal tumor (GIST)
• Leiomyosarcoma
• Liposarcoma
• Desmoid tumor
Primary mesenchymal neoplasms
• Lymphangiomas
• Lipomas
• Solitary fibrous tumor
• Perivascular epithelioid cell neoplasms (PEComas)
• Desmoplastic small round cell tumors
Lymphomas
Secondary tumors

Modified from WHO classification of tumors of the digestive system, IARC, Lyon 2010

Pancreatic Intraepithelial Neoplasia

Epidemiology, Radiology, and Macroscopic Findings

Pancreatic intraepithelial neoplasia (PanIN) is a mucinous intraductal epithelial proliferation that by definition involves ducts that are less than 1 cm in diameter (most less than 0.5 cm). Of note, the normal pancreatic ductal cells do not show visible cytoplasmic mucin on H&E-stained sections, except the large interlobular ducts.

Low-grade PanIN is a relatively common incidental finding that is present in 50% of older adults [7]. In contrast, high-grade PanIN is a recognized precursor lesion to invasive pancreatic ductal adenocarcinoma.

Due to their small size, PanIN is typically appreciated on microscopic slides rather than from gross or radiological examination. However, subtle radiographic findings of localized lobular atrophy may be a clue for the finding of PanIN in patients with a strong family history of pancreatic carcinoma [8].

Grading

The original three-tiered grading system for dysplasia (low-, intermediate-, and high-grade dysplasia) in PanINs, intraductal papillary mucinous neoplasms (IPMNs), and mucinous cystic neoplasms (MCNs) has been recently revised to a two-tiered grading system (low- and high-grade dysplasia) [9]. This is because many of the low- or intermediate-grade lesions have revealed a very low risk of progression to invasive cancer [10]; therefore, it is more clinically relevant to group them together as a low-grade category, reflecting their less aggressive biology and need for conservative management of these lesions. The term high-grade dysplasia is reserved for those lesions at the uppermost end of the spectrum and is equivalent to "carcinoma in situ."

Because low-grade PanIN lesions (PanIN-1 and PanIN-2 in WHO 2010 classification) are so common and of no proven clinical significance, there is no need to report them in the pathology reports, especially in patients with an invasive adenocarcinoma [9]. In contrast, high-grade PanINs (PanIN-3 in WHO 2010) should always be reported, especially in the absence of an invasive carcinoma as they may serve as surrogate markers for invasion elsewhere in the pancreas [11].

This revised two-tiered grading system is based solely on histology, and the lesions are graded on the basis of the highest degree of architectural and cytologic atypia identified anywhere within the lesion. The following terminology is recommended for grading and reporting dysplasia in PanIN according to the Baltimore consensus [9]:

Low-grade PanIN
High-grade PanIN ("carcinoma in situ")

Histology

Histologically, the mucinous epithelium in PanIN is either flat or papillary in configuration. Both the main pancreatic duct and peripheral pancreatic lobules can be involved by PanIN. PanIN is frequently multifocal with varying degrees of dysplasia within the gland.

Low-grade PanIN includes the former PanIN-1 and PanIN-2 in WHO 2010 classification. PanIN-1 demonstrates flat or papillary mucinous epithelium that lacks cytologic atypia (Fig. 3.2a and b). PanIN-2 typically shows papillary mucinous epithelium that always harbors nuclear atypia including loss of polarity, nuclear crowding, nuclear enlargement, and hyperchromasia (Fig. 3.2c and d). Mitoses are rare and without atypical forms.

High-grade PanIN refers to the former PanIN-3/carcinoma in situ and is assigned as pTis in the pTNM staging. They typically show papillary and micropapillary architecture with variable cribriforming, budding, and luminal necrosis and are characterized by severe cytologic atypia (macronucleoli and frequent/abnormal mitosis) (Fig. 3.2e and f).

Resection Margins

In the absence of invasive carcinoma, high-grade PanIN at the resection margin may warrant additional surgery, since high-grade PanIN lesions are often associated with an invasive carcinoma [12]. On the other hand, in patients with invasive carcinoma, the presence of PanINs of any grade at the resection margin does not seem to affect patient survival [13].

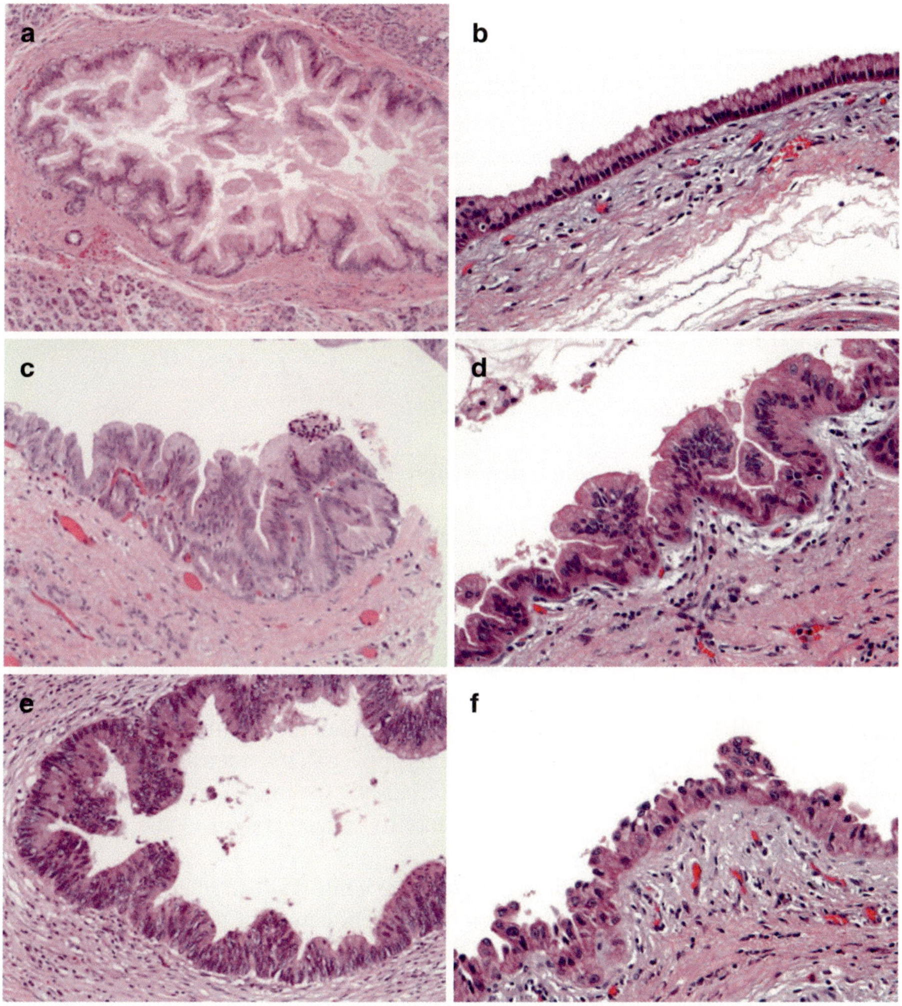

Fig. 3.2 Pancreatic intraductal neoplasia (PanIN) with various degrees of dysplasia. According to 2015 Baltimore consensus, low-grade dysplasia includes the former PanIN-1 (**a** and **b**) and PanIN-2 (**c** and **d**) of WHO 2010 classification, and high-grade dysplasia refers to the former PanIN-3/carcinoma in situ (**e** and **f**). When compared to low-grade dysplasia, high-grade dysplasia shows high-grade architectural and cytologic atypia and frequent mitotic figures (**a**, **c**, **e**, 200×; **b**, **d**, **f**, 400×)

Molecular Genetics

As a precursor lesion to invasive ductal carcinoma, PanIN shares remarkably similar molecular abnormalities as the carcinoma. *KRAS* oncogene activation appears to occur early in the sequence, while mutation of tumor suppressor genes takes place later (loss of *CDKN2A* in the middle stage, *SMAD4* and *TP53* mutations in the late stage) [14, 15].

Pancreatic Ductal Adenocarcinoma

Conventional Ductal Adenocarcinoma

Epidemiology, Radiology, and Macroscopic Findings

More than 90% of pancreatic neoplasms have a ductal origin, and 80–90% of these lesions are invasive ductal adenocarcinomas. Most patients are between 60 and 80 years of age. Incidence is about 50% higher in men than in women. In the USA, the rate of pancreatic ductal adenocarcinoma is 50–100% higher in African Americans than in whites living in the same areas. The best known risk factors for pancreatic cancers are tobacco smoking, high intake of dietary saturated fat, chronic pancreatitis, diabetes, and obesity [16–20]; heavy drinking of alcohol may weakly increase the risk.

Radiographically, ductal adenocarcinomas appear as hypodense masses on computed tomography (CT) imaging in 92% of cases. "Double-duct" sign (dilation of both the biliary and pancreatic ducts) points to cancer arising in the head of the pancreas.

Macroscopically, ductal adenocarcinomas are white-yellow, sclerotic, and poorly defined masses that efface the normal lobular architecture of the pancreatic gland. More than 75% of ductal adenocarcinomas are solid tumors. Most arise in the head of the pancreas (60–70%), and the rest are located in the body (5–15%) and the tail (10–15%). Very rarely, heterotopic pancreatic tissue in the gastrointestinal tract can give rise to pancreatic carcinoma. Tumors involving the pancreatic body/tail are typically larger than that involving the head of the pancreas. The mean diameter of pancreatic head tumor is 2.5–3.5 cm.

Histology

Microscopically, pancreatic ductal adenocarcinomas form well- to poorly differentiated glandular or ductal structures (Fig. 3.3) that diffusely infiltrate the pancreatic parenchyma and elicit florid desmoplastic stromal reaction. Compared to the poorly differentiated ones, the well- to moderately differentiated carcinomas show better glandular differentiation, more mucin production, less mitoses, and less nuclear atypia and polymorphism.

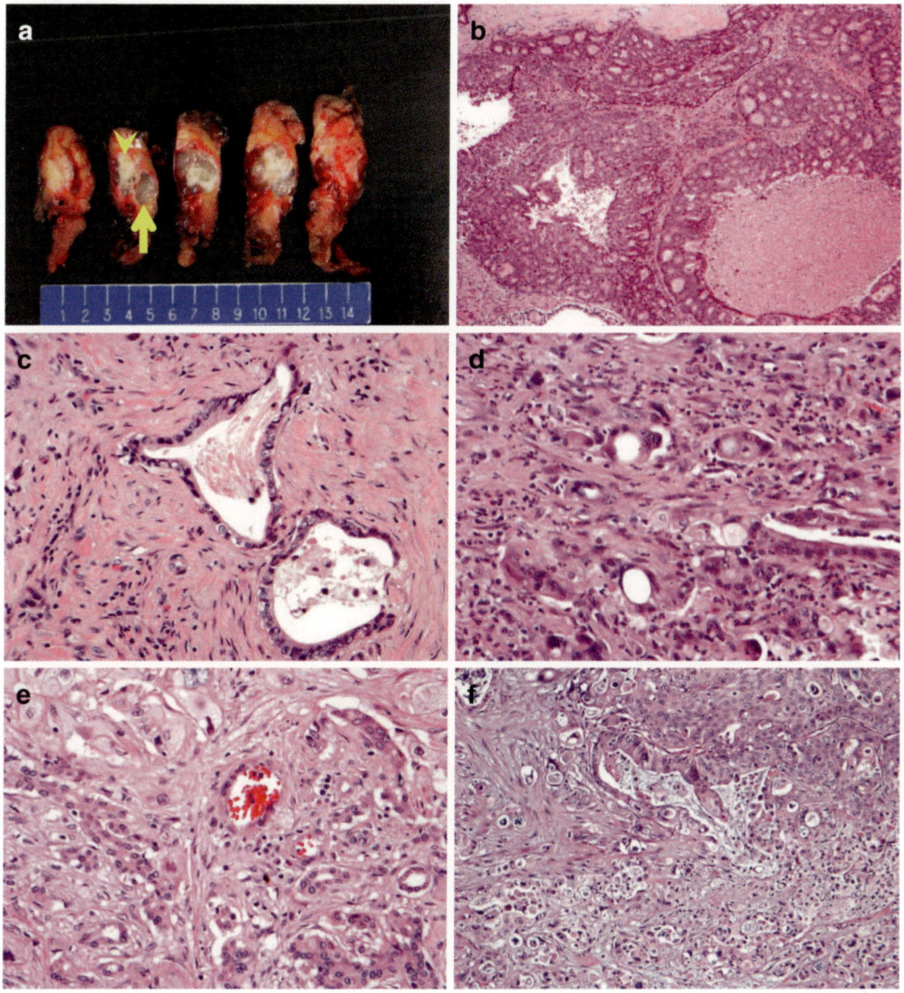

Fig. 3.3 Pancreatic ductal adenocarcinoma. Gross photo (**a**) shows cut surfaces of a pancreas containing invasive carcinoma (*arrowhead*) arising in an intraductal papillary mucinous neoplasm (*arrow*). Examples of various morphologies of pancreatic ductal adenocarcinoma range from cribriforming glands (**b**, 200×), duct-like structures (**c**, 400×), and abortive/poorly formed glands to cords and single infiltrating cells (**d**–**f**, 200×). Note the prominent stromal desmoplastic reaction to the invasive carcinoma in **c** (**a**–**f**: H&E stain)

Perineural invasion (Fig. 3.4a and b) and lymphovascular invasion (Fig. 3.4c) are the two major mechanisms for tumor spread, and both are diagnostic of an invasive carcinoma. Other clues for diagnosing pancreatic adenocarcinoma include "naked" tumor glands in peripancreatic fat (Fig. 3.4d), glands directly adjacent to vascular structures (Fig. 3.4e), and glands containing epithelial cells with greater than four times variation of nuclear size (Fig. 3.4f).

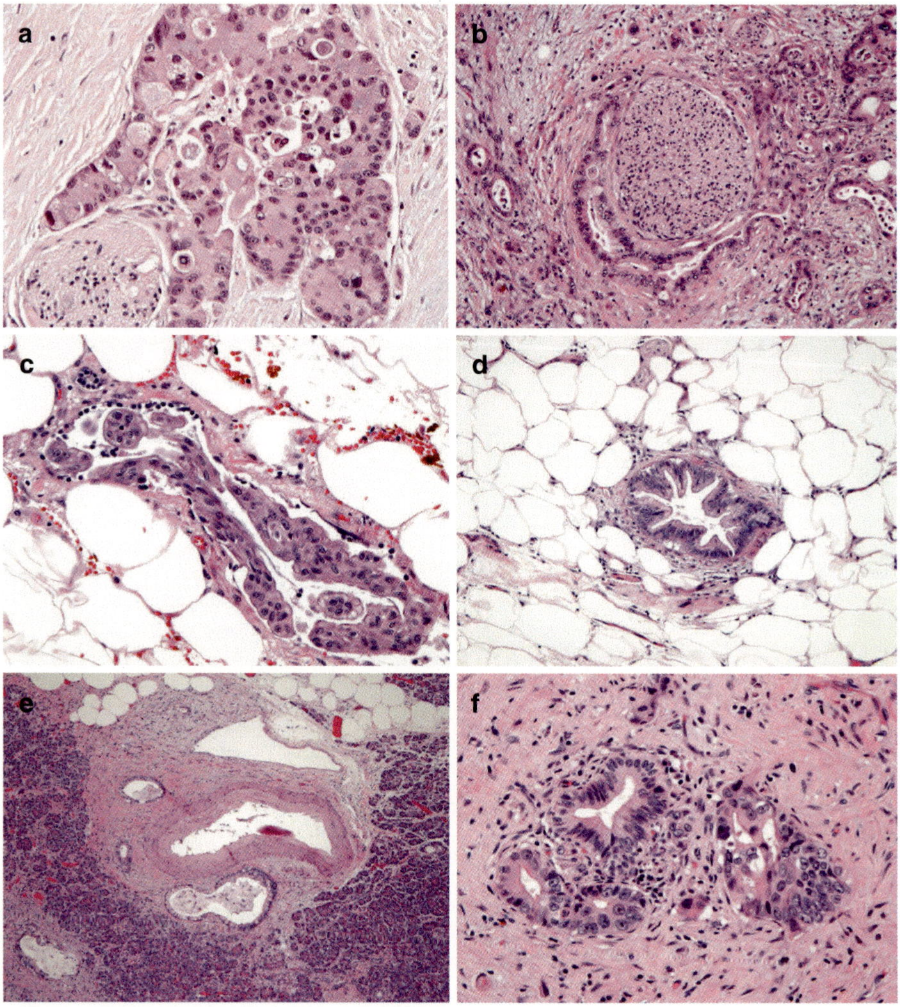

Fig. 3.4 Diagnostic features of invasive pancreatic ductal adenocarcinoma. Perineural invasion (**a**, 400×; **b**, 200×), lymphovascular invasion (**c**, 400×), isolated gland in peripancreatic fat (**d**, 200×), atypical gland immediately adjacent to blood vessel (**e**, 100×), and pleomorphism of tumor nuclei/four times variation of nuclear size (f, 400×) (**a–f**: H&E stain)

The following histological types of pancreatic ductal adenocarcinomas appear to have no prognostic significance: foamy gland pattern (Fig. 3.5a), clear cell features (Fig. 3.5b and c), and large duct features. In contrast, some histologic variants of ductal adenocarcinoma are of more significant prognostic value, and these will be discussed in the section "ductal adenocarcinoma variants and mixed neoplasms of the pancreas."

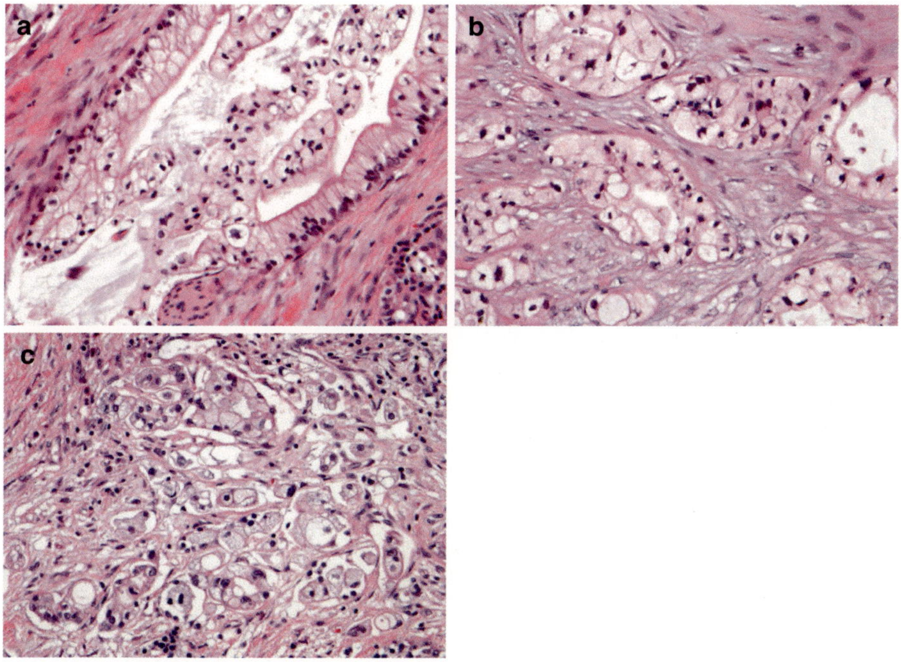

Fig. 3.5 Common histologic features of pancreatic ductal adenocarcinomas. Foamy gland pattern (**a**) and clear cell features (Figs. **b** and **c**) (**a**–**c**: H&E stain, 400×)

Differential Diagnosis

Chronic pancreatitis may mimic pancreatic ductal carcinoma on clinical and pathologic examination. The former often affects younger patients (<40 years) and diffusely involves the gland without a discrete mass. Groove pancreatitis may be indistinguishable from pancreatic carcinoma clinically and radiologically. Histologically, no malignant cells are found, but reactive stoma is common. Groove pancreatitis also shows characteristic thickening and fibrosis of the duodenal wall around the minor ampulla, with frequent cyst formation that is lined by inflamed granulation tissue. The fibrosis may extend into the head of the pancreas and may involve the common bile duct.

Sometimes, ampullary/periampullary carcinomas and cholangiocarcinomas of the distal common bile duct may mimic ductal adenocarcinoma of the pancreatic head. Careful examination of the epicenter of the mass and the identification of precursor lesions are essential.

Staging and Grading

According to the new eighth edition of American Joint Committee on Cancer (AJCC) staging, pT1 to pT3 tumors are staged primarily based on tumor size, and pT4 tumor is based on invasion of large vessels (Table 3.2). This change from AJCC

Table 3.2 AJCC eighth edition pTNM definitions of carcinoma of exocrine pancreas and poorly differentiated neuroendocrine carcinoma

pTX	Primary tumor cannot be assessed
pT0	No evidence of primary tumor
pTis	Carcinoma in situ
pT1	Tumor ≤2 cm in greatest dimension
pT1a	Tumor ≤0.5 cm in greatest dimension
pT1b	Tumor >0.5 cm and <1 cm in greatest dimension
pT1c	Tumor 1–2 cm in greatest dimension
pT2	Tumor >2 cm and ≤4 cm in greatest dimension
pT3	Tumor >4 cm in greatest dimension
pT4	Tumor involves celiac axis, superior mesenteric artery, and/or common hepatic artery, regardless of size
pNX	Regional lymph nodes cannot be assessed
pN0	No regional lymph node metastasis
pN1	Metastasis in one to three regional lymph nodes
pN2	Metastasis in four or more regional lymph nodes
pM0	No distant metastasis
pM1	Distant metastasis

seventh edition alleviates the difficulty in histologic evaluation of extrapancreatic extension in the prior staging edition. The pancreas does not have a capsule, and the distinction between the pancreas and extrapancreatic soft tissue often is obscured by fibrosis as part of the tumor or chronic pancreatitis.

While WHO endorses the sophisticated Klöppel's grading scheme that is based on glandular differentiation, mucin production, mitoses, and nuclear atypia, such grading system is not widely used by practicing pathologists. A four-tiered grading system, recommended by AJCC, is most commonly used for the grading of pancreatic ductal adenocarcinoma. It is based solely on glandular differentiation, similar to that used in the grading of bowel adenocarcinomas:

G1 Well differentiated
G2 Moderately differentiated
G3 Poorly differentiated
G4 Undifferentiated

Ductal Adenocarcinoma Variants

Some histologic variants of pancreatic ductal adenocarcinoma show prognostic value. Colloid carcinomas and medullary carcinomas tend to have better prognosis than conventional ductal adenocarcinoma, whereas the other histologic variants (adenosquamous carcinoma, signet ring cell carcinoma, hepatoid carcinoma, and undifferentiated carcinoma) appear to pursue a more aggressive clinical course.

Adenosquamous Carcinoma

Adenosquamous carcinoma represents 1–4% of exocrine pancreatic malignancies. This neoplasm shows both ductal and squamous differentiation (Fig. 3.6a), and by definition, each component should account for at least 30% of the neoplasm. Patients with resected adenosquamous carcinoma have a poorer prognosis (median survival 7–11 months) than those with pure adenocarcinoma. Furthermore, the presence of any squamous component in the neoplasm appears to portend a worse prognosis [21].

Colloid Carcinoma

Colloid carcinoma often arises from IPMN and MCN, and it is characterized by large extracellular stromal mucin pools (at least 80% of the neoplasm) with floating neoplastic cells (Fig. 3.6b). Colloid carcinomas seem to have a more favorable prognosis than conventional ductal adenocarcinomas [22]. Unlike conventional ductal adenocarcinomas, loss of *SMAD4* is not usually seen in colloid carcinoma.

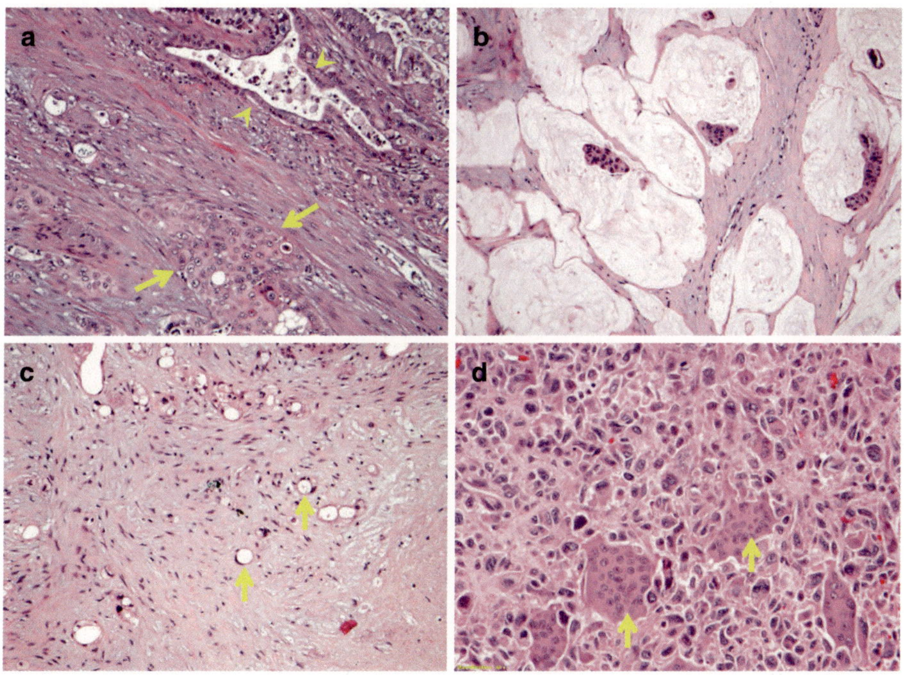

Fig. 3.6 Histologic variants of pancreatic ductal adenocarcinoma. Adenosquamous carcinoma (**a**) consists of both glandular (*arrowheads*) and squamous (*arrows*) differentiation. Colloid carcinoma (**b**) shows large stromal mucin pools with floating neoplastic cells. Signet ring cell carcinoma (**c**) is composed of discohesive cells with large intracytoplasmic mucin and eccentric crescent-shaped nuclei (*arrows*). Undifferentiated carcinoma (**d**) demonstrates sheets of malignant cells and may contain osteoclast-like giant cells (*arrows*) (**a**–**d**: H&E stain, 200×)

Signet Ring Cell Carcinoma

Signet ring cell carcinoma is extremely rare in the pancreas and the prognosis is very poor. By definition, at least 50% of the neoplasm is composed of discohesive cells with large intracytoplasmic mucin and eccentric crescent-shaped nuclei (Fig. 3.6c). A gastric or breast primary should be considered before making this diagnosis.

Medullary Carcinoma

Medullary carcinoma is a poorly differentiated carcinoma with characteristic syncytial growth pattern, pushing borders and increased numbers of tumor-infiltrating lymphocytes. Some are associated with microsatellite instability and Lynch syndrome and have better prognosis than conventional ductal adenocarcinoma.

Hepatoid Carcinoma

Hepatoid carcinoma of the pancreas is extremely rare. Pancreatic metastases from an occult hepatocellular carcinoma should be excluded before rendering this diagnosis.

Undifferentiated (Anaplastic) Carcinomas

Undifferentiated carcinomas occur in elderly patients and have poor prognosis. The median survival time is only 5 months after surgical resection. There is often an associated in situ or invasive adenocarcinoma or an associated MCN. A subset of undifferentiated carcinomas have osteoclast-like giant cells (Fig. 3.6d).

Carcinomas with Mixed Differentiation

These are neoplasms that have significant (>30%) components of more than one distinct direction of differentiation (ductal, neuroendocrine, or acinar). The neoplastic neuroendocrine cells are typically high grade, and the mixed ductal-neuroendocrine carcinomas behave like the usual ductal adenocarcinoma. Mixed acinar-neuroendocrine carcinoma and mixed acinar-ductal carcinoma are rare neoplasms. Mixed acinar-neuroendocrine-ductal carcinoma is extremely rare.

Molecular Genetics

Genetic abnormalities involving four genes (*KRAS*, *CDKN2A*, *TP53*, *SMAD4*) have been found in most pancreatic ductal adenocarcinomas [23, 24] (Table 3).

Table 3 Common gene mutations associated with pancreatic ductal adenocarcinomas

Genes	Mutation frequency in pancreatic ductal adenocarcinoma
KRAS	>95%
CDKN2A (formerly known as *p16*, *INK4A*, *CDKN*)	95%
TP53	50–80%
SMAD4	55%

Table 4 Hereditary syndromes and pancreatic cancer

Genes	Associated hereditary syndromes	Mode of inheritance	Increased risk of pancreatic cancer	Histology
STK11 (19p)	Peutz-Jeghers syndrome	Autosomal dominant	132-fold	IPMN
PRSS1 (7q), *SPINK1* (5q)	Hereditary pancreatitis	Autosomal dominant (*PRSS1*); autosomal recessive (*SPINK1*)	53-fold	Ductal adenocarcinoma
CDKN2A (9p)	Familial atypical multiple mole melanoma (FAMMM)	Autosomal dominant	13–22-fold	Ductal adenocarcinoma
Unknown	Familial pancreatic cancer (three or more relatives with pancreatic cancer)	Autosomal dominant	9–32-fold	
MSH2 (2p), *MLH1* (3p), and others	Lynch syndrome	Autosomal dominant	Ninefold	Medullary carcinoma
BRCA2 (13q), *PALB2* (16p), *FANCC* (9q), *FANCG* (9p), and possibly *BRCA1* (17q)	Familial breast cancer and other Fanconi anemia genes	Autosomal dominant	Three- to tenfold (*BRCA2*), twofold (*BRCA1*)	Ductal adenocarcinoma
APC	Familial adenomatous polyposis (FAP)	Autosomal dominant	fourfold	Ductal adenocarcinoma; IPMN

Data source from WHO classification of tumors of the digestive system, IARC, Lyon 2010; Shi et al. Arch Pathol Lab Med 2009, 133:365-374

Approximately 10% of pancreatic cancers have a familial basis [25]. Table 4 lists select genetic abnormalities and their associated hereditary syndromes that are implicated in pancreatic cancers [26–34].

In addition, alternations of many other core signaling pathways have also been found in pancreatic ductal adenocarcinoma [35], including apoptosis, G1/S phase transition, DNA damage control, hedgehog signaling, cell adhesion/invasion, integrin signaling, MAPK8 (JNK) signaling, GTPase signaling, transforming growth factor-β (TGF-β) signaling, and NOTCH signaling. Epigenetic changes have been described in pancreatic cancer, including DNA hyper- or hypo-methylation and aberrant microRNA expression.

Intraductal Neoplasms of the Pancreas

Intraductal neoplasms of the pancreas are defined as macroscopic cystic or mass-forming epithelial neoplasms with ductal differentiation that grow primarily within the ductal systems of the pancreas. The minimal size of 1 cm separates intraductal neoplasms from PanIN (less than 0.5 cm). Intraductal neoplasms include intraductal papillary mucinous neoplasm (IPMN) and intraductal tubulopapillary neoplasm (ITPN), both are slow-growing intraductal tumors that are radiologically and grossly detectable [4].

Intraductal Papillary Mucinous Neoplasm

Epidemiology, Radiology, and Macroscopic Findings

Increasing numbers of intraductal neoplasms are detected due to the increased use of cross-sectional imaging in recent years. IPMN accounts for at least 5% of all pancreatic neoplasms. The average patient age is in the seventh to eighth decade. The majority of IPMN (80%) are located in the head of the pancreas.

IPMNs are radiographically and grossly cystic (dilated ducts), with variable amounts of intraluminal mucin. Based on the involvement of the ductal system, IPMNs can be divided into main duct type, branch duct type, and combined type. Main duct type IPMNs are more likely to harbor high-grade dysplasia and invasive carcinoma than branch duct type. The clinical behavior of combined duct type mirrors that of main duct type.

Histology

As its name suggests, the microscopic appearance of IPMN is that of cystically dilated ducts lined by flat to papillary epithelium with variable amounts of intracytoplasmic mucin. Depending on the histomorphology and differentiation, IPMN can be divided into four major epithelial subtypes (WHO 2010): gastric type (50%), intestinal type (35%), pancreatobiliary type (15%), and oncocytic type (rare) [36–40].

Gastric type resembles gastric foveolar epithelium with tall columnar mucinous cells (Fig. 3.7a). It is the most common subtype, usually located in branch ducts, and is associated with low-grade dysplasia. **Intestinal type** resembles adenomas of

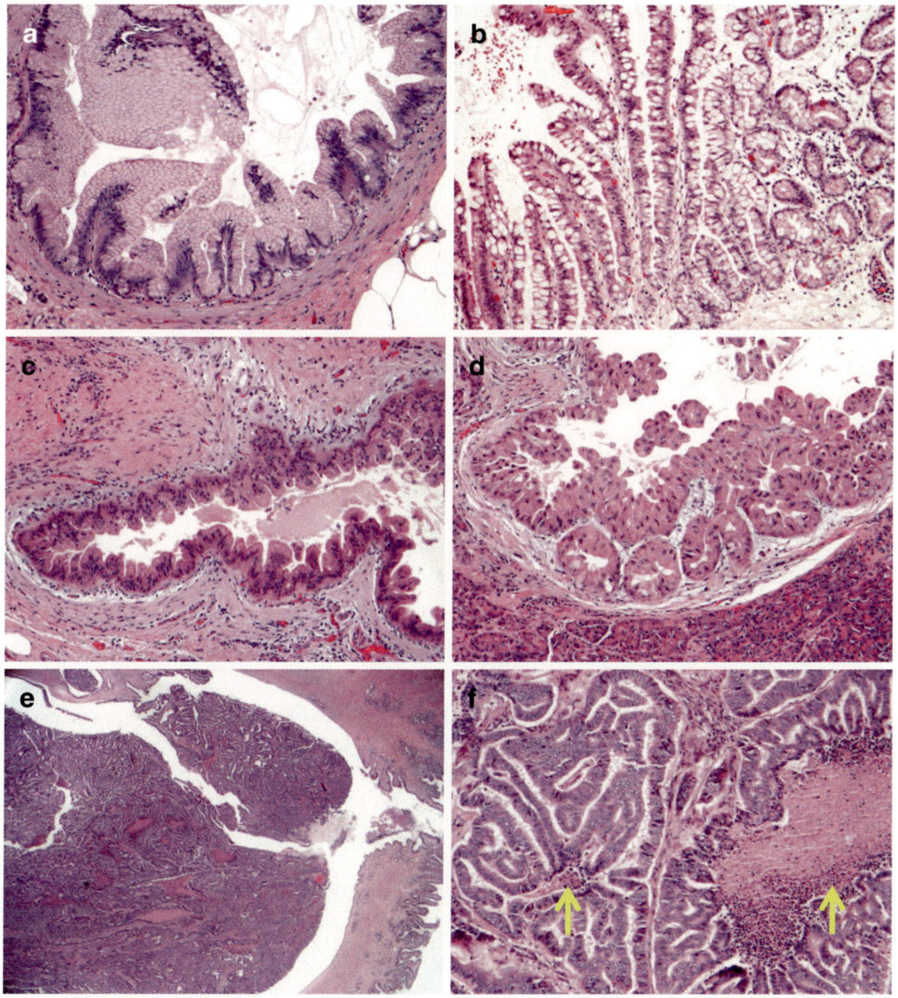

Fig. 3.7 Histological types of intraductal papillary mucinous neoplasm (IPMN). The gastric type (**a**) contains tall columnar foveolar mucin cells. Intestinal type (**b**) demonstrates intestinal epithelium with goblet cells. Pancreatobiliary type (**c**) is composed of cuboidal cells arranged in complex papillae. Oncocytic type (**d**) is characterized by cells with prominent nucleoli and abundant eosinophilic cytoplasms that are arranged into complex, multilayered epithelium. Intraductal papillary neoplasms (ITPN) (**e** and **f**) lack visible mucin and are composed of tubulopapillary structures with extensive high-grade dysplasia and foci of necrosis (**f**, *arrows*) (**a–f**: H&E stain, **a**, **b**, **c**, **d**, **f**, 200x; **e**, 20×)

gastrointestinal tract (Fig. 3.7b); it is mainly found in the main duct and is often associated with intermediate- to high-grade dysplasia. **Pancreatobiliary type** is composed of cuboidal cells arranged in complex papillae (Fig. 3.7c); it is typically found in the main duct and frequently harbors high-grade dysplasia. **Oncocytic type** is characterized by cells with abundant eosinophilic cytoplasms that are arranged into complex, multilayered, focally cribriforming epithelium (Fig. 3.7d); high-grade dysplasia is the rule.

The oncocytic variant of IPMN is also termed intraductal oncocytic papillary neoplasm (IOPN) by some authorities, due to its differing molecular characteristics and better prognosis than conventional IPMN [41–43].

Immunohistochemistry for mucin glycoproteins (MUCs) is useful in distinguishing morphological subtypes [4, 37]. In general, gastric-type IPMNs express MUC5AC, but not MUC1 or MUC2. Intestinal-type IPMNs are known for strong and diffuse expression of intestinal markers MUC2 and CDX2, in addition to MUC5AC. Pancreatobiliary-type IPMNs express MUC1 and MUC5AC, but not intestinal markers (MUC2 and CDX2). Oncocytic-type IPMNs express MUC6 (pyloric-type mucin) and MUC5AC (focal), as well as diffuse reactivity to mitochondrial elements.

Grading

As discussed previously in PanIN grading, the original three-tiered grading system for dysplasia (low-, intermediate-, and high-grade dysplasia) IPMNs has been recently revised to a two-tiered grading system (low- and high-grade dysplasia) [9]. The former low- and intermediate-grade dysplasia is now to be categorized as low grade, which is in line with the more indolent biologic behavior of these lesions in contrast to the high-grade dysplasia ones. The following terminology is recommended for grading dysplasia in IPMN [9]:

For tumor-forming intraepithelial neoplasm without invasion:

IPMN, low-grade
IPMN, high- grade

For IPMN with an associated invasive carcinoma:

IPMN, __ grade, with an associated invasive carcinoma

Invasive Carcinoma Arising in IPMN

One third of IPMNs are associated with invasive adenocarcinoma. There are two distinct types of invasive adenocarcinoma arising in IPMN: tubular adenocarcinoma and colloid carcinoma. Tubular (conventional ductal) adenocarcinomas often arise in pancreatobiliary-type, intestinal-type, and less commonly gastric-type IPMN. Colloid carcinoma is mostly associated with intestinal-type IPMN and is characterized by abundant stromal mucin pools with floating malignant epithelium. Colloid carcinoma seems to portend a better prognosis than tubular adenocarcinoma [22, 44].

Resection Margins

In the absence of invasive carcinoma, the clinical significance of the presence of IPMN at a resection margin is debatable. There are conflicting data regarding association between recurrences and the presence of IPMN at a margin, although high-grade dysplasia at the margin is reported and may have significance [45–49]. Regardless of the margin status, careful clinical follow-up after resection of IPMN of any grade is important due to the multifocal nature of IPMNs [50].

Intraductal Tubulopapillary Neoplasm

Intraductal tubulopapillary neoplasms (ITPNs) account for less than 1% of all pancreatic exocrine neoplasms and only 3% of intraductal neoplasms of the pancreas [51–53]. Patients with ITPNs are a decade younger than patients with IPMNs. ITPNs are often indistinguishable from IPMNs preoperatively. About half of ITPNs occur in the head of the pancreas, a third diffusely involve the gland, and 15% are localized to the tail.

Macroscopically, ITPNs represent neoplastic proliferation within dilated pancreatic ducts; however, they do not produce mucin and do not have cystic change.

Microscopically, ITPNs are composed of tubulopapillary structures with extensive high-grade dysplasia (Figs. 3.7e and f). Approximately 40% of cases have an associated invasive adenocarcinoma. Immunohistochemically, ITPNs express MUC1 (90%) and MUC6 (60%) while lacking MUC2 and MUC5AC. ITPNs are thought to have different molecular tumorigenesis and have a better prognosis than IPMNs. The major histologic differential diagnosis includes IPMN (pancreatobiliary type) and intraductal acinar cell carcinoma.

Molecular Genetics

IPMN shares similar, but not identical, mutation profiles as pancreatic ductal adenocarcinoma. Similar to ductal adenocarcinoma, activating point mutations in codon 12 of *KRAS* are present in 30–80% of IPMNs [54, 55]. Allelic losses of *CDKN2A*, *TP53*, and *SMAD4* are found in up to 40% of IPMNs, and these losses increase with increasing degree of dysplasia [56–58].

The following genes are mutated in IPMNs but not in pancreatic ductal adenocarcinomas [59–61]: *RNF43* (75% of IPMNs), *GNAS* (60%), *APC* (25%), and *PIK3CA* (10%). *BRAF* mutation is seen in a small number of IPMNs [54].

ITPN shows different mutation profile than IPMN, which potentially could explain their differing histomorphology and prognosis. Studies have found that ITPNs typically lack *KRAS* or *TP53* mutations, while abnormal nuclear accumulation of *β-catenin* is observed in some cases [51].

Pancreatic Neuroendocrine Neoplasms

Epidemiology, Radiology, and Macroscopic Findings

Pancreatic neuroendocrine tumors (PanNETs) are uncommon and represent 1–2% of all pancreatic neoplasms. The peak incidence is between 30 and 60 years, and the mean age at presentation is 50 years. The majority of cases are non-syndromic and sporadic; rare cases are associated with multiple endocrine neoplasia syndrome (MEN1), von Hippel-Lindau syndrome, and tuberous sclerosis.

About 60–70% of all pancreatic NETs are functioning tumors. The most common type is insulinoma, followed by glucagonoma, gastrinoma, and somatostatinoma [62]. Serotonin-producing tumors account for about 25% of PanNETs, and they uniquely involve main pancreatic ducts [63]. It is important to note that positive immunohistochemical staining for peptide hormone does not correlate with the tumor functional type; nonfunctional tumors may stain for multiple peptides. Therefore, immunostains for specific hormones are not routinely performed in PanNET specimens.

Macroscopically, PanNETs are well demarcated, solitary, and white-yellow to pink-brown in color. Rare cystic PanNETs are present. Nonfunctioning NETs are generally larger than functioning PanNETs likely due to later detection. PanNETs are typically >2 cm in diameter (often 5 cm or more).

Histology

Well-Differentiated Pancreatic Neuroendocrine Tumor

Well-differentiated PanNETs are composed of a monotonous population of round cells arranged in nests, trabeculae, pseudoacinar, and solid patterns (Fig. 3.8a–c). The nuclear chromatin is dispersed and classically described as "salt and pepper" (Fig. 3.8d). The morphological appearance generally does not predict functional status with two exceptions: amyloid deposits may be seen with insulinoma, and glandular structures containing psammoma bodies are often seen with somatostatin cell tumors. Diffuse positivity for synaptophysin and chromogranin (Fig. 3.8e) immunostains is typical for well-differentiated PanNET. The Ki-67 proliferation index is low (Fig. 3.8f). Occasionally, well-differentiated PanNET may show less common histologic features, such as oncocytes, rhabdoid cells, clear cells, and vacuolated lipid-rich cells. A subset of well-differentiated neoplasms has a high proliferative index but is still considered well differentiated [64, 65].

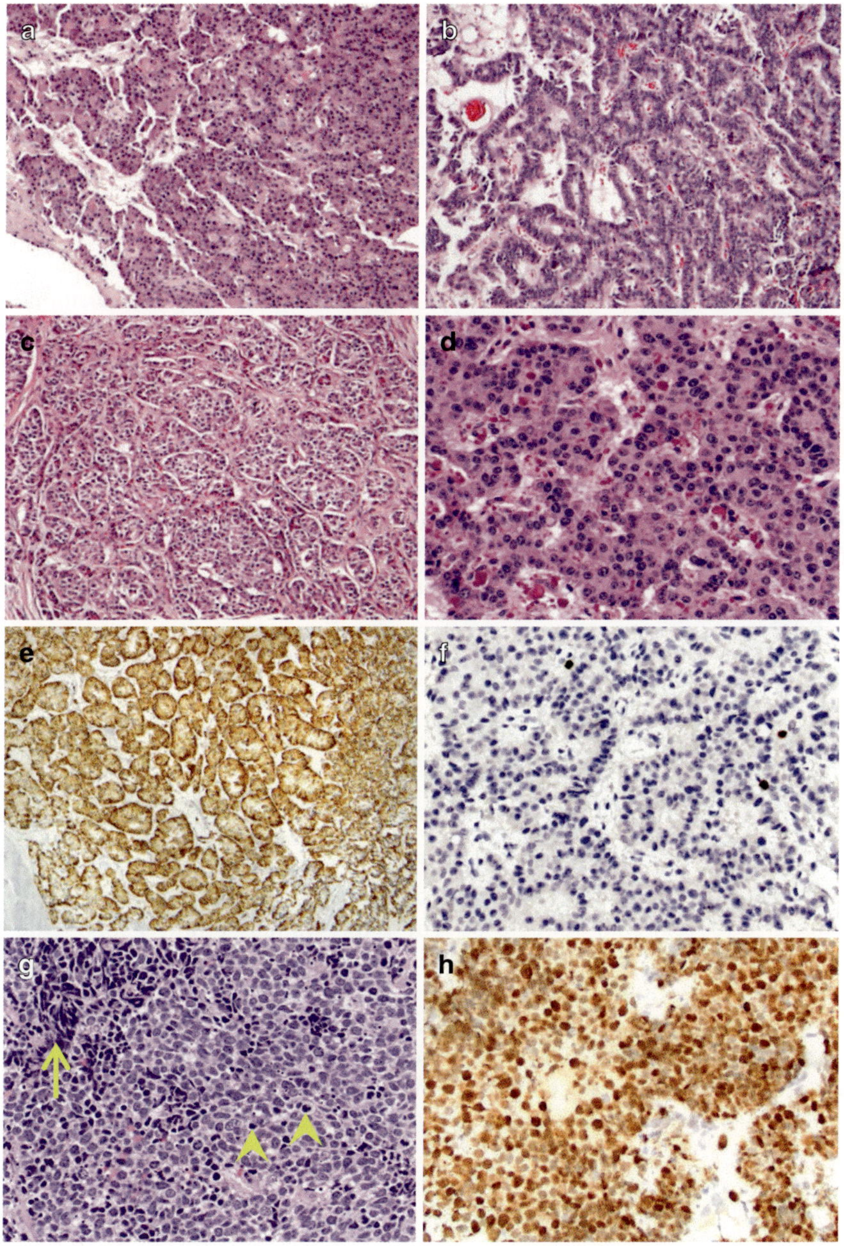

Fig. 3.8 Pancreatic neuroendocrine tumors. Well-differentiated pancreatic neuroendocrine tumors are composed of monotonous population of round cells arranged in pseudoacini (**a**, 200×), trabeculae (**b**, 200×), and nests (**c**, 200×). The nuclear chromatin is dispersed and classically described as "salt-and-pepper" pattern (**d**, 400×). A chromogranin immunostain is diffusely positive (**e**, 200×). Ki-67 labeling index is low (**f**, 400×). **g** and **h** demonstrate a poorly differentiated neuroendocrine carcinoma, small cell type. It is characterized by sheets of cells with high nuclear cytoplasmic ratio, frequent apoptosis (**g**, arrowheads; 400×) and a characteristic of crush artifact (**g**, *arrow*; 400×). Ki-67 labeling index is high (**h**, 400×) (**a–d**, **e** and **g**: H&E stain)

Poorly Differentiated Pancreatic Neuroendocrine Carcinoma

Poorly differentiated neuroendocrine carcinomas (NEC) are high-grade neuroendocrine tumors that are either small cell type (Fig. 3.8g and h) or large cell type. They constitute 2–3% of all pancreatic endocrine neoplasms and are characterized by the lack of a low-grade organoid appearance and the presence of >20 mitoses per 10 high-power fields (HPF). In the pancreas, large cell carcinomas are more common than small cell carcinomas [66]. Aggressive features such as brisk mitoses, tumor necrosis, perineural invasion, and lymphovascular invasion are often present. Typically, no reactivity for peptide hormones is found in pancreatic NECs.

The small cell variant is morphologically similar to small cell carcinoma of the lung, composed of small- to medium-sized cells with high nuclear-cytoplasmic ratio and prominent nuclear molding. Synaptophysin and chromogranin stains are typically very focal and weak.

The large cell variant resembles large cell neuroendocrine carcinoma of the lung, composed of large cells with abundant eosinophilic cytoplasm and prominent nucleoli. Synaptophysin and chromogranin stains typically show more reactivity than that seen in the small cell variant. The mitotic count is typically greater than 10 per 10 HPF.

Differential Diagnosis

Acinar Cell Carcinoma

Acinar cell carcinoma represents 1–2% of pancreatic neoplasms and is characterized by exocrine/acinar cell differentiation. It typically follows an aggressive course (5-year survival of 6%). These tumors may mimic PanNET due to the similar nested to solid growth pattern. Careful examination of nuclear features may be helpful in the distinction: NET shows stippled chromatin without prominent nucleoli, whereas acinar cell carcinoma demonstrates vesicular nuclei with prominent nucleoli. Unlike ductal adenocarcinoma, stromal desmoplasia is absent in acinar cell carcinoma. Immunohistochemistry is also valuable in the differential diagnosis. Acinar cell carcinoma is positive for trypsin and chymotrypsin and negative for chromogranin, whereas neuroendocrine tumor is negative for trypsin and chymotrypsin and diffusely positive for synaptophysin and chromogranin. Acinar cell carcinoma appears to have different molecular genetics than pancreatic ductal adenocarcinoma.

Solid Pseudopapillary Tumor

Solid pseudopapillary tumor (Fig. 3.9a) is a rare pancreatic neoplasm of unclear cellular origin and shows unique demographic features. Patients are usually 20–30 years old and usually women. The prognosis is excellent with >80% of patients cured with surgical resection, although metastasis and recurrence occur in up to 10% of cases. Histologically, the bland cytology mimics neuroendocrine tumor (uniform round to oval nuclei with finely dispersed chromatin). However, the architecture reveals the "solid pseudopapillary" nature of the tumor secondary to preservation of perivascular neoplastic cells and loss of tumor cells away from the vessels (Fig. 3.9b). By immunohistochemistry, solid pseudopapillary tumor is positive for β-catenin (nuclear reactivity), CD10, and α-1-antitrypsin and negative for chromogranin. Pancreatic neuroendocrine tumors show the opposite pattern of staining.

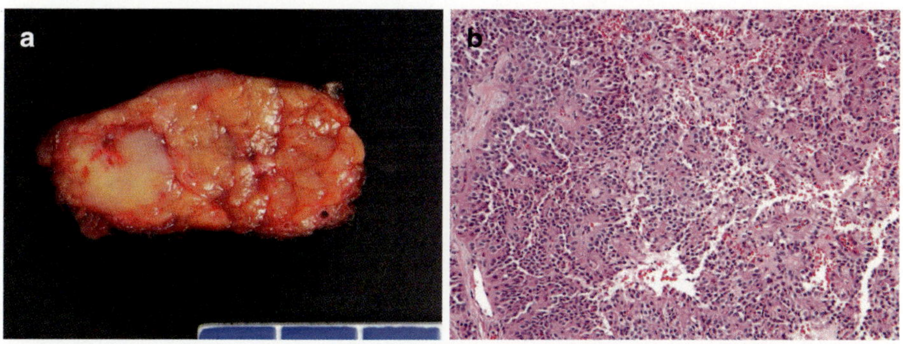

Fig. 3.9 Solid pseudopapillary neoplasm. Gross appearance (**a**) is a well-circumscribed tumor. Histologic sections (**b**, 200×) show papillary structures composed of bland neoplastic cells arranged around the fibrovascular core (**b**: H&E stain)

Pancreatoblastoma

Pancreatoblastoma is the most common malignant pancreatic neoplasm of childhood, but it is a rare tumor in adults. It is comprised of a variable mixture of acinar, endocrine, squamoid nests, and stromal components. Loss of 11p is the hallmark genetic alteration in these tumors. In contrast, PanNET shows uniform endocrine differentiation and lacks squamoid nests.

Grading and Staging

Pancreatic neuroendocrine tumors are histologically graded into three categories according to the current (2010) WHO classification, based on mitotic count and Ki-67 labeling index (Table 5).

This classification is straightforward in most cases; however, it is important to point out that not all G3 tumors are poorly differentiated. A subset is well differentiated but with increased Ki-67 (>20%), with or without increased mitotic count. These well-differentiated G3 NETs have a lower average Ki-67 than poorly differentiated NEC (40% vs. 70%) and show better outcome (2- and 5-year survivals of 74.9 and 29.1% vs. 22.5 and 16.1%) [64].

According to the new eighth edition of AJCC cancer staging, well-differentiated PanNET is staged using similar criteria as pancreatic ductal carcinoma (Table 3.2), primarily based on tumor size (pT1–pT3) and invasion of large vessels (pT4). For pT staging, the tumor size cutoffs for pT1, pT2, and pT3 tumors are <2, 2–4, and >4 cm. Unique to the PanNET staging criteria is that invasion of adjacent organs is also part of the staging of pT3 and pT4 tumors. If PanNET invades into duodenum or bile duct, it is classified as pT3 regardless of the tumor size. If PanNET involves the stomach, spleen, colon, or adrenal gland, it is considered pT4.

Table 5 Grading criteria of pancreatic neuroendocrine tumors (WHO 2010)

Classification	WHO grade	Mitotic count	Ki-67 labeling index
Well-differentiated neuroendocrine tumor, grade 1	G1	<2 per 10 high-power fields (HPF)	and ≤2%
Well-differentiated neuroendocrine tumor, grade 2	G2	2–20 per 10 HPF	or 3–20%
Poorly differentiated neuroendocrine carcinoma (small cell carcinoma or large cell endocrine carcinoma), grade 3	G3	>20 per 10 HPF	or >20%

Modified from WHO classification of tumors of the digestive system, IARC, Lyon 2010

Molecular Genetics

The molecular alterations in PanNETs are different from those of pancreatic ductal adenocarcinoma; common genetic mutations associated with the latter (*TP53*, *KRAS*, *CDKN2A*, *SMAD4*) are not found with significant frequency in pancreatic NETs [67–70]. *DAXX* and *ATRX* mutations, as well as mTOR pathway (*PTEN*, *TSC2*, *PIK3CA*) abnormalities, are found in 43% and 14% of PanNET, respectively [71]. Chromatin remodeling and PI3K/Akt/mTOR pathways are involved in most well-differentiated PanNET, while mutations in *TP53* and *RB* may contribute to the development of poorly differentiated NECs [72].

Of particular interest is the utilization of unique molecular signatures in distinguishing high-grade (G3) well-differentiated PanNET from poorly differentiated NECs, since the prognosis and treatment differ. For example, *DAXX* and *ATRX* mutations are present in most well-differentiated PanNET, but not seen in poorly differentiated NECs. In contrast, alterations in *RB*, *TP53*, or *SMAD* genes are seen in poorly differentiated NEC, but not in well-differentiated NETs [64, 65, 71, 73].

Somatic *MEN1* mutations are seen in about 20% of sporadic PanNETs [74–78]. Loss of 11q13 or more distal parts of the long arm of chromosome 11 appears to be a frequent event in PanNET tumorigenesis [79–81].

Cystic Lesions

Pseudocyst

Pseudocyst is a peripancreatic unilocular cyst containing necrotic contents rich in pancreatic enzymes. The cyst is lined by a thick fibrous pseudocapsule without lining epithelium. Pseudocysts range from a few to 20 cm and occasionally are multiple. They are typically associated with history of acute pancreatitis and elevated serum amylase levels.

Histologic sections of the pseudocyst demonstrate an inflamed fibrotic pseudocapsule surrounding necrotic adipocytes and debris. Extensive sampling of the cyst is usually required before rendering the diagnosis of pseudocyst, to exclude the possibility of other neoplastic epithelial cysts.

Intraductal Papillary Mucinous Neoplasm

For detailed discussions, please see above section "intraductal neoplasms of the pancreas."

Serous Cystic Neoplasm

Serous cystadenoma is a relatively uncommon neoplasm, accounting for 1–2% of all pancreatic neoplasms [4]. Serous cystadenocarcinoma is even rarer, representing 1–3% of serous cystic neoplasms. These lesions usually occur in the body/tail of the pancreas and show a female predominance (female to male ratio of 3:1). Patient's mean age is 66 years.

The characteristic gross/radiological appearance is a well-circumscribed tumor composed of numerous small cysts (>1 mm to 1 cm in diameter) and contains central fibrous scar (Fig. 3.10a). These tumors less often show a macrocys-

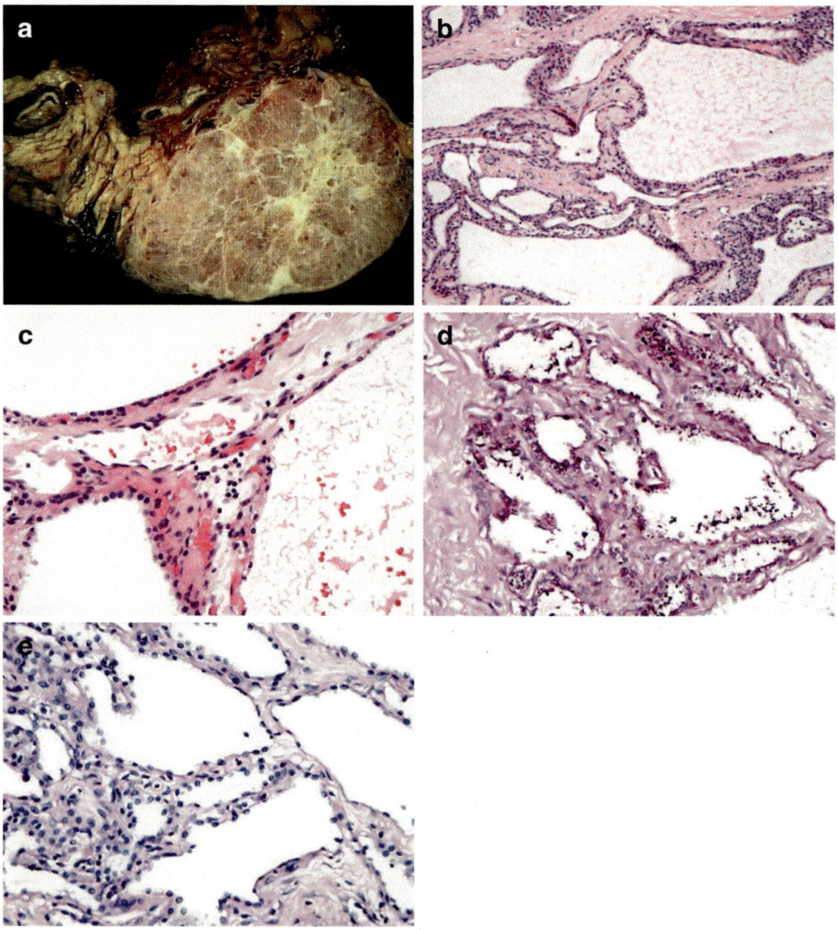

Fig. 3.10 Serous microcystic adenoma. Gross appearance (**a**) is a well-circumscribed tumor with central fibrous scar and numerous small cysts. The cysts are lined by cuboidal clear cells (**b**, 200×; **c**, 400×, H&E stain) due to cytoplasmic accumulation of glycogen. The glycogen can be highlighted by periodic acid-Schiff (PAS) stain (**d**, magenta granules; 400×) and will be digested by diastase (**e**, PAS with diastase; 400×)

tic or solid configuration. Serous cystic neoplasm may be associated with *VHL* gene mutation.

Microscopically, the cyst epithelium is composed of single layer of flat to cuboidal clear cells (Fig. 3.10b and c), with no or little cytologic atypia. Interestingly, the clearing of the cytoplasm is due to cytoplasmic glycogen accumulation, not mucin, as demonstrated by periodic acid-Schiff (PAS) stain with and without diastase (Fig. 3.10d and e). Due to the bland morphology/similarity to serous adenoma, malignancy (serous cystadenocarcinoma) is defined by the presence of distant metastasis.

Mucinous Cystic Neoplasm

Mucinous cystic neoplasm (MCN) accounts for about 8% of surgically resected cystic lesions of the pancreas [4]. It occurs almost exclusively in women (female to male ratio of 20:1). The mean patient age is 50 years. MCN with an associated invasive carcinoma occurs in patients who are 5–10 years older than patients with noninvasive MCNs. Greater than 95% of MCNs occur in the body and tail of the pancreas.

Microscopically, MCNs resemble mucinous neoplasms of the ovary. The cyst lining is classically composed of tall columnar mucinous cells, although some cases show predominantly cuboidal cells with no obvious mucin. The hallmark of MCNs is the subepithelial, cellular, spindle cell stroma (Fig. 3.11a–c), which is diagnostically crucial to establish the correct diagnosis of MCN in cases that have extensive epithelial denudation. This ovarian-type stroma is found at least focally in all MCNs and is regarded as diagnostic prerequisite for MCN. The ovarian-type stroma demonstrates sex cord stromal differentiation and is positive for progesterone receptor (Fig. 3.11b), estrogen receptor, calretinin, CD99, and inhibin. MCNs may exhibit variable epithelial dysplasia (Fig. 3.11d).

As discussed previously in PanIN and IPMN grading, the original three-tiered grading system for dysplasia (low-, intermediate-, and high-grade dysplasia) has been recently revised to a two-tiered grading system (low- and high-grade dysplasia), with merging of low- and intermediate-grade dysplasia [9]. The morphologic types of MCN include gastric, intestinal, pancreatobiliary, and oncocytic [36].

The following terminology is recommended for grading dysplasia in MCN:

For tumor-forming intraepithelial neoplasm without invasion:

MCN, low-grade
MCN, high-grade

For MCN with an associated invasive carcinoma:

MCN, __ grade, with an associated invasive carcinoma

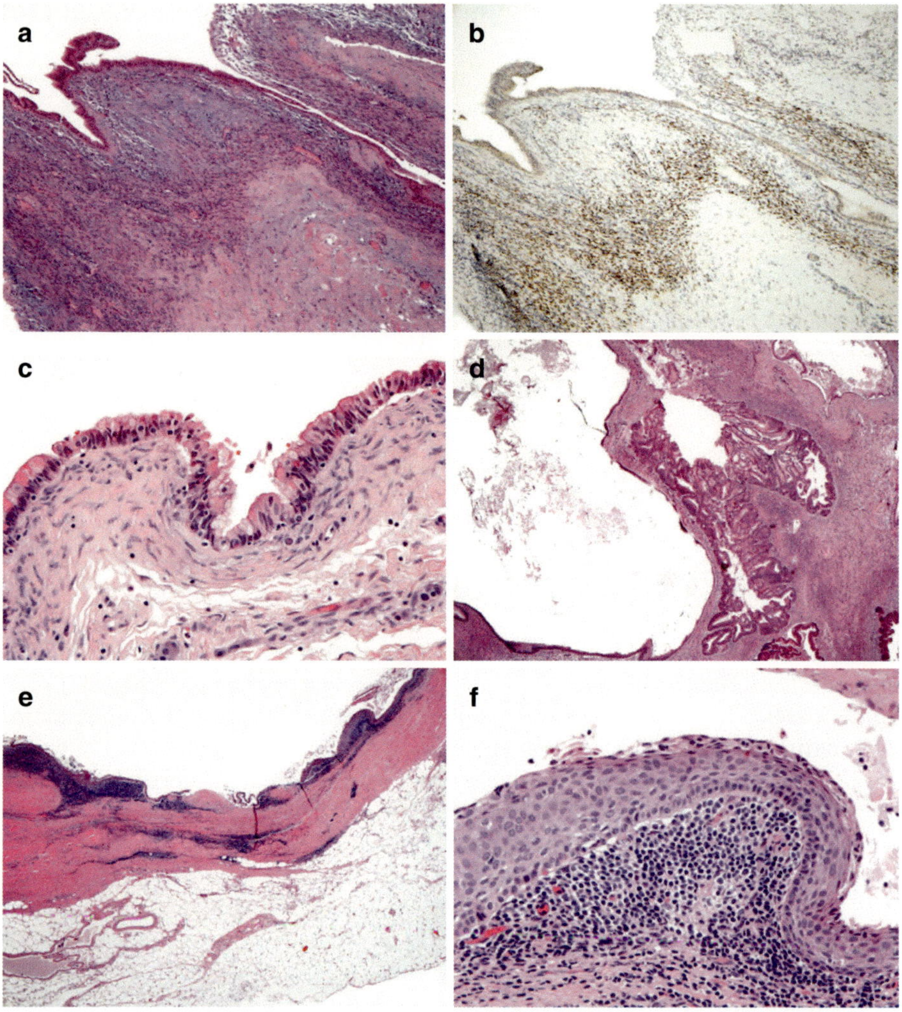

Fig. 3.11 Mucinous cystic neoplasm (MCN) (**a–d**) and lymphoepithelial cyst (**e–f**). MCN shows characteristic of subepithelial ovarian-type stroma (**a**, 100×), which is positive for estrogen and progesterone receptor (**b**, 100×). The cyst lining consists of variable mucinous epithelium (**c**, 400×) that may develop epithelial dysplasia (**d**, 100×). In contrast, the cyst wall of a lymphoepithelial cyst contains lymphoid follicles (**e**, 40×) which underlie a stratified squamous epithelium (**f**, 400×) (**a** and **c–f**: H&E stain)

Lymphoepithelial Cyst

Lymphoepithelial cyst is a rare cystic neoplasm of the pancreas. It occurs predominantly in men in the fifth to sixth decade. Unlike its counterpart in the salivary gland, lymphoepithelial cyst of the pancreas does not have association with HIV infection, lymphoma, and autoimmune conditions. It most often occurs in the periphery of the pancreas in the body or tail region or in peripancreatic soft tissue. Grossly, the thin-walled cyst contains serous to caseous cyst contents and has a smooth cyst lining.

Microscopically, the cyst is lined by a stratified squamous epithelium with variable amount of keratinization. Lymphoid tissue with lymphoid follicles surrounds the squamous epithelium (Fig. 3.11e and f).

Cystic Change in Typically Solid Tumors

Occasionally, some solid tumors of the pancreas may undergo cystic degeneration and bear a cystic gross appearance. The cystic change may be related to central necrosis of the tumor. Grossly, the cyst may contain serous to serosanguinous fluid with or without necrotic debris. Pancreatic tumors that may have cystic change include ductal adenocarcinoma, pancreatic neuroendocrine tumor, acinar neoplasms, solid cystic pseudopapillary neoplasms, and metastatic tumors.

Careful microscopic examination of the periphery of the cyst usually identifies recognizable neoplastic cells. Extensive sampling of the cyst may be needed before establishing a correct diagnosis.

Cytology Overview

Indication and Cytology Sample Procuring

The primary indication for pancreatic biopsy is a mass or biliary duct stricture with clinical suspicion of neoplasm. While NCCN and surgical guidelines state that biopsy proof of malignancy is not required before surgical resection for resectable patients when the clinical suspicion of cancer is high [82, 83], many clinicians request a cytology or tissue diagnosis before surgical intervention. For unresectable tumors, a positive biopsy or aspirate is usually required before administration of chemotherapy.

Fine needle aspiration (FNA) biopsy, particularly endoscopic ultrasound-guided FNA (EUS-FNA) biopsy, has become a well-established diagnostic tool and technique of choice for the diagnosis of pancreatic lesions [84–86]. Tissue biopsy is less often used by some due to the difficulty in interpretation, relatively lower diagnostic accuracy, and higher complication rates. FNA biopsy can be obtained by a variety of imaging guiding techniques. EUS-FNA biopsy is simple, accurate, and safe. In most institutions, it has essentially replaced tissue biopsy and other image-guided FNA techniques. To date, the vast majority of EUS-FNA needles are designed to obtain cytologic specimens. It has been highly effective for most pancreatic tumors with reliable diagnostic accuracy, but some authors believe it can be of limited value in disease entities whose diagnosis relies on tissue architecture or ancillary studies.

Recently, needles with novel tip shapes have been designed to attempt to obtain a core biopsy in addition to cytology [87–89]. Many controversial questions remain as to the actual effectiveness of obtaining true core tissue, sample preparation, ease of interpretation, etc.

In addition, pancreatobiliary tract brushing by endoscopic retrograde cholangiography (ERCP) is a useful diagnostic modality for biliary stricture rather than a distinct mass lesion.

Sample Preparation and Rapid On-Site Evaluation

Cytology sample preparation is different from routine H&E histologic preparation. FNA and biliary brushing specimens can be prepared by conventional smear, liquid-based preparation, cytocentrifugation (cytospin), and cell block. In most institutions, a combination of preparation methods is used to maximize the diagnostic yield. Conventional smear combined with cell block preparation is most commonly used for FNA specimens. Usually, half of conventional smear slides are stained with Diff-Quik staining method at the time of on-site evaluation, and the other half are stained with Papanicolaou staining method (either alcohol fixed or air-dried followed by rehydration) after the procedure. The purpose of cell block preparation is to have the ability to perform ancillary studies when necessary including immunohistochemistry stains, special stains, and molecular testing. Liquid-based preparation or cytocentrifugation instead of conventional smear is mostly used for biliary brushing samples.

Many studies have shown that rapid on-site evaluation for solid pancreatic lesions is helpful for overall diagnostic yield and appropriate sample triage [90, 91]. However, there are studies indicating that it has limited value with experienced operators performing the procedure [92]. It is generally accepted that on-site evaluation offers limited value for cystic lesions.

Diagnostic Accuracy and Reporting Terminology

EUS-FNA has high diagnostic sensitivity and specificity for pancreatic solid lesions. The false negative rate varies depending on its definition [93]. Sampling error is more common than interpretation error. The broadly accepted false positive rate is approximately 0–1% [94–96]; however, there are reports indicating higher rate (as high as 4–5%). The diagnostic accuracy for cystic lesions is much lower.

Conventional cytology reporting categories (including nondiagnostic, negative for malignancy, atypical, suspicious, and malignant) apply to pancreatic cytology. In 2014, Papanicolaou Society of Cytopathology developed a set of guidelines for pancreatobiliary cytology (Table 3.6) [97–99]. The proposed terminology scheme

Table 3.6 Papanicolaou Society of Cytopathology guidelines for pancreatobiliary cytology (2014)

I. Nondiagnostic
II. Negative for malignancy
III. Atypical
IV. Neoplastic
• Benign
– Serous cystadenoma
• Other
– Premalignant mucinous cyst
Intraductal papillary mucinous neoplasm (IPMN)
Mucinous cystic neoplasm (MCN)
– Neoplasm of low-grade malignant behavior
Pancreatic neuroendocrine tumor (PanNET)
Solid pseudopapillary tumor (SPT)
V. Suspicious
VI. Positive/malignant

recommends a six-tiered system: **nondiagnostic, negative for malignancy, atypical, neoplastic, suspicious, and positive/malignant**. The guidelines are designed to stratify the risk of malignancy with diagnostic categories for guiding appropriate management algorithms. Unique to this scheme is the "neoplastic" category, which is separated into "benign" (serous cystadenoma) and "other" (premalignant mucinous cyst including IPMN and MCN and neoplasm of low-grade malignant behavior including NET and solid pseudopapillary tumor).

Normal Pancreas and Benign Gastrointestinal (GI) Tract Contamination

Being able to identify normal pancreatic elements and benign GI tract contamination is essential for pancreatic cytology interpretation. The vast majority of the normal pancreas consists of acinar cells.

Benign biliary ductal cells and normal islets of Langerhans, even if sampled, should be in the minority. The FNA of normal pancreas is often cellular. The acinar cells typically exhibit tight/cohesive clusters with two-dimensional microacinar and/or three-dimensional grape-like clusters, pyramidal or polygonal cell borders, basally oriented nuclei, and apical cytoplasmic zymogen granules (better appreciated on Diff-Quik-stained smears) (Fig. 3.12). Normal islet cells are rarely appreciated.

Benign ductal epithelial cells display cohesive, flat, well-organized, evenly spaced, and monolayer sheets with "honeycomb" appearance. The cells are cuboidal to columnar, have round and regular nuclei, have evenly distributed chromatin, and have inconspicuous nucleoli. Benign GI tract ductal epithelial cell contamina-

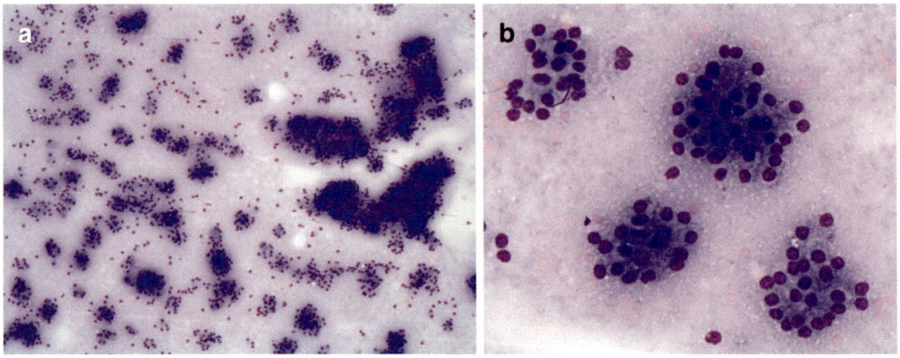

Fig. 3.12 Benign acinar cells exhibit tight/cohesive clusters with two-dimensional microacinar and/or three-dimensional grape-like clusters [**a**: Diff-Quik (DQ) stain, 40×; **b**: DQ stain, 400×]

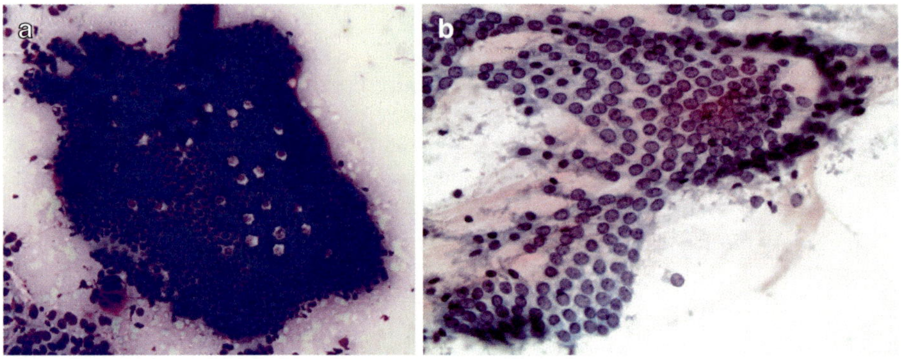

Fig. 3.13 Benign gastrointestinal tract ductal epithelial cells display well-organized monolayer sheets with "honeycomb" appearance. Characteristics of the duodenal epithelium are the scattered distinct goblet cells within the sheets (**a**: DQ stain, 200×). Characteristics of the gastric epithelium is the presence of foveolar cells with intracellular mucin cups and distinct cell borders [**b**: Papanicolaou (Pap) stain, 200×]

tion is unavoidable and very common in pancreatic FNA. Pancreatic head lesions are sampled through duodenal wall, and body/tail lesions are sampled through gastric wall. Both duodenal and gastric ductal contamination appears flat, well-organized architecture similar to normal biliary ductal epithelial cells and can be difficult to distinguish. Characteristics of the duodenal epithelium are the scattered distinct goblet cells within the sheets (Fig. 3.13a). Characteristics of the gastric epithelium is the presence of foveolar cells with intracellular mucin cups and distinct cell borders (Fig. 3.13b). Benign GI tract ductal epithelial cell contamination can be difficult to distinguish from biliary ductal epithelium with low-grade PanIN or low-grade premalignant mucinous cyst. The distinction from high-grade lesions is usually not difficult.

Pancreatic Ductal Adenocarcinoma

Most conventional pancreatic ductal adenocarcinoma is readily recognizable, and EUS-FNA diagnosis is straightforward. On low power, the cellularity is typically moderate to high (Fig. 3.14a). On high power, ductal epithelial cells demonstrate architectural crowding, overlapping, and three-dimensional clusters (Fig. 3.14b). Some authors describe the disorganized groups as "drunken honeycomb" arrangement. The most consistent nuclear features include nuclear enlargement, nuclear membrane irregularity, and anisonucleosis with 4:1 variation within the same group. Intracellular mucin, signet ring cells, and mitosis are not always present but helpful if they are. Poorly differentiated ductal adenocarcinoma can show dyshesive or isolated cells and hyperchromasia (Fig. 3.14c). In well- and moderately differentiated tumors, it is not uncommon to see pale chromatin with small eccentrically located

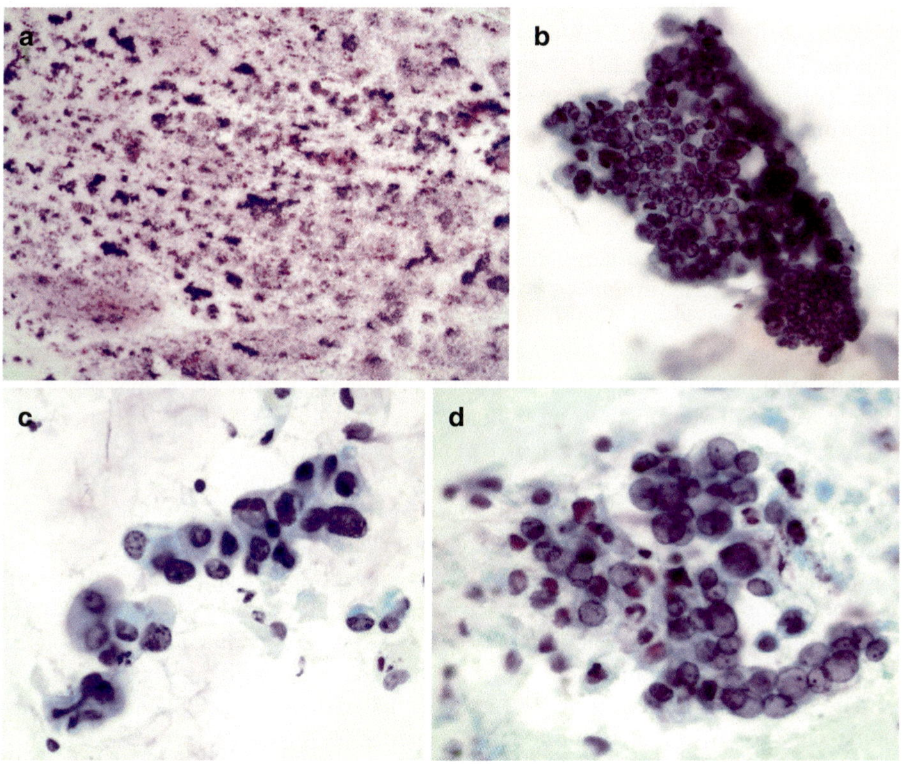

Fig. 3.14 Example of pancreatic ductal adenocarcinoma. Cellular aspirate (**a**: DQ stain, 20×) demonstrates architectural crowding and overlapping with nuclear enlargement, nuclear membrane irregularity, and anisonucleosis with 4:1 variation within the same group (**b**: Pap stain, 400×). Poorly differentiated ductal adenocarcinoma can show dyshesion and hyperchromasia (**c**: Pap stain, 400×), but in well- to moderately differentiated tumors, it is not uncommon to see pale chromatin with small eccentrically located nucleoli (**d**: Pap stain, 400×)

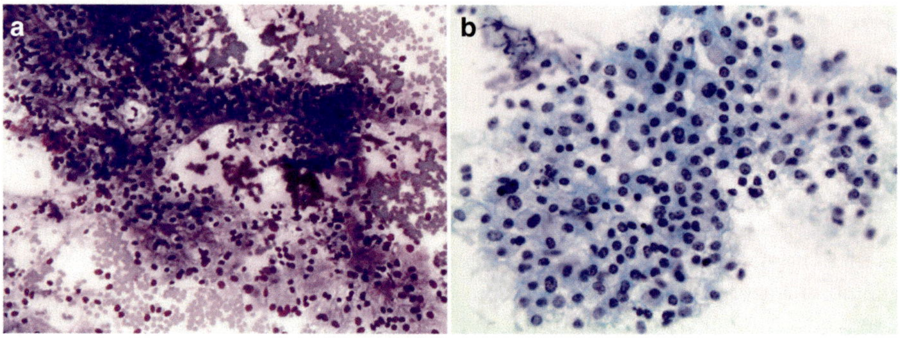

Fig. 3.15 Foamy gland pattern pancreatic ductal adenocarcinoma. It is deceptively benign appearing with low nuclear/cytoplasmic ratio and abundant foamy cytoplasm, closely resembling gastric foveolar epithelium (**a**: DQ stain, 400×; **b**: Pap stain, 400×)

nucleoli (Fig. 3.14d). Background desmoplastic stroma is very common in resection specimens of pancreatic ductal adenocarcinoma, but this stroma is not always aspirated on FNA. Necrosis can be seen. Pancreatic ductal adenocarcinoma with foamy gland pattern can become a diagnostic pitfall because it is deceptively benign looking with low nuclear/cytoplasmic ratio and abundant foamy cytoplasm (Fig. 3.15). It closely resembles gastric foveolar epithelium. Pure foamy gland pattern is not common; this pattern typically intermingles with conventional ductal adenocarcinoma. Stelow et al. reported that 23% of pancreatic ductal adenocarcinoma FNA had a variable degree of foamy changes [100].

There are several variants of pancreatic ductal adenocarcinoma listed in WHO (2010). The most relevant variants for cytology diagnosis are adenosquamous cell carcinoma and anaplastic/undifferentiated carcinoma, because different treatment options or clinical trials may apply. For adenosquamous cell carcinoma, one component often predominates and features of dual differentiation may be focal (Fig. 3.16). By definition, at least 30% of each component is required for diagnosis. A pure squamous carcinoma should raise the suspicion of a metastasis but may also represent under-sampling of an adenosquamous cell carcinoma. In a case of adenocarcinoma predominating, careful evaluation of cytomorphology helps to exclude squamous contamination [101]. In contrast to conventional pancreatic ductal adenocarcinoma, undifferentiated carcinoma is poorly cohesive, is cellular with scant stroma, and has marked pleomorphism (Fig. 3.17). Accurate diagnosis relies on the exclusion of metastatic undifferentiated/high-grade tumor from another site.

The differential diagnosis of pancreatic ductal adenocarcinoma includes conventional chronic pancreatitis, autoimmune pancreatitis, groove pancreatitis, reactive ductal atypia, incidentally sampled PanIN, and metastatic adenocarcinoma from other sites. Various types of chronic pancreatitis may lead to an atypical diagnosis [102, 103] and typically feature low cellularity, mild ductal atypia (Fig. 3.18), fibrous tissue fragments, variable acinar component, and background chronic inflammatory cells. Certainly, a combined evaluation of cellularity and cytomorphology is important. Type 1 autoimmune pancreatitis (lymphoplasmacytic sclerosing pancreatitis) deserves particular consideration and should be excluded preoperatively, because a simple course of steroids has both diagnostic and treatment value [12, 13]. Clinical-radiological

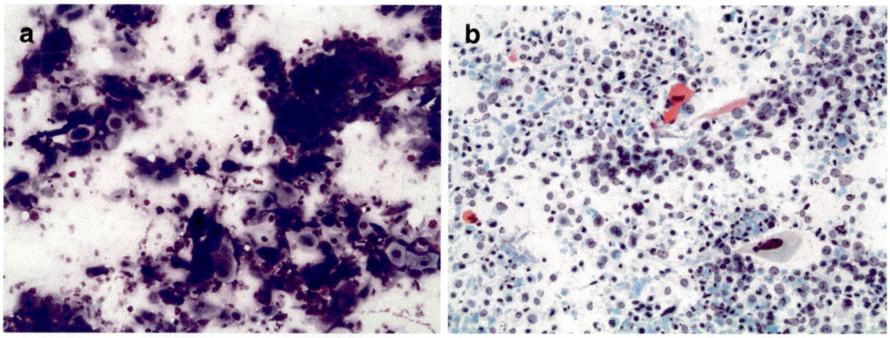

Fig. 3.16 Adenosquamous cell carcinoma.One component often predominates and features of dual differentiation may be focal. **a** (DQ stain, 400×): Squamous carcinoma predominates; **b** (Pap stain, 200×): adenocarcinoma predominates

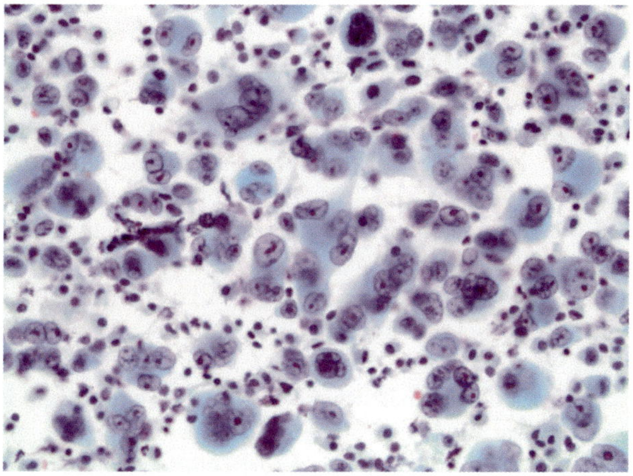

Fig. 3.17 Undifferentiated carcinoma is poorly cohesive, is cellular with scant stroma, and has marked pleomorphism (Pap stain, 400×)

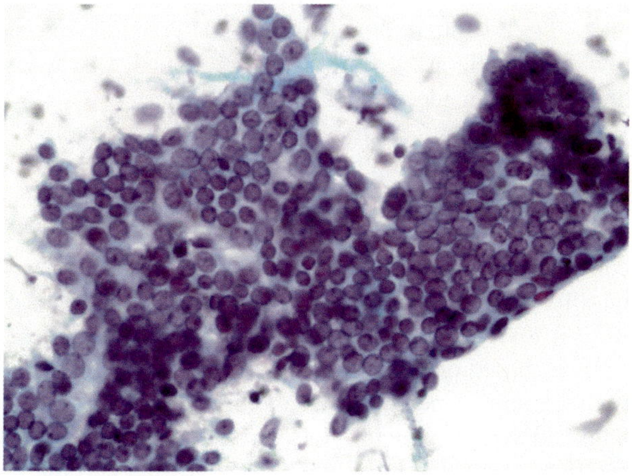

Fig. 3.18 Reactive ductal epithelia atypia that can be seen in the setting of chronic pancreatitis (Pap stain, 400×)

correlation is essential for the diagnosis, and elevated serum IgG4 is the most sensitive and specific laboratory indicator. Incidentally sampled PanIN can contaminate the aspirate, but the quantity of neoplastic cells from PanIN should be much less than those in pancreatic ductal adenocarcinoma [104]. Isolated low-grade PanIN is not uncommon, and the clinical significance is regarded to be negligible. For metastatic adenocarcinoma, knowing the history and an adequate and cellular cell block for immunohistochemical stains are crucial for definitive diagnosis.

Pancreatic Neuroendocrine Tumor (PanNET)

Similar to pancreatic ductal adenocarcinoma, EUS-FNA diagnosis of PanNET has high sensitivity and specificity [105, 106].

Well-differentiated PanNET comprises most PanNET and is the second most common solid neoplasm in the pancreas. The aspirate smear is typically moderate to high in cellularity with loosely cohesive, pseudo-rosette forming or single monotonous small cells (Fig. 3.19). The nuclei are uniform and round to oval and may appear eccentric with plasmacytoid appearance. The chromatin is finely stippled (salt and pepper) (better highlighted by Papanicolaou stain). The cytoplasm is moderate to abundant and granular. Vacuolated and oncocytic PanNETs have been described [107, 108]. Oncocytic variant of PanNET can have abundant cytoplasm, prominent nucleoli, and more anisonucleosis than conventional NET (Fig. 3.20). Poorly differentiated PanNEC is much less common than PanNET. The aspirate smears demonstrate either typical small cell neuroendocrine carcinoma as seen in the lung (Fig. 3.21) or high-grade neuroendocrine carcinoma defined by high Ki-67 labeling or mitotic count. Immunohistochemical stains performed on the cell block section are usually performed to confirm the neuroendocrine differentiation. Studies have shown that Ki-67 labeling performed on cell blocks can be used to grade PanNETs, but limitations exist particularly for grade 2 tumors. The major reasons for discordance include non-tumor cell contamination and insufficient sampling [109].

The reported false negative rate in PanNET is about 10% [105, 106]. The main factors causing inadequate sampling include location in the pancreatic head, presence of rich stromal fibrosis, and cystic PanNET. Interpretation errors are caused by low tumor cellularity, diluting benign acinar cells, and lack of material for confirmatory immunohistochemical stains.

The false positive rate is reported to be less than 1%. The benign mimics include benign acinar cells and florid islet cell aggregation in the setting of chronic pancreatitis. Normal acinar cells are the most common diagnostic pitfall of PanNET. In contrast to loose clusters or single cells in PanNET, the clusters of normal acinar cells are tighter with microacinar and/or grape-like architecture, the nuclei are basally located, and the cytoplasm shows zymogen granules. When acinar cells exhibit loss of apical cytoplasmic zymogen granules, the distinction can be very difficult based on individual cell cytomorphology. Islet cell aggregation associated with chronic pancreatitis is another benign mimic. The relative low cellularity, admixed reactive ductal cells and lymphocytes, and background fibrotic stromal fragments are all helpful features suggesting chronic pancreatitis.

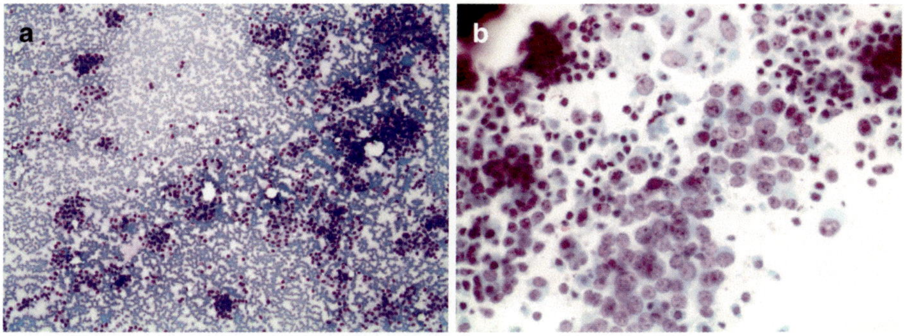

Fig. 3.19 Well-differentiated pancreatic neuroendocrine tumor is characterized by moderate to high cellular smear with loosely cohesive, pseudo-rosette forming or single monotonous small cells (**a**: DQ stain, 200×; **b**: Pap stain, 400×)

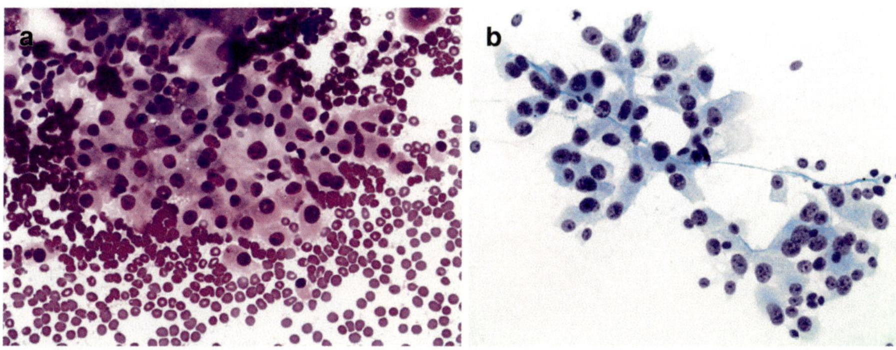

Fig. 3.20 Oncocytic variant of pancreatic neuroendocrine tumor shows abundant cytoplasm, prominent nucleoli, and more anisonucleosis than conventional well-differentiated neuroendocrine tumor (**a**: DQ stain, 200×; **b**: Pap stain, 400×)

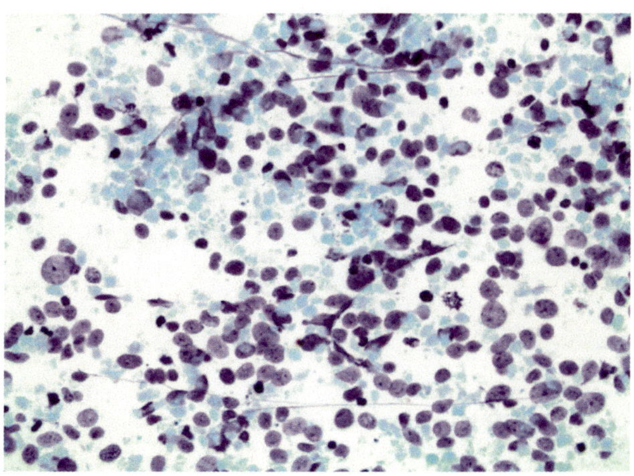

Fig. 3.21 Poorly differentiated pancreatic neuroendocrine carcinoma (Pap stain, 400×) with high-grade cytomorphologic features and background necrosis, apoptosis, and mitosis

The major entities causing misclassification include solid pseudopapillary tumor and acinar cell carcinoma. Because of the overlapping cytomorphology among these entities, immunohistochemical stains as previously described are often required for the distinction.

Classic solid pseudopapillary tumor demonstrates pseudo-papillae with myxoid or hyalinized vascular stalks (Fig. 3.22a). The neoplastic cells are monotonous and have round to oval nuclei often with nuclear grooves, finely textured chromatin, and granular cytoplasm. Compared to PanNET, the smears are more cellular, and the cells are more oval than round with more clustering. Marked degenerative change can be seen. Extracellular metachromatic globules are a characteristic feature (Fig. 3.22b). Slender cytoplasmic processes (cercariform) and clear cytoplasmic vacuoles have been described [110, 111]. Immunohistochemical stain evaluation (β-catenin most important) on cell block section is crucial for definitive diagnosis.

Acinar cell carcinoma has a distinctive cytological appearance but is frequently misdiagnosed on cytology, probably due to the extreme rareness and lack of awareness [112]. FNA smears are highly cellular with loosely cohesive clusters or isolated/naked tumor nuclei (Fig. 3.23). Microacinar structure recapitulates normal acinar architecture. The tumor cells have round to oval nuclei, smooth nuclear contour, and delicate granular cytoplasm. Prominent nucleoli are the characteristic. Immunohistochemical stains are essential for correct diagnosis.

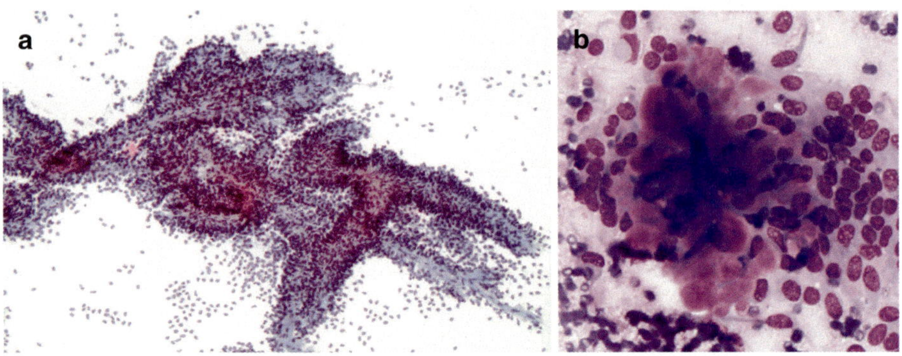

Fig. 3.22 Classic solid pseudopapillary tumor demonstrates pseudo-papillae with vascular stalks (**a**: Pap stain, 200×). Extracellular metachromatic globules are characteristic (**b**, DQ stain, 400×)

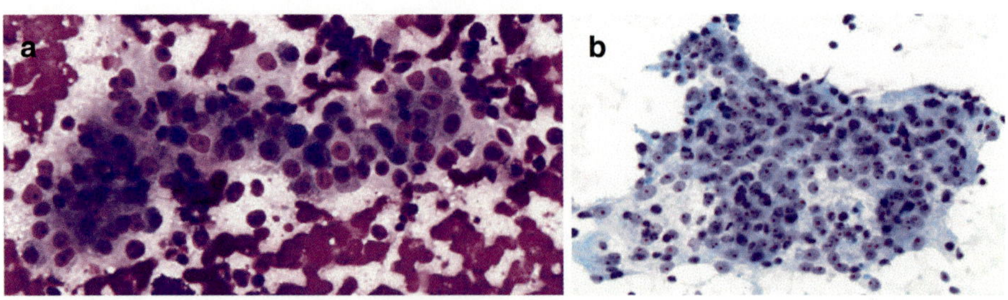

Fig. 3.23 Acinar cell carcinoma smears are highly cellular with loosely cohesive clusters or isolated/naked tumor nuclei. Prominent nucleoli are characteristic (**a**: DQ stain, 400×; **b**: Pap stain, 400×)

Cystic Lesions of the Pancreas

The cytologic diagnostic approach for pancreatic cystic lesions is very different from solid lesions. While cytomorphology evaluation is important, it is a component of multifactorial overall assessment which also includes clinical-radiological findings and cystic fluid analysis [113–115]. For the management of pancreatic cysts, the first question is whether the cyst is a premalignant mucinous cyst, and the second is whether there is high-grade epithelial dysplasia.

Cyst Fluid Analysis

Cyst fluid analysis is often prioritized over cytology preparation for cystic lesions with no solid features by imaging, because of the low diagnostic yield on cytology preparation alone.

The first step is cyst fluid analysis by traditional biochemistry (Table 3.7). Studies have shown that the most reliable indicator to distinguish mucinous from nonmucinous pancreatic cysts is carcinoembryonic antigen (CEA) (a cut-off value ≥192–200 ng/ml), with approximately 80% accuracy in the diagnosis of a mucinous pancreatic cyst [114, 116]. However, cyst fluid analysis has no role in distinguishing the grade of epithelial dysplasia. Amylase can be elevated in both pseudocysts and cystic mucinous neoplasms but is typically not elevated in serous cystadenoma. New molecular testing has become available, but the practical utility remains controversial [117]. KRAS mutation is an early oncogenic mutation in the adenoma-carcinoma sequence, commonly seen in cystic mucinous neoplasms, but does not distinguish low-grade PanIN, which is very common and can be seen in otherwise unremarkable pancreas. It adds no value if CEA is elevated. GNAS mutation has been shown helpful in distinguishing IPMN from MCN.

To date, cytomorphology evaluation is still the most accurate test for the detection of high-grade dysplasia/malignancy in pancreatic cystic mucinous neoplasms. Similar to CEA levels, the presence of KRAS mutation and GNAS mutation has no established value in distinguishing premalignant from malignant lesions. Newer molecular testing panels/DNA profiling will continue to evolve.

Table 3.7 Cyst fluid analysis for pancreatic cystic lesions

Cyst type	Amylase	CEA	KRAS	GNAS
IPMN	High	High	+	+
MCN	High/low	High	+	–
Pseudocyst	High/low	Low	–	–
Serous cystadenoma	Low	Low	–	–

Premalignant Mucinous Cyst: Intraductal Papillary Mucinous Neoplasm (IPMN) and Mucinous Cystic Neoplasm (MCN)

Surgical resection of all pancreatic cysts is not necessary, and surgical resection of all pancreatic mucinous cysts is logistically not possible. Therefore, the goal of management is detection of high risk mucinous cysts before the development of invasive carcinoma.

In general, cytologic distinction between IPMN and MCN is not possible on FNA aspirate. The subepithelial ovarian-type stroma seen in MCN is usually not appreciated on cytology. The goal of cytologic evaluation is to identify the presence or absence of thick neoplastic mucin and high-grade epithelial dysplasia or carcinoma. Thick, colloidal-like mucin with or without mucinous epithelium is diagnostic of a neoplastic mucinous cyst (Fig. 3.24a). The distinction between low-grade dysplasia and GI tract contamination is not possible by cytology in most cases (Fig. 3.24b). High-grade epithelial dysplasia is characterized by tight clusters or isolated cells with nuclear enlargement, high nuclear-cytoplasmic ratio, irregular nuclear contour, and variably vacuolated cytoplasm (Fig. 3.24c–d).

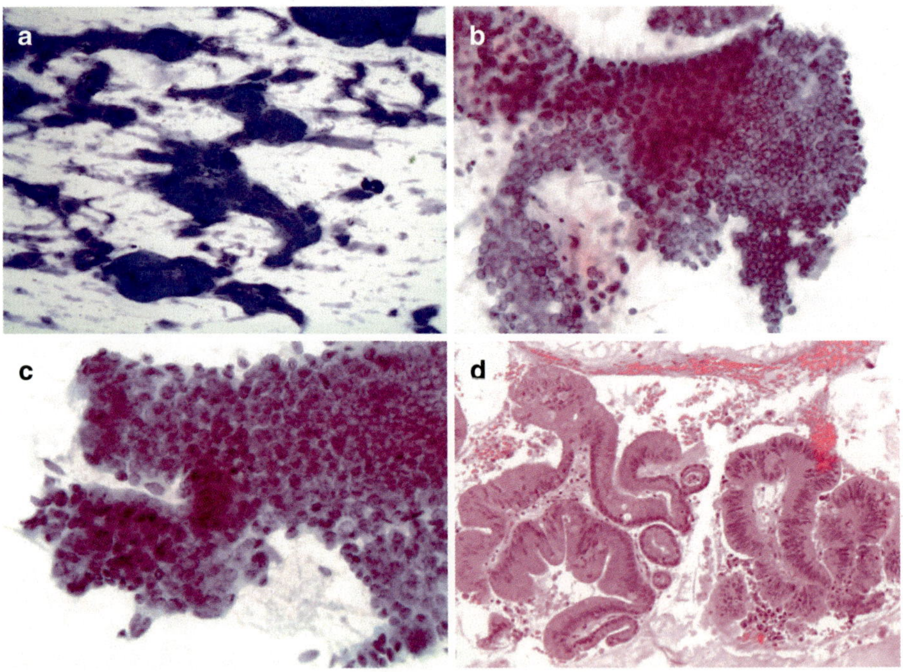

Fig. 3.24 Premalignant mucinous cyst. Thick, colloidal-like mucin with or without mucinous epithelium is diagnostic of a neoplastic mucinous cyst (**a**: DQ stain, 200×). (**b**) (Pap stain, 400×): low-grade dysplasia is difficult to distinguish from benign gastrointestinal tract mucosal contamination. (**c**) (Pap stain, 400×): high-grade dysplasia. (**d**): (cell block preparation, H&E stain, 400×): an area containing both low-grade dysplasia (*left*) and high-grade dysplasia (*right*)

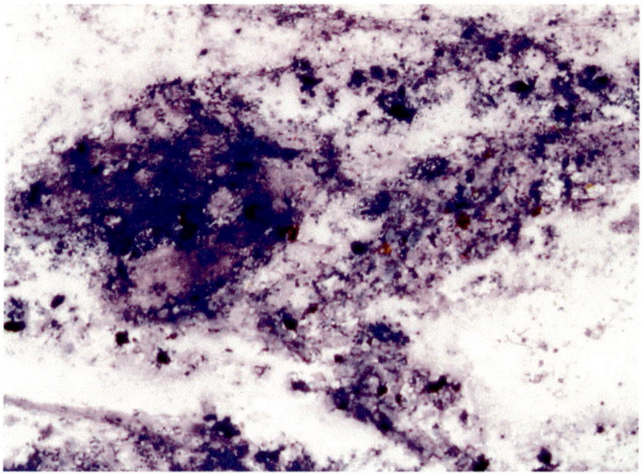

Fig. 3.25 Pseudocyst with debris and pigment (DQ stain, 200×)

Pseudocyst

The typical cytomorphologic features of pseudocyst include nonmucinous turbid fluid with admixed inflammatory cells, histiocytes, yellow pigment and debris (Fig. 3.25). No epithelial lining cells are present; however, benign GI tract contamination can be seen. The cyst fluid analysis shows high amylase without elevated CEA.

Serous Cystadenoma

The cytologic diagnosis of serous cystadenoma is challenging. An FNA diagnosis of nondiagnostic or nonspecific/negative for malignancy interpretation is common because the aspirate is often hypocellular. When the neoplastic cells are present, they are cuboidal and bland appearing with clear and finely vacuolated cytoplasm in a background of clean or bloody fluid. The cyst fluid analysis is low in amylase and CEA.

Lymphoepithelial Cyst

The FNA aspirate of lymphoepithelial cyst is characterized by anucleated and nucleated squamous cells and variable keratin debris and cholesterol clefts (Fig. 3.26). The lymphocytes within the cystic wall are not always sampled. The cyst fluid analysis is unremarkable.

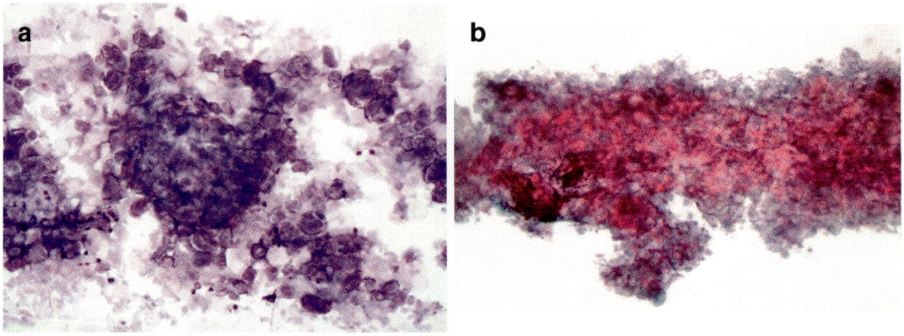

Fig. 3.26 Lymphoepithelial cyst with anucleated keratin debris and nucleated squamous cells (**a**: DQ stain, 200×; **b**: Pap stain, 200×). The lymphocytes within the cystic wall are often not sampled

References

1. Siegel RL, Miller KD, Jemal A. Cancer statistics, 2016. CA Cancer J Clin. 2016;66(1):7–30.
2. Matrisian LM, Berlin JD. The past, present, and future of pancreatic cancer clinical trials. Am Soc Clin Oncol Educ Book. 2016;35:e205–15.
3. Rahib L, Smith BD, Aizenberg R, Rosenzweig AB, Fleshman JM, Matrisian LM. Projecting cancer incidence and deaths to 2030: the unexpected burden of thyroid, liver, and pancreas cancers in the United States. Cancer Res. 2014;74(11):2913–21.
4. Bosman FCF, Hruban R, Theise N. World health organization classification of tumours of the digestive system. 4th ed. Lyon: International Agency for Research on Cancer (IARC) Press; 2010. p. 279–337.
5. Adsay NV, Andea A, Basturk O, Kilinc N, Nassar H, Cheng JD. Secondary tumors of the pancreas: an analysis of a surgical and autopsy database and review of the literature. Virchows Arch. 2004;444(6):527–35.
6. Nakamura E, Shimizu M, Itoh T, Manabe T. Secondary tumors of the pancreas: clinicopathological study of 103 autopsy cases of Japanese patients. Pathol Int. 2001;51(9):686–90.
7. Andea A, Sarkar F, Adsay VN. Clinicopathological correlates of pancreatic intraepithelial neoplasia: a comparative analysis of 82 cases with and 152 cases without pancreatic ductal adenocarcinoma. Mod Pathol. 2003;16(10):996–1006.
8. Brune K, Abe T, Canto M, O'Malley L, Klein AP, Maitra A, Volkan Adsay N, Fishman EK, Cameron JL, Yeo CJ, et al. Multifocal neoplastic precursor lesions associated with lobular atrophy of the pancreas in patients having a strong family history of pancreatic cancer. Am J Surg Pathol. 2006;30(9):1067–76.
9. Basturk O, Hong SM, Wood LD, Adsay NV, Albores-Saavedra J, Biankin AV, Brosens LA, Fukushima N, Goggins M, Hruban RH, et al. A revised classification system and recommendations from the Baltimore consensus meeting for neoplastic precursor lesions in the pancreas. Am J Surg Pathol. 2015;39(12):1730–41.
10. Allen PJ, D'Angelica M, Gonen M, Jaques DP, Coit DG, Jarnagin WR, DeMatteo R, Fong Y, Blumgart LH, Brennan MF. A selective approach to the resection of cystic lesions of the pancreas: results from 539 consecutive patients. Ann Surg. 2006;244(4):572–82.
11. Brat DJ, Lillemoe KD, Yeo CJ, Warfield PB, Hruban RH. Progression of pancreatic intraductal neoplasias to infiltrating adenocarcinoma of the pancreas. Am J Surg Pathol. 1998;22(2):163–9.
12. McCarthy DM, Brat DJ, Wilentz RE, Yeo CJ, Cameron JL, Kern SE, Hruban RH. Pancreatic intraepithelial neoplasia and infiltrating adenocarcinoma: analysis of progression and recurrence by DPC4 immunohistochemical labeling. Hum Pathol. 2001;32(6):638–42.

13. Matthaei H, Schulick RD, Hruban RH, Maitra A. Cystic precursors to invasive pancreatic cancer. Nat Rev Gastroenterol Hepatol. 2011;8(3):141–50.
14. Lemoine NR, Jain S, Hughes CM, Staddon SL, Maillet B, Hall PA, Kloppel G. Ki-ras oncogene activation in preinvasive pancreatic cancer. Gastroenterology. 1992;102(1):230–6.
15. Moskaluk CA, Hruban RH, Kern SE. p16 and K-ras gene mutations in the intraductal precursors of human pancreatic adenocarcinoma. Cancer Res. 1997;57(11):2140–3.
16. Ahlgren JD. Epidemiology and risk factors in pancreatic cancer. Semin Oncol. 1996;23(2):241–50.
17. Cuzick J, Babiker AG. Pancreatic cancer, alcohol, diabetes mellitus and gall-bladder disease. Int J Cancer. 1989;43(3):415–21.
18. Ekbom A, McLaughlin JK, Karlsson BM, Nyren O, Gridley G, Adami HO, Fraumeni JF Jr. Pancreatitis and pancreatic cancer: a population-based study. J Natl Cancer Inst. 1994;86(8):625–7.
19. Ghadirian P, Simard A, Baillargeon J. Tobacco, alcohol, and coffee and cancer of the pancreas. A population-based, case-control study in Quebec, Canada. Cancer. 1991;67(10):2664–70.
20. Lowenfels AB, Maisonneuve P, Cavallini G, Ammann RW, Lankisch PG, Andersen JR, Dimagno EP, Andren-Sandberg A, Domellof L. Pancreatitis and the risk of pancreatic cancer. International Pancreatitis Study Group. N Engl J Med. 1993;328(20):1433–7.
21. Voong KR, Davison J, Pawlik TM, Uy MO, Hsu CC, Winter J, Hruban RH, Laheru D, Rudra S, Swartz MJ, et al. Resected pancreatic adenosquamous carcinoma: clinicopathologic review and evaluation of adjuvant chemotherapy and radiation in 38 patients. Hum Pathol. 2010;41(1):113–22.
22. Poultsides GA, Reddy S, Cameron JL, Hruban RH, Pawlik TM, Ahuja N, Jain A, Edil BH, Iacobuzio-Donahue CA, Schulick RD, et al. Histopathologic basis for the favorable survival after resection of intraductal papillary mucinous neoplasm-associated invasive adenocarcinoma of the pancreas. Ann Surg. 2010;251(3):470–6.
23. Hong SM, Park JY, Hruban RH, Goggins M. Molecular signatures of pancreatic cancer. Arch Pathol Lab Med. 2011;135(6):716–27.
24. Hruban RH, Adsay NV. Molecular classification of neoplasms of the pancreas. Hum Pathol. 2009;40(5):612–23.
25. Shi C, Hruban RH, Klein AP. Familial pancreatic cancer. Arch Pathol Lab Med. 2009;133(3):365–74.
26. Yeo TP. Demographics, epidemiology, and inheritance of pancreatic ductal adenocarcinoma. Semin Oncol. 2015;42(1):8–18.
27. Bergman W, Watson P, de Jong J, Lynch HT, Fusaro RM. Systemic cancer and the FAMMM syndrome. Br J Cancer. 1990;61(6):932–6.
28. Berman DB, Costalas J, Schultz DC, Grana G, Daly M, Godwin AK. A common mutation in BRCA2 that predisposes to a variety of cancers is found in both Jewish Ashkenazi and non-Jewish individuals. Cancer Res. 1996;56(15):3409–14.
29. Couch FJ, Johnson MR, Rabe K, Boardman L, McWilliams R, de Andrade M, Petersen G. Germ line Fanconi anemia complementation group C mutations and pancreatic cancer. Cancer Res. 2005;65(2):383–6.
30. Lal G, Liu G, Schmocker B, Kaurah P, Ozcelik H, Narod SA, Redston M, Gallinger S. Inherited predisposition to pancreatic adenocarcinoma: role of family history and germline p16, BRCA1, and BRCA2 mutations. Cancer Res. 2000;60(2):409–16.
31. Liede A, Karlan BY, Narod SA. Cancer risks for male carriers of germline mutations in BRCA1 or BRCA2: a review of the literature. J Clin Oncol. 2004;22(4):735–42.
32. Mahlamaki EH, Hoglund M, Gorunova L, Karhu R, Dawiskiba S, Andren-Sandberg A, Kallioniemi OP, Johansson B. Comparative genomic hybridization reveals frequent gains of 20q, 8q, 11q, 12p, and 17q, and losses of 18q, 9p, and 15q in pancreatic cancer. Genes Chromosomes Cancer. 1997;20(4):383–91.
33. Su GH, Hruban RH, Bansal RK, Bova GS, Tang DJ, Shekher MC, Westerman AM, Entius MM, Goggins M, Yeo CJ, et al. Germline and somatic mutations of the STK11/LKB1 Peutz-Jeghers gene in pancreatic and biliary cancers. Am J Pathol. 1999;154(6):1835–40.

34. van der Heijden MS, Yeo CJ, Hruban RH, Kern SE. Fanconi anemia gene mutations in young-onset pancreatic cancer. Cancer Res. 2003;63(10):2585–8.
35. Jones S, Zhang X, Parsons DW, Lin JC, Leary RJ, Angenendt P, Mankoo P, Carter H, Kamiyama H, Jimeno A, et al. Core signaling pathways in human pancreatic cancers revealed by global genomic analyses. Science. 2008;321(5897):1801–6.
36. Furukawa T, Kloppel G, Volkan Adsay N, Albores-Saavedra J, Fukushima N, Horii A, Hruban RH, Kato Y, Klimstra DS, Longnecker DS, et al. Classification of types of intraductal papillary-mucinous neoplasm of the pancreas: a consensus study. Virchows Arch. 2005;447(5):794–9.
37. Kwak HA, Liu X, Allende DS, Pai RK, Hart J, Xiao SY. Interobserver variability in intraductal papillary mucinous neoplasm subtypes and application of their mucin immunoprofiles. Mod Pathol. 2016;29(9):977–84.
38. Adsay NV, Conlon KC, Zee SY, Brennan MF, Klimstra DS. Intraductal papillary-mucinous neoplasms of the pancreas: an analysis of in situ and invasive carcinomas in 28 patients. Cancer. 2002;94(1):62–77.
39. Adsay NV, Longnecker DS, Klimstra DS. Pancreatic tumors with cystic dilatation of the ducts: intraductal papillary mucinous neoplasms and intraductal oncocytic papillary neoplasms. Semin Diagn Pathol. 2000;17(1):16–30.
40. Adsay NV, Merati K, Andea A, Sarkar F, Hruban RH, Wilentz RE, Goggins M, Iocobuzio-Donahue C, Longnecker DS, Klimstra DS. The dichotomy in the preinvasive neoplasia to invasive carcinoma sequence in the pancreas: differential expression of MUC1 and MUC2 supports the existence of two separate pathways of carcinogenesis. Mod Pathol. 2002;15(10):1087–95.
41. Basturk O, Chung SM, Hruban RH, Adsay NV, Askan G, Iacobuzio-Donahue C, Balci S, Zee SY, Memis B, Shia J, et al. Distinct pathways of pathogenesis of intraductal oncocytic papillary neoplasms and intraductal papillary mucinous neoplasms of the pancreas. Virchows Arch. 2016;469(5):523–32.
42. Reid MD, Stallworth CR, Lewis MM, Akkas G, Memis B, Basturk O, Adsay V. Cytopathologic diagnosis of oncocytic type intraductal papillary mucinous neoplasm: criteria and clinical implications of accurate diagnosis. Cancer Cytopathol. 2016;124(2):122–34.
43. Marchegiani G, Mino-Kenudson M, Ferrone CR, Warshaw AL, Lillemoe KD, Fernandez-del Castillo C. Oncocytic-type intraductal papillary mucinous neoplasms: a unique malignant pancreatic tumor with good long-term prognosis. J Am Coll Surg. 2015;220(5):839–44.
44. Adsay NV, Merati K, Basturk O, Iacobuzio-Donahue C, Levi E, Cheng JD, Sarkar FH, Hruban RH, Klimstra DS. Pathologically and biologically distinct types of epithelium in intraductal papillary mucinous neoplasms: delineation of an "intestinal" pathway of carcinogenesis in the pancreas. Am J Surg Pathol. 2004;28(7):839–48.
45. Frankel TL, LaFemina J, Bamboat ZM, D'Angelica MI, DeMatteo RP, Fong Y, Kingham TP, Jarnagin WR, Allen PJ. Dysplasia at the surgical margin is associated with recurrence after resection of non-invasive intraductal papillary mucinous neoplasms. HPB (Oxford). 2013;15(10):814–21.
46. Fujii T, Kato K, Kodera Y, Kanda M, Nagai S, Yamada S, Kanzaki A, Sugimoto H, Nomoto S, Takeda S, et al. Prognostic impact of pancreatic margin status in the intraductal papillary mucinous neoplasms of the pancreas. Surgery. 2010;148(2):285–90.
47. Leng KM, Wang ZD, Zhao JB, Cui YF, Zhong XY. Impact of pancreatic margin status and lymph node metastases on recurrence after resection for invasive and noninvasive intraductal papillary mucinous neoplasms of the pancreas: a meta-analysis. Dig Surg. 2012;29(3):213–25.
48. Nakagohri T, Kinoshita T, Konishi M, Takahashi S, Gotohda N. Surgical outcome of intraductal papillary mucinous neoplasms of the pancreas. Ann Surg Oncol. 2007;14(11):3174–80.
49. Raut CP, Cleary KR, Staerkel GA, Abbruzzese JL, Wolff RA, Lee JH, Vauthey JN, Lee JE, Pisters PW, Evans DB. Intraductal papillary mucinous neoplasms of the pancreas: effect of invasion and pancreatic margin status on recurrence and survival. Ann Surg Oncol. 2006;13(4):582–94.

50. Eguchi H, Ishikawa O, Ohigashi H, Sasaki Y, Yamada T, Nakaizumi A, Uehara H, Takenaka A, Kasugai T, Imaoka S. Role of intraoperative cytology combined with histology in detecting continuous and skip type intraductal cancer existence for intraductal papillary mucinous carcinoma of the pancreas. Cancer. 2006;107(11):2567–75.
51. Yamaguchi H, Shimizu M, Ban S, Koyama I, Hatori T, Fujita I, Yamamoto M, Kawamura S, Kobayashi M, Ishida K, et al. Intraductal tubulopapillary neoplasms of the pancreas distinct from pancreatic intraepithelial neoplasia and intraductal papillary mucinous neoplasms. Am J Surg Pathol. 2009;33(8):1164–72.
52. Date K, Okabayashi T, Shima Y, Iwata J, Sumiyoshi T, Kozuki A, Morita S, Hata Y, Noda Y, Nishioka A, et al. Clinicopathological features and surgical outcomes of intraductal tubulopapillary neoplasm of the pancreas: a systematic review. Langenbeck's Arch Surg. 2016;401(4):439–47.
53. Rooney SL, Shi J. Intraductal tubulopapillary neoplasm of the pancreas: an update from a pathologist's perspective. Arch Pathol Lab Med. 2016;140(10):1068–73.
54. Schonleben F, Qiu W, Bruckman KC, Ciau NT, Li X, Lauerman MH, Frucht H, Chabot JA, Allendorf JD, Remotti HE, et al. BRAF and KRAS gene mutations in intraductal papillary mucinous neoplasm/carcinoma (IPMN/IPMC) of the pancreas. Cancer Lett. 2007;249(2):242–8.
55. Uemura K, Hiyama E, Murakami Y, Kanehiro T, Ohge H, Sueda T, Yokoyama T. Comparative analysis of K-ras point mutation, telomerase activity, and p53 overexpression in pancreatic tumours. Oncol Rep. 2003;10(2):277–83.
56. Abe T, Fukushima N, Brune K, Boehm C, Sato N, Matsubayashi H, Canto M, Petersen GM, Hruban RH, Goggins M. Genome-wide allelotypes of familial pancreatic adenocarcinomas and familial and sporadic intraductal papillary mucinous neoplasms. Clin Cancer Res. 2007;13(20):6019–25.
57. Fujii H, Inagaki M, Kasai S, Miyokawa N, Tokusashi Y, Gabrielson E, Hruban RH. Genetic progression and heterogeneity in intraductal papillary-mucinous neoplasms of the pancreas. Am J Pathol. 1997;151(5):1447–54.
58. Wada K. p16 and p53 gene alterations and accumulations in the malignant evolution of intraductal papillary-mucinous tumors of the pancreas. J Hepato-Biliary-Pancreat Surg. 2002;9(1):76–85.
59. Wu J, Jiao Y, Dal Molin M, Maitra A, de Wilde RF, Wood LD, Eshleman JR, Goggins MG, Wolfgang CL, Canto MI, et al. Whole-exome sequencing of neoplastic cysts of the pancreas reveals recurrent mutations in components of ubiquitin-dependent pathways. Proc Natl Acad Sci U S A. 2011;108(52):21188–93.
60. Wu J, Matthaei H, Maitra A, Dal Molin M, Wood LD, Eshleman JR, Goggins M, Canto MI, Schulick RD, Edil BH, et al. Recurrent GNAS mutations define an unexpected pathway for pancreatic cyst development. Sci Transl Med. 2011;3(92):92ra66.
61. Schonleben F, Qiu W, Ciau NT, Ho DJ, Li X, Allendorf JD, Remotti HE, Su GH. PIK3CA mutations in intraductal papillary mucinous neoplasm/carcinoma of the pancreas. Clin Cancer Res. 2006;12(12):3851–5.
62. Kim JY, Hong SM. Recent updates on neuroendocrine tumors from the gastrointestinal and pancreatobiliary tracts. Arch Pathol Lab Med. 2016;140(5):437–48.
63. McCall CM, Shi C, Klein AP, Konukiewitz B, Edil BH, Ellison TA, Wolfgang CL, Schulick RD, Kloppel G, Hruban RH. Serotonin expression in pancreatic neuroendocrine tumors correlates with a trabecular histologic pattern and large duct involvement. Hum Pathol. 2012;43(8):1169–76.
64. Basturk O, Yang Z, Tang LH, Hruban RH, Adsay V, McCall CM, Krasinskas AM, Jang KT, Frankel WL, Balci S, et al. The high-grade (WHO G3) pancreatic neuroendocrine tumor category is morphologically and biologically heterogenous and includes both well differentiated and poorly differentiated neoplasms. Am J Surg Pathol. 2015;39(5):683–90.
65. Tang LH, Basturk O, Sue JJ, Klimstra DS. A practical approach to the classification of WHO Grade 3 (G3) well-differentiated neuroendocrine tumor (WD-NET) and poorly

differentiated neuroendocrine carcinoma (PD-NEC) of the pancreas. Am J Surg Pathol. 2016;40(9):1192–202.
66. Basturk O, Tang L, Hruban RH, Adsay V, Yang Z, Krasinskas AM, Vakiani E, La Rosa S, Jang KT, Frankel WL, et al. Poorly differentiated neuroendocrine carcinomas of the pancreas: a clinicopathologic analysis of 44 cases. Am J Surg Pathol. 2014;38(4):437–47.
67. Hruban RH, Iacobuzio-Donahue C, Wilentz RE, Goggins M, Kern SE. Molecular pathology of pancreatic cancer. Cancer J. 2001;7(4):251–8.
68. Moore PS, Orlandini S, Zamboni G, Capelli P, Rigaud G, Falconi M, Bassi C, Lemoine NR, Scarpa A. Pancreatic tumours: molecular pathways implicated in ductal cancer are involved in ampullary but not in exocrine nonductal or endocrine tumorigenesis. Br J Cancer. 2001;84(2):253–62.
69. Perren A, Komminoth P, Saremaslani P, Matter C, Feurer S, Lees JA, Heitz PU, Eng C. Mutation and expression analyses reveal differential subcellular compartmentalization of PTEN in endocrine pancreatic tumors compared to normal islet cells. Am J Pathol. 2000;157(4):1097–103.
70. Serrano J, Goebel SU, Peghini PL, Lubensky IA, Gibril F, Jensen RT. Alterations in the p16INK4a/CDKN2A tumor suppressor gene in gastrinomas. J Clin Endocrinol Metab. 2000;85(11):4146–56.
71. Jiao Y, Shi C, Edil BH, de Wilde RF, Klimstra DS, Maitra A, Schulick RD, Tang LH, Wolfgang CL, Choti MA, et al. DAXX/ATRX, MEN1, and mTOR pathway genes are frequently altered in pancreatic neuroendocrine tumors. Science. 2011;331(6021):1199–203.
72. Shi C, Klimstra DS. Pancreatic neuroendocrine tumors: pathologic and molecular characteristics. Semin Diagn Pathol. 2014;31(6):498–511.
73. Yachida S, Vakiani E, White CM, Zhong Y, Saunders T, Morgan R, de Wilde RF, Maitra A, Hicks J, Demarzo AM, et al. Small cell and large cell neuroendocrine carcinomas of the pancreas are genetically similar and distinct from well-differentiated pancreatic neuroendocrine tumors. Am J Surg Pathol. 2012;36(2):173–84.
74. Gortz B, Roth J, Krahenmann A, de Krijger RR, Muletta-Feurer S, Rutimann K, Saremaslani P, Speel EJ, Heitz PU, Komminoth P. Mutations and allelic deletions of the MEN1 gene are associated with a subset of sporadic endocrine pancreatic and neuroendocrine tumors and not restricted to foregut neoplasms. Am J Pathol. 1999;154(2):429–36.
75. Moore PS, Missiaglia E, Antonello D, Zamo A, Zamboni G, Corleto V, Falconi M, Scarpa A. Role of disease-causing genes in sporadic pancreatic endocrine tumors: MEN1 and VHL. Genes Chromosomes Cancer. 2001;32(2):177–81.
76. Shan L, Nakamura Y, Nakamura M, Yokoi T, Tsujimoto M, Arima R, Kameya T, Kakudo K. Somatic mutations of multiple endocrine neoplasia type 1 gene in the sporadic endocrine tumors. Lab Investig. 1998;78(4):471–5.
77. Wang EH, Ebrahimi SA, Wu AY, Kashefi C, Passaro E Jr, Sawicki MP. Mutation of the MENIN gene in sporadic pancreatic endocrine tumors. Cancer Res. 1998;58(19):4417–20.
78. Zhuang Z, Vortmeyer AO, Pack S, Huang S, Pham TA, Wang C, Park WS, Agarwal SK, Debelenko LV, Kester M, et al. Somatic mutations of the MEN1 tumor suppressor gene in sporadic gastrinomas and insulinomas. Cancer Res. 1997;57(21):4682–6.
79. D'Adda T, Pizzi S, Azzoni C, Bottarelli L, Crafa P, Pasquali C, Davoli C, Corleto VD, Delle Fave G, Bordi C. Different patterns of 11q allelic losses in digestive endocrine tumors. Hum Pathol. 2002;33(3):322–9.
80. Hessman O, Lindberg D, Einarsson A, Lillhager P, Carling T, Grimelius L, Eriksson B, Akerstrom G, Westin G, Skogseid B. Genetic alterations on 3p, 11q13, and 18q in nonfamilial and MEN 1-associated pancreatic endocrine tumors. Genes Chromosomes Cancer. 1999;26(3):258–64.
81. Hessman O, Lindberg D, Skogseid B, Carling T, Hellman P, Rastad J, Akerstrom G, Westin G. Mutation of the multiple endocrine neoplasia type 1 gene in nonfamilial, malignant tumors of the endocrine pancreas. Cancer Res. 1998;58(3):377–9.
82. Asbun HJ, Conlon K, Fernandez-Cruz L, Friess H, Shrikhande SV, Adham M, Bassi C, Bockhorn M, Buchler M, Charnley RM, et al. When to perform a pancreatoduodenectomy in

the absence of positive histology? A consensus statement by the International Study Group of Pancreatic Surgery. Surgery. 2014;155(5):887–92.
83. Bockhorn M, Uzunoglu FG, Adham M, Imrie C, Milicevic M, Sandberg AA, Asbun HJ, Bassi C, Buchler M, Charnley RM, et al. Borderline resectable pancreatic cancer: a consensus statement by the International Study Group of Pancreatic Surgery (ISGPS). Surgery. 2014;155(6):977–88.
84. Eltoum IA, Alston EA, Roberson J. Trends in pancreatic pathology practice before and after implementation of endoscopic ultrasound-guided fine-needle aspiration: an example of disruptive innovation effect? Arch Pathol Lab Med. 2012;136(4):447–53.
85. Jhala NC, Jhala D, Eltoum I, Vickers SM, Wilcox CM, Chhieng DC, Eloubeidi MA. Endoscopic ultrasound-guided fine-needle aspiration biopsy: a powerful tool to obtain samples from small lesions. Cancer. 2004;102(4):239–46.
86. Volmar KE, Vollmer RT, Routbort MJ, Creager AJ. Pancreatic and bile duct brushing cytology in 1000 cases: review of findings and comparison of preparation methods. Cancer. 2006;108(4):231–8.
87. Adler DG, Witt B, Chadwick B, Wells J, Taylor LJ, Dimaio C, Schmidt R. Pathologic evaluation of a new endoscopic ultrasound needle designed to obtain core tissue samples: a pilot study. Endosc Ultrasound. 2016;5(3):178–83.
88. Dwyer J, Pantanowitz L, Ohori NP, Pai RK, Vrbin C, Brand RE, Monaco SE. Endoscopic ultrasound-guided FNA and ProCore biopsy in sampling pancreatic and intra-abdominal masses. Cancer Cytopathol. 2016;124(2):110–21.
89. Kamata K, Kitano M, Yasukawa S, Kudo M, Chiba Y, Ogura T, Higuchi K, Fukutake N, Ashida R, Yamasaki T, et al. Histologic diagnosis of pancreatic masses using 25-gauge endoscopic ultrasound needles with and without a core trap: a multicenter randomized trial. Endoscopy. 2016;48(7):632–8.
90. da Cunha SG, Ko HM, Saieg MA. Geddie WR: "The petals and thorns" of ROSE (rapid on-site evaluation). Cancer Cytopathol. 2013;121(1):4–8.
91. Jhala NC, Eltoum IA, Eloubeidi MA, Meara R, Chhieng DC, Crowe DR, Jhala D. Providing on-site diagnosis of malignancy on endoscopic-ultrasound-guided fine-needle aspirates: should it be done? Ann Diagn Pathol. 2007;11(3):176–81.
92. Cermak TS, Wang B, DeBrito P, Carroll J, Haddad N, Sidawy MK. Does on-site adequacy evaluation reduce the nondiagnostic rate in endoscopic ultrasound-guided fine-needle aspiration of pancreatic lesions? Cancer Cytopathol. 2012;120(5):319–25.
93. Woolf KM, Liang H, Sletten ZJ, Russell DK, Bonfiglio TA, Zhou Z. False-negative rate of endoscopic ultrasound-guided fine-needle aspiration for pancreatic solid and cystic lesions with matched surgical resections as the gold standard: one institution's experience. Cancer Cytopathol. 2013;121(8):449–58.
94. Gleeson FC, Kipp BR, Caudill JL, Clain JE, Clayton AC, Halling KC, Henry MR, Rajan E, Topazian MD, Wang KK, et al. False positive endoscopic ultrasound fine needle aspiration cytology: incidence and risk factors. Gut. 2010;59(5):586–93.
95. Schwartz DA, Unni KK, Levy MJ, Clain JE, Wiersema MJ. The rate of false-positive results with EUS-guided fine-needle aspiration. Gastrointest Endosc. 2002;56(6):868–72.
96. Siddiqui AA, Kowalski TE, Shahid H, O'Donnell S, Tolin J, Loren DE, Infantolino A, Hong SK, Eloubeidi MA. False-positive EUS-guided FNA cytology for solid pancreatic lesions. Gastrointest Endosc. 2011;74(3):535–40.
97. Pitman MB, Centeno BA, Ali SZ, Genevay M, Stelow E, Mino-Kenudson M, Castillo CF, Schmidt CM, Brugge WR, Layfield LJ. Standardized terminology and nomenclature for pancreatobiliary cytology: the Papanicolaou Society of Cytopathology Guidelines. Cytojournal. 2014;11(Suppl 1):3.
98. Pitman MB, Centeno BA, Ali SZ, Genevay M, Stelow E, Mino-Kenudson M, Fernandez-del Castillo C, Max Schmidt C, Brugge W, Layfield L. Standardized terminology and nomenclature for pancreatobiliary cytology: the Papanicolaou Society of Cytopathology guidelines. Diagn Cytopathol. 2014;42(4):338–50.

99. Pitman MB, Layfield LJ. Guidelines for pancreaticobiliary cytology from the Papanicolaou Society of Cytopathology: a review. Cancer Cytopathol. 2014;122(6):399–411.
100. Stelow EB, Pambuccian SE, Bardales RH, et al. The cytology of pancreatic foamy gland adenocarcinoma. Am J Clin Pathol. 2004;121(6):893–7.
101. Olson MT, Siddiqui MT, Ali SZ. The differential diagnosis of squamous cells in pancreatic aspirates: from contamination to adenosquamous carcinoma. Acta Cytol. 2013;57(2):139–46.
102. Chute DJ, Stelow EB. Fine-needle aspiration features of paraduodenal pancreatitis (groove pancreatitis): a report of three cases. Diagn Cytopathol. 2012;40(12):1116–21.
103. Holmes BJ, Hruban RH, Wolfgang CL, Ali SZ. Fine needle aspirate of autoimmune pancreatitis (lymphoplasmacytic sclerosing pancreatitis): cytomorphologic characteristics and clinical correlates. Acta Cytol. 2012;56(3):228–32.
104. Jarboe EA, Layfield LJ. Cytologic features of pancreatic intraepithelial neoplasia and pancreatitis: potential pitfalls in the diagnosis of pancreatic ductal carcinoma. Diagn Cytopathol. 2011;39(8):575–81.
105. Hijioka S, Hara K, Mizuno N, Imaoka H, Bhatia V, Mekky MA, Yoshimura K, Yoshida T, Okuno N, Hieda N, et al. Diagnostic performance and factors influencing the accuracy of EUS-FNA of pancreatic neuroendocrine neoplasms. J Gastroenterol. 2016 Sep;51(9):923–30.
106. Hooper K, Mukhtar F, Li S, Eltoum IA. Diagnostic error assessment and associated harm of endoscopic ultrasound-guided fine-needle aspiration of neuroendocrine neoplasms of the pancreas. Cancer Cytopathol. 2013;121(11):653–60.
107. Chen S, Wang X, Lin J. Fine needle aspiration of oncocytic variants of pancreatic neuroendocrine tumor: a report of three misdiagnosed cases. Acta Cytol. 2014;58(2):131–7.
108. Levy GH, Finkelstein A, Harigopal M, Chhieng D, Cai G. Cytoplasmic vacuolization: an under-recognized cytomorphologic feature in endocrine tumors of the pancreas. Diagn Cytopathol. 2013;41(7):623–8.
109. Jin M, Roth R, Gayetsky V, Niederberger N, Lehman A, Wakely PE. Grading pancreatic neuroendocrine neoplasms by Ki-67 staining on cytology cell blocks: manual count and digital image analysis of 58 cases. JASC. 2016;5(5):286–95.
110. Samad A, Shah AA, Stelow EB, Alsharif M, Cameron SE, Pambuccian SE. Cercariform cells: another cytologic feature distinguishing solid pseudopapillary neoplasms from pancreatic endocrine neoplasms and acinar cell carcinomas in endoscopic ultrasound-guided fine-needle aspirates. Cancer Cytopathol. 2013;121(6):298–310.
111. Zhao P, deBrito P, Ozdemirli M, Sidawy MK. Solid-pseudopapillary neoplasm of the pancreas: awareness of unusual clinical presentations and morphology of the clear cell variant can prevent diagnostic errors. Diagn Cytopathol. 2013;41(10):889–95.
112. Sigel CS, Klimstra DS. Cytomorphologic and immunophenotypical features of acinar cell neoplasms of the pancreas. Cancer Cytopathol. 2013;121(8):459–70.
113. Pitman MB. Revised international consensus guidelines for the management of patients with mucinous cysts. Cancer Cytopathol. 2012;120(6):361–5.
114. Pitman MB. Pancreatic cyst fluid triage: a critical component of the preoperative evaluation of pancreatic cysts. Cancer Cytopathol. 2013;121(2):57–60.
115. Pitman MB, Yaeger KA, Brugge WR, Mino-Kenudson M. Prospective analysis of atypical epithelial cells as a high-risk cytologic feature for malignancy in pancreatic cysts. Cancer Cytopathol. 2013;121(1):29–36.
116. Cizginer S, Turner BG, Bilge AR, Karaca C, Pitman MB, Brugge WR. Cyst fluid carcinoembryonic antigen is an accurate diagnostic marker of pancreatic mucinous cysts. Pancreas. 2011;40(7):1024–8.
117. Khalid A, Zahid M, Finkelstein SD, LeBlanc JK, Kaushik N, Ahmad N, Brugge WR, Edmundowicz SA, Hawes RH, McGrath KM. Pancreatic cyst fluid DNA analysis in evaluating pancreatic cysts: a report of the PANDA study. Gastrointest Endosc. 2009;69(6):1095–102.

Chapter 4
Screening for Pancreatic Cancer: Who to Screen and How to Follow-Up?

Phil A. Hart, Peter P. Stanich, and Heather Hampel

Abbreviations

CAPS	Cancer of the Pancreas Screening Consortium
DM	Diabetes mellitus
EUS	Endoscopic ultrasound
FDR	First-degree relative
FNA	Fine needle aspiration
FPC	Familial pancreatic cancer
PDAC	Pancreatic ductal adenocarcinoma
SDR	Second-degree relative

Introduction

Pancreatic cancer (i.e., pancreatic ductal adenocarcinoma (PDAC)) is now the third most common cause of cancer-related death in the United States [1]. The annual incidence of PDAC is approximately 40,000 cases, with projections that PDAC will become the second most common cause of cancer death by 2030 [2]. There have been only small improvements in the 5-year survival rate over the last two decades,

P.A. Hart, M.D. (✉) • P.P. Stanich, M.D.
Division of Gastroenterology, Hepatology, and Nutrition, The Ohio State University Wexner Medical Center, 410 West Tenth Avenue, Columbus, OH 43210, USA
e-mail: philip.hart@osumc.edu

H. Hampel, M.S., C.G.C.
Division of Human Genetics, The Ohio State University Wexner Medical Center, Columbus, OH, USA

T. Bekaii-Saab, B. El-Rayes (eds.), *Current and Emerging Therapies in Pancreatic Cancer*, DOI 10.1007/978-3-319-58256-6_4

which remains <10%. The majority of patients are diagnosed at a late stage of disease, which is unfortunate as the 5-year survival rate for patients diagnosed with an earlier stage of disease that permits surgical resection is much higher at approximately 25%. Thus, early detection of PDAC has the potential to improve outcomes by allowing more patients to receive potentially curative therapies that already exist. Considering the relatively low prevalence of PDAC, it is not currently feasible to screen the general population, so testing is concentrated on those at increased risk. This is most accurately referred to as "surveillance" indicating that testing is performed in patients at increased risk for the disease of interest; however, in this chapter we use the phrase "screening" to be consistent with previously published literature. This chapter further reviews the rationale for PDAC screening, including clinical challenges and current approaches.

Rationale for PDAC Screening

PDAC is one of the most aggressive solid tumors due to a combination of delayed cancer stage at the time of diagnosis, aggressive tumor biology, and ineffective therapies. At the time of cancer diagnosis, >50% have metastatic disease, with <10% having localized disease [1]. There are multiple explanations for the delayed stage at cancer diagnosis, including the nonspecific nature of symptoms, including abdominal pain, back pain, and weight loss. Furthermore, these symptoms typically do not begin until later in the disease progression, which is particularly true for localizing symptoms such as jaundice. In the absence of an accurate disease biomarker, early detection using current strategies requires the use of cross-sectional imaging (using CT or MRI) and/or endoscopic ultrasonography (EUS). Thus, early detection of PDAC requires testing asymptomatic patients with imaging and/or EUS.

True screening of asymptomatic patients in the general population for PDAC is challenging due to the low disease prevalence. The following scenario illustrates the futility of general population screening using a single hypothetical screening test with excellent diagnostic accuracy:

> Based on the 2010 census there were slightly over 40 million adults in the US who were 65 or older. Assuming that all 53,000 of the estimated new PDAC cases in 2016 occurred within this population demographic a hypothetical screening test that was 98% sensitive and 98% specific would detect 51,940 cancers. However, in the process this would also produce 798,940 false positive screening results with a meager positive predictive value of 6.1%. In addition to the potential for test-related anxiety, each false positive result would generate unnecessary, and costly, cross-sectional imaging and/or invasive endoscopic assessment of the pancreas.

Based on this example, it is clear that even a cheap, noninvasive test satisfying this hypothetical test's diagnostic accuracy would lead to an unacceptable number of false-positive results requiring unnecessary additional testing and, therefore, would not be effective. Thus, it is necessary to further enrich the "screening population" with patients who are more likely to develop PDAC [3]. The various nongenetic risk factors for developing PDAC, including obesity, diabetes mellitus (DM), cigarette smoking, and chronic pancreatitis, are discussed in detail in Chap. 1. It is notable, however, that the majority of identified risk factors only confer a moderately increased risk (RR ~1.5–2.5) [4]. Although it is important to consider the influence of these factors when considering the disease pathogenesis, the relatively small increased risk remains inadequate to accomplish successful early detection. Most experts agree that screening should be considered in those with a risk factor associated with a relative risk ≥5 or with a combination of factors resulting in a cumulative lifetime risk for PDAC of ≥5% [5]. The risks associated with new-onset DM after age 50 and/or family history of PDAC fulfill these thresholds for which PDAC screening may be effective.

Risk of PDAC Associated with New-Onset DM

Diabetes is a complex risk factor for PDAC with a bidirectional association and different magnitude of risk based on the DM duration [6]. Additionally, emerging data suggest that different antidiabetic therapies can increase or decrease PDAC risk. The prevalence of DM in those diagnosed with PDAC is high and exceeds that observed in other common cancers [7]. Interestingly, the DM often develops within 36 months of PDAC diagnosis and precedes the onset of cancer-related symptoms by >12 months [8, 9]. The risk for PDAC in those with long-standing DM is only modest (RR 1.5) in comparison to the risk associated with new-onset DM (RR 5.4) [9]. There is accumulating evidence suggesting that new-onset DM may represent a paraneoplastic syndrome for many patients with PDAC, which has been reviewed elsewhere [9].

The magnitude of increased risk for new-onset DM suggests this may be useful to include as a criterion for PDAC screening. A population-based cohort study demonstrated that indeed the risk for PDAC is increased in those with new-onset DM (observed: expected ratio of 7.94) [10]. However, in this study of the 2122 subjects with new-onset diabetes, only 0.85% had underlying PDAC. Even though new-onset DM may be incorporated into a PDAC screening algorithm, additional filters are needed to minimize false positives and improve the cost-effectiveness. Recent small studies have demonstrated that weight loss at the time of DM onset and a blunted pancreatic polypeptide response to mixed meal can help discriminate between new-onset DM secondary to PDAC and presumed type 2 DM [11, 12]. At least one clinical trial to validate these findings is currently enrolling subjects (NCT02001337). In the interim, it is recommended that new-onset DM in a high-risk individual should lead to initiation of screening [5].

Risk of PDAC Associated with Family History of PDAC

In addition to these modifiable risk factors, family history is important to consider regarding the risk for PDAC. It is estimated that 5–10% of patients with PDAC have a positive family history of PDAC in either a first- or second-degree relative [4]. The relative risk for development of PDAC varies depending on the number of affected relatives, the relatedness of relatives (i.e., first vs. second degree), and/or the presence of germline mutations associated with a hereditary cancer syndrome. The lifetime cumulative risk for PDAC in the general population is approximately 1.5%, and relative risk for PDAC is approximately 4.6, 6.4, and 32.0 based on the presence of one, two, or three affected first-degree relatives, respectively (when studied in those with a familial pancreatic cancer kindred) [13]. The familial pancreatic cancer (FPC) syndrome has been defined as a family with ≥2 first-degree relatives with PDAC who do not meet criteria for a known PDAC-associated hereditary syndrome [5]. The onset of PDAC at an age < 50 within an FPC kindred appears to further increase the risk for PDAC, an effect that was not observed in families not fulfilling FPC criteria (i.e., sporadic PDAC kindreds) [14].

Risk of PDAC Associated with Germline Mutations

In addition to the number of affected relatives, it is important to consider whether or not an identifiable hereditary cancer syndrome is present. In recent large studies, the frequency of germline mutations for all patients with PDAC (irrespective of family history) is approximately 3–5% [15, 16]. In these studies, the most commonly identified mutations were in the *BRCA2* and *ATM* genes. Other less common genes which have also implicated in the genetic predisposition for PDAC include *BRCA1*, *PALB2*, *STK11*, *APC*, *TP53*, and *CDK2NA* (which encodes the *p16* gene). Further discussion of these genetic defects is provided in Chap. 1 and elsewhere [17]. The *PRSS1* gene mutation does not cause a hereditary cancer syndrome, but is associated with hereditary pancreatitis and a dramatically elevated risk for PDAC.

There are few data and no current universal consensus to guide which patients should be screened for a potential germline mutation. For example, the updated NCCN guidelines (2016) for PDAC recommend considering a referral for genetic counseling "for PDAC patients who are young or who have a family history of cancer," but no further guidance is provided. Based on the increased probability of having abnormal genetic testing, we recommend genetic counseling and consideration of testing in selected scenarios, as well as in all affected individuals with an Ashkenazi Jewish ancestry (Box 4.1) [18]. When testing is performed, we recommend a genetic testing panel including analysis for hereditary breast-ovarian cancer syndromes (*BRCA1/2* and *PALB2*), familial atypical mole melanoma syndrome (*CDKN2A*), and ataxia-telangiectasia mutation (*ATM*) carriers as well as testing for Peutz-Jeghers syndrome (*STK11*), Lynch syndrome (*MLH1*, *MSH2*, *MSH6*, *PMS2*, and *EPCAM*), and hereditary (*PRSS1*) pancreatitis if there is suggestive personal or family history present [17]. The risk for PDAC associated with familial adenomatosis polyposis syndrome and Li-Fraumeni syndrome is believed to be increased but has not been well characterized, and these conditions can be readily identified clinically.

Box 4.1 Referral for genetics evaluation should be considered in the following patient scenarios:

- PDAC patient with ≥1 affected relatives (any relationship)
- PDAC patient with a personal or family history of extrapancreatic cancer associated with a hereditary PDAC syndrome (e.g., breast, ovarian, colon, or melanoma)
- PDAC patient with cancer diagnosis ≤40 years old
- Unaffected patient with ≥2 affected relatives (at least one first-degree relative)

There are several important considerations that will likely further expand the indications for genetic screening. In addition to the practical considerations of decreased testing costs and increased accessibility, the genetic contribution within the seemingly "sporadic" cases of PDAC is increasingly recognized, as illustrated above. Importantly, the genetic profile of a patient affected with PDAC may influence treatment decisions. The primary example is the use of poly(ADP-ribose) polymerase (PARP) inhibitors or platinum-based chemotherapy for patients with BRCA1/2 or PALB2 mutations [19]. Similarly, patients with Lynch syndrome may potentially be candidates for novel immune therapy [20]. The potential to develop more personalized treatment approaches and increased accessibility suggests that in the future universal screening may become a reality in clinical practice.

Indications for PDAC Screening

The rationale for PDAC screening (i.e., "surveillance") is primarily based on the estimated increased risk for PDAC rather than demonstration of survival benefit from screening. Accordingly it is recommended that PDAC screening in those at increased risk should be performed in experienced centers under research conditions. Different combinations of risk factors may be present depending on the presence of modifiable risk factors, family history, and any potential genetic mutations. Since nonfamilial/genetic risk factors only confer a weak to moderate risk for PDAC, they do not currently play a major role in the decision to initiate a PDAC screening program but likely modify the risk. Current risk prediction models are available to assess the risk based on family history but do not incorporate the patient's lifestyle risk factors or genetic profile [21].

The appropriateness of potential combinations of germline mutations and family history has been thoughtfully reviewed by the International Cancer of the Pancreas Screening (CAPS) Consortium [5]. This ongoing consortium consists of a multidisciplinary team seeking to further improve our approach to PDAC screening. The Table 4.1 summarizes the degree of agreement to offer screening for different combinations of genetic profiles and family history. In large part, the consensus recommendations reflect the cumulative lifetime risk for PDAC due to these risk factors. In summary, screening should be considered for those fulfilling one of the criteria shown in Box 4.2 [17].

Table 4.1 Recommendation for pancreatic cancer screening based on the combination of family history and genetic profile

# Affected relatives	0	1		2		≥3	
# Affected FDRs	0	1	0	≥1	0	≥1	0
No germline mutation	No	No	No	Yes	No	Yes	–
BRCA1	–	Indeterminate	–	Yes	Indeterminate	Yes	–
BRCA2	Indeterminate	Yes	–	Yes	Yes	Yes	Yes[a]
PALB2	No	Yes	–	Yes	–	Yes	–
STK11	Yes	Yes	Yes	Yes	Yes	Yes	Yes
CDK2NA	Indeterminate	Yes	Indeterminate	Yes	Indeterminate	Yes	Indeterminate
Lynch syndrome[b]	No	Yes	No	Yes	Indeterminate	Yes	Indeterminate

The color coding reflects the proportion of international experts (among 49 voting participants) in the CAPS Consortium who agreed with screening for the respective combination of family history and genetic mutations (*green* ≥75%; *yellow* 50–74%; *red* <50%) [5]. Blank boxes indicate no vote was reported for the combination. FDR, first-degree relative

[a]Although no formal vote was reported for patients with a BRCA2 mutation and three or more affected distant relatives, it can be assumed screening is recommended based on the high level of agreement for those with the same mutation and fewer affected relatives

[b]Associated with *MLH1*, *MSH2*, *MSH6*, *PMS2*, or *EPCAM* gene mutations

Box 4.2 Pancreatic cancer screening should be considered for those fulfilling any of the following criteria:

1. Mutation carrier of a hereditary PDAC syndrome with substantial increased risk, irrespective of family history (Peutz-Jeghers syndrome (*STK11*), hereditary (*PRSS1*) pancreatitis, and familial atypical mole melanoma syndrome (*CDKN2A*))
2. Mutation carrier of a hereditary PDAC syndrome with some increased risk and at least one affected first- or second-degree relative (breast and ovarian cancer syndromes (*BRCA1*, *BRCA2*, *PALB2*), *ATM*, and Lynch syndrome)
3. All members of an FPC kindred with a first-degree relationship to a relative with PDAC

Practical Clinical Considerations

There are multiple clinical factors to be considered in patients felt to be appropriate for PDAC screening, including the optimal screening protocol, the age to start screening, and the risks of screening. One of the challenges to overcome in screening for PDAC is there is a small window of opportunity for early detection. The ideal lesion to identify would be either a PanIN-3 lesion or T1 tumor. However, the PanIN-3 lesion by definition is radiographically occult using traditional imaging techniques. Therefore, the ideal lesion to detect in a PDAC screening program would be a T1 tumor that hasn't invaded into the local tissue. The ability to detect a small tumor requires advanced imaging techniques.

Screening Test Modalities

Current imaging modalities include CT, MRI, and EUS. Additionally, there is an emerging role of screening for diabetes mellitus as a means of facilitating early detection. Although a CA19-9 level may be helpful if it is elevated, the overall accuracy is low, and the only definitive preoperative means of establishing a diagnosis of PDAC is fine needle aspiration (FNA) of the pancreas.

In the sporadic PDAC literature, there is emerging support for the concept of DM developing as a paraneoplastic syndrome in the majority of patients preceding a PDAC diagnosis. Importantly, the onset of this DM is approximately 2–3 years prior to diagnosis at a point when no radiographic abnormalities can be identified [22]. The mechanism of this DM is unclear, but there are initial data suggesting this is likely the consequence of beta cell dysfunction induced by the primary tumor [23]. Although this relationship has not been examined in patients with familial PDAC, the ease and low cost of diabetes screening make this an easy intervention to implement. The frequency of DM screening hasn't been defined, but annual fasting blood glucose and hemoglobin A1c currently seem reasonable.

Of the cross-sectional imaging modalities, MRI with contrast and MRCP (MRI/MRCP) is the preferred modality among experts [5]. MRI/MRCP is preferred over CT for PDAC screening due to improved sensitivity for detection of small pancreatic tumors and improved sensitivity for abnormal changes in the pancreatic duct, which occur prior to the onset of PDAC [24, 25]. An additional benefit of MRI/MRCP is the avoidance of radiation for those undergoing serial imaging studies. There are a small number of situations in which MRI/MRCP is contraindicated, including previous placement of a cardiac device, body habitus that doesn't permit access to the scanner, and claustrophobia that cannot be palliated with routine measures. It is unclear whether CT imaging is a sufficient replacement in these instances but could be considered on an individual basis.

EUS affords the greater sensitivity for detection of small tumors compared to CT and MRI/MRCP and is therefore the preferred diagnostic modality to screen for PDAC. Unfortunately, the high resolution must be balanced with the need for sedation, cost, and invasiveness of the test. Advantages over MRI/MRCP include the ability to detect smaller tumors and to obtain tissue from any areas of radiographic concern (e.g., pancreatic duct cutoff) [26]. However, there are currently no studies demonstrating superiority of EUS over MRI/MRCP for PDAC screening, and most experts consider the tests complimentary for this clinical scenario.

Age to Start Screening

There is no consensus regarding the age to begin screening, but age 50 years or 10 years prior to the age of onset for any affected first-degree relatives is often considered (Box 4.3) [5, 17]. This recommendation is primarily based on the epidemiology of PDAC in which the incidence in those younger than 40 years of age is exceedingly low. Additionally, multiple studies have demonstrated an increased likelihood of detecting abnormalities in a PDAC screening program for older compared to younger subjects [27, 28]. One exception to this recommendation is in those with Peutz-Jeghers syndrome, in which it is recommended to start screening at age 35 years due to the markedly increased risk. At the time of the initial clinical evaluation of patients with possible increased risk for PDAC, it is reasonable to obtain baseline cross-sectional imaging (i.e., MRI/MRCP) to assess for the possibility of clinically silent chronic pancreatitis or pancreatic cysts in an effort to provide a comprehensive risk assessment.

Box 4.3 PDAC screening recommendations
Beginning at age 50 or 10 years earlier than the youngest diagnosis in the family:

1. Annual fasting glucose and hemoglobin A1c testing
2. Annual MRI/MRCP*
3. Annual EUS*

*Consider alternating the MRI/MRCP and EUS every 6 months.

Frequency of Screening

The most commonly recommended frequency of screening test(s) is every 12 months [5]. This recommendation is heavily influenced by the desire to avoid excessive health-care utilization. However, based on the observation that patients with PDAC may not have any visible abnormalities within 6 months of cancer diagnosis, a 12-month duration may be too long in some cases. Thus, an alternate strategy for those undergoing annual testing with both MRI/MRCP and EUS is to stagger the tests and perform one or the other every 6 months to minimize the interval between each test.

In summary, those undergoing screening for PDAC should likely receive annual MRI/MRCP and/or EUS. The addition of annual screening for diabetes mellitus and staggering the screening test interval to every 6 months may further improve the detection of early PDAC, but requires further investigation to confirm.

Patient Counseling and Genetic Counseling

Prior to undergoing testing, patients should undergo a genetics evaluation to obtain a detailed family history and obtain pretest estimation of the likelihood of harboring a germline mutation in a genetic syndrome associated with PDAC. Similarly, potential implications for the patient, patient's spouse, and family of potential test results should be discussed prior to testing. The results of genetic testing of a proband with PDAC are primarily for the purposes of family counseling. There is, however, the emerging possibility that genetic test results may guide treatment options. A current example of this is the use of poly(ADP-ribose) polymerase (PARP) inhibitors for those with BRCA-mutated PDAC [19]. Additionally, assessment for somatic mutations is being increasingly performed for guidance of refractory chemotherapy regimens but is beyond the scope of this article.

Although it is always preferable to perform genetic testing in an affected proband with PDAC, there are several circumstances in which this is not possible. Possibilities include the proband's unwillingness to undergo testing, family estrangement, or the patient's death prior to undergoing testing. In these situations, the closest family member to the proband, preferably a first-degree relative, is the optimal person to undergo testing. Many patients seek to undergo testing to gain a better understanding of their (or their family member's) cancer risks. For those who do undergo testing, the results may or may not be informative to guide the decision regarding whether or not to screen for PDAC or other extrapancreatic malignancies (when the mutation is part of a hereditary cancer syndrome). Unaffected individuals, who test negative for a pancreatic cancer susceptibility gene mutation, may still be at increased risk for pancreatic cancer since it is not known that their affected relative had a mutation in the first place. This is called an "uninformative negative," and PDAC screening may still be justified for these individuals. However, if another unaffected individual in the same family is subsequently found to have a mutation in one of the genes known to cause pancreatic cancer, then the original unaffected individual who tested negative has a "true negative" result and would not need to continue PDAC screening.

Risks/Benefits of PDAC Screening

Prior to enrolling a patient in a PDAC screening program, it is important they are provided with a detailed explanation of the potential benefits and risks. Specifically, it should be highlighted that there is a higher likelihood of detecting a false-positive result than a true positive result considering the low incidence of PDAC. A false-positive test has been variably defined in previous studies, but practically this can be defined as any abnormality of the pancreas that cannot be explained as a normal variant or necessitates additional testing (including FNA). There is a high prevalence of pancreatic cysts (which generally represent branch-duct intraductal papillary mucinous neoplasms (IPMNs)) of approximately 2–30% of the general population [29–31]. In a multicenter study of high-risk individuals for PDAC, 42% (92/216) were found to have at least one pancreatic lesion, which was typically a small cyst [27]. Thus, patients should be mentally prepared for a diagnosis of a pancreatic lesion (cystic or solid) prior to embarking on initial testing.

In addition to the risk of false-positive screening results, many patients may experience test-related anxiety. Efforts should be made to minimize any delays in communication of test results in this setting. It is reassuring that a recent study demonstrated the overall psychologic burden of participating in a screening program is relatively low [32]. Otherwise, the direct risks from the screening tests are fairly low. The risks of MRI/MRCP are negligible and are limited to patient discomfort during the test and contrast exposure. Although EUS is an invasive test, the risks of EUS without FNA are minimal and essentially limited to the risk of sedation. For those with an abnormality requiring FNA, the overall risks are slightly increased, but remain low, including bleeding, post-FNA pancreatitis, and infection [33].

Summary

The outcomes of PDAC remain poor for multiple reasons, including diagnosis at a late stage of disease. For patients with a substantially increased risk of developing PDAC, periodic screening with a combination of MRI/MRCP and/or EUS may allow for earlier detection. The effectiveness of PDAC screening remains unproven and is a continued area of research. Similarly, multiple questions remain regarding the optimal age to start screening, frequency of screening, and whether screening should be offered for those with genetic mutations but without a family history of PDAC. Ongoing multinational studies are underway and will hopefully inform these knowledge gaps.

Conflicts of Interest/Disclosures No conflicts of interest exist.

References

1. Siegel RL, Miller KD, Jemal A. Cancer statistics, 2016. CA Cancer J Clin. 2016;66:7–30.
2. Rahib L, Smith BD, Aizenberg R, et al. Projecting cancer incidence and deaths to 2030: the unexpected burden of thyroid, liver, and pancreas cancers in the United States. Cancer Res. 2014;74:2913–21.

3. Pannala R, Basu A, Petersen GM, et al. New-onset diabetes: a potential clue to the early diagnosis of pancreatic cancer. Lancet Oncol. 2009;10:88–95.
4. Ryan DP, Hong TS, Bardeesy N. Pancreatic adenocarcinoma. N Engl J Med. 2014;371:1039–49.
5. Canto MI, Harinck F, Hruban RH, et al. International cancer of the pancreas screening (CAPS) consortium summit on the management of patients with increased risk for familial pancreatic cancer. Gut. 2013;62:339–47.
6. Hart PA, Chari ST. Diabetes mellitus and pancreatic cancer: why the association matters? Pancreas. 2013;42:1207–9.
7. Aggarwal G, Kamada P, Chari ST. Prevalence of diabetes mellitus in pancreatic cancer compared to common cancers. Pancreas. 2013;42:198–201.
8. Chari ST, Leibson CL, Rabe KG, et al. Pancreatic cancer-associated diabetes mellitus: prevalence and temporal association with diagnosis of cancer. Gastroenterology. 2008;134:95–101.
9. Sah RP, Nagpal SJ, Mukhopadhyay D, et al. New insights into pancreatic cancer-induced paraneoplastic diabetes. Nat Rev Gastroenterol Hepatol. 2013;10:423–33.
10. Chari ST, Leibson CL, Rabe KG, et al. Probability of pancreatic cancer following diabetes: a population-based study. Gastroenterology. 2005;129:504–11.
11. Hart PA, Baichoo E, Bi Y, et al. Pancreatic polypeptide response to a mixed meal is blunted in pancreatic head cancer associated with diabetes mellitus. Pancreatology. 2015;15:162–6.
12. Hart PA, Kamada P, Rabe KG, et al. Weight loss precedes cancer-specific symptoms in pancreatic cancer-associated diabetes mellitus. Pancreas. 2011;40:768–72.
13. Klein AP, Brune KA, Petersen GM, et al. Prospective risk of pancreatic cancer in familial pancreatic cancer kindreds. Cancer Res. 2004;64:2634–8.
14. Brune KA, Lau B, Palmisano E, et al. Importance of age of onset in pancreatic cancer kindreds. J Natl Cancer Inst. 2010;102:119–26.
15. Grant RC, Selander I, Connor AA, et al. Prevalence of germline mutations in cancer predisposition genes in patients with pancreatic cancer. Gastroenterology. 2015;148:556–64.
16. Zhen DB, Rabe KG, Gallinger S, et al. BRCA1, BRCA2, PALB2, and CDKN2A mutations in familial pancreatic cancer: a PACGENE study. Genet Med. 2015;17:569–77.
17. Syngal S, Brand RE, Church JM, et al. ACG clinical guideline: genetic testing and management of hereditary gastrointestinal cancer syndromes. Am J Gastroenterol. 2015;110:223–62. quiz 263
18. Hampel H, Bennett RL, Buchanan A, et al. A practice guideline from the American College of Medical Genetics and Genomics and the National Society of genetic counselors: referral indications for cancer predisposition assessment. Genet Med. 2015;17:70–87.
19. Bhalla A, Saif MW. PARP-inhibitors in BRCA-associated pancreatic cancer. JOP. 2014;15:340–3.
20. Le DT, Uram JN, Wang H, et al. PD-1 blockade in tumors with mismatch-repair deficiency. N Engl J Med. 2015;372:2509–20.
21. Wang W, Chen S, Brune KA, et al. PancPRO: risk assessment for individuals with a family history of pancreatic cancer. J Clin Oncol. 2007;25:1417–22.
22. Pelaez-Luna M, Takahashi N, Fletcher JG, et al. Resectability of presymptomatic pancreatic cancer and its relationship to onset of diabetes: a retrospective review of CT scans and fasting glucose values prior to diagnosis. Am J Gastroenterol. 2007;102:2157–63.
23. Hart PA, Bellin M, Andersen DK. Type 3c (pancreatogenic) diabetes mellitus secondary to chronic pancreatitis and pancreatic cancer. Lancet Gastroenterol Hepatol. 2016;1:226–37.
24. Gangi S, Fletcher JG, Nathan MA, et al. Time interval between abnormalities seen on CT and the clinical diagnosis of pancreatic cancer: retrospective review of CT scans obtained before diagnosis. AJR Am J Roentgenol. 2004;182:897–903.
25. DeWitt J, Devereaux B, Chriswell M, et al. Comparison of endoscopic ultrasonography and multidetector computed tomography for detecting and staging pancreatic cancer. Ann Intern Med. 2004;141:753–63.
26. Krishna S. Diagnostic performance of endoscopic ultrasound for detection of pancreatic malignancy following an indeterminate multidetector CT scan: a systemic review and meta-analysis. Surg Endosc. 2016; doi:10.1007/s00464-017-5516-y.

27. Canto MI, Hruban RH, Fishman EK, et al. Frequent detection of pancreatic lesions in asymptomatic high-risk individuals. Gastroenterology. 2012;142:796–804. quiz e14-5
28. Ludwig E, Olson SH, Bayuga S, et al. Feasibility and yield of screening in relatives from familial pancreatic cancer families. Am J Gastroenterol. 2011;106:946–54.
29. Lee KS, Sekhar A, Rofsky NM, et al. Prevalence of incidental pancreatic cysts in the adult population on MR imaging. Am J Gastroenterol. 2010;105:2079–84.
30. Laffan TA, Horton KM, Klein AP, et al. Prevalence of unsuspected pancreatic cysts on MDCT. AJR Am J Roentgenol. 2008;191:802–7.
31. Moris M, Bridges MD, Pooley RA, et al. Association between advances in high-resolution cross-section imaging technologies and increase in prevalence of pancreatic cysts from 2005 to 2014. Clin Gastroenterol Hepatol. 2016;14:585–593 e3.
32. Konings IC, Sidharta GN, Harinck F, et al. Repeated participation in pancreatic cancer surveillance by high-risk individuals imposes low psychological burden. Psychooncology. 2016;25:971–8.
33. Committee ASoP, Early DS, Acosta RD, et al. Adverse events associated with EUS and EUS with FNA. Gastrointest Endosc. 2013;77:839–43.

Chapter 5
Staging and Prognostic Implications

Amit Mahipal and Richard Kim

Introduction

Pancreatic ductal adenocarcinoma accounts for 90% of the tumors in the pancreas. Pancreatic adenocarcinoma is the fourth most common cause of cancer deaths in the United States with estimated 41,780 deaths and 53,070 new cases in 2016 [1]. The aggressive nature of this cancer is confirmed by the fact that the 5-year survival rate remains approximately 6%. The cornerstone of curative approach for patients with pancreatic cancer involved radical resection with negative microscopic margins (defined as R0 resection). Even among patients who undergo potentially curative resection, the 5-year survival is only 20%. With the improvements in modern surgical techniques and adjuvant chemotherapeutic regimens, the median survival in clinical trials has increased to 28 months. Notably, the perioperative morbidity and mortality has substantially decreased especially at high-volume centers making surgical resections feasible for higher proportion of patients. The selection of patients for surgical resection is of utmost importance as the benefit of surgery in patients with metastatic disease or R2 (macroscopic disease at surgical margins) is highly limited.

Staging on pancreatic cancer has prognostic and predictive implications. There are two types of staging system typically used: TNM staging by American Joint Committee on Cancer (AJCC) and clinical classification system based on imaging studies [2]. The accurate staging of pancreatic cancer is extremely important for treatment recommendations.

A. Mahipal, M.B.B.S., M.P.H.
Department of Oncology, Mayo Clinic, Rochester, MN, USA

R. Kim, M.D. (✉)
Department of Gastrointestinal Oncology, Moffitt Cancer Center,
12902 Magnolia Drive FOB-2, Tampa, FL 33612, USA
e-mail: richard.kim@moffitt.org

T. Bekaii-Saab, B. El-Rayes (eds.), *Current and Emerging Therapies in Pancreatic Cancer*, DOI 10.1007/978-3-319-58256-6_5

TNM Staging

TNM staging is detailed in Table 5.1 [2]. The "T stage" is dependent upon the tumor size and involvement of blood vessels, in particular, celiac axis or superior mesenteric artery. "N stage" and "M stage" are determined by involvement of regional lymph node or presence of distant metastases. This staging system requires assessment of regional lymph nodes that sometimes requires pathologic confirmation for accuracy, as radiologic imaging may not be able to clarify if the enlarged lymph nodes are reactive or malignant. Since only minority of patients with pancreatic cancer undergo resection, staging is primarily performed based on clinical imaging rather than on pathology.

The prognostic significance of TNM staging was validated using the National Cancer Database (NCDB) [3]. In this study of > 120,000 patients, approximately 15% of the

Table 5.1 TNM staging for pancreatic cancer

a. Classification of pancreatic cancer by TNM staging [2]					
T (primary tumor)		*N (regional lymph nodes)*		*M (distant metastases)*	
Tx	Primary tumor not assessable	Nx	Not assessable	M0	No metastases
T0	No evidence of primary tumor	N0	No lymph node metastasis	M1	Distant metastases
Tis	Carcinoma in situ	N1	Lymph node metastases		
T1	Tumor ≤ 2 cm, confined to the pancreas				
T2	Tumor > 2 cm, confined to the pancreas				
T3	Extension of tumor beyond the pancreas without involvement of the celiac axis or superior mesenteric artery				
T4	Tumor involves the celiac axis or superior mesenteric artery				

b. Stage grouping for pancreatic cancer			
Stage	*T (primary tumor)*	*N (regional lymph nodes)*	*M (distant metastases)*
0	Tis	N0	M0
IA	T1	N0	M0
IB	T2	N0	M0
IIA	T3	N 0	M0
IIB	T1–T3	N1	M0
III	T4	N0–N1	M0
IV	T0–T4	N0–N1	M1

patients underwent surgical resection. The median overall survival for all patients was 10 months for stage IA patients compared to only 2.5 months for stage IV pancreatic cancers. Among patients who underwent pancreatectomy, the median overall survival for patients with stages IA, IIA, III, and IV was 24.1, 15.4, 10.6, and 4.5 months, respectively. The median survival for respective stages among non-resected patients was 6.8, 6.2, 7.2, and 2.5 months. The differences in survival between patients who underwent surgery and patients who didn't undergo pancreatectomy reflect the benefits of surgery as well as the patient's baseline characteristics including performance status, comorbidities that would make patients for surgery, and access to medical centers with specialized surgical capabilities. This study included patients who were diagnosed prior to 2000 before the advent of modern chemotherapeutic regimens that have likely improved outcomes. This study suggests that the TNM stagingsystem is an effective prognostic tool for patients that are staged clinically and pathologically. There was one discrepancy found in this staging system, where patients with stage IIb disease had better survival than patients with stage IIb disease during the first 2 years of diagnosis among nonsurgical patients. This discrepancy may be due to the fact that CT scan or other staging modalities could be inconsistent in differentiating lymph node involvement.

Clinical Classification

The clinical classification system divides the patients into four distinct groups: resectable, borderline resectable, locally advanced, and metastatic. Approximately 20% of the patients present with resectable stage, 30% with borderline resectable or locally advanced, and 50% with metastatic stage [4]. This classification system is more geared toward different treatment modalities for various stages. However, this staging system has prognostic implications as well.

The definition of resectable, borderline resectable, and locally advanced disease is not uniform, and there are variations in definitions between the different medical societies (Table 5.2). Moreover, there is variation among surgeons as well as different medical centers. A patient considered unresectable at a center may be considered for curative resection at a high-volume center. This makes it difficult to group patients and compare outcomes and optimal treatment strategy. Involvement of blood vessels and ability to obtain R0 resection are the distinguishing factors for clinical staging.

National Comprehensive Care Network (NCCN) clinical classification criteria are as follows for the four groups:

(1) Resectable
   a. Arterial: No arterial tumor contact
   b. Venous: No tumor contact with superior mesenteric vein or portal vein or ≤ 180° without vein contour irregularity

Table 5.2 Resectability criteria for pancreatic cancer

Vessel	NCCN	Intergroup (Alliance)	AHPBA/ SSO/SSAT	MD Anderson
Celiac axis	No solid tumor contact for pancreatic head; ≤ 180° for body/tail	Tumor-vessel interface < 180°	No abutment	Abutment
Superior mesenteric artery	Solid tumor contact ≤ 180°	Tumor-vessel interface < 180°	Abutment	Abutment
Common hepatic artery	Solid tumor contact ≤ 180° allowing for safe reconstruction	Reconstructible involvement by tumor	Abutment or short-segment encasement	Abutment or short-segment encasement
Superior mesenteric vein or portal vein	Solid tumor contact ≤ 180° with contour irregularity or thrombosis or > 180° allowing for safe reconstruction	Tumor-vessel interface ≥ 180° and/or reconstructible occlusion	Occlusion	Occlusion

(2) Borderline resectable

a. Arterial:
   Pancreatic head/uncinate tumor
   i. Tumor contact with common hepatic artery without involvement of celiac axis
   ii. Tumor contact with the superior mesenteric artery ≤ 180°
   Pancreatic body/tail tumor
   i. Tumor contact with celiac axis ≤ 180°
   ii. Tumor contact with celiac axis > 180° without gastroduodenal artery or aorta involvement
b. Venous: Suitable vessel proximal and distal to site of involvement for safe resection and reconstruction
   i. Tumor contact with superior mesenteric vein or portal vein ≤ 180° with contour irregularity of the vein
   ii. Tumor contact with superior mesenteric vein or portal vein > 180°

(3) Locally advanced

a. Arterial:
   Pancreatic head/uncinate tumor
   i. Tumor contact with celiac axis or superior mesenteric artery > 180°
   ii. Tumor contact with the first jejunal branch of superior mesenteric artery
   Pancreatic body/tail tumor
      i. Tumor contact with superior mesenteric artery or celiac axis > 180°
      ii. Tumor contact with celiac axis and aorta

b. Venous:
   i. Unreconstructible superior mesenteric vein or portal vein
   ii. Tumor contact with proximal jejunal branch into superior mesenteric vein

(4) Metastatic
Presence of distant metastases

Vascular Involvement for Staging

The importance of arterial and venous involvement for staging of pancreatic cancer is due to the differential outcomes of surgical resection with vascular involvement and ability to perform vascular resection. Vascular resection had consistently demonstrated to increase the probability of R1 resection compared to pancreatic cancer resection without vascular involvement [5]. Patients with R0 resection have consistently demonstrated to have better survival than patients with margin-positive disease at the time of resection [6]. Cancer in uncinate process of the pancreas has higher chances of vascular involvement with tumor resulting in higher rates of venous resection [7, 8]. Patients with vascular involvement are classified into borderline resectable or locally advanced group. One of the issues in evaluating outcomes for patients with vascular involvement is that patients are frequently treated with neoadjuvant therapy consisting of chemotherapy and/or radiation therapy [9]. Only patients who have good performance status and who do not develop metastatic disease are subsequently taken for surgery leading to selection bias.

Venous Involvement

Involvement of the portal vein or superior mesenteric vein by tumor may require venous resection along with removal of primary tumor to achieve clear margins. Siriwardana et al. in 2006 published one of the largest systematic review involving 1646 patients from 52 studies who underwent portal vein and/or superior mesenteric vein along with pancreatic cancer surgery [10]. The median survival was only 13 months with 5-year survival rate of 7%. The median postoperative morbidity and mortality was 42% and 5.9%, respectively. This study suggested that concomitant venous resection leads to poor outcomes. However, multiple contradictory reports, primarily single-institution studies, have been published since then. Zhou et al. reported an updated meta-analysis in 2012 involving 19 nonrandomized studies comprising 2247 patients [11]. There were 661 patients that underwent portomesenteric venous resection. There were no significant differences in perioperative morbidity or overall survival between patients who underwent pancreatic resection with or without venous resections. The 5-year overall survival was 12.3% in patients with venous resection. In contrast to reports from single-institutional experiences, the data from inpatient hospital database (Nationwide Inpatient Sample) in the United States involving more than 10,000 patients demonstrated contradictory results [12]. Vascular resection in patients undergoing pancreatectomy was associated with increase in perioperative morbidity, but there were no significant differences in perioperative mortality. In this study, the hospital charges were used to evaluate the adverse outcomes and included patients with both arterial and venous resections. Moreover, the operative re-intervention was similar between the two groups.

One of the limiting factors of the above studies is the lack of data on the type of venous resection [13]. The various categories of venous reconstruction including venography, segmental resection with vein-to-vein anastomosis, and venous conduits may have different perioperative risks and thus lead to varied outcomes. Other issue is that decision regarding venous resection is frequently based on preoperative imaging. Even during surgical resection, it can be difficult to distinguish between peritumoral inflammation and venous invasion by cancer. Venous resection is frequently performed to achieve R0 resection if there is any doubt about microscopic venous invasion.

Thus, the results of multiple studies suggest that venous resection can be performed along with pancreatectomy safely at high-volume centers without adversely affecting the outcomes. There seems to be no increase in perioperative mortality, although the perioperative morbidity might be slightly higher. Although the results are inconsistent, it seems that pancreatic resection even with venous resection is associated with improved survival in patients with pancreatic cancer compared to patients who do not undergo surgery. Further, the 5-year survival of approximately 10–20% in the surgery group with venous resections suggests that a small proportion of patients are cured.

Arterial Involvement

The goal of arterial resection in patients undergoing pancreatic resection is to obtain negative retroperitoneal margins during pancreatic cancer surgery. Arterial resection is less common than venous resection with pancreatectomy. The outcomes for arterial resection with pancreatectomy are difficult to determine as it is frequently combined with venous resection. As with venous resections, majority of the data for arterial resections is derived from retrospective cohorts. Mollberg et al. reported a meta-analysis of 26 studies including 366 and 2243 patients who underwent pancreatectomy with and without arterial resection, respectively [14]. Significantly, increased risk for perioperative mortality was associated with arterial resection (odds ratio (OR), 5.05; 95% CI, 2.69–9.45%). The median perioperative morbidity and mortality with arterial resection was 53.6% and 11.8%, respectively. The 1-year

(OR, 0.49) and 3-year (OR, 0.39) survival was poorer as well with arterial resection. The probability of 5-year survival was zero. Even compared to venous resection with pancreatectomy, arterial resection was associated with increased perioperative mortality and lower 1-year survival. The authors concluded that arterial resection was associated with poor short-term and long-term survival, and arterial resection should be restricted to highly selected patients. In contrast, similar 1-year and 3-year survival with and without arterial resection was reported in a case-controlled study by Bachellier et al. [15]. The arterial wall invasion at the site of arterial resection was an independent prognostic marker. In this study, patients did not receive any neoadjuvant study. Frequently, patients with arterial involvement are treated with neoadjuvant therapy prior to surgery to increase the R0 resection as well as to prevent futile surgery in patients who would develop metastatic disease during preoperative treatment. The lack of standard neoadjuvant treatment can make it difficult to evaluate the outcomes of patients with arterial involvement who underwent pancreatic resection.

Thus, at this time in cases of arterial involvement, only highly selected patients should be considered for pancreatic resection, as the benefit of surgery is unclear.

Clinical Implication of Staging Systems

The two different staging systems, TNM and clinical classification, have prognostic implications as well, useful for treatment recommendations. In the TNM staging, patients with borderline resectable and locally advanced pancreatic cancer are clubbed together in stage III. Patients with stage I and II cancer will typically fall in resectable group, but there are few patients with borderline resectable pancreatic cancer who may be classified in stage II, especially with involvement of the superior mesenteric or portal vein. Thus, the clinical classification is more helpful to make therapeutic decisions.

The accurate staging and differentiation between resectable and unresectable pancreatic cancer are of utmost importance. Workup at diagnosis includes measurement of tumor markers, endoscopic ultrasound, computed tomography (CT), and magnetic resonance imaging (MRI). Many centers have developed multiphase dedicated pancreatic protocol CT scan for more accurate determination of blood vessel involvement with malignancy. In addition, laparotomy and/or positron-emission tomography (PET) scan may help detect metastases in additional patients initially considered to have early-stage disease and thus prevent futile pancreatic resection. The tumor marker, CA 19-9, is elevated in approximately 80% of the patients with pancreatic cancer and seems to correlate with staging. CA 19-9 levels can help provide additional information for resectability and response to therapy. As the imaging modalities continue to improve, the staging of pancreatic cancer would become more accurate letting clinicians and patients make better, informed decisions regarding therapy.

The role of diagnostic laparoscopy in initial staging of patients with potentially resectable pancreatic cancer continues to evolve. Some institutions selectively incorporate laparoscopy as a preoperative staging procedure, while other centers do not use it. In a meta-analysis of 16 studies involving 1146 patients, diagnostic laparoscopy in addition to CT scan decreased the probability of finding unresectable disease at surgical resection from 41% with CT scan alone to 20% with combined modality [16]. According to this study, diagnostic laparoscopy can potentially help identify the presence of metastatic disease and prevent unnecessary laparotomy in 21% of the patients. However, with the advent of modern imaging studies, including multiphase CT scan, MRI, and/or PET scan, the diagnostic yield of laparoscopy is probably lower. Larger studies involving current imaging techniques are needed to address the role of diagnostic laparoscopy in preoperative setting in patients with pancreatic cancer. Other option includes the use of diagnostic laparoscopy in selected resectable patients with high levels of tumor markers as they are otherwise considered to have high risk of metastatic disease.

The therapeutic strategy and goals of treatment for patients with various stages are different. For fit patients with resectable stage pancreatic cancer, upfront surgery is typically recommended. However, at some centers, neoadjuvant treatment is preferred even for this subgroup. The goal of resection in pancreatic cancer patients is to achieve R0 resection. Patients who undergo surgery but have macroscopic disease at margins likely do not derive any survival benefit [6]. The definition of R1 resection varies between different studies, which usually suggest the presence of microscopic disease at or near the surgical margins. Some studies have limited definition of R1 resection margins if tumor is present at the margins, while in other studies, the presence of microscopic tumor cells within 1 mm of surgical margins is considered R1 resection [17–19]. The Union for International Cancer Control (UICC) typically requires the absence of cancer cells within 1 mm of margins for R0 resection. In contrast, Chang et al. demonstrated that the presence of tumor cells within 1.5 mm of retroperitoneal margin was an independent predictor of survival [20]. In the retrospective series, patients who undergo R0 resection seem to have better overall survival with median overall survival in the range of 18–28 months compared to 14–21 months among patients with R1 resection [17, 21–24].

Patients with borderline resectable pancreatic cancer are suggested to receive neoadjuvant treatment typically consisting of chemotherapy and/or concurrent chemotherapy and radiation therapy followed by possible surgical resection [9]. Patients with metastatic disease usually undergo palliative systemic chemotherapy [25, 26]. Chemotherapy is recommended for patients with locally advanced pancreatic cancer. The role of radiation therapy in these patients is somewhat controversial [27]. In selected patients with a very good response to treatment, 10–20% of the patients with locally advanced disease are able to undergo potentially curative pancreatic resection. This is in contrast to patients with borderline resectable pancreatic cancer, where approximately half of the patients may be able to undergo surgical resection after neoadjuvant therapy. Although there is a lack of prospective trial data demonstrating the benefit of neoadjuvant therapy in patients with borderline resectable pancreatic cancer, there is some indication that R0 resection rates may be higher with preoperative therapy [9]. With the advent of more aggressive modern chemotherapeutic regimens including the combination of gemcitabine and nab-paclitaxel and combination of 5-fluorouracil, folinic acid, irinotecan, and oxaliplatin (FOLFIRINOX), it is quite possible that pancreatic resection rates for both borderline resectable and locally advanced pancreatic cancer may increase [28–30].

References

1. Siegel RL, Miller KD, Jemal A. Cancer statistics, 2016. CA Cancer J Clin. 2016;66(1):7–30.
2. Edge S, Byrd D, Compton C, Fritz A, Greene F, Trotti A. AJCC cancer staging handbook: from the AJCC cancer staging manual 7th edition. New York: Springer; 2009.
3. Bilimoria KY, Bentrem DJ, Ko CY, Ritchey J, Stewart AK, Winchester DP, et al. Validation of the 6th edition AJCC pancreatic cancer staging system: report from the National Cancer Database. Cancer. [Research Support, Non-US Gov't ValidationStudies]. 2007;110(4):738–44.
4. Stathis A, Moore MJ. Advanced pancreatic carcinoma: current treatment and future challenges. Nat Rev Clin Oncol. [Review]. 2010;7(3):163–72.
5. Katz MH, Crane CH, Varadhachary G. Management of borderline resectable pancreatic cancer. Semin Radiat Oncol. [Review]. 2014;24(2):105–12.
6. Liles JS, Katz MH. Pancreaticoduodenectomy with vascular resection for pancreatic head adenocarcinoma. Expert Rev Anticancer Ther. [Review]. 2014;14(8):919–29.
7. Ouaissi M, Hubert C, Verhelst R, Astarci P, Sempoux C, Jouret-Mourin A, et al. Vascular reconstruction during pancreatoduodenectomy for ductal adenocarcinoma of the pancreas improves resectability but does not achieve cure. World J Surg. [Comparative Study]. 2010;34(11):2648–61.
8. Padilla-Thornton AE, Willmann JK, Jeffrey RB. Adenocarcinoma of the uncinate process of the pancreas: MDCT patterns of local invasion and clinical features at presentation. Eur Radiol. [Comparative Study]. 2012;22(5):1067–74.
9. Mahipal A, Frakes J, Hoffe S, Kim R. Management of borderline resectable pancreatic cancer. World J Gastrointest Oncol. [Review]. 2015;7(10):241–9.
10. Siriwardana HP, Siriwardena AK. Systematic review of outcome of synchronous portal-superior mesenteric vein resection during pancreatectomy for cancer. Br J Surg. [Review]. 2006;93(6):662–73.
11. Zhou Y, Zhang Z, Liu Y, Li B, Xu D. Pancreatectomy combined with superior mesenteric vein-portal vein resection for pancreatic cancer: a meta-analysis. World J Surg. [Meta-Analysis]. 2012;36(4):884–91.
12. Worni M, Castleberry AW, Clary BM, Gloor B, Carvalho E, Jacobs DO, et al. Concomitant vascular reconstruction during pancreatectomy for malignant disease: a propensity score-adjusted, population-based trend analysis involving 10,206 patients. JAMA Surg. 2013;148(4):331–8.
13. Bockhorn M, Uzunoglu FG, Adham M, Imrie C, Milicevic M, Sandberg AA, et al. Borderline resectable pancreatic cancer: a consensus statement by the international study Group of Pancreatic Surgery (ISGPS). Surgery. [Consensus Development Conference Practice Guideline]. 2014;155(6):977–88.
14. Mollberg N, Rahbari NN, Koch M, Hartwig W, Hoeger Y, Buchler MW, et al. Arterial resection during pancreatectomy for pancreatic cancer: a systematic review and meta-analysis. Ann Surg. [Comparative Study Meta-Analysis Review]. 2011;254(6):882–93.
15. Bachellier P, Rosso E, Lucescu I, Oussoultzoglou E, Tracey J, Pessaux P, et al. Is the need for an arterial resection a contraindication to pancreatic resection for locally advanced pancreatic adenocarcinoma? A case-matched controlled study. J Surg Oncol. 2011;103(1):75–84.

16. Allen VB, Gurusamy KS, Takwoingi Y, Kalia A, Davidson BR. Diagnostic accuracy of laparoscopy following computed tomography (CT) scanning for assessing the resectability with curative intent in pancreatic and periampullary cancer. Cochrane Database Syst Rev. [Meta-Analysis Research Support, Non-US Gov't Review]. 2016;7:CD009323.
17. Raut CP, Tseng JF, Sun CC, Wang H, Wolff RA, Crane CH, et al. Impact of resection status on pattern of failure and survival after pancreaticoduodenectomy for pancreatic adenocarcinoma. Ann Surg. [Research Support, NIH, Extramural Research Support, Non-US Gov't]. 2007;246(1):52–60.
18. Verbeke CS, Leitch D, Menon KV, McMahon MJ, Guillou PJ, Anthoney A. Redefining the R1 resection in pancreatic cancer. Br J Surg. 2006;93(10):1232–7.
19. Esposito I, Kleeff J, Bergmann F, Reiser C, Herpel E, Friess H, et al. Most pancreatic cancer resections are R1 resections. Ann Surg Oncol. 2008;15(6):1651–60.
20. Chang DK, Johns AL, Merrett ND, Gill AJ, Colvin EK, Scarlett CJ, et al. Margin clearance and outcome in resected pancreatic cancer. J Clin Oncol. [Research Support, Non-US Gov't]. 2009;27(17):2855–62.
21. Fatima J, Schnelldorfer T, Barton J, Wood CM, Wiste HJ, Smyrk TC, et al. Pancreatoduodenectomy for ductal adenocarcinoma: implications of positive margin on survival. Arch Surg. 2010;145(2):167–72.
22. Hsu CC, Herman JM, Corsini MM, Winter JM, Callister MD, Haddock MG, et al. Adjuvant chemoradiation for pancreatic adenocarcinoma: the Johns Hopkins Hospital-Mayo Clinic collaborative study. Ann Surg Oncol. [Multicenter Study]. 2010;17(4):981–90.
23. Schnelldorfer T, Ware AL, Sarr MG, Smyrk TC, Zhang L, Qin R, et al. Long-term survival after pancreatoduodenectomy for pancreatic adenocarcinoma: is cure possible? Ann Surg. 2008;247(3):456–62.
24. Winter JM, Cameron JL, Campbell KA, Arnold MA, Chang DC, Coleman J, et al. 1423 pancreaticoduodenectomies for pancreatic cancer: a single-institution experience. J Gastrointest Surg. 2006;10(9):1199–210. discussion 210-1
25. Von Hoff DD, Ervin T, Arena FP, Chiorean EG, Infante J, Moore M, et al. Increased survival in pancreatic cancer with nab-paclitaxel plus gemcitabine. N Engl J Med. [Clinical Trial, Phase III Multicenter Study Randomized Controlled Trial Research Support, Non-US Gov't]. 2013;369(18):1691–703.
26. Conroy T, Desseigne F, Ychou M, Bouche O, Guimbaud R, Becouarn Y, et al. FOLFIRINOX versus gemcitabine for metastatic pancreatic cancer. N Engl J Med. [Clinical Trial, Phase II Clinical Trial, Phase III Comparative Study Multicenter Study Randomized Controlled Trial Research Support, Non-US Gov't]. 2011;364(19):1817–25.
27. Sajjad M, Batra S, Hoffe S, Kim R, Springett G, Mahipal A. Use of radiation therapy in locally advanced pancreatic cancer improves survival: a SEER database analysis. Am J Clin Oncol. 2016; doi:10.1097/COC.0000000000000261.
28. Blazer M, Wu C, Goldberg RM, Phillips G, Schmidt C, Muscarella P, et al. Neoadjuvant modified (m) FOLFIRINOX for locally advanced unresectable (LAPC) and borderline resectable (BRPC) adenocarcinoma of the pancreas. Ann Surg Oncol. 2015;22(4):1153–9.
29. Boone BA, Steve J, Krasinskas AM, Zureikat AH, Lembersky BC, Gibson MK, et al. Outcomes with FOLFIRINOX for borderline resectable and locally unresectable pancreatic cancer. J Surg Oncol. [Research Support, NIH, Extramural]. 2013;108(4):236–41.
30. Suker M, Beumer BR, Sadot E, Marthey L, Faris JE, Mellon EA, et al. FOLFIRINOX for locally advanced pancreatic cancer: a systematic review and patient-level meta-analysis. Lancet Oncol. 2016;17(6):801–10.

Chapter 6
Current and Emerging Therapies in Pancreatic Cancer

Maria Diab and Philip A. Philip

Introduction

The FDA-NIH Biomarker Working Group defines a biomarker as "a defined characteristic that is measured as an indicator of normal biological processes, pathogenic processes, or response to an exposure or intervention, including therapeutic interventions" [1]. Biomarkers can be diagnostic, predictive, or prognostic, although these connotations often overlap [1]. Among the features of an attractive biomarker are abundance, high sensitivity and specificity to the disease or aspect studied, feasibility of collection in a noninvasive or minimally invasive manner, and reasonable cost. In a disease with such poor prognosis as pancreatic cancer (PC), a screening tool for early detection remains to be identified. Furthermore, reliable biomarkers that guide the best course of treatment for individualized patients are still lacking, and monitoring response to therapy remains heavily dependent on imaging. Despite extensive efforts invested in identifying an effective biomarker, CA19-9 remains the only FDA-approved biomarker in clinical practice for the management of pancreatic cancer [2]. The aim of this chapter is to give an overview of biomarkers evaluated in pancreatic cancer, with a special focus on those utilized in treatment.

M. Diab
Wayne State University, Detroit, MI, USA

P.A. Philip, M.D. (✉)
Karmanos Cancer Institute, Wayne State University, Detroit, MI, USA
e-mail: philipp@karmanos.org

T. Bekaii-Saab, B. El-Rayes (eds.), *Current and Emerging Therapies in Pancreatic Cancer*, DOI 10.1007/978-3-319-58256-6_6

CA19-9

CA19-9 is one of the earliest and most validated markers in PC. It requires the presence of sialylated Lewis (Le)a blood group antigen to be expressed [3]. It was first described as a tumor-associated carbohydrate in colorectal cancer cells by Koprowski in 1979 [4, 5] and was subsequently described in other tissues, including the pancreas [3]. Using ELISA, serum CA19-9 level is frequently obtained as part of standard of care for patients with PC. It is typically elevated in patients with pancreatic cancer with the exception of Lewis negative blood type (Le a-b-) patients, as they are unable to synthesize the molecule [6]. CA19-9 may be elevated in nonmalignant pancreatic conditions, such as chronic pancreatitis [7], as well as in other malignancies [8]. It is also elevated in obstructive jaundice [9]. It might therefore be judicious to check the CA19-9 level after decompression of an obstructed bile duct for better accuracy in a jaundiced patient. CA19-9 levels can be prognostic in patients considered for resection; higher CA19-9 levels (>1000 U/mL) at diagnosis are associated with larger masses (>5 cm) [6], of which only approximately 5% are resectable. Other lower cutoffs of serum CA19-9 were reported for the prediction of operability and long-term survival [9–12]. Patients with resectable PC on imaging but with high serum concentrations of CA19-9 may be spared futile radical surgery or at a minimum started on preoperative systemic therapy in lieu of immediate surgery.

CA19-9 levels are monitored throughout the disease course and are expected to decrease and normalize with successful surgical resection. Patients whose levels decrease after surgical resection but do not return to normal may have shorter survival times compared to patients whose values drop to normal [6, 13–15]. The same held true for patients with unresectable disease, as those who had normalization of their CA19-9 levels post-neoadjuvant chemotherapy had longer overall survival [16]. CA19-9 can also aid in predicting response to chemotherapy. Patients with resectable disease who had postoperative CA19-9 values >90 U/mL did not benefit from adjuvant chemotherapy compared to those with postoperative CA19-9 values lower than or equal to 90 U/mL [17]. Interestingly, one study showed that early decreases of CA19-9 (defined as decreases occurring after two cycles of chemotherapy) do not convey a lengthened survival compared to patients who did not have a corresponding decrease [18]. Increasing levels of CA19-9 while on neoadjuvant therapy are usually associated with local progression and/or distal metastases [19]. Despite the extensive investigations on CA19-9, we still cannot solely rely upon it in the management of PC, be it in diagnosis, predicting resectability, or monitoring for recurrence or response to therapy, without also relying on imaging [20].

C-Reactive Protein

The C-reactive protein (CRP) is a member of the pentraxin family of proteins, which are secreted by the liver in response to a myriad of inflammatory cytokines [21]. Similar to immunoglobulins, CRP binds to Fc receptors, the interaction of which leads to the production of proinflammatory cytokines, namely, interleukin (IL- 6), which further feeds the generation of CRP [21, 22]. Serum levels of CRP might assist in discriminating patients with PC from those with benign pancreatic pathologies [23]. Elevated CRP levels in the serum of PC patients are associated with shorter survival rates [24, 25], irrespective of the effects of biliary tract obstruction on the levels of CRP [26]. In one study, Falconer showed that patients with unresectable disease who had a serum CRP level of >10 mg/L had median survival of 66 days compared to 222 days for patients with lower levels of CRP [27]. In another study, elevated preoperative CRP levels (≥4.5 mg/L) significantly correlated with higher tumor stage, unresectability of primary tumor, and poor performance status that was independent of age, gender, and administration of chemotherapy [28]. A low Karnofsky Performance Status, hypoalbuminemia, anemia, and large tumor burden were more frequent in patients with CRP levels of >2.0 mg/dL compared to those with a low CRP level (<0.5 mg/dL) [29]. An elevated CRP level was an independent prognostic factor for cancer-specific survival [28] and was associated with shorter times to progression [30].

Different prognostic scoring systems that take into account preoperative CRP levels can be utilized to estimate survival benefit from surgical approaches in the management of PC and may assist in selection of patients for surgery [31, 32]. One example is the Preoperative Prognostic Score (PPS) which takes into account preoperative platelet count, CRP levels, and CA19-9 levels in patients with locally advanced disease undergoing distal pancreatectomy with en bloc celiac axis resection [32]. The PPS scoring system showed a decreased 1- and 5-year survival rates with higher PPS scores [32]. Another scoring system, the modified Glasgow Prognostic Score (mGPS), takes into account preoperative albumin and CRP levels in patients undergoing expandable metal stent placement for unresectable malignant biliary obstruction [31]. Similar to the PPS, higher mGPS scores were associated with poorer postoperative survival [31]. Elevated CRP/albumin ratios (>0.03) were associated with poorer outcomes in PC patients undergoing pancreatic resection [33]. Lower preoperative CRP levels and neutrophil/lymphocyte ratios were independent prognostic factors in predicting postsurgical survival for patients with resectable PC undergoing pancreatic resection [34]. In patients with locally advanced disease receiving chemoradiotherapy, an elevated pretreatment CRP level (>3.0 mg/L) was associated with higher rates of treatment failure, distant metastases, and shorter survival [35]. Finally, CRP levels might have a role in early detection of inflammatory changes following surgery [24, 36].

KRAS

The *KRAS* oncogene is a GTPase protein belonging to the Ras family and is located on chromosome 12p; activating mutations are described in >90% of PC [37]. Those mutations are believed to be early events in the malignant transformation and may be associated with poor survival [38]. The mutated gene also plays a role in altered metabolism in the tumor niche, metastases, and drug resistance [39]. It is also involved in angiogenesis through CXC chemokines and vascular endothelial growth factor [40]. Through activating the downstream pathways RAF/MEK/ERK and PI3K/Akt/mTOR, the activated oncogene promotes cell proliferation and inhibits apoptosis [37].

KRAS mutations in pancreatic juice were suggested as a biomarker to differentiate pancreatic cancer from nonmalignant pancreatic diseases, an attractive aspect to screen patients who are at high risk of developing pancreatic cancer [41, 42]. In a study of 22 patients with pancreatic cancer, *KRAS* mutations were detected in 17 of 22 patients, compared with none detected in 24 and 29 with healthy pancreatic tissue and nonmalignant pancreatic disease, respectively [41]. Interestingly, *KRAS* mutations detected in the pancreatic juice can precede clinical evidence of pancreatic cancer [41]. In the treatment setting, tracking circulating mutated *KRAS* in the peripheral blood of patients receiving therapy might be used as a measure of response to therapy [43]. In patients with locally advanced disease receiving gefitinib, paclitaxel, and radiation therapy who had detectable plasma *KRAS* mutation pretreatment, undetectable plasma *KRAS* mutations posttreatment correlated with more favorable survival [43]. Nonetheless, the utility of *KRAS* evaluation in the management of pancreatic cancer warrants further investigation.

Unfortunately, despite its ubiquity, extensive attempts to target *KRAS* with drugs have not been successful [44, 45]. This has to do in part with the heterogenous mutations that affect *KRAS*, most of which occur at—but not restricted to—codon 12, and in part to the myriad of links *KRAS* has with up- and downstream pathways. This has directed the focus to targeting pathways downstream of *KRAS*, namely, RAF/MEK/ERK and PI3K/Akt/mTOR. Selumetinib and trametinib are two oral inhibitors of mitogen-activated protein kinase kinases 1 and 2 (MEK1/2). Administration of selumetinib in addition to capecitabine in the setting of advanced disease resulted in a longer overall survival (OS) compared to capecitabine alone (5.4 vs 5.0 months) [46]. This difference, however, was not statistically significant [46]. Combining trametinib to gemcitabine in chemonaïve patients with metastatic disease didn't yield any survival benefit [47].

Rigosertib is a first-in-class RAS mimetic and a small-molecule inhibitor of multiple signaling pathways including polo-like kinase 1 (PLK1) and phosphoinositide 3-kinase (PI3K). Combining rigosertib with gemcitabine in treatment-naïve patients with metastatic disease did not demonstrate a survival benefit [48]. The combination of trametinib with buparlisib, a pan-PI3K inhibitor, also failed to show a survival benefit [49], as did the combination of enzastaurin, an inhibitor of PI3K/AKT and PKCβ, with gemcitabine for locally advanced/metastatic disease [50]. Other ongoing trials include investigating RX-0201 (an Akt antisense oligonucleotide) in combination with GEM [51], as well as BEZ235 (an inhibitor of PI3K and mTOR) in combination with the MEK inhibitor MEK162 [52] and buparlisib (BMK120) in combination mFOLFOX-6 [53].

Attempts to target mTOR include utilizing everolimus and temsirolimus. Single-agent everolimus showed minimal to no efficacy in patients with gemcitabine-refractory metastatic disease [54, 55]. The combination everolimus/capecitabine was associated with a progression-free survival (PFS) and OS of

3.6 and 8.9 months, respectively [56]. Combining temsirolimus with erlotinib also showed unencouraging results [55].

The targeting of p21-activated kinases (PAKs) using glaucarubinone, in combination with gemcitabine, showed some promising results [57, 58]. Most recently, the advent of small interfering RNAs (siRNA) is becoming an attractive approach to target KRAS. A phase 1/2a trial combined siG12D-*LODER*™ with gemcitabine for patients with locally advanced disease; the recommended dose was further investigated with modified FOLFIRINOX [59]. The majority of patients had stable disease; 2 of 12 patients had a partial response. Median overall survival was 15.12 months, with an 18-month survival of 38.5% [59].

SMAD4

The *SMAD4* gene (previously known as DPC4) is a tumor suppressor gene located on chromosome 18q and is inactivated in approximately 50% of cases of pancreatic cancer [44]. SMAD4 serves as a central mediator of the canonical transforming growth factor (TGF)-β signaling pathway which regulates cell proliferation, differentiation, apoptosis, and migration [60].

Loss of *SMAD4* expression is an independent prognostic marker, associated with lymphovascular invasion, tumor progression, local and distant metastases, and shorter survival [61–63]. Some studies show that patients with an intact *SMAD4* more commonly have local disease progression, while those with *SMAD4* loss have more distant progression [64].

Negative preoperative *SMAD4* status in patients with locally advanced disease undergoing pancreaticoduodenectomy with en bloc resection correlated with earlier time to metastatic disease postsurgically and with six times higher likelihood of developing metastases [65]. Therefore, preoperative *SMAD4* status might assist in stratifying patients who might benefit from such an extensive surgical approach. Postsurgically, loss of *SMAD4* expression may be utilized as a positive predictive marker for benefit from adjuvant gemcitabine-based chemotherapy [66].

DNA Repair Defects and Microsatellite Instability

BRCA2 is a tumor suppressor gene located on chromosome 13q and regulates processes of DNA damage repair [67]. Germline mutations in *BRCA2* are implicated in hereditary breast and ovarian cancers and in approximately 5% of pancreatic cancers [67, 68]. Normally, inhibiting the poly (ADP-ribose) polymerase (PARP) family leads to the accumulation of double-strand DNA breaks that are subsequently repaired through *BRCA*-dependent homologous recombination [69]. This has led to the idea that tumors harboring mutated DNA repair proteins (including *BRCA1/2* mutations) might be more susceptible to agents that result in DNA cross-linking damage, such as platinum agents [70], and therapies that disable rescue DNA repair pathways, such as PARP inhibitors, which would collectively trigger the apoptosis cascade. DNA repair gene mutations, in that sense, could be used as predictive markers to stratify patients who might favorably respond to those therapies [71, 72]. For instance, patients with *BRCA*-mutated pancreatic cancer (one with resectable, one with locally advanced, and three with metastatic disease) who were treated with platinum-based chemotherapy achieved partial and complete responses and had longer PFS [73]. Furthermore, patients with *BRCA*-mutated, stage III/IV disease who were treated with platinum-based chemotherapy had longer OS compared to those who received nonplatinum therapy [74]. Similarly, olaparib, an oral PARP inhibitor investigated in breast and ovarian cancers [75–77], was associated with a response rate of 21.7% when administered as a single agent in patients with advanced, gemcitabine-refractory PDAC [78]. Trials investigating olaparib and veliparib, another PAPR inhibitor, in combination therapy to other treatments, such as gemcitabine, are being undertaken [79, 80].

Microsatellites, located most commonly in noncoding regions of the genome, are short, repetitive sequences of base pairs of DNA, and those repeats constitute single, double, or greater combinations of base pairs [81]. Replication errors occur due to strand slippage resulting in insertions or deletions within the microsatellite regions [81]. Those errors are typically detected by the DNA mismatch repair proteins [81]. Microsatellite instability (MSI) is related to defective DNA mismatch repair function and is a feature of familial and sporadic cancers of multiple sites [81]. Lynch syndrome is a familial form of DNA mismatch repair deficiency that manifests with a spectrum of MSI-positive tumors, including gastrointestinal (a subset of which are extracolonic) malignancies [82]. Major components of the DNA mismatch repair system include the MutS heterodimers (MSH2 combined with MSH3 or MSH6) and the MutL heterodimers (MLH1 combined with MLH3, PMS1, or PMS2) [83]. Mutations in MMR such as *MLH1* and *MSH2* are present in approximately 4% of pancreatic cancer [84]. Tumors are classified as MSI-high (MSI-H) or MSI-low (MSI-L) or microsatellite stable (MSS) based on the number of anomalies detected using the National Cancer Institute panel or immunohistochemistry. MSI-H status is associated with a poorly differentiated, medullary tumor phenotype, wild-type *KRAS*, and a better overall survival compared to patients with MSI-L or MSS tumors [84, 85], and can therefore be used as prognostic markers for OS [86].

MicroRNAs

MicroRNAs (miRs) are small (19–25 nucleotides) noncoding ribonucleic acids (RNAs) that interact with messenger RNA and serve as negative regulators of gene expression by binding to imperfect complementary regions in the 3′ untranslated region of the target messenger RNA, inhibiting their translation or leading to their degradation [87, 88]. MiRs regulate, and are in turn regulated by, many key pathways involved in cell differentiation, proliferation, and apoptosis that eventually control the expression of both oncogenes and tumor suppressor genes [89, 90]. They can be isolated from a number of sources, including the serum, stool, and pancreatic juice, and are abundant, making them very attractive potential biomarkers [91]. Differential expression of a number of miRs, including miR-200a/200b and miR-1290, helped distinguish normal, nonmalignant, and malignant pancreatic conditions [92–94]. Furthermore, certain miR profiles have been associated with chemoresistance. For instance, downregulation of the miR-200 family was observed in gemcitabine-resistant pancreatic cancer cells [95]. Overexpression of miR-365 induced gemcitabine resistance through directly targeting the adaptor protein Src homology 2 domain containing 1 (SHC1) and apoptosis-promoting protein BAX [96]. Additionally, pancreatic cancer stem cells, which are crucial for tumor self-renewal and chemoresistance, were found to differentially express miR-99a, miR-100, miR-125b, miR-192, and miR-429 [97]. Approaches to target miRs therapeutically included introducing a miR antagonist or use of a miR mimic agent [98]. In preclinical models, transfecting gemcitabine-resistant pancreatic cells with miR-205 and miR-7 reduced the expression of TUBB3 and Pak-1, respectively, and reduced the cancer stem cell population [99]. Similar results were achieved with administering complexed micelles of gemcitabine and the tumor suppressor miR-205 [100]. Finally, monitoring miRNA levels during therapy might have some utility in gauging treatment response as well as the development of resistance. Postsurgical levels of plasma miR-18a and 221 were reduced compared to presurgical levels [101, 102]; a resurgence of miRNA-18a level was associated with recurrence [102]. In preclinical models, mice with KRAS-mutated pancreatic tumors treated with gemcitabine had significantly lower serum levels of miR-155 compared to healthy mice (also treated with gemcitabine), suggesting miR-155 as a potential indicator of tumor-specific effects of the treatment [103].

Circulating Tumor DNA

Cell-free nucleic acids are DNA fragments of 70–100 base pairs detected physiologically in the serum of healthy hosts, also known as "liquid biopsy" [104]. They originate from apoptotic and necrotic cells, but the exact mechanism of their release to the bloodstream has yet to be elucidated [105]. In cancer patients, circulating tumor DNA (ctDNA), released from cancer cells, represents variable fractions of the cell-free DNA that can be distinguished from physiologic cell-free DNA by the presence of cancer-related mutations since ctDNA displays the same genetic alterations harbored by the tumor, e.g., *KRAS*-mutated tumors shed ctDNA harboring *KRAS* mutations [106]. Higher levels of ctDNA correlate with tumor burden [107], vascular encasement [108], and metastatic disease [109]. Higher levels at diagnosis correlated with worse PFS and OS [110]. Persistently detectable *KRAS*-mutated ctDNA following surgical resection was associated with higher rates of relapse, even before detection of relapse on standard imaging [111]. Undetectable circulating *KRAS* mutations following treatment with gefitinib and chemoradiotherapy were associated with improved OS [43]. Similarly, low levels of *KRAS* ctDNA during treatment with gemcitabine or FOLFIRINOX were associated with longer OS compared to higher levels of *KRAS* ctDNA in the setting of nonresectable disease [112]. However, more research is needed to further elucidate the role of ctDNA in response to therapy.

Circulating Tumor Cells

Similar to ctDNA, circulating tumor cells (CTC) are shed from solid tumors into circulation and are detected on liquid biopsies [110]. CTC positivity was correlated with poor tumor differentiation [113] and demonstrated an independent prognostic impact on OS [113]. In one report, median survival rates of CTC-positive (11 of 26 patients) and CTC-negative patients were 110.5 and 375.8 days, respectively [114]. In the setting of operable disease, CTC detection in the portal vein, during surgery, was marginally associated with the development of liver metastases later in the course [115]. Additionally, detection of CTCs harboring markers of tumor-initiating cells (such as CD133 and CD44) was associated with disease recurrence [116]. Profiling the mutational status of CTC and detecting any changes from that of the primary tumor might correlate with developing metastases and with treatment resistance [117]. Therefore, CTC may have a role in monitoring response to therapy [118]. In preclinical models, a reduction in CTC burden following treatment with a PI3K inhibitor correlated with tumor growth inhibition [118]. Furthermore, CTC profiling might have a role in predicting the optimal treatment regimen based on prespecified models derived from previous patient-derived grafts [119]. In a study by Yu et al., for instance, three patients received FOLFIRINOX; longer PFS was observed in one patient whose CTC profiling predicted sensitivity to FOLFIRINOX compared to the remaining two patients whose CTC profiling predicted intermediate and low sensitivity (7.3 month vs 2.1 and 1.7 months, respectively) [119]. However, large-scale clinical trials are greatly needed to confirm this.

SPARC

The intricate stroma of pancreatic cancer is one of the contributing factors to its chemoresistance. SPARC (secreted protein acidic and rich in cysteine) is a protein involved in cell matrix interactions, angiogenesis, and cell migration and has been reported to inhibit cancer growth [120]. Although it undergoes epigenetic silencing in pancreatic cancer, stromal fibroblasts adjacent to infiltrating pancreatic adenocarcinomas frequently express SPARC [120]. This increased expression of SPARC in peritumoral fibroblasts, but not in cancer cells, has been linked to poor prognosis [120, 121]. Similarly, SPARC expression in distal stroma was inversely correlated with OS [122]. SPARC displays high affinity to albumin, which has led to the idea that administering nab-paclitaxel in tumors with high expression of SPARC would result in depletion of the stroma and improved delivery of chemotherapy [123]. Furthermore, co-administration of gemcitabine and nab-paclitaxel reduced levels of the gemcitabine metabolizing enzyme cytidine deaminase, rendering cancer cells more sensitive to gemcitabine treatment [124]. Results from the MPACT trial, comparing the combination of gemcitabine/nab-paclitaxel to single-agent gemcitabine, showed a more preferable OS of 8.5 months in the combination arm compared to 6.7 months in the single-agent gemcitabine arm [125] in patients with metastatic disease. This could make SPARC a positive predictive marker for treatment with nab-paclitaxel-based therapies, although conflicting reports showed no association between SPARC levels and treatment efficacy in preclinical and clinical models [126, 127].

hENT

The human equilibrative nucleoside transporter (hENT) represents a major membrane route for the cellular uptake of gemcitabine, which is necessary owing to gemcitabine's hydrophilicity and, hence, slow diffusion through the lipid layer of the plasma membrane [128]. Low expression of hENT1 renders tumor cells resistant to gemcitabine due to poor intracellular accumulation of gemcitabine [129]. This observation was reproduced in preclinical studies that showed induced gemcitabine resistance in tumor cells with pharmacological inhibition of hENT1 [130]. Patients receiving palliative gemcitabine whose tumors expressed hENT1 had significantly longer survival compared to those with low or absent hENT1 expression (13 vs 4 months, respectively) [131]. Furthermore, reports from the ESPAC-3 trial reproduced the potential use for hENT1 as a predictive marker for the use of gemcitabine (median overall survival of 26.2 vs 17.1 months for patients with high and low hENT1 expression, respectively); however, hENT1 did not predict survival in 5-fluorouracil-treated patients [132]. This suggests that evaluation of hENT1 in the work-up of pancreatic cancer patients might be of benefit, and those with high hENT1 expression would preferentially receive gemcitabine-based therapy.

Conclusion

CA19-9 remains the only FDA-approved biomarker for the management of pancreatic cancer despite, however, not without downsides. For instance, CA19-9 cannot reliably differentiate pancreatic cancer from other pancreatic pathologies because its levels are affected by other pathological processes, such as inflammatory pancreatobiliary mechanisms. Other biomarkers have been identified that might be of potential utility in screening for as well as in the management of pancreatic cancer, including hENT1 and SPARC, both of which may have the capability of stratifying patients based on predicted benefit from specific chemotherapeutic agents. Other biomarkers, such as microRNAs, ctDNA, and CTCs, might play a role in monitoring response to therapy and assist in recognizing development of resistance. However, large-scale prospective trials are needed to further validate these roles.

References

1. Group, F.-N.B.W. BEST (Biomarkers, EndpointS, and other tools) resource [Internet]. Silver Spring (MD): Food and Drug Administration (US); 2016. https://www.ncbi.nlm.nih.gov/books/NBK326791/Co-published by National Institutes of Health (US), Bethesda (MD)
2. Winter JM, Yeo CJ, Brody JR. Diagnostic, prognostic, and predictive biomarkers in pancreatic cancer. J Surg Oncol. 2013;107(1):15–22.
3. Eskelinen M, Haglund U. Developments in serologic detection of human pancreatic adenocarcinoma. Scand J Gastroenterol. 1999;34(9):833–44.
4. Koprowski H, et al. Specific antigen in serum of patients with colon carcinoma. Science. 1981;212(4490):53–5.
5. Koprowski H, et al. Colorectal carcinoma antigens detected by hybridoma antibodies. Somatic Cell Genet. 1979;5(6):957–71.
6. Tian F, et al. Prognostic value of serum CA 19-9 levels in pancreatic adenocarcinoma. Ann Surg. 1992;215(4):350–5.
7. Steinberg W. The clinical utility of the CA 19-9 tumor-associated antigen. Am J Gastroenterol. 1990;85(4):350–5.
8. Duffy MJ. CA 19-9 as a marker for gastrointestinal cancers: a review. Ann Clin Biochem. 1998;35(Pt 3):364–70.
9. Ballehaninna UK, Chamberlain RS. The clinical utility of serum CA 19-9 in the diagnosis, prognosis and management of pancreatic adenocarcinoma: an evidence based appraisal. J Gastrointest Oncol. 2012;3(2):105–19.
10. Forsmark CE, Lambiase L, Vogel SB. Diagnosis of pancreatic cancer and prediction of unresectability using the tumor-associated antigen CA19-9. Pancreas. 1994;9(6):731–4.
11. Zhang S, et al. Clinical value of serum CA19-9 levels in evaluating resectability of pancreatic carcinoma. World J Gastroenterol. 2008;14(23):3750–3.
12. Hartwig W, et al. CA19-9 in potentially resectable pancreatic cancer: perspective to adjust surgical and perioperative therapy. Ann Surg Oncol. 2013;20(7):2188–96.
13. Berger AC, et al. Postresection CA 19-9 predicts overall survival in patients with pancreatic cancer treated with adjuvant chemoradiation: a prospective validation by RTOG 9704. J Clin Oncol. 2008;26(36):5918–22.
14. Glenn J, et al. Evaluation of the utility of a radioimmunoassay for serum CA 19-9 levels in patients before and after treatment of carcinoma of the pancreas. J Clin Oncol. 1988;6(3):462–8.
15. Montgomery RC, et al. Prediction of recurrence and survival by post-resection CA 19-9 values in patients with adenocarcinoma of the pancreas. Ann Surg Oncol. 1997;4(7):551–6.
16. Tzeng CW, et al. Serum carbohydrate antigen 19-9 represents a marker of response to neoadjuvant therapy in patients with borderline resectable pancreatic cancer. HPB (Oxford). 2014;16(5):430–8.
17. Humphris JL, et al. The prognostic and predictive value of serum CA19.9 in pancreatic cancer. Ann Oncol. 2012;23(7):1713–22.
18. Hess V, et al. CA 19-9 tumour-marker response to chemotherapy in patients with advanced pancreatic cancer enrolled in a randomised controlled trial. Lancet Oncol. 2008;9(2):132–8.

19. Willett CG, Daly WJ, Warshaw AL. CA 19-9 is an index of response to neoadjunctive chemoradiation therapy in pancreatic cancer. Am J Surg. 1996;172(4):350–2.
20. Locker GY, et al. ASCO 2006 update of recommendations for the use of tumor markers in gastrointestinal cancer. J Clin Oncol. 2006;24(33):5313–27.
21. Du Clos TW. Function of C-reactive protein. Ann Med. 2000;32(4):274–8.
22. Moses AG, et al. Pro-inflammatory cytokine release by peripheral blood mononuclear cells from patients with advanced pancreatic cancer: relationship to acute phase response and survival. Oncol Rep. 2009;21(4):1091–5.
23. Zhang P, et al. Development of serum parameters panels for the early detection of pancreatic cancer. Int J Cancer. 2014;134(11):2646–55.
24. Tingstedt B, et al. Predictive factors in pancreatic ductal adenocarcinoma: role of the inflammatory response. Scand J Gastroenterol. 2007;42(6):754–9.
25. Alkhateeb A, et al. Elevation in multiple serum inflammatory biomarkers predicts survival of pancreatic cancer patients with inoperable disease. J Gastrointest Cancer. 2014;45(2):161–7.
26. Pine JK, et al. Serum C-reactive protein concentration and the prognosis of ductal adenocarcinoma of the head of pancreas. Eur J Surg Oncol. 2009;35(6):605–10.
27. Falconer JS, et al. Acute-phase protein response and survival duration of patients with pancreatic cancer. Cancer. 1995;75(8):2077–82.
28. Szkandera J, et al. Validation of C-reactive protein levels as a prognostic indicator for survival in a large cohort of pancreatic cancer patients. Br J Cancer. 2014;110(1):183–8.
29. Mitsunaga S, et al. C-reactive protein level is an indicator of the aggressiveness of advanced pancreatic cancer. Pancreas. 2016;45(1):110–6.
30. Haas M, et al. Prognostic value of CA 19-9, CEA, CRP, LDH and bilirubin levels in locally advanced and metastatic pancreatic cancer: results from a multicenter, pooled analysis of patients receiving palliative chemotherapy. J Cancer Res Clin Oncol. 2013;139(4):681–9.
31. Iwasaki Y, et al. Usefulness of an inflammation-based prognostic score (mGPS) for predicting survival in patients with unresectable malignant biliary obstruction. World J Surg. 2013;37(9):2222–8.
32. Miura T, et al. A new preoperative prognostic scoring system to predict prognosis in patients with locally advanced pancreatic body cancer who undergo distal pancreatectomy with en bloc celiac axis resection: a retrospective cohort study. Surgery. 2014;155(3):457–67.
33. Haruki K, et al. The C-reactive protein to albumin ratio predicts long-term outcomes in patients with pancreatic cancer after pancreatic resection. World J Surg. 2016;40(9):2254–60.
34. Stevens L, et al. Prognostic significance of pre-operative C-reactive protein and the neutrophil-lymphocyte ratio in resectable pancreatic cancer: a systematic review. HPB (Oxford). 2015;17(4):285–91.
35. Kishi T, et al. Pretreatment C-reactive protein level predicts outcome and patterns of failure after chemoradiotherapy for locally advanced pancreatic cancer. Pancreatology. 2015;15(6):694–700.
36. Warschkow R, et al. Diagnostic study and meta-analysis of C-reactive protein as a predictor of postoperative inflammatory complications after pancreatic surgery. J Hepatobiliary Pancreat Sci. 2012;19(4):492–500.
37. Almoguera C, et al. Most human carcinomas of the exocrine pancreas contain mutant c-K-ras genes. Cell. 1988;53(4):549–54.
38. Rachakonda PS, et al. Somatic mutations in exocrine pancreatic tumors: association with patient survival. PLoS One. 2013;8(4):e60870.
39. Mann KM, et al. KRAS-related proteins in pancreatic cancer. Pharmacol Ther. 2016;168:29–42.
40. Matsuo Y, et al. K-Ras promotes angiogenesis mediated by immortalized human pancreatic epithelial cells through mitogen-activated protein kinase signaling pathways. Mol Cancer Res. 2009;7(6):799–808.
41. Berthelemy P, et al. Identification of K-ras mutations in pancreatic juice in the early diagnosis of pancreatic cancer. Ann Intern Med. 1995;123(3):188–91.

42. Boadas J, et al. Clinical usefulness of K-ras gene mutation detection and cytology in pancreatic juice in the diagnosis and screening of pancreatic cancer. Eur J Gastroenterol Hepatol. 2001;13(10):1153–9.
43. Olsen CC, et al. Results of a phase I trial of 12 patients with locally advanced pancreatic carcinoma combining gefitinib, paclitaxel, and 3-dimensional conformal radiation: report of toxicity and evaluation of circulating K-ras as a potential biomarker of response to therapy. Am J Clin Oncol. 2009;32(2):115–21.
44. Jones S, et al. Core signaling pathways in human pancreatic cancers revealed by global genomic analyses. Science. 2008;321(5897):1801–6.
45. Van Cutsem E, et al. Phase III trial of gemcitabine plus tipifarnib compared with gemcitabine plus placebo in advanced pancreatic cancer. J Clin Oncol. 2004;22(8):1430–8.
46. Bodoky G, et al. A phase II open-label randomized study to assess the efficacy and safety of selumetinib (AZD6244 [ARRY-142886]) versus capecitabine in patients with advanced or metastatic pancreatic cancer who have failed first-line gemcitabine therapy. Investig New Drugs. 2012;30(3):1216–23.
47. Infante JR, et al. A phase 1b study of trametinib, an oral mitogen-activated protein kinase kinase (MEK) inhibitor, in combination with gemcitabine in advanced solid tumours. Eur J Cancer. 2013;49(9):2077–85.
48. O'Neil BH, et al. A phase II/III randomized study to compare the efficacy and safety of rigosertib plus gemcitabine versus gemcitabine alone in patients with previously untreated metastatic pancreatic cancer. Ann Oncol. 2015;26(12):2505.
49. Bedard PL, et al. A phase Ib dose-escalation study of the oral pan-PI3K inhibitor buparlisib (BKM120) in combination with the oral MEK1/2 inhibitor trametinib (GSK1120212) in patients with selected advanced solid tumors. Clin Cancer Res. 2015;21(4):730–8.
50. Richards DA, et al. Gemcitabine plus enzastaurin or single-agent gemcitabine in locally advanced or metastatic pancreatic cancer: results of a phase II, randomized, noncomparative study. Investig New Drugs. 2011;29(1):144–53.
51. Rexahn Pharmaceuticals Inc. A safety and efficacy study of RX-0201 plus gemcitabine in metastatic pancreatic cancer. https://clinicaltrials.gov/ct2/show/NCT01028495.
52. Array BioPharma. safety, pharmacokinetics and pharmacodynamics of BEZ235 Plus MEK162 in selected advanced solid tumor patients. https://clinicaltrials.gov/ct2/show/NCT01337765.
53. UNC Lineberger Comprehensive Cancer Center. BKM120 + mFOLFOX6 in advanced solid tumors with expansion cohort pancreatic cancer. https://clinicaltrials.gov/ct2/show/NCT01571024.
54. Wolpin BM, et al. Oral mTOR inhibitor everolimus in patients with gemcitabine-refractory metastatic pancreatic cancer. J Clin Oncol. 2009;27(2):193–8.
55. Javle MM, et al. Inhibition of the mammalian target of rapamycin (mTOR) in advanced pancreatic cancer: results of two phase II studies. BMC Cancer. 2010;10:368.
56. Kordes S, et al. Phase II study of capecitabine and the oral mTOR inhibitor everolimus in patients with advanced pancreatic cancer. Cancer Chemother Pharmacol. 2015;75(6):1135–41.
57. Yeo D, et al. Glaucarubinone combined with gemcitabine improves pancreatic cancer survival in an Immunocompetent Orthotopic murine model. J Investig Surg. 2016;29(6):366–72.
58. Yeo D, et al. Glaucarubinone and gemcitabine synergistically reduce pancreatic cancer growth via down-regulation of P21-activated kinases. Cancer Lett. 2014;346(2):264–72.
59. Golan T, et al. RNAi therapy targeting KRAS in combination with chemotherapy for locally advanced pancreatic cancer patients. Oncotarget. 2015;6(27):24560–70.
60. Iacobuzio-Donahue CA, et al. DPC4 gene status of the primary carcinoma correlates with patterns of failure in patients with pancreatic cancer. J Clin Oncol. 2009;27(11):1806–13.
61. Yamada S, et al. SMAD4 expression predicts local spread and treatment failure in resected pancreatic cancer. Pancreas. 2015;44(4):660–4.
62. Oshima M, et al. Immunohistochemically detected expression of 3 major genes (CDKN2A/p16, TP53, and SMAD4/DPC4) strongly predicts survival in patients with resectable pancreatic cancer. Ann Surg. 2013;258(2):336–46.

63. Ottenhof NA, et al. Multivariate analysis of immunohistochemical evaluation of protein expression in pancreatic ductal adenocarcinoma reveals prognostic significance for persistent Smad4 expression only. Cell Oncol (Dordr). 2012;35(2):119–26.
64. Crane CH, et al. Phase II trial of cetuximab, gemcitabine, and oxaliplatin followed by chemoradiation with cetuximab for locally advanced (T4) pancreatic adenocarcinoma: correlation of Smad4(Dpc4) immunostaining with pattern of disease progression. J Clin Oncol. 2011;29(22):3037–43.
65. Boone BA, et al. Loss of SMAD4 staining in pre-operative cell blocks is associated with distant metastases following pancreaticoduodenectomy with venous resection for pancreatic cancer. J Surg Oncol. 2014;110(2):171–5.
66. Bachet JB, et al. Contribution of CXCR4 and SMAD4 in predicting disease progression pattern and benefit from adjuvant chemotherapy in resected pancreatic adenocarcinoma. Ann Oncol. 2012;23(9):2327–35.
67. Goggins M, et al. Germline BRCA2 gene mutations in patients with apparently sporadic pancreatic carcinomas. Cancer Res. 1996;56(23):5360–4.
68. Lal G, et al. Inherited predisposition to pancreatic adenocarcinoma: role of family history and germ-line p16, BRCA1, and BRCA2 mutations. Cancer Res. 2000;60(2):409–16.
69. Tentori L, Graziani G. Chemopotentiation by PARP inhibitors in cancer therapy. Pharmacol Res. 2005;52(1):25–33.
70. Waddell N, et al. Whole genomes redefine the mutational landscape of pancreatic cancer. Nature. 2015;518(7540):495–501.
71. Martinez-Useros J, Garcia-Foncillas J. The role of BRCA2 mutation status as diagnostic, predictive, and prognosis biomarker for pancreatic cancer. Biomed Res Int. 2016;2016:1869304.
72. Luo G, et al. Pancreatic cancer: BRCA mutation and personalized treatment. Expert Rev Anticancer Ther. 2015;15(10):1223–31.
73. Tran BZ, Zogopoulos G, Borgida A, Holter S, Gallinger S, Moore MJ. Platinum-based chemotherapy (pt-chemo) in pancreatic adenocarcinoma (pc) associated with brca mutations: a translational case series. J Clin Oncol. 2012;30. (suppl 4; abstr 217), 2012. Abstract available at: http://meetinglibrary.asco.org/content/87854-115
74. Golan T, et al. Overall survival and clinical characteristics of pancreatic cancer in BRCA mutation carriers. Br J Cancer. 2014;111(6):1132–8.
75. Audeh MW, et al. Oral poly(ADP-ribose) polymerase inhibitor olaparib in patients with BRCA1 or BRCA2 mutations and recurrent ovarian cancer: a proof-of-concept trial. Lancet. 2010;376(9737):245–51.
76. Tutt A, et al. Oral poly(ADP-ribose) polymerase inhibitor olaparib in patients with BRCA1 or BRCA2 mutations and advanced breast cancer: a proof-of-concept trial. Lancet. 2010;376(9737):235–44.
77. Fong PC, et al. Poly(ADP)-ribose polymerase inhibition: frequent durable responses in BRCA carrier ovarian cancer correlating with platinum-free interval. J Clin Oncol. 2010;28(15):2512–9.
78. Kaufman B, et al. Olaparib monotherapy in patients with advanced cancer and a germline BRCA1/2 mutation. J Clin Oncol. 2015;33(3):244–50.
79. NCI. Gemcitabine hydrochloride and cisplatin with or without veliparib or veliparib alone in treating patients with locally advanced or metastatic pancreatic cancer. Identifier NCT01585805. https://clinicaltrials.gov/ct2/show/NCT01585805.
80. AstraZeneca. Study to assess the safety & tolerability of a PARP inhibitor in combination with gemcitabine in pancreatic cancer. Identifier: NCT01585805. https://clinicaltrials.gov/ct2/show/NCT00515866.
81. Shah SN, Hile SE, Eckert KA. Defective mismatch repair, microsatellite mutation bias, and variability in clinical cancer phenotypes. Cancer Res. 2010;70(2):431–5.
82. Gologan A, Sepulveda AR. Microsatellite instability and DNA mismatch repair deficiency testing in hereditary and sporadic gastrointestinal cancers. Clin Lab Med. 2005;25(1):179–96.

83. Kunkel TA, Erie DA. DNA mismatch repair. Annu Rev Biochem. 2005;74:681–710.
84. Goggins M, et al. Pancreatic adenocarcinomas with DNA replication errors (RER+) are associated with wild-type K-ras and characteristic histopathology. Poor differentiation, a syncytial growth pattern, and pushing borders suggest RER+. Am J Pathol. 1998;152(6):1501–7.
85. Yamamoto H, et al. Genetic and clinical features of human pancreatic ductal adenocarcinomas with widespread microsatellite instability. Cancer Res. 2001;61(7):3139–44.
86. Dong X, et al. DNA mismatch repair gene polymorphisms affect survival in pancreatic cancer. Oncologist. 2011;16(1):61–70.
87. Galasso M, Sandhu SK, Volinia S. MicroRNA expression signatures in solid malignancies. Cancer J. 2012;18(3):238–43.
88. Zhang B, et al. microRNAs as oncogenes and tumor suppressors. Dev Biol. 2007;302(1):1–12.
89. Torrisani J, et al. Let-7 MicroRNA transfer in pancreatic cancer-derived cells inhibits in vitro cell proliferation but fails to alter tumor progression. Hum Gene Ther. 2009;20(8):831–44.
90. Iorio MV, Croce CM. MicroRNAs in cancer: small molecules with a huge impact. J Clin Oncol. 2009;27(34):5848–56.
91. Diab M, et al. The role of microRNAs in the diagnosis and treatment of pancreatic adenocarcinoma. J Clin Med. 2016;5(6):E59.
92. Li A, et al. Pancreatic cancers epigenetically silence SIP1 and hypomethylate and overexpress miR-200a/200b in association with elevated circulating miR-200a and miR-200b levels. Cancer Res. 2010;70(13):5226–37.
93. Li A, et al. MicroRNA array analysis finds elevated serum miR-1290 accurately distinguishes patients with low-stage pancreatic cancer from healthy and disease controls. Clin Cancer Res. 2013;19(13):3600–10.
94. Liu J, et al. Combination of plasma microRNAs with serum CA19-9 for early detection of pancreatic cancer. Int J Cancer. 2012;131(3):683–91.
95. Park JK, et al. Antisense inhibition of microRNA-21 or −221 arrests cell cycle, induces apoptosis, and sensitizes the effects of gemcitabine in pancreatic adenocarcinoma. Pancreas. 2009;38(7):e190–9.
96. Hamada S, et al. MiR-365 induces gemcitabine resistance in pancreatic cancer cells by targeting the adaptor protein SHC1 and pro-apoptotic regulator BAX. Cell Signal. 2014;26(2):179–85.
97. Jung DE, et al. Differentially expressed microRNAs in pancreatic cancer stem cells. Pancreas. 2011;40(8):1180–7.
98. Rosenfeld N, et al. MicroRNAs accurately identify cancer tissue origin. Nat Biotechnol. 2008;26(4):462–9.
99. Singh S, et al. miRNA profiling in pancreatic cancer and restoration of chemosensitivity. Cancer Lett. 2013;334(2):211–20.
100. Mittal A, et al. Efficacy of gemcitabine conjugated and miRNA-205 complexed micelles for treatment of advanced pancreatic cancer. Biomaterials. 2014;35(25):7077–87.
101. Kawaguchi T, et al. Clinical impact of circulating miR-221 in plasma of patients with pancreatic cancer. Br J Cancer. 2013;108(2):361–9.
102. Morimura R, et al. Novel diagnostic value of circulating miR-18a in plasma of patients with pancreatic cancer. Br J Cancer. 2011;105(11):1733–40.
103. LaConti JJ, et al. Tissue and serum microRNAs in the Kras(G12D) transgenic animal model and in patients with pancreatic cancer. PLoS One. 2011;6(6):e20687.
104. Riva F, et al. Clinical applications of circulating tumor DNA and circulating tumor cells in pancreatic cancer. Mol Oncol. 2016;10(3):481–93.
105. Jahr JS, et al. A novel approach to measuring circulating blood volume: the use of a hemoglobin-based oxygen carrier in a rabbit model. Anesth Analg. 2001;92(3):609–14.
106. Kinugasa H, et al. Detection of K-ras gene mutation by liquid biopsy in patients with pancreatic cancer. Cancer. 2015;121(13):2271–80.

107. Schwarzenbach H, et al. Detection and monitoring of cell-free DNA in blood of patients with colorectal cancer. Ann N Y Acad Sci. 2008;1137:190–6.
108. Singh N, et al. High levels of cell-free circulating nucleic acids in pancreatic cancer are associated with vascular encasement, metastasis and poor survival. Cancer Investig. 2015;33(3):78–85.
109. Bettegowda C, et al. Detection of circulating tumor DNA in early- and late-stage human malignancies. Sci Transl Med. 2014;6(224):224ra24.
110. Tjensvoll K, et al. Clinical relevance of circulating KRAS mutated DNA in plasma from patients with advanced pancreatic cancer. Mol Oncol. 2016;10(4):635–43.
111. Sausen M, et al. Clinical implications of genomic alterations in the tumour and circulation of pancreatic cancer patients. Nat Commun. 2015;6:7686.
112. Johansen JSV, Vibat CRT, Calatayud D, Jensen BV, Hasselby JP, Collisson EA, Lu T, Poole JC, Erlander M. Comparative circulating tumor DNA levels for KRAS mutations in patients with nonresectable pancreatic cancer. J Clin Oncol. 2015;33. (suppl 3; abstr 288). Abstract available through http://meetinglibrary.asco.org/content/140281-158, 2015
113. Bidard FC, et al. Circulating tumor cells in locally advanced pancreatic adenocarcinoma: the ancillary CirCe 07 study to the LAP 07 trial. Ann Oncol. 2013;24(8):2057–61.
114. Kurihara T, et al. Detection of circulating tumor cells in patients with pancreatic cancer: a preliminary result. J Hepato-Biliary-Pancreat Surg. 2008;15(2):189–95.
115. Bissolati M, et al. Portal vein-circulating tumor cells predict liver metastases in patients with resectable pancreatic cancer. Tumour Biol. 2015;36(2):991–6.
116. Poruk KE, et al. Circulating tumor cells expressing markers of tumor initiating cells predict poor survival and cancer recurrence in patients with pancreatic ductal adenocarcinoma. Clin Cancer Res. 2016; doi:10.1158/1078-0432.CCR-16-1467.
117. Yu M, et al. RNA sequencing of pancreatic circulating tumour cells implicates WNT signalling in metastasis. Nature. 2012;487(7408):510–3.
118. Torphy RJ, et al. Circulating tumor cells as a biomarker of response to treatment in patient-derived xenograft mouse models of pancreatic adenocarcinoma. PLoS One. 2014;9(2):e89474.
119. Yu KH, et al. Pharmacogenomic modeling of circulating tumor and invasive cells for prediction of chemotherapy response and resistance in pancreatic cancer. Clin Cancer Res. 2014;20(20):5281–9.
120. Infante JR, et al. Peritumoral fibroblast SPARC expression and patient outcome with resectable pancreatic adenocarcinoma. J Clin Oncol. 2007;25(3):319–25.
121. Han W, et al. Prognostic value of SPARC in patients with pancreatic cancer: a systematic review and meta-analysis. PLoS One. 2016;11(1):e0145803.
122. Mantoni TS, et al. Stromal SPARC expression and patient survival after chemoradiation for non-resectable pancreatic adenocarcinoma. Cancer Biol Ther. 2008;7(11):1806–15.
123. Garber K. Stromal depletion goes on trial in pancreatic cancer. J Natl Cancer Inst. 2010;102(7):448–50.
124. Frese KK, et al. Nab-paclitaxel potentiates gemcitabine activity by reducing cytidine deaminase levels in a mouse model of pancreatic cancer. Cancer Discov. 2012;2(3):260–9.
125. Von Hoff DD, et al. Increased survival in pancreatic cancer with nab-paclitaxel plus gemcitabine. N Engl J Med. 2013;369(18):1691–703.
126. Hidalgo M, et al. SPARC expression did not predict efficacy of nab-paclitaxel plus gemcitabine or gemcitabine alone for metastatic pancreatic cancer in an exploratory analysis of the phase III MPACT trial. Clin Cancer Res. 2015;21(21):4811–8.
127. Kim H, et al. SPARC-independent delivery of nab-paclitaxel without depleting tumor Stroma in patient-derived pancreatic cancer Xenografts. Mol Cancer Ther. 2016;15(4):680–8.
128. Mackey JR, et al. Functional nucleoside transporters are required for gemcitabine influx and manifestation of toxicity in cancer cell lines. Cancer Res. 1998;58(19):4349–57.

129. Nakano Y, et al. Gemcitabine chemoresistance and molecular markers associated with gemcitabine transport and metabolism in human pancreatic cancer cells. Br J Cancer. 2007;96(3):457–63.
130. Mackey JR, et al. Gemcitabine transport in xenopus oocytes expressing recombinant plasma membrane mammalian nucleoside transporters. J Natl Cancer Inst. 1999;91(21):1876–81.
131. Spratlin J, et al. The absence of human equilibrative nucleoside transporter 1 is associated with reduced survival in patients with gemcitabine-treated pancreas adenocarcinoma. Clin Cancer Res. 2004;10(20):6956–61.
132. Greenhalf W, et al. Pancreatic cancer hENT1 expression and survival from gemcitabine in patients from the ESPAC-3 trial. J Natl Cancer Inst. 2014;106(1):djt347.

Chapter 7
Imaging of Pancreatic Malignancies

Ferenc Czeyda-Pommersheim, Bobby Kalb, and Diego Martin

MRI Methodology

Magnetic Resonance Cholangiopancreatography

Magnetic resonance cholangiopancreatography (MRCP) is the key MRI sequence for luminal imaging of the pancreatic ductal system. By utilizing a heavily T2-weighted (T2W) sequence with echo times in excess of 700 ms, MRCP provides excellent anatomic detail of the fluid-containing structures of the abdomen and is ideally suited for imaging of the pancreatic duct. Several different technical approaches to MRCP may be pursued. Conventional two-dimensional (2D) MRCP sequences constitute the fastest and most frequently employed method. Three-dimensional (3D) acquisition MRCP methods are also available that produce high-quality, near-isotropic resolution images of the pancreatic ductal system. The criteria for selection of a 3D or 2D MRCP technique may vary from center to center. Three-dimensional acquisition methods offer the strengths of excellent contrast and improved signal to noise ratios relative to the 2D techniques. In addition, the high-resolution acquisition method of a 3D acquisition allows for more reliable distinction of small calculi from flow artifacts that may be seen with the 2D method. However, the larger time investment required for 3D image acquisition may discourage some centers from routine use of this technique. While 3D MRCP may provide better delineation of the pancreatic ductal anatomy in comparison with the 2D technique, additional soft tissue imaging that is required for a comprehensive MR examination of the pancreas provides additional diagnostic

F. Czeyda-Pommersheim, M.D. (✉) • B. Kalb, M.D. • D. Martin, M.D., Ph.D.
Department of Medical Imaging, Banner University Medical Center, 1501 North Campbell Avenue, PO Box 245067, Tucson, AZ 85724, USA
e-mail: POMMERSHEIMF@radiology.arizona.edu

T. Bekaii-Saab, B. El-Rayes (eds.), *Current and Emerging Therapies in Pancreatic Cancer*, DOI 10.1007/978-3-319-58256-6_7

information that may obviate some of the benefits of the 3D MRCP technique. In patients with irregular respiratory cycles that are difficult to capture by the navigator pulse, there may be a significant time investment in a 3D image acquisition that is ultimately deteriorated by artifacts such as ghosting and blurring; 2D methods, in comparison, tend to be much more robust methods that are resistant to this type of motion degradation.

Soft Tissue Imaging

Despite the many benefits of MRCP, obtaining this sequence alone is insufficient for a comprehensive analysis of the pancreas. MRCP is a luminal technique and does not provide adequate analysis of the surrounding soft tissues that are frequently a contributor to pancreatic pathology, and imaging evaluation of pancreatic disease is incomplete without dynamic, T1-weighted (T1W) contrast-enhanced 3D gradient echo (GRE) sequences coupled with shorter echo, single-shot T2W sequences to assess to surrounding soft tissues.

T2-Weighted and Steady-State Free Precession Imaging

When acquired with a single-shot technique, these sequences are motion insensitive and produce consistently high image quality. The single-shot technique, however, is prone to through-plane flow artifacts, most often in the extrahepatic bile duct. Steady-state free precession sequences (SSFP), like T2W sequences, produce bright signal in fluid-containing structures. However, SSFP sequences are less prone to this flow void artifact, even when acquired with a single-shot technique.

T1-Weighted Imaging

Dynamic, fat-saturated gadolinium chelate-enhanced T1W 3D GRE imaging is a critical portion of a comprehensive MR evaluation of the pancreas. This technique is performed during a single breath hold and is thus sensitive to motion artifact. Recently, newer T1W 3D GRE sequences have been developed utilizing a radial pattern of k-space filling, reducing flip angle inaccuracies and motion artifacts; this has the effect of preserving image quality even in freely breathing patients [1].

Precontrast T1W images are important to evaluate the background pancreatic parenchyma; normal pancreas is intrinsically bright on T1W images (due to proteins within the pancreatic acina), and loss of this normal T1 signal is a marker of background pancreatic parenchymal disease. A dynamic, arterial phase sequence acquired with a bolus tracking method [2] demonstrates robust, early enhancement of the pancreatic parenchyma. Solid neoplasms in the pancreas are reliably identified on dynamic post-contrast images.

Evolving Role of MRI and ERCP

Endoscopic retrograde cholangiopancreatography (ERCP) is a commonly utilized procedure for evaluation of the pancreas. Advantages of ERCP include the ability to perform a therapeutic intervention, including cytological brushings, stone extraction, and stent placement for ductal obstructive diseases. However, as a diagnostic imaging modality, ERCP has several disadvantages compared to MRI. ERCP is an invasive methodology, and complications include post-procedure pancreatitis, bleeding, cholangitis, and perforation. A large, multicenter review found the overall ERCP complication rate to be 6.85% [3] and the ERCP-related mortality rate to be 0.33%; the mortality rate has been reported as high as 1% [4]. Performed by opacifying the pancreatic ductal system with contrast, ERCP only provides a luminal evaluation of the pancreatic duct. In the evaluation of malignant pancreatic disease, ERCP cannot assess for extraductal disease and is limited in tumor staging. In contrast, MRI is a noninvasive imaging technique with no radiation or need for moderate sedation and provides a comprehensive assessment of not only the lumen of the pancreatic duct but also the surrounding soft tissues.

Pancreatic Adenocarcinoma

Pancreatic adenocarcinoma is the most common exocrine pancreatic tumor and the 12th most common cancer worldwide. In the United States, it accounts for approximately 3% of new cancers diagnosed annually and 7% of all cancer deaths. Most cases occur sporadically; up to 10% are caused by germ line mutations. Of the sporadic cases, environmental exposures have been shown to play a role in tumor development. Smoking is the most common known environmental risk factor [5].

Ductal adenocarcinoma originates in the pancreatic duct epithelium and in most cases results in obstruction of the upstream pancreatic duct by the time it is of sufficient size to be detectable on imaging, a characteristic that can help pinpoint the location of the tumor on CT and MRI. Surgical resection offers the only potential cure; however, as the tumor usually presents at an advanced stage, only up to 20% of patients are candidates for surgery. Five-year survival in patients who undergo tumor resection is 10% for those with lymph node metastases and approximately 30% for patients with node-negative disease.

MRI has been shown to have superior sensitivity compared to CT in detecting lesions of adenocarcinoma in the pancreas [6]. Pancreatic adenocarcinoma is most commonly a solid soft tissue mass T1 hypointense to the normal pancreas on T1-weighed fat-suppressed imaging and shows progressive enhancement on dynamic post-contrast images (Fig. 7.1). The lesion is most conspicuous in the early arterial phase where it is markedly hypointense compared to the adjacent normal pancreas [7]. The tumor contains cystic elements in less than 10% of cases mimicking a cystic pancreatic neoplasm (Fig. 7.2); however, a soft tissue mass should be the predominant finding on MRI for adenocarcinoma to be considered [8].

The most common benign mimic of pancreatic adenocarcinoma on CT is focal fatty infiltration and focal pancreatitis. MRI can reliably distinguish both from adenocarcinoma. In focal lipomatosis, chemical shift imaging will show the presence of microscopic lipid as signal drop on the opposed phase sequence compared to the

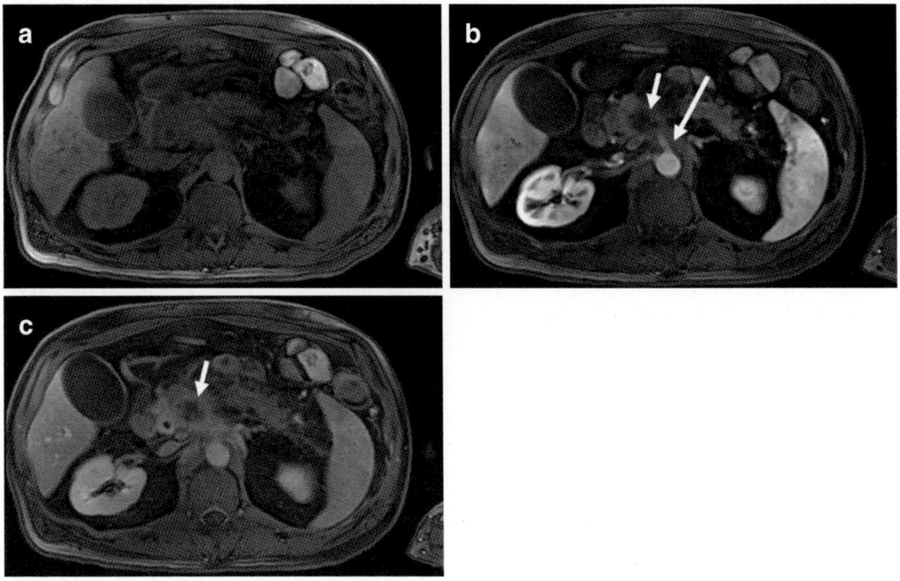

Fig. 7.1 Pancreatic adenocarcinoma with imaging evidence of invasion of the superior mesenteric artery (SMA). T1WFS (**a**), T1WFS post-contrast arterial (**b**), and portal venous phase (**c**) images show a hypoenhancing mass in the uncinate process of the pancreas (*arrow* in **b**, **c**) that near completely encases the superior mesenteric artery (*long arrow* in **b**)

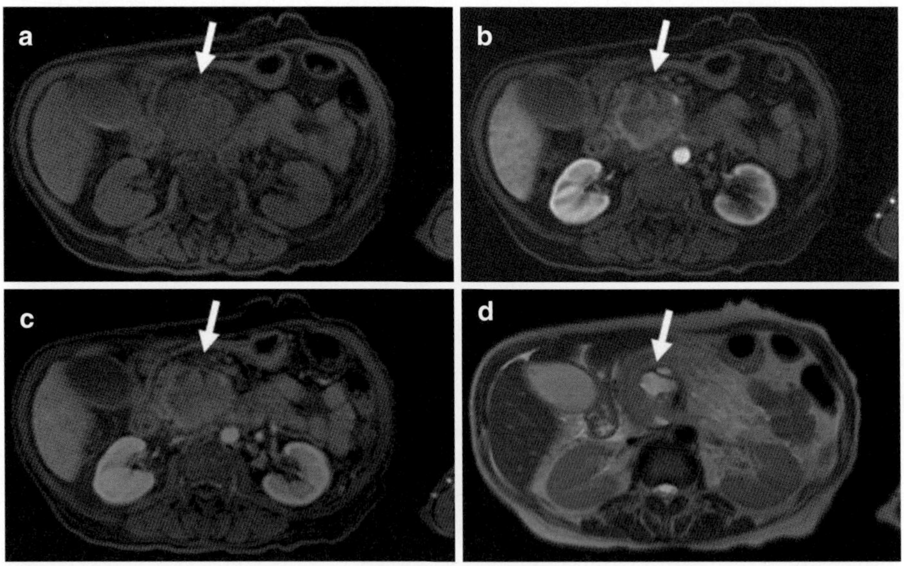

Fig. 7.2 Adenocarcinoma with cystic changes. MRI (**a**, T1WFS; **b**, T1WFS w/gad arterial phase; **c**, T1WFS w/gad portal venous phase; **d**, T2W) shows a predominantly solid mass in the head of the pancreas with delayed enhancement (*arrow* in **a**, **b**, **c**) and a cystic region (*arrow* in **d**)

in phase (Fig. 7.3). Focal pancreatitis will show increased T2 signal in the involved pancreas best seen on T2-weighed fat-suppressed sequences (Fig. 7.4). Both in focal lipomatosis and focal pancreatitis, a normal caliber duct will be seen coursing through the lesion, a finding extremely unusual in adenocarcinoma, which in almost all cases will cause marked narrowing and upstream dilation of the pancreatic duct.

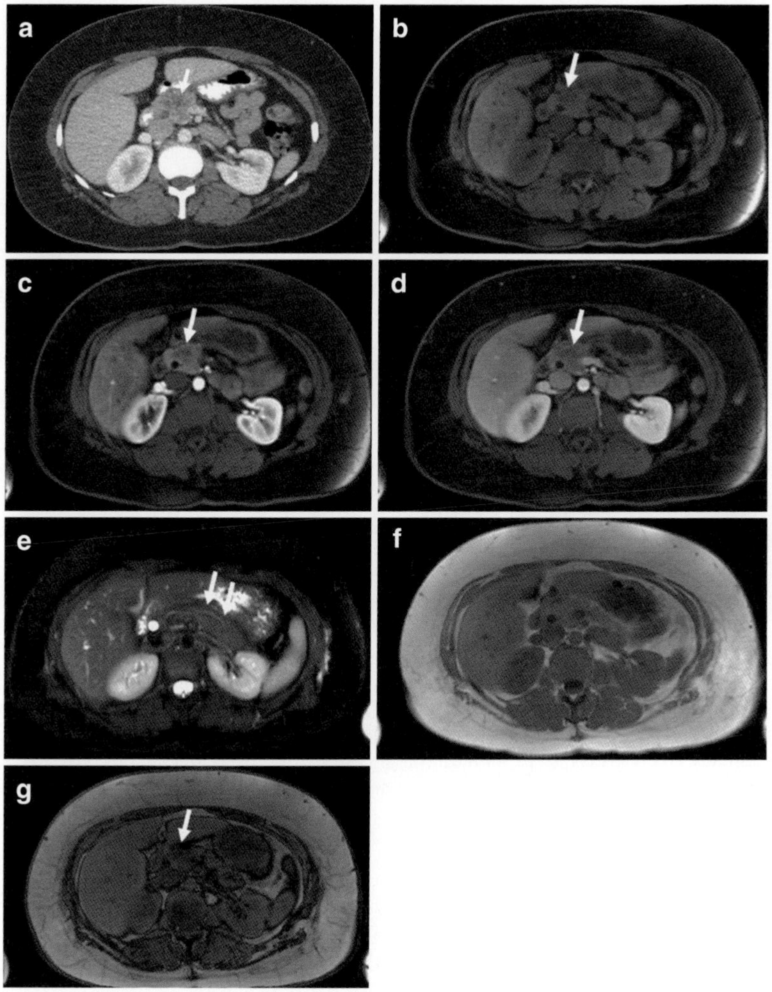

Fig. 7.3 Focal steatosis in the pancreatic head in a 38-year-old woman who presented with peri-umbilical pain. CT scan showed a hypoenhancing mass in the pancreatic head (*arrow*). MRI performed subsequently (**b**, T1W FS; **c**, T1WFS with contrast arterial phase; **d**, T1WFS portal venous phase; **e**, T2WFS; **f**, T1W in phase; **g**, T1W opposed phase) shows a T1 hypointense region (*arrow* in **b**) that shows relative hypoenhancement (*arrow* in **c**, **d**) corresponding to the abnormality on the CT. The pancreatic duct is not dilated (*double arrow* in **e**); this would be unusual in pancreatic adenocarcinoma which characteristically obstructs the duct when it reaches this size. On chemical shift imaging, there is signal dropout on the opposed phase image (*arrow* in **g**) corresponding to this lesion, in keeping with focal fatty infiltration mimicking adenocarcinoma

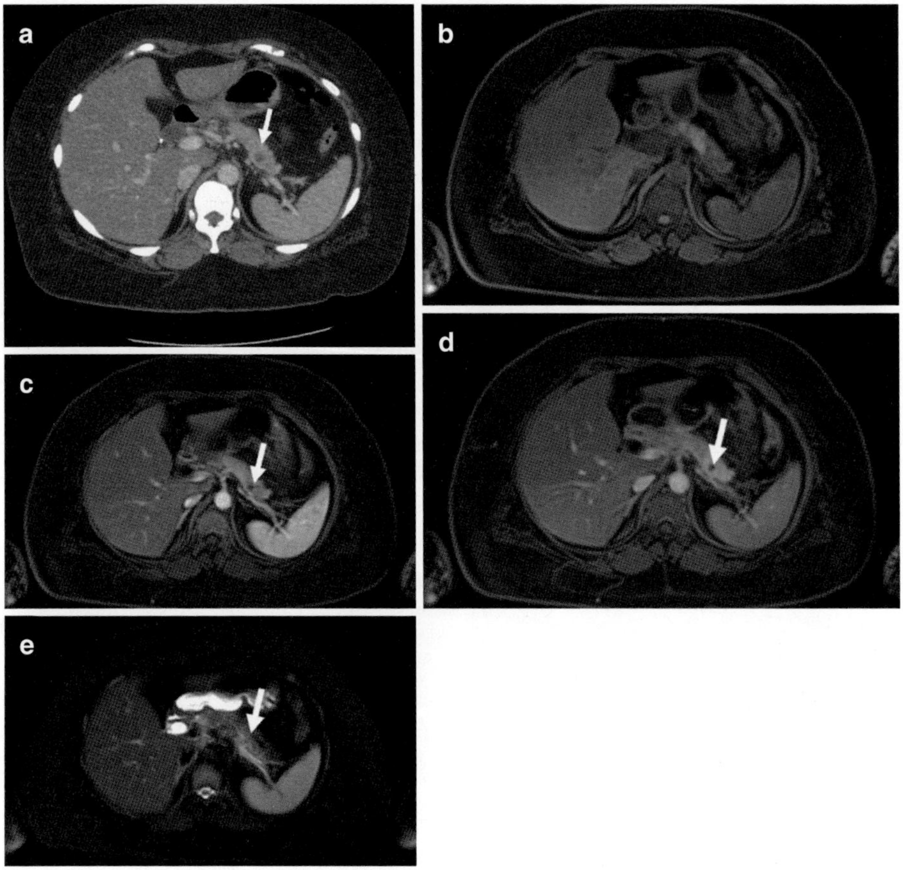

Fig. 7.4 Focal pancreatitis mimicking a lesion in a 35-year-old woman with abdominal pain. CT scan showed a hypoenhancing, solid-appearing lesion in the tail of the pancreas (*arrow* in **a**). Subsequent MRI (**b**, T1WFS; **c**, T1WFS arterial phase; **d**, T1WFS portal venous phase; **e**, T2WFS) shows that the lesion shows relative hypoenhancement on the dynamic post-contrast images (*arrow* in **c**, **d**), with edema in the tail of the pancreas (*arrow* in **e**) in keeping with a pseudolesion of focal pancreatitis

The majority of patients with pancreatic adenocarcinoma are not surgical candidates at the time of diagnosis. While indications for resection vary at different centers, universal signs of unresectability on imaging are infiltration of adjacent organs, invasion of the peripancreatic arteries, and distant metastases. Extensive involvement of the peripancreatic veins is also usually a contraindication although at some centers limited invasion of the portal vein or the superior mesenteric vein does not preclude surgery. A modified surgical approach may be used in these cases where the invaded vein segment is resected and the vessel is repaired with a graft.

MRI can accurately exclude vascular involvement by showing lack of direct contact of the lesion with vessels. In cases where there is direct contact, tumor encasement of less than 90° of the vessel circumference denotes a very low likelihood of vascular invasion, while a greater than 90° of contact has a high (40% or higher) likelihood of tumor vascular invasion [9] (see Fig. 7.1). MRI has been shown superior to CT in detecting distant metastatic disease [6].

Pancreatic Cystic Neoplasms

Intraductal Papillary Mucinous Neoplasm

IPMN is an intraductal papillary mucin-producing cystic neoplasm that arises from the main pancreatic duct or its branches. There are three subtypes depending on the anatomic site of origin: main branch, side branch, and mixed. Histologically, IPMN may harbor varying degrees of dysplasia with malignant potential; they most often progress into ductal adenocarcinoma or colloid carcinoma. Main branch and mixed types have a higher risk of malignancy (approximately 70%) and require surgical referral, while small (<1 cm) side branch IPMN carries an extremely low risk of progressing to malignancy [10, 11]. Based on cohort studies, the lag time of progression from IPMN adenoma to adenocarcinoma is at least several years [12]. Patients who undergo resection of invasive adenocarcinoma that arose from an IPMN have a more favorable long-term prognosis (5-year survival of approximately 40%) than those with adenocarcinoma without a preceding IPMN.

MRI has been shown to be as reliable as CT and EUS for detection and characterization of pancreas IPMN, without the need for an invasive procedure or exposure to ionizing radiation which is important as many of these lesions will require imaging follow-up [13, 14].

Main duct IPMN appears as diffuse or focal dilation of the pancreatic duct to 5 mm or greater in the absence of other etiologies such as an obstructing mass, ductal stone, or chronic pancreatitis. Side branch IPMN appears on MRI as a cystic lesion in the pancreas with direct communication to the main pancreatic duct (Fig. 7.5). High-risk imaging characteristics of side branch IPMN are a dilated main duct of greater than 1 cm (indicating mixed type IPMN) internal septa or mural nodules (Fig. 7.6). Lesions with these characteristics warrant surgical referral

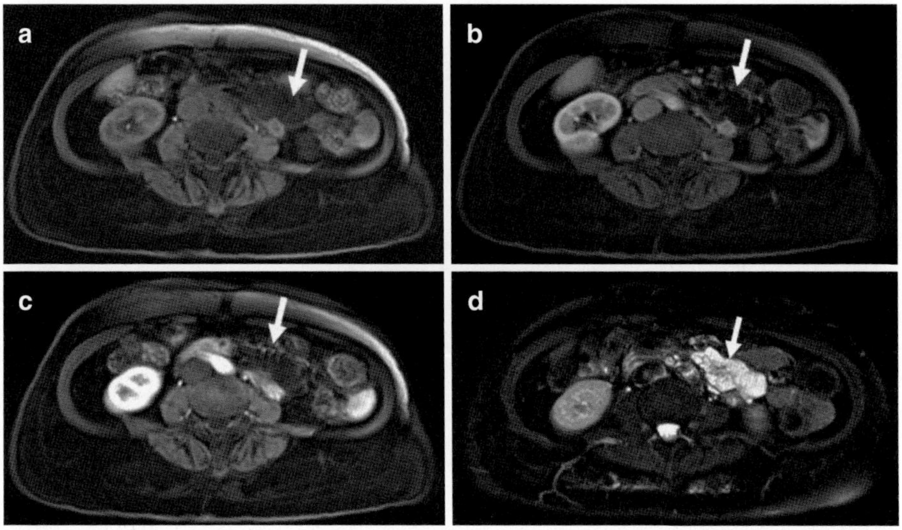

Fig. 7.5 Side branch IPMN. MRI (**a**, T1WFS; **b**, T1WFS w/gad arterial phase; **c**, T1WFS w/gad portal venous phase; **d**, T2WFS) shows a mildly complex cystic lesion with enhancing thin septations but no nodularity or soft tissue component in the uncinate process of the pancreas (*arrows*)

and are often resected without further testing. Main duct dilation of 5–9 mm or a simple side branch IPMN with a diameter of >3 cm is considered worrisome features [15].

Imaging follow-up of asymptomatic IPMN without high-risk features that would warrant intervention has been controversial. Recent recommendations for side branch IPMN with no concerning imaging characteristics suggest a total of 5-year follow-up with MRI at 1 and then 2-year intervals in patients who are candidates for surgery. IPMN with one worrisome imaging feature, or those that develop such characteristics on follow-up, should be evaluated with EUS/FNA. If more than one worrisome characteristics are present, evaluation for surgical resection is recommended [11, 16]. Once the initial diagnosis of a low-risk side branch IPMN has been established, there is recent evidence supporting the effectiveness of a simplified IPMN follow-up MRI protocol without gadolinium with substantial time savings compared to a full abdomen MRI examination [17].

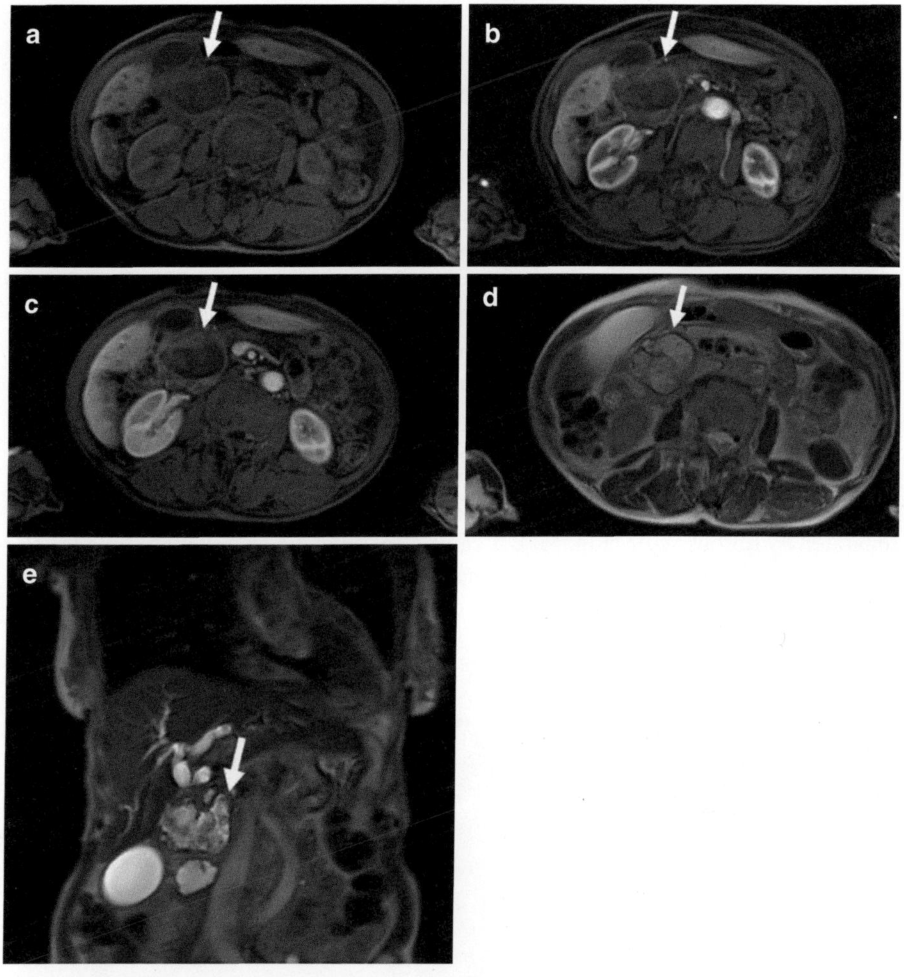

Fig. 7.6 IPMN with malignant degeneration into pancreatic adenocarcinoma. MRI (**a**, T1WFS; **b**, T1WFS w/gad arterial phase; **c**, T1WFS w/gad portal venous phase; **d**, T2W axial; **e**, T2W coronal) shows a complex but primarily cystic mass in the head of the pancreas with irregular, nodular-enhancing internal septations (*arrows*)

Serous Cystadenoma

Pancreatic serous cystadenomas most frequently occur in middle-aged to older women and are often incidentally detected on imaging, although when large enough (>4 cm in greatest diameter) may present with symptoms due to mass effect. On microscopic examination these lesions are composed of multiple small cysts lined with cuboidal cells containing glycogen but no mucin. Cyst contents are characterized by the absence of amylase (unlike pseudocysts), CA19-9, or CEA (unlike adenocarcinoma with cystic degeneration). Malignant transformation into serous cystadenocarcinoma is extremely rare [18]. Diagnosis is often suggested based on imaging findings and patient demographics. Cases with characteristic findings do not require further treatment or imaging follow-up unless the diagnosis remains in doubt or the patient has significant symptoms [19].

MRI has been shown to have higher accuracy in diagnosing serous cystadenoma compared to ultrasound or CT [20]. Three types of serous cystadenoma have been described based on imaging appearance: polycystic, oligocystic, and honeycomb. Over 70% are the polycystic type composed of multiple cysts of <2 cm in diameter separated by fibrous septa (Fig. 7.7). A central scar may be observed in some lesions and may calcify. The honeycomb pattern accounts for approximately 20% of lesions and is characterized by small cysts that cannot be distinguished by imaging; these lesions therefore appear as a solid mass. Oligocystic tumors account for 10% of serous cystadenoma and are unilocular or composed of a few cysts >2 cm in diameter.

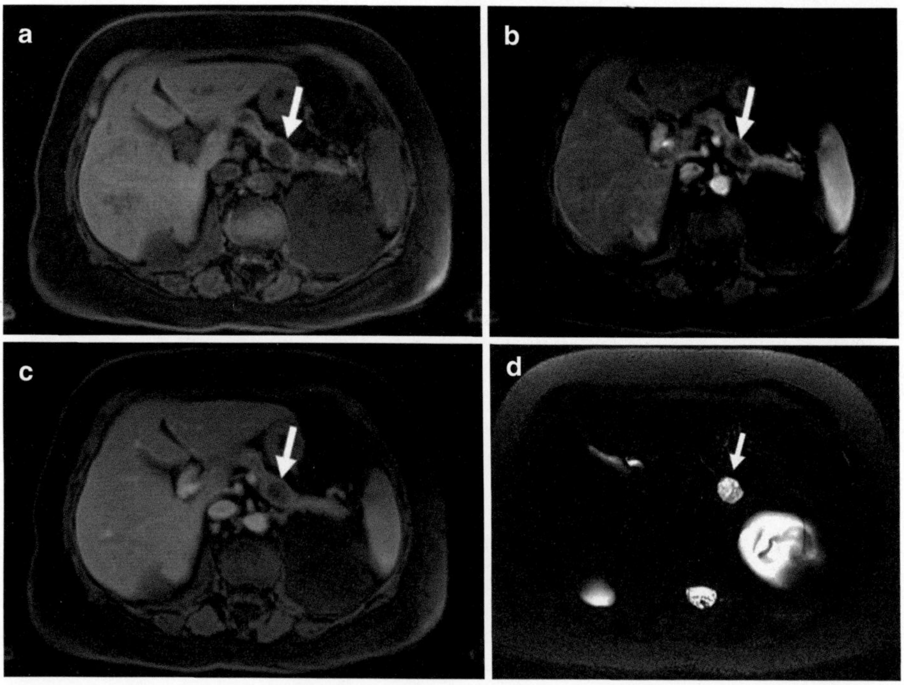

Fig. 7.7 Serous cystadenoma. MRI (**a**, T1WFS; **b**, T1WFS w/gad arterial phase; **c**, T1WFS w/gad portal venous phase; **d**, T2W axial MRCP) shows a lesion composed of small cysts in the tail of the pancreas (*arrow*). The lesion has thin, enhancing septa but no nodularity or soft tissue component

It is often not possible to distinguish oligocystic serous cystadenomas based on imaging alone from other cystic neoplasms such as pseudocyst, IPMN, or mucinous cystadenoma although serous cystadenomas are more often multilocular or lobulated, while mucinous tumors more commonly have a smooth contour. Unlike IPMN these tumors are not connected to the main pancreatic duct [21].

Mucinous Cystic Neoplasm

Mucinous cystic neoplasms (MCN) of the pancreas are composed of mucinous epithelium and ovarian-type stroma, similar to MCN of hepatobiliary or ovarian origin. These tumors are thought to arise from intrapancreatic rests of ovarian epithelium; they almost exclusively occur in women and have significant malignant potential [22]. The prevalence of cancer in resected lesions varies widely (6–36%) and is thought to be overestimated as many small simple pancreatic cystic lesions are never resected and may represent benign MCN. The risk of malignancy in smaller lesions (<5 cm) is relatively low [23]. Due to the high risk of malignant degeneration, most MCN are surgically removed unless the patient is a poor operative candidate. The risk of recurrence following resection is low.

MCN appear on MRI as large, uni- or multilocular thick-walled cystic lesions that do not communicate with the pancreatic duct (Fig. 7.8). Due to the cystic nature of the tumor, MRI is well suited for imaging evaluation of MCN, the cystic component is well seen on heavily T2-weighted sequences, and any soft tissue component

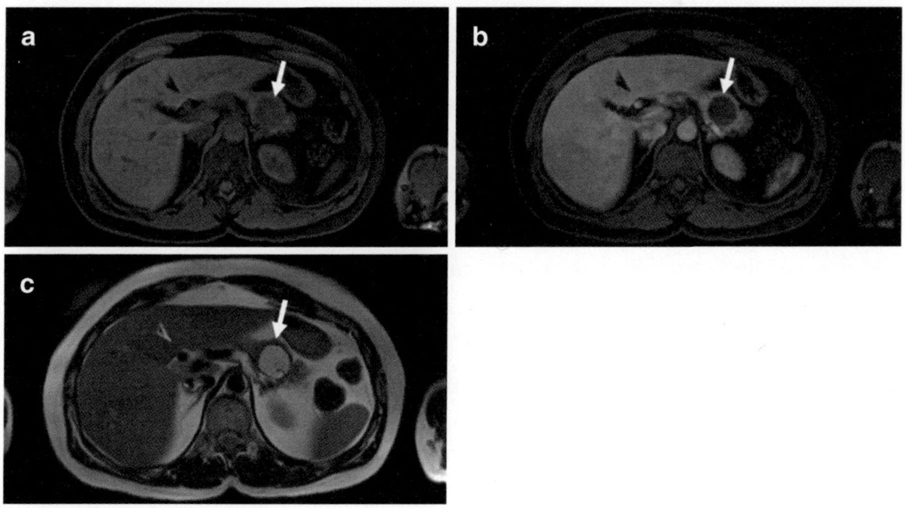

Fig. 7.8 Mucinous cystadenoma in a 46-year-old woman. MRI (**a**, T1WFS; **b**, T1WFS w/gad portal venous phase; **c**, T2WTSE) shows a multilocular cystic lesion in the tail of the pancreas (*arrow*) composed of large cysts with at least one internal septation. No communication with the main duct could be found. The internal septa are smoothly and uniformly enhancing (*arrow* in **b**). There is no soft tissue component or enhancing nodules. Endoscopic ultrasound and cyst aspiration confirmed mucinous cystadenoma

or septa can be evaluated on T1-weighted pre- and post-contrast images. Individual cysts within the tumor are typically larger than those of serous cystadenomas. MCN are usually solitary and are most commonly located in the pancreatic body or tail. While most MCN are resected in patients who are high-risk operative candidates, small (<3 cm) tumors without enhancing mural nodules or a soft tissue component may be followed with imaging.

Solid Pseudopapillary Neoplasm

SPN, the least common of the pancreatic exocrine tumors discussed, typically occurs in women in their third or fourth decade. The pathogenesis and the cell of origin are uncertain. Clinical presentation is often nonspecific and is related to mass effect from the tumor although many patients are asymptomatic. With the increasing use of cross-sectional imaging done for other reasons, these tumors are now incidentally detected at an earlier stage [24]. On gross examination, many tumors show cystic areas or hemorrhagic cystic degeneration and also have a significant soft tissue component. A tumor capsule is often seen in larger lesions. SPN is a premalignant or low-grade malignant tumor with an excellent prognosis, even in cases when metastases are present. Surgical resection is usually curative [25].

On MRI SPN appears as a heterogenous, often T2 hyperintense mass. Regions of high T1 signal can be seen on precontrast images due to hemorrhagic cystic areas. Solid components show heterogenous early enhancement with delayed fill-in and often an enhancing tumor capsule. The tumor typically enhances less in the arterial phase than normal pancreas which distinguishes these lesions from pancreatic neuroendocrine tumors that are typically strongly arterial enhancing [26]. While the imaging appearance of SPN may be similar to other cystic pancreatic neoplasms, those are much less common in the typical demographic group of SPN patients. Pseudocyst also may appear similar; however, these lack an enhancing soft tissue component and usually have either a history of or imaging evidence of acute pancreatitis. In cases where the imaging diagnosis is in doubt, endoscopic ultrasound and fine needle aspiration may be performed prior to surgical therapy.

Endocrine Tumors of the Pancreas

Pancreatic neuroendocrine tumors (PNET) are rare neoplasms that arise from the endocrine pancreas, more specifically from pluripotent cells in the pancreatic ductal/acinar system [27]. PNET accounts for <5% of pancreatic tumors [28], though the incidence of PNETs may be increasing due to improved noninvasive imaging diagnostics that are able to detect small lesions incidentally, prior to tumors causing clinical symptoms. While PNETs are less aggressive with an improved prognosis compared to the more common ductal adenocarcinoma, these tumors exhibit a wide range of biological behavior. The 2010 World Health Organization classification of tumor biology is dependent on tumor proliferative index as measured by Ki-67 and mitotic rate. A majority (60–70%) of patients present with metastatic disease, and the 5-year survival for PNET (excluding insulinoma) is approximately 65%.

While approximately 90% of PNETs occur sporadically, several familial syndromes are associated with an increased risk for the development of PNET. These syndromes are multiple endocrine neoplasia type 1 (MEN1), von Hippel-Lindau syndrome (vHL), neurofibromatosis type 1 (NF1), and tuberous sclerosis. The occurrence of PNET is most common in MEN1 (approximately 80–100% of patients develop PNET), while the incidence is much lower in the remaining syndromes (ranging from 20% to <1%).

PNET may be categorized as functioning or nonfunctioning, based on the presence or absence of associated hormonal hypersecretion. The vast majority (>90%) of PNETs are nonfunctioning and thus present at a later stage of disease, often with compression of adjacent anatomic structures (such as the biliary and pancreatic ductal system) or with metastatic disease. Functional PNETs are divided into insulinomas (40–60%), gastrinomas (20–50%), glucagonomas, somatostatinomas, and VIPomas; each functional tumor is associated with the hypersecretion of its own specific secretory hormone which causes a specific clinical syndrome that typically allows for earlier detection compared to nonfunctional tumors (age 55 years for functioning tumors versus 65 years for nonfunctioning).

Imaging

MRI is the imaging method of choice for the diagnosis of solid pancreatic tumors. Dynamic, contrast-enhanced MRI has been shown to provide superior tumor conspicuity compared to MDCT for pancreatic cancer in general [29] and is ideal for screening patients with familial syndromes at risk for development of PNET, due to the lack of ionizing radiation. The soft tissue resolution of MRI allows for a high sensitivity for tumor detection and staging [14] including evaluation of both the pancreas and the liver.

In distinction from ductal adenocarcinoma, PNET are well-circumscribed tumors. On T1W images, PNETs are hypointense, contrasting well with the background high-signal pancreatic parenchyma. T2 signal is variable and is typically moderately elevated (Fig. 7.9). Dynamic, post-contrast images demonstrate intense early enhancement which may be homogeneous, ringlike, or heterogeneous. PNET may undergo cystic degeneration, demonstrating a core of high-signal fluid on T2W sequences. However, dynamic enhanced images will still demonstrate a well-

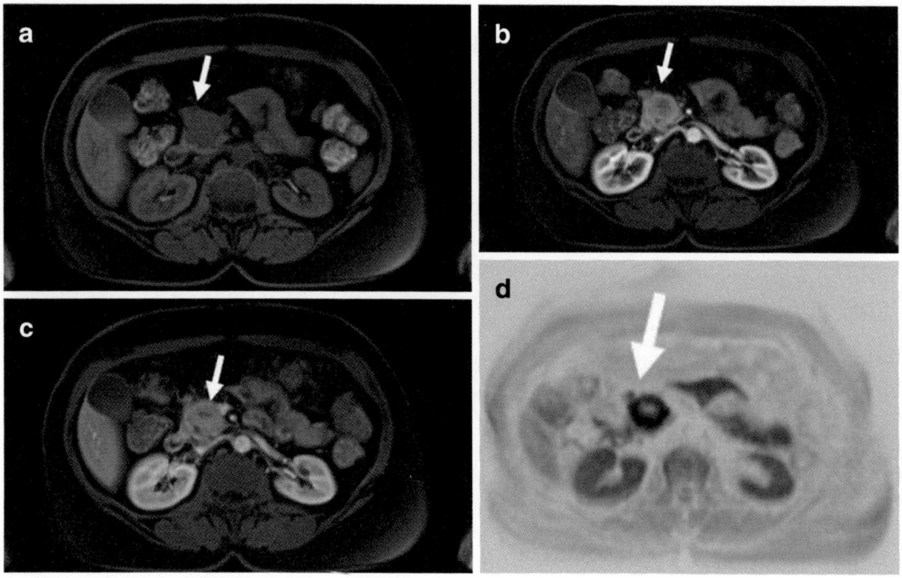

Fig. 7.9 Pancreatic neuroendocrine tumor. MRI (**a**, T1WFS; **b**, T1WFS w/gad arterial phase; **c**, T1WFS w/gad portal venous phase; **d**, DWI $b = 500$) shows a solid mass in the head of the pancreas that enhances most on the arterial phase image (*arrow* in **b**) and shows diffusion restriction (*arrow* in **d**)

vascularized rim or internal nodularity that is indicative of a neoplastic process. Diffusion-weighted imaging (DWI) has been demonstrated by some authors to improve the detection of PNET and may also aid in the detection of hepatic metastatic disease [30].

References

1. Chandarana H, et al. Free-breathing radial 3D fat-suppressed T1-weighted gradient Echo sequence: a viable alternative for contrast-enhanced liver imaging in patients unable to suspend respiration. Investig Radiol. 2011;46(10):648–53.
2. Sharma P, et al. Optimization of single injection liver arterial phase gadolinium enhanced MRI using bolus track real-time imaging. J Magn Reson Imaging. 2011;33(1):110–8.
3. Andriulli A, et al. Incidence rates of post-ERCP complications: a systematic survey of prospective studies. Am J Gastroenterol. 2007;102(8):1781–8.
4. Christensen M, et al. Complications of ERCP: a prospective study. Gastrointest Endosc. 2004;60(5):721–31.
5. Raimondi S, Maisonneuve P, Lowenfels AB. Epidemiology of pancreatic cancer: an overview. Nat Rev Gastroenterol Hepatol. 2009;6(12):699–708.
6. Schima W, et al. Pancreatic adenocarcinoma. Eur Radiol. 2007;17(3):638–49.
7. Miller FH, Rini NJ, Keppke AL. MRI of adenocarcinoma of the pancreas. Am J Roentgenol. 2006;187(4):W365–74.

8. Yoon S, et al. Pancreatic ductal adenocarcinoma with intratumoral cystic lesions on MRI: correlation with histopathological findings. Br J Radiol. 2014;83(988):318–26.
9. Lu D, et al. Local staging of pancreatic cancer: criteria for unresectability of major vessels as revealed by pancreatic-phase, thin-section helical CT. AJR Am J Roentgenol. 1997;168(6):1439–43.
10. Shi C, Hruban RH. Intraductal papillary mucinous neoplasm. Hum Pathol. 2012;43(1):1–16.
11. Tanaka M, et al. International consensus guidelines 2012 for the management of IPMN and MCN of the pancreas. Pancreatology. 2012;12(3):183–97.
12. Sohn TA, et al. Intraductal papillary mucinous neoplasms of the pancreas: an updated experience. Ann Surg. 2004;239(6):788–99.
13. Sainani NI, et al. Comparative performance of MDCT and MRI with MR cholangiopancreatography in characterizing small pancreatic cysts. Am J Roentgenol. 2009;193(3):722–31.
14. Kim JH, et al. Diagnostic performance of MRI and EUS in the differentiation of benign from malignant pancreatic cyst and cyst communication with the main duct. Eur J Radiol. 2012;81(11):2927–35.
15. Machado NO, al Qadhi H, al Wahibi K. Intraductal papillary mucinous neoplasm of pancreas. N Am J Med Sci. 2015;7(5):160–75.
16. Vege SS, et al. American gastroenterological association institute guideline on the diagnosis and management of asymptomatic neoplastic pancreatic cysts. Gastroenterology. 2015;148(4):819.
17. Nougaret S, et al. Incidental pancreatic cysts: natural history and diagnostic accuracy of a limited serial pancreatic cyst MRI protocol. Eur Radiol. 2014;24(5):1020–9.
18. Pyke CM, et al. The spectrum of serous cystadenoma of the pancreas. Clinical, pathologic, and surgical aspects. Ann Surg. 1992;215(2):132.
19. Scheiman JM, Hwang JH, Moayyedi P. American Gastroenterological Association technical review on the diagnosis and management of asymptomatic neoplastic pancreatic cysts. Gastroenterology. 2015;148(4):824–848.e22.
20. Bassi C, et al. Management of 100 consecutive cases of pancreatic serous cystadenoma: wait for symptoms and see at imaging or vice versa? World J Surg. 2003;27(3):319–23.
21. Choi J-Y, et al. Typical and atypical manifestations of serous cystadenoma of the pancreas: imaging findings with pathologic correlation. Am J Roentgenol. 2009;193(1):136–42.
22. Zamboni G, et al. Mucinous cystic tumors of the pancreas: clinicopathological features, prognosis, and relationship to other mucinous cystic tumors. Am J Surg Pathol. 1999;23(4):410–22.
23. Reddy RP, et al. Pancreatic mucinous cystic neoplasm defined by ovarian stroma: demographics, clinical features, and prevalence of cancer. Clin Gastroenterol Hepatol. 2004;2(11):1026–31.
24. Romics L, et al. Solid pseudopapillary neoplasm of the pancreas—proposed algorithms for diagnosis and surgical treatment. Langenbeck's Arch Surg. 2010;395(6):747–55.
25. Papavramidis T, Papavramidis S. Solid pseudopapillary tumors of the pancreas: review of 718 patients reported in English literature. J Am Coll Surg. 2005;200(6):965–72.
26. Cantisani V, et al. MR imaging features of solid pseudopapillary tumor of the pancreas in adult and pediatric patients. AJR Am J Roentgenol. 2003;181(2):395–401.
27. Kuo JH, Lee JA, Chabot JA. Nonfunctional pancreatic neuroendocrine tumors. Surg Clin N Am. 2014;94(3):689–708.
28. Amin S, Kim MK. Islet cell tumors of the pancreas. Gastroenterol Clin N Am. 2016;45(1):83–100.
29. Park HS, et al. Preoperative evaluation of pancreatic cancer: comparison of gadolinium-enhanced dynamic MRI with MR cholangiopancreatography versus MDCT. J Magn Reson Imaging. 2009;30(3):586–95.
30. Farchione A, et al. Evaluation of the added value of diffusion-weighted imaging to conventional magnetic resonance imaging in pancreatic neuroendocrine tumors and comparison with 68Ga-DOTANOC positron emission tomography/computed tomography. Pancreas. 2016;45(3):345–54.

Chapter 8
Advanced Endoscopic Procedures

James J. Farrell

Introduction

Advanced endoscopic procedures defined as endoscopic ultrasound (EUS), endoscopic retrograde cholangiopancreatography (ERCP), and endoscopic enteral stent placement have a very central and important role in the diagnosis, treatment, and palliation of patients with pancreatic cancer. They are used as part of a multidisciplinary management approach which also includes both radiologic and surgical approaches to management of patients with pancreatic cancer. This chapter will review the role of these advanced endoscopic procedures in pancreatic cancer.

Endoscopic Ultrasound

EUS combines regular flexible endoscopy with ultrasound to provide superior imaging of the pancreas compared with high-quality CT or MRI [1]. It has practical applications in early detection of pancreatic masses as well as in the evaluation of patients with pancreatic cysts and pancreatic masses [2]. Importantly, the ability to safely direct a fine needle biopsy under ultrasound guidance into the pancreas has expanded the indications for EUS in pancreatic cancer not just in the realm of diagnosis to confirm a suspected pancreatic malignancy but also for EUS-guided therapeutic interventions for pancreatic disease [3].

J.J. Farrell, M.D.
Yale Pancreatic Disease Program, Interventional Endoscopy, Yale University School of Medicine, LMP 1080, 15 York Street, New Haven, CT 06510-3221, USA
e-mail: james.j.farrell@yale.edu

T. Bekaii-Saab, B. El-Rayes (eds.), *Current and Emerging Therapies in Pancreatic Cancer*, DOI 10.1007/978-3-319-58256-6_8

Early Detection of Pancreatic Malignancy

High-Risk Pancreatic Cancer Screening

Due to the rising prevalence of pancreatic cancer and the limited treatment options for patients with pancreatic cancer, there is an increasing emphasis on the value of pancreatic cancer screening. As no simple blood tests or other noninvasive tests currently exist for the effective early detection of both pancreatic cancer and its early preinvasive forms (so-called PanIN lesions), current screening studies have focused on combination of high-quality noninvasive imaging with CT or MRI with endoscopic ultrasound [4]. Most studies have targeted groups of patients considered to be at increased risk of developing pancreatic cancer such as familial pancreatic cancer kindred (FPC, defined as having two or more first-degree relatives with pancreatic cancer) or those with specific genetic mutations or syndromes such as a BRCA2 or BRCA1 mutations [5]. Typically EUS has been shown to be as sensitive as MRI for the diagnosis of pancreatic cysts, likely IPMNs, in these patients with the added advantage of being able to image chronic pancreatitis-like changes in the pancreatic parenchyma [6]. Chronic pancreatitis-like change seen on EUS imaging in individuals with FPC has been associated with lobulocentric atrophy and may be a marker for multifocal PanIN lesions [7]. EUS findings including heterogeneous parenchyma, hypoechoic nodules, hyperechoic main duct walls, and discrete masses have a high positive predictive value for PanIN in high-risk individuals [7, 8]. Current consensus recommendations favor the use of alternating MRI and EUS for screening of high-risk patients, although the true outcome of this approach is still unclear [5]. The use of endoscopy and endoscopic ultrasound in these patients also allows for the collection of pancreatic juice for the assay of early detection biomarkers such as K-ras, GNAS, P53, and SMAD4 mutations [9, 10].

Pancreatic Cyst Evaluation

Incidental pancreatic cysts are increasingly diagnosed through the widespread use of cross-sectional imaging. The clinical differential ranges from benign pseudocysts and serous cystadenomas to premalignant or even malignant mucinous lesions such as mucinous cystic neoplasm (MCN) and intraductal papillary mucinous neoplasm (IPMN) [11, 12]. While the majority of these lesions, including the majority of mucinous lesion, will not evolve into a pancreatic malignancy, detailed clinical and radiologic evaluation is necessary not only to help separate out the mucinous from the non-mucinous cysts but also to differentiate concerning mucinous lesions which may require surgical management from those which will require just surveillance alone [11]. For example, patients with presumed mucinous lesions with jaundice, a solid component on noninvasive imaging, or a pancreatic duct greater than 10 mm in diameter are at high risk of having malignancy and will likely require surgical management [13, 14]. Endoscopic ultrasound can be useful in this group of patients to confirm the diagnosis and the extent of the disease. For patients with presumed mucinous lesions with worrisome features (cyst size > 3 cm, main pancreatic duct diameter between 5 and 9 mm, rapidly enlarging cyst and/or abrupt change in caliber of the main pancreatic duct), EUS can be helpful in further evaluating for evidence of malignancy [13, 14]. Even in groups of patients with mucinous lesions who are considered to be low risk for malignancy, long-term surveillance is often performed using a combination of both MRI and EUS imaging.

Evaluation of Pancreatic Masses

Diagnosis and Differential Diagnosis

EUS is useful in the detection and evaluation of pancreatic masses, especially very small masses (ranging in size from 0.5 cm to 2 cm). In patients with suspected pancreatic masses (e.g., jaundice, chronic pancreatitis [15], increased PET-FDG imaging uptake) but no definite masses on cross-sectional images such as CT or MRI, endoscopic ultrasound has been shown to be very effective in identifying a focal mass often amenable to EUS biopsy for tissue confirmation [1]. EUS imaging alone can also be very effective in differentiating the etiology of pancreatic masses. For example, pancreatic adenocarcinoma is typically irregular and hypoechoic, compared with normal surrounding pancreatic parenchyma, whereas a pancreatic endocrine neoplasm is typically more well circumscribed and normoechoic. While patients with chronic pancreatitis are at increased risk of developing pancreatic cancer, it is often very difficult to differentiate between mass-forming pancreatitis and pancreatic cancer, due to the irregular heterogeneous nature of the surrounding chronic pancreatitis. Some EUS features (e.g., less severe main pancreatic duct dilatation, a more irregular main pancreatic duct, and more dilated side branches) favor a diagnosis of mass-forming chronic pancreatitis with features favoring malignancy including size larger than 2 cm, vessel ingrowth, an absence of cystic spaces, and an absence of diffuse pancreatitis, vascular involvement, and enlarged lymph nodes [2, 15, 16].

Similarly autoimmune pancreatitis, a specific form of chronic pancreatitis which is typically responsive to steroids, may present as a focal mass which can be difficult to differentiate from pancreatic ductal adenocarcinoma [17]. Although the EUS features in AIP show characteristic features such as echo-poor pancreatic parenchyma with echogenic interlobular septa, a thickened border (in the diffuse type), as well as more lobularity and hyperechoic pancreatic duct margin detected at a higher frequency in early stage compared with advanced stage AIP, it is generally accepted that one cannot rely entirely on EUS imaging to make a diagnosis and differentiate from pancreatic cancer [18]. Whereas tissue diagnosis is the gold standard, a variety of other clinical and imaging features (including EUS features) are often combined to make a diagnosis of AIP [19–21]. Other pancreatic masses which are difficult to easily confirm using EUS imaging alone and often require a tissue diagnosis include primary pancreatic lymphoma, microcystic serous cystadenoma (SCA), and metastases to the pancreas [22, 23].

Staging of Pancreatic Cancer

For patients with suspected or diagnosed pancreatic malignancy, EUS can be very effective in tumor staging and assessing the patient for surgical resectability. A recent meta-analysis reported a sensitivity of 71 vs. 67% for high-quality pancreatic CT vs. MRI in the staging of pancreatic cancer but with a relatively high specificity of 90% [24]. While currently the majority of pancreatic malignancy staging is performed with high-quality pancreatic CT or MRI, EUS can still be very helpful in assisting with vascular staging (e.g., portal vein, SMA, SMV involvement) in patients with small masses, inflammation, or poor-quality imaging studies and especially in patients who are not candidates for contrast-enhanced CT or MR [24–27]. Overall EUS has been reported to have a higher sensitivity for diagnosing portal vein and portal confluence invasion, especially when certain EUS features such as visualization of tumor in the vessel lumen, complete obstruction, or collateral vessels are present. In addition to assessment of vessel involvement, perivascular cuffing, malignant-appearing lymph nodes, and liver masses may be evaluated with EUS-FNA to provide more objective information for staging [28]. With the increasing use of neoadjuvant treatment strategies for clearly resectable, borderline, and even locally advanced pancreatic cancer, there is a need for more accurate staging after treatment to guide surgical resection decision. Often regular staging with non-invasive imaging after treatment is less accurate than in treatment naïve patients [29, 30]. Increasingly, EUS is used to assist in the preoperative evaluation of this subgroup of patients with pancreatic cancer [31].

Tissue Diagnosis

EUS-Fine Needle Aspiration

Whereas EUS imaging is very sensitive to diagnose pancreatic malignancy, (about 95%) it is not specific. Prior to the advent of EUS, pancreatic cancer tissue diagnosis was done either at the time of surgical exploration or by bile duct brushings at ERCP or by percutaneous biopsy using either abdominal ultrasound guidance or CT guidance. ERCP brushing biopsy has a sensitivity of 20–71% in the diagnosis of pancreatic malignancy [32]. However, EUS-FNA (fine needle aspiration) biopsy has now typically replaced these methods as the test of choice for primary pancreatic tissue diagnosis [33]. Meta-analyses have shown a pooled sensitivity of between 85 and 87% and a specificity of 96–98% for EUS-FNA in diagnosing pancreatic cancer [3, 34].

EUS-FNA refers to techniques used to acquire tissue primarily for cytologic evaluation, and EUS-FNAB (fine needle biopsy) refers to techniques used to acquire tissue for histologic evaluation. Both are performed using a linear echoendoscope. Typically, the linear echoendoscope needs to be positioned in the second and third portion of the duodenum to biopsy uncinate lesions, in the second portion and the duodenal bulb for pancreatic head and neck lesions, and in the stomach for pancreatic neck, body, and tail lesions. Apposition between the linear echoendoscope and either the gastric or duodenal wall is necessary with continuous endoscopic suction to decrease the amount of air intervening and so improving the EUS imaging. Under direct EUS guidance, a needle may be passed into the target lesion within the pancreas, with fanning recommended through at least four different areas to sample most pancreatic masses [35, 36]. A variety of different gauge needles are available for EUS-FNA ranging in size from 25 gauge to 19 gauge. Most endosonographers use either a 25G or a 22G needle, and although there has been conflicting information about the yield, it is felt that the smaller needle is more easily passed through desmoplastic tissue and induces less bleeding.

The recognized benefits of EUS-FNA in the evaluation of pancreatic masses include its high yield compared with alternative methods of diagnosis, the ability to detect small lesions, a low risk of seeding, and the overall cost-effectiveness. Although no definitive randomized clinical trial data exist, EUS-FNA does appear to be superior after nondiagnostic CT-guided biopsy or ERCP with cytologic brushing [37, 38]. The theoretical benefit of EUS in detecting and so biopsying small pancreatic masses less than 2 cm has been borne out by several large studies showing the superior accuracy of EUS-FNA compared with either CT-FNA or abdominal ultrasound FNA for pancreatic masses less than 3 cm (86 vs. 62%) and even for masses not seen on multidetector CT [39, 40]. This is then in the setting of decreased risk and clinical significance of peritoneal seeding associated with EUS-FNA compared with percutaneous biopsy in patients with pancreatic masses (2.2 vs. 16.3%) [41]. Overall, EUS-FNA of pancreatic masses is considered very safe with an overall pancreatitis risk rate between 0.3 and 0.9% and overall complication rate of 2.5%. These are compared with high rates of pancreatitis of up to 4% with percutaneous biopsies and between 5 and15% for ERCP-guided biopsies [42, 43]. EUS-FNA biopsy of the pancreas in the diagnosis can result in less invasive additional procedures and more cost-effective management of pancreatic cancer, especially by avoiding unnecessary surgeries [44, 45].

EUS-FNA remains operator dependent with a very significant learning curve, requiring additional focused training [46]. Sampling error due to pancreatic cancer desmoplastic reaction and necrosis, especially in aggressive tumors, is associated with the suboptimal performance of EUS-FNA. The use of rapid on-site cytology evaluation, whereby pathologists present during the EUS-FNA procedure advise about adequacy and diagnosis, results in improved overall accuracy, fewer needle passes necessary to make a diagnosis, and decreased need for repeat diagnostic procedures [47, 48]. Several studies have shown a decreased sensitivity of EUS in identification of pancreatic malignant masses in the setting of chronic pancreatitis due to the difficulty in distinguishing the mass from the surrounding abnormal pancreatic parenchyma [48]. In addition, however, EUS-FNA has a lower sensitivity between 53 and 71% in the setting of chronic pancreatitis even when additional passes and the use of an on-site cytologist [49, 50]. Although original studies seem to suggest the inferior diagnostic yields of EUS and EUS-FNA in the diagnosis of other nonadenocarcinoma such as PNET, lymphoma, and metastatic lesions to the pancreas, most recent work seems to suggest a higher sensitivity comparable to that seen in pancreatic ductal adenocarcinoma probably related to the use of ROSE and special cytologic stains [51].

EUS-Fine Needle Biopsy

The current diagnostic yield for EUS-FNA cytology of pancreatic masses is high, better than for non-pancreatic indications, but not perfect [52–56]. There are several reasons for the suboptimal diagnostic results including variable operator-dependent EUS imaging and technique, the lack of local available cytologic expertise, poor specimen cellularity, and lack of detail on the tissue architecture and morphology. This latter issue is particularly problematic for separating out well-differentiated pancreatic ductal adenocarcinoma from normal pancreatic tissue, as well as trying to diagnose pancreatic malignancy in the setting of chronic pancreatitis [49, 57]. Often there is just not enough tissue with EUS-FNA for additional ancillary studies, leading to lack of a definite diagnosis and the need for repeat tissue acquisition. Trying to make a diagnosis using hypocellular samples is a common cause for a false diagnosis.

Hence, there are several potential and theoretical benefits to endoscopically pursuing a pancreatic histology or core biopsy (EUS-FNB). Firstly, the ability to assess tissue architecture may improve the ability to diagnose well-differentiated pancreatic adenocarcinoma where the cytologic findings (lack of the typical hyperchromasia of malignancy, minimal architectural disorder, and modestly increased nuclear-cytoplasmic ratios) may be similar to normal appearing pancreas and malignancy in the setting of chronic pancreatitis. The second reason to consider a core biopsy for histology is the need to get a more representative sample of the pancreatic mass. For example, due to the dense stromal proliferation seen in pancreatic ductal adenocarcinoma, it is possible that core histologic tissue would allow for further study of the stroma which is typically not commented on or assessed during regular pancreatic FNA cytology. Another reason to pursue histologic tissue is to allow for immunohistochemistry or additional marker studies. With our increased understanding of the molecular basis for pancreatic disease, and the role in which molecular markers (e.g., protein, DNA, or RNA based) may be helpful in making a diagnosis, such as separating primary pancreatic ductal adenocarcinoma from similar-looking metastases to the pancreas, or even predicting a response to treatment, there is a need for greater volumes of tissue which can be processed in the appropriate way to study and quantify these markers. While this may be possible with cytology, the specimens are typically small, and quantitation of immunocytochemistry markers is difficult if there is limited cytologic specimen. A histologic core of tissue allows the pathologist to obtain several sections for IHC analysis and likely quantitate the tissue-based marker used. Under these circumstances, both stroma and epithelial markers may be assessed [58, 59]. In addition, the ability to microdissect out epithelial tissue may facilitate more accurate DNA or RNA analysis of the pancreatic specimen, through being able to identify the cell-based origin of the marker in question [60]. Finally, it is possible that with the known limitation of EUS-FNA cytology, the availability of reliable pancreatic histologic biopsy and core biopsy may remove the need for on-site cytologic evaluation and multiple FNA needle passes.

Whether using a regular FNA needle or a dedicated FNAB needle, there are some similarities between the EUS-FNA and EUS-FNB needle biopsy technique. A variety of dedicated needles ranging in sizes from19 G to 25 G are available including a standard spring-loaded Trucut needle. While no direct comparison exists between all the different needle types, both needle size and processing of the specimens all play an important role in improving yield and diagnosis. Whereas the relative merits of one needle size over another, the use of suction over no suction, and the use of a stylet have been evaluated in detail for regular EUS-FNA, currently there is no randomized comparative data for EUS-FNB available to address these questions. One study suggests that size does matter when it comes to histologic yield with one study showing the histologic yield of the 19G "ProCore" needle is 89.5% compared with 82.5 and 63% for the 22G and 25G "ProCore" needles, respectively [57]. Recently published data has reported an overall diagnostic accuracy of 96% using a 25G "ProCore" needle and a "slow pull" or "capillary technique," compared with the published literature using standard suction which reported a yield of 89% [61, 62].

A variety of additional strategies exist to overcome the current limitation of both EUS and EUS-FNA or EUS-FNB. The use of contrast-enhanced EUS and EUS elastography are two new supplemental imaging technologies which may improve diagnostic yield of EUS imaging and help target EUS-FNA and EUS-FNB more precisely. Contrast-enhanced EUS employs oscillation of microbubbles using ultrasound waves after injection of intravenous contrast containing microbubbles to enhance imaging of lesions associated with hypervascular structures such as endocrine neoplasms. EUS elastography uses assessment of tissue stiffness to help differentiate between malignant and nonmalignant masses [63]. In addition, a variety of molecular markers including immunocytochemical markers, FISH analysis, DNA mutational analysis including whole exome sequencing, and microRNA analysis have been proposed to improve the diagnostic yield of EUS-FNA cytology, but most are not in routine clinical use [64].

EUS-Guided Interventions

EUS-Celiac Plexus Neurolysis (EUS-CPN)

EUS-guided celiac nerve block is now a well-accepted treatment for the management of pain associated with pancreatic cancer. While similar in technique to either CT or fluoroscopically guided plexus neurolysis, the ability of the EUS linear echoendoscope to accurately identify the celiac plexus and directly guide injection with a local anesthetic (e.g., bupivacaine) and alcohol makes this an easy and safe alternative to standard pain management [65, 66]. A meta-analysis of 119 patients showed the success rate for EUS-guided plexus neurolysis (EUS-CPN) in managing pain in patients with pancreatic cancer of 72% [67]. EUS-guided direct celiac ganglion injection has also been used for the management of pain, but its superiority is unclear [68]. In one small study, positive and complete response rates were significantly higher in the EUS-guided direct celiac ganglia neurolysis group than in the EUS-CPN group [68].

EUS-Fine Needle Injection

EUS-fine needle injection (EUS-FNI) refers using EUS for direct injection or implantation into the pancreas. The use of EUS-guided fiducial marker implantation to help guide stereotactic body radiation therapy (SBRT) is now currently routinely performed. Fiducial markers are radiopaque seeds which can be placed with a 19G or 22G needle with technical success rates of 85–100% and without serious complications. They are implanted in or near the tumor to demarcate its border and facilitate image-guided radiation therapy and so minimize unnecessary radiation to healthy-bordering tissue [69–72].

EUS-guided tattooing of the pancreas is also now increasingly used clinically. With improved invasive and noninvasive imaging, ever-small pancreatic adenocarcinomas and other neoplasms, especially PNETs, are being identified. To assist with perioperative localization, often as these operations are being performed laparoscopically, EUS-guided tattooing using India ink, indocyanine green, and carbon particles is often employed [73–75]. This may be performed several weeks prior to surgical management due to the chronicity of the tattoo.

EUS-guided interventions have now also emerged as management and treatment options for patients with pancreatic cancer. A variety of direct injection treatments have been performed experimentally in humans including alcohol, gemcitabine, paclitaxel (OncoGel), oncolytic adenovirus (ONYX-015), and immunoreactive agents such as cytoplants, dendritic cells, and TNFerade. Whereas alcohol injection has been most studied for the management of symptomatic nonoperable insulinomas, the most widely studied EUS-FNI treatment for pancreatic cancer was TNFerade in a multicenter randomized clinical trial for patients with locally advanced pancreatic cancer [76–78]. While safe with multiple repeat injections, it was not shown to be more effective than standard treatment [76]. EUS-guided ablations with more directed treatments such as radiofrequency ablation and brachytherapy implantation have also been tried in patients with pancreatic cancer. There are at least two clinical studies of the role of EUS implantation of iodine-125 under EUS guidance for unresectable pancreatic cancer in combination with chemotherapy. Both studies of EUS-guided brachytherapy showed an improvement in pain symptoms but not overall survival [79, 80].

EUS-Guided Biliary Drainage

Finally, although percutaneous transhepatic biliary drainage or surgical decompression is typically formed for biliary drainage after a failed ERCP, there is increasing data supporting the safety and efficacy of EUS-guided biliary drainage as an alternative, especially in the 3–10% of patients with pancreatic cancer who cannot undergo ERCP biliary decompression, typically due to tumor infiltration in the region of the ampulla. These techniques include EUS-guided rendezvous technique, EUS-guided choledochoduodenostomy, EUS-guided hepaticogastrostomy, and even EUS-guided gallbladder drainage. Typically, either a dilated extrahepatic biliary duct or intrahepatic duct radicle is identified and accessed with a needle under direct EUS guidance. After the tract is dilated, a fully covered metal biliary stent or lumen-apposing stent can be deployed for biliary drainage. Technical success rates for this procedure are quoted at over 90%, but it is associated with a 5–10% risk of complications including bile leak and perforation, requiring that this be performed at expert centers [81, 82].

Endoscopic Retrograde Cholangiopancreatography

Diagnosis

ERCP involves the passage of a flexible duodenoscope to the level of the major ampulla, and cannulating either the bile duct or pancreatic duct (or both), using specialized catheters. Through a combination of endoscopic and fluoroscopic imaging, ERCP can provide very detailed images of both the biliary and pancreatic ductal systems. For example, a "double duct" sign on ERCP with stricturing and dilatation involving both the bile duct and the pancreatic duct is caused by pancreatic malignancy in up to 90% of patients. The sensitivity and specificity of the "double duct sign" observed by ERCP for pancreatic cancer vary between 50–76% and 63–80%, respectively [83].

However, ERCP is also associated with significant risks, especially pancreatitis. For this reason and due to the increasing use of EUS for the effective cytologic diagnosis of pancreatic malignancy, there has been a decrease in the use of pure diagnostic ERCP [84]. In view of its therapeutic possibilities, it still does play a role in tissue diagnosis, especially in the setting of obstructive jaundice in the setting of a known or suspected pancreatic mass, where ERCP-guided biliary stent placement is likely for management of obstructive jaundice. Under these circumstances, ERCP is capable of cytologic sampling via brush cytology, forceps biopsy, and/or needle aspiration. Typically, the yield of cytologic brushing of a biliary stricture for the diagnosis of pancreatic cancer is around 56% with a specificity of 90%. The sensitivity of all three cytological sampling methods is 62% with a negative predictive value of 39% [85]. The results are typically higher for malignancy of bile duct origin rather than malignancy [86]. Pancreatic duct stricture brushings are not recommended routinely due to the high risk of complication.

The increasing availability of reliable high-quality ERCP-guided cholangioscopy and pancreatoscopy has increased the role for diagnostic ERCP [87]. For indeterminate biliary strictures (those without an associated pancreatic mass on imaging), cholangioscopic targeted biopsies have an increased diagnostic yield. Although typically not performed during the routine evaluation of pancreatic cancer, ERCP-guided pancreatoscopy may have a role in the diagnosis and staging of a premalignant pancreatic main duct lesion, IPMN. The direct visualization and biopsy of papillary fronds associated with this disease can be helpful in confirming the diagnosis.

Biliary Decompression

Whereas ERCP has a decreasing diagnostic role in pancreatic malignancy (due to the advent of improve CT and MRI, as well as endoscopic ultrasound), it does play a critical role in palliative treatment, especially for patients with unresectable pancreatic malignancy, through biliary stent placement for obstructive jaundice. However, its role in preoperative drainage for potentially resectable pancreatic malignancy is unclear.

The technical success of biliary stenting by ERCP is over 90%. As the majority of pancreatic cancers present in the head of the pancreas, and the majority of these will present with obstructive jaundice, often resulting in progressive liver dysfunction, pruritus, coagulopathy, and malabsorption, biliary decompression becomes an important treatment goal. As only up to 15% of these patients are potentially surgical resection candidates, the majority of them then rely on some form of biliary decompression. Endoscopic biliary decompression has been shown to be less invasive, safer, and more convenient than surgical bypass. Especially for patients with unresectable pancreatic malignancy, it is important in maintaining quality of life and continued medical treatments such as chemotherapy.

Type of Biliary Stents

Initially, plastic biliary stents were used ranging in sizes from 7 to 11.5Fr, with the increasing diameter being associated with less stent occlusion. Studies have demonstrated the superiority of biliary stenting with these plastic stents compared with surgical biliary decompression with fewer complications, shorter hospital stays, and lower costs [88–90]. The development of endoscopic biliary self-expandable metal stents (SEMS) offers larger diameter which is associated with reduced risk of occlusion and longer duration of patency. The original biliary SEMS were uncovered which were associated with tumor ingrowth (and associated occlusion) and were not easily removed (if needs be). More recently partially covered and now fully covered biliary SEMS are associated with less tumor ingrowth and are considered to be more easily removed. However, there have been concerns about increased rates of cholecystitis (related to cystic duct occlusion), pancreatitis (related to pancreatic duct obstruction), and migration, with these covered biliary SEMS.

Multiple studies including a meta-analysis of several RCTs comparing plastic stenting with uncovered SEMS, while showing no significant difference in technical success, therapeutic success rates, or 30-day mortality or complication rate, did show a lower 4-month stent occlusion rate and overall risk of obstruction for uncovered SEMS compared with plastic stent [91]. Although the cost of the SEMS and the ERCP procedure itself influence the analysis, several studies suggest that uncovered SEMS are more cost-effective if the patient's life expectancy is longer than 4–6 months [91, 92].

As tumor ingrowth is a major reason for early occlusion in uncovered SEMS, SEMS covered with a membrane either fully or partially were developed to address this issue. One meta-analysis comprising 1061 patients showed no difference in patency between covered and uncovered SEMS after 6 and 12 months and no difference in rates of pancreatitis, cholecystitis, perforation, bleeding, cholangitis, length of hospital stay, or number of recurrent biliary obstruction [93]. However, covered SEMS did have a higher migration rate (OR 7.13; 95% CI 0.07–0.55) and a higher rate of tumor overgrowth (OR 1.88, 95% CI 1.02–3.45). Another meta-analysis on five fully published RCT comprising 781 patients showed that while stent dysfunction occurred at a similar rate, there is a trend toward later obstruction with the covered SEMS [94] which also have a significantly longer patency duration and lower frequency of blockage from tumor ingrowth compared with U-SEMS. Although there was no difference in the rates of pancreatitis and cholecystitis between covered SEMS and uncovered SEMS in this analysis, the rate of stent migration, tumor ingrowth, and sludge formation were all significantly higher in the covered SEMS groups. Overall, the clinical decision-making about deciding which type of biliary stent to use needs to balance the risks of migration but ability to reintervene if necessary and replace the biliary stents with the likely improved patency rates due to less tumor ingrowth of covered SEMS.

Preoperative Biliary Drainage

For patients with clearly resectable pancreatic malignancy, the role of preoperative biliary drainage remains controversial. Clinical and experimental data had long supported the concept that preoperative hyperbilirubinemia predicted increased postoperative complications, possibly related to affecting nutritional status and immune function. In fact, early studies suggested that there was a link between increased levels of serum bilirubin and an increased incidence of postoperative infectious, renal, and nutritional complications as well as postoperative mortality [95]. However, more recently, several studies including a randomized controlled trial suggested that preoperative biliary drainage should be avoided in patients with potentially resectable pancreatic cancer because it is associated with increased morbidity [96]. This multicenter randomized clinical trial compared outcomes of preoperative biliary drainage in a group of patients with clearly resectable disease and those who underwent early surgery and did not have preoperative drainage. The technical success of the preoperative endoscopic biliary drainage was successful in 94% but with a very high complication rate of 46% including stent occlusion and cholangitis. The overall rate of postsurgical complications was similar, but the rate of serious postoperative complications was significantly higher in the preoperative biliary drainage group [96]. This has then been further supported by a meta-analysis of six RCTs to compare the outcomes of surgery done for biliary obstruction with and without preoperative biliary decompression which demonstrated significantly higher levels of serious postoperative morbidity in the preoperative biliary drainage group compared with the direct surgery group but without a significant difference in terms of postoperative mortality or length of hospitalization [97]. However, it needs to be remembered that many of these studies did not include patients with marked hyperbilirubinemia. For example, in the RCT by van der Gaag, patients with severe jaundice (total bilirubin >14.6 mg/dL) were excluded from the study [96]. Therefore, the role of preoperative biliary drainage in patients with marked jaundice is unclear. Overall, if the patient is severely jaundiced, or symptomatic with, for example, pruritus, or surgery needs to be delayed to optimize medical comorbidities or to administer neoadjuvant therapy, then preoperative biliary drainage may well be justified.

Role of Biliary Stenting in Neoadjuvant Treatment of Pancreatic Cancer

With evolving data supporting neoadjuvant chemo- or chemoradiation therapy for potentially resectable patients with pancreatic cancer resulting in improved postsurgical outcomes, and its increasing role in borderline resectable pancreatic cancer, the role for preoperative biliary decompression in this subgroup of patients is becoming better defined [98]. Reliable biliary drainage is required to prevent liver toxicity from some of the chemotherapeutic agents used, which may be required for a period of up to 3 months, before surgery is contemplated. For patients with resectable pancreatic cancer with anticipated surgical resection in less than 3 months, the placement of a plastic biliary stent has often been deemed adequate. The advent of newer neoadjuvant treatment for locally advanced and borderline resectable patients now requires at least 3–4 months of treatment before the patient is reassessed for surgical management. These patients also require increased assurance of prolonged biliary drainage to avoid interruption of medical treatment due to episodes of biliary obstruction or cholangitis. Hence, it does seem reasonable to consider the use of SEMS in this group. However, this is balanced by the issue of cost and the embedding of these stents in the biliary tissue making their removal at surgery more difficult. SEMS have also been associated with the development of a hyperplastic reaction which may interfere with surgical resection, although there is growing evidence that the use of properly placed covered SEMS (due to the ability to prevent tumor ingrowth and hyperplasia, and so be removed easily) do not result in increased operative or postoperative complications [99, 100].

Gastric Outlet Obstruction

Approximately 15–20% of patients with pancreatic cancer develop GOO [101–103]. Clinical symptoms of GOO include vomiting, nausea, malnutrition, and dehydration. Most patients with GOO are therefore in a poor clinical condition at presentation and have a short life expectancy if left untreated [104, 105]. Traditionally, open gastrojejunostomy (GJJ) has been the standard palliative treatment in these patients. Laparoscopic GJJ has been introduced as an alternative to open GJJ to relieve symptoms of malignant GOO. Laparoscopic GJJ has been reported to be less invasive and was associated with a faster recovery compared to open GJJ; however, morbidity and mortality of the procedure remained high [103, 105–107].

Enteral stent placement is an attractive alternative treatment [108–111]. It typically involves the placement of a wire across the malignant stricture, followed by a through-the-scope deployment of either a covered or uncovered stent typically ranging in diameter from 18 to 22 mm and in length from 60 to 120 mm. In the case of pancreatic malignancy, often both biliary stenting and duodenal stenting are required. The technical challenges for this are dependent on the level of the duodenal obstruction. If the level of duodenal obstruction is proximal to the major papilla, often passage of the duodenoscope through the duodenal stricture is possible (often with dilatation), in order to perform biliary stenting prior to placement of the duodenal stent. Other approaches in this setting include placement of a duodenal stent followed either immediately or after a few days by advancement of the duodenoscope through the duodenal stent for placement of the biliary stent. Alternatively, EUS-guided biliary drainage or a percutaneous biliary decompression may be necessary. When the obstruction in the second duodenum also involves the major papilla, it can be very difficult to place a biliary stent by ERCP. Under these circumstances, a duodenal stent is placed followed by either EUS-guided biliary drainage via a hepaticojejunostomy or choledochoduodenostomy or percutaneous biliary drainage. For the scenario of duodenal obstruction distal to the papilla, the sequence of placement of both the duodenal and biliary stent is not critical.

Several studies have demonstrated that SEMS placement is associated with faster resumption of oral intake, shorter post procedural hospital stays, lesser morbidity, and lower costs compared with gastrojejunostomy [75, 112–114]. In a systemic review, we compared the outcome of GJJ with that of duodenal stent placement [115]. A total of 44 studies were selected including only 2 randomized trials (with 27 and 18 patients) [116, 117]. A total of 1046 patients received a duodenal stent, which, in most cases, was an uncovered enteral metal stent, with a stent diameter of 20–24 mm, whereas 297 patients underwent GJJ. This review showed that initial clinical success was higher after stent placement (89% vs. 72%). Major complication rates were however similar (early, 7 vs. 6%, respectively, and late, 18 vs. 17%, respectively). Recurrent obstructive symptoms were more commonly seen after stent placement, whereas hospital stay was shorter after stent placement. The results of this review suggested that stent placement is associated with more favorable results in patients with a relatively short life expectancy, while GJJ is preferable in patients with a better prognosis [115].

References

1. DeWitt J, et al. Comparison of endoscopic ultrasonography and multidetector computed tomography for detecting and staging pancreatic cancer. Ann Intern Med. 2004;141(10):753–63.
2. Brand B, et al. Endoscopic ultrasound for differential diagnosis of focal pancreatic lesions, confirmed by surgery. Scand J Gastroenterol. 2000;35(11):1221–8.
3. Hewitt MJ, et al. EUS-guided FNA for diagnosis of solid pancreatic neoplasms: a meta-analysis. Gastrointest Endosc. 2012;75(2):319–31.
4. Chari ST, et al. Early detection of sporadic pancreatic cancer: summative review. Pancreas. 2015;44(5):693–712.
5. Canto MI, et al. International cancer of the pancreas screening (CAPS) consortium summit on the management of patients with increased risk for familial pancreatic cancer. Gut. 2013;62(3):339–47.
6. Canto MI, et al. Frequent detection of pancreatic lesions in asymptomatic high-risk individuals. Gastroenterology. 2012;142(4):796–804. quiz e14-5
7. Brune K, et al. Multifocal neoplastic precursor lesions associated with lobular atrophy of the pancreas in patients having a strong family history of pancreatic cancer. Am J Surg Pathol. 2006;30(9):1067–76.
8. Brentnall TA, et al. Early diagnosis and treatment of pancreatic dysplasia in patients with a family history of pancreatic cancer. Ann Intern Med. 1999;131(4):247–55.
9. Kanda M, et al. Mutant GNAS detected in duodenal collections of secretin-stimulated pancreatic juice indicates the presence or emergence of pancreatic cysts. Gut. 2013;62(7):1024–33.
10. Eshleman JR, et al. KRAS and guanine nucleotide-binding protein mutations in pancreatic juice collected from the duodenum of patients at high risk for neoplasia undergoing endoscopic ultrasound. Clin Gastroenterol Hepatol. 2015;13(5):963–9. e4
11. Farrell JJ, Fernandez-del Castillo C. Pancreatic cystic neoplasms: management and unanswered questions. Gastroenterology. 2013;144(6):1303–15.
12. Farrell JJ. Prevalence, diagnosis and Management of Pancreatic Cystic Neoplasms: current status and future directions. Gut Liver. 2015;9(5):571–89.
13. Tanaka M, et al. International consensus guidelines 2012 for the management of IPMN and MCN of the pancreas. Pancreatology. 2012;12(3):183–97.
14. Vege SS, et al. American gastroenterological association institute guideline on the diagnosis and management of asymptomatic neoplastic pancreatic cysts. Gastroenterology. 2015;148(4):819–22. quize12-3
15. Perez-Johnston R, Sainani NI, Sahani DV. Imaging of chronic pancreatitis (including groove and autoimmune pancreatitis). Radiol Clin N Am. 2012;50(3):447–66.
16. Rosch T, et al. Endoscopic ultrasound in pancreatic tumor diagnosis. Gastrointest Endosc. 1991;37(3):347–52.
17. Madhani K, Farrell JJ. Autoimmune pancreatitis: an update on diagnosis and management. Gastroenterol Clin N Am. 2016;45(1):29–43.
18. Takuma K, et al. Strategy to differentiate autoimmune pancreatitis from pancreas cancer. World J Gastroenterol. 2012;18(10):1015–20.
19. Kubota K, et al. A proposal for differentiation between early- and advanced-stage autoimmune pancreatitis by endoscopic ultrasonography. Dig Endosc. 2009;21(3):162–9.
20. Farrell JJ, et al. EUS findings in patients with autoimmune pancreatitis. Gastrointest Endosc. 2004;60(6):927–36.
21. Buscarini E, et al. Endoscopic ultrasonography findings in autoimmune pancreatitis. World J Gastroenterol. 2011;17(16):2080–5.
22. El H II, et al. Endoscopic ultrasound-guided biopsy of pancreatic metastases: a large single-center experience. Pancreas. 2013;42(3):524–30.
23. DeWitt J, et al. EUS-guided FNA of pancreatic metastases: a multicenter experience. Gastrointest Endosc. 2005;61(6):689–96.

24. Zhang Y, et al. Preoperative vascular evaluation with computed tomography and magnetic resonance imaging for pancreatic cancer: a meta-analysis. Pancreatology. 2012;12(3):227–33.
25. Brugge WR, et al. The use of EUS to diagnose malignant portal venous system invasion by pancreatic cancer. Gastrointest Endosc. 1996;43(6):561–7.
26. Rosch T, et al. Endoscopic ultrasound criteria for vascular invasion in the staging of cancer of the head of the pancreas: a blind reevaluation of videotapes. Gastrointest Endosc. 2000;52(4):469–77.
27. Dewitt J, et al. Comparison of endoscopic ultrasound and computed tomography for the preoperative evaluation of pancreatic cancer: a systematic review. Clin Gastroenterol Hepatol. 2006;4(6):717–25. quiz 664
28. tenBerge J, et al. EUS-guided fine needle aspiration of the liver: indications, yield, and safety based on an international survey of 167 cases. Gastrointest Endosc. 2002;55(7):859–62.
29. Wagner M, et al. CT evaluation after neoadjuvant FOLFIRINOX chemotherapy for borderline and locally advanced pancreatic adenocarcinoma. Eur Radiol. 2017;27(7):3104–16.
30. Xia, B.T., et al., Does radiologic response correlate to pathologic response in patients undergoing neoadjuvant therapy for borderline respectable pancreatic malignancy? J Surg Oncol, 2017; 115(4):376–383.
31. Donahue TR, et al. Downstaging chemotherapy and alteration in the classic computed tomography/magnetic resonance imaging signs of vascular involvement in patients with pancreaticobiliary malignant tumors: influence on patient selection for surgery. Arch Surg. 2011;146(7):836–43.
32. Lee JG, Leung J. Tissue sampling at ERCP in suspected pancreatic cancer. Gastrointest Endosc Clin N Am. 1998;8(1):221–35.
33. Wiersema MJ, et al. Endosonography-guided fine-needle aspiration biopsy: diagnostic accuracy and complication assessment. Gastroenterology. 1997;112(4):1087–95.
34. Puli SR, et al. How good is endoscopic ultrasound-guided fine-needle aspiration in diagnosing the correct etiology for a solid pancreatic mass?: a meta-analysis and systematic review. Pancreas. 2013;42(1):20–6.
35. Savides TJ. Tricks for improving EUS-FNA accuracy and maximizing cellular yield. Gastrointest Endosc. 2009;69(2 Suppl):S130–3.
36. Varadarajulu S, Bang JY, Hebert-Magee S. Assessment of the technical performance of the flexible 19-gauge EUS-FNA needle. Gastrointest Endosc. 2012;76(2):336–43.
37. Harewood GC, Wiersema MJ. Endosonography-guided fine needle aspiration biopsy in the evaluation of pancreatic masses. Am J Gastroenterol. 2002;97(6):1386–91.
38. Horwhat JD, et al. A randomized comparison of EUS-guided FNA versus CT or US-guided FNA for the evaluation of pancreatic mass lesions. Gastrointest Endosc. 2006;63(7):966–75.
39. Volmar KE, et al. Pancreatic FNA in 1000 cases: a comparison of imaging modalities. Gastrointest Endosc. 2005;61(7):854–61.
40. Wang W, et al. Use of EUS-FNA in diagnosing pancreatic neoplasm without a definitive mass on CT. Gastrointest Endosc. 2013;78(1):73–80.
41. Micames C, et al. Lower frequency of peritoneal carcinomatosis in patients with pancreatic cancer diagnosed by EUS-guided FNA vs. percutaneous FNA. Gastrointest Endosc. 2003;58(5):690–5.
42. Eloubeidi MA, et al. Acute pancreatitis after EUS-guided FNA of solid pancreatic masses: a pooled analysis from EUS centers in the United States. Gastrointest Endosc. 2004;60(3):385–9.
43. Eloubeidi MA, et al. Frequency of major complications after EUS-guided FNA of solid pancreatic masses: a prospective evaluation. Gastrointest Endosc. 2006;63(4):622–9.
44. Tierney WM, et al. The clinical and economic impact of alternative staging strategies for adenocarcinoma of the pancreas. Am J Gastroenterol. 2000;95(7):1708–13.
45. Harewood GC, Wiersema MJ. A cost analysis of endoscopic ultrasound in the evaluation of pancreatic head adenocarcinoma. Am J Gastroenterol. 2001;96(9):2651–6.

46. Mertz H, Gautam S. The learning curve for EUS-guided FNA of pancreatic cancer. Gastrointest Endosc. 2004;59(1):33–7.
47. Klapman JB, et al. Clinical impact of on-site cytopathology interpretation on endoscopic ultrasound-guided fine needle aspiration. Am J Gastroenterol. 2003;98(6):1289–94.
48. Farrell JJ. Diagnosing pancreatic malignancy in the setting of chronic pancreatitis: is there room for improvement? Gastrointest Endosc. 2005;62(5):737–41.
49. Varadarajulu S, Tamhane A, Eloubeidi MA. Yield of EUS-guided FNA of pancreatic masses in the presence or the absence of chronic pancreatitis. Gastrointest Endosc. 2005;62(5):728–36; quiz 751, 753.
50. Fritscher-Ravens A, et al. Comparison of endoscopic ultrasound-guided fine needle aspiration for focal pancreatic lesions in patients with normal parenchyma and chronic pancreatitis. Am J Gastroenterol. 2002;97(11):2768–75.
51. Atiq M, et al. Role of endoscopic ultrasonography in evaluation of metastatic lesions to the pancreas: a tertiary cancer center experience. Pancreas. 2013;42(3):516–23.
52. Tharian B, et al. Endoscopic ultrasound fine needle aspiration: technique and applications in clinical practice. World J Gastrointest Endosc. 2012;4(12):532–44.
53. Varadarajulu S, Fockens P, Hawes RH. Best practices in endoscopic ultrasound-guided fine-needle aspiration. Clin Gastroenterol Hepatol. 2012;10(7):697–703.
54. Weston BR, Bhutani MS. Optimizing diagnostic yield for EUS-guided sampling of solid pancreatic lesions: a technical review. Gastroenterol Hepatol (N Y). 2013;9(6):352–63.
55. Polkowski M, et al. Learning, techniques, and complications of endoscopic ultrasound (EUS)-guided sampling in gastroenterology: European Society of Gastrointestinal Endoscopy (ESGE) technical guideline. Endoscopy. 2012;44(2):190–206.
56. Varadarajulu S, et al. Endoscopic ultrasound-guided tissue acquisition. Dig Endosc. 2014;26(Suppl 1):62–9.
57. Panic N, Larghi A. Techniques for endoscopic ultrasound-guided fine-needle biopsy. Gastrointest Endosc Clin N Am. 2014;24(1):83–107.
58. Donahue TR, et al. Stromal MicroRNA-21 levels predict response to 5-fluorouracil in patients with pancreatic cancer. J Surg Oncol. 2014;110(8):952–9.
59. Neuzillet C, et al. Stromal expression of SPARC in pancreatic adenocarcinoma. Cancer Metastasis Rev. 2013;32(3–4):585–602.
60. Simone NL, et al. Laser capture microdissection: beyond functional genomics to proteomics. Mol Diagn. 2000;5(4):301–7.
61. Larghi A, et al. Feasibility and yield of a novel 22-gauge histology EUS needle in patients with pancreatic masses: a multicenter prospective cohort study. Surg Endosc. 2013;27(10):3733–8.
62. Iwashita T, et al. High single-pass diagnostic yield of a new 25-gauge core biopsy needle for EUS-guided FNA biopsy in solid pancreatic lesions. Gastrointest Endosc. 2013;77(6):909–15.
63. Saftoiu A, et al. Neural network analysis of dynamic sequences of EUS elastography used for the differential diagnosis of chronic pancreatitis and pancreatic cancer. Gastrointest Endosc. 2008;68(6):1086–94.
64. Fuccio L, et al. The role of K-ras gene mutation analysis in EUS-guided FNA cytology specimens for the differential diagnosis of pancreatic solid masses: a meta-analysis of prospective studies. Gastrointest Endosc. 2013;78(4):596–608.
65. Luz LP, Al-Haddad MA, DeWitt JA. EUS-guided celiac plexus interventions in pancreatic cancer pain: an update and controversies for the endosonographer. Endosc Ultrasound. 2014;3(4):213–20.
66. Fujii-Lau LL, et al. Impact of celiac neurolysis on survival in patients with pancreatic cancer. Gastrointest Endosc. 2015;82(1):46–56. e2
67. Kaufman M, et al. Efficacy of endoscopic ultrasound-guided celiac plexus block and celiac plexus neurolysis for managing abdominal pain associated with chronic pancreatitis and pancreatic cancer. J Clin Gastroenterol. 2010;44(2):127–34.
68. Doi S, et al. Endoscopic ultrasound-guided celiac ganglia neurolysis vs. celiac plexus neurolysis: a randomized multicenter trial. Endoscopy. 2013;45(5):362–9.

69. DiMaio CJ, et al. EUS-guided fiducial placement for image-guided radiation therapy in GI malignancies by using a 22-gauge needle (with videos). Gastrointest Endosc. 2010;71(7):1204–10.
70. Pishvaian AC, et al. EUS-guided fiducial placement for CyberKnife radiotherapy of mediastinal and abdominal malignancies. Gastrointest Endosc. 2006;64(3):412–7.
71. Park WG, et al. EUS-guided gold fiducial insertion for image-guided radiation therapy of pancreatic cancer: 50 successful cases without fluoroscopy. Gastrointest Endosc. 2010;71(3):513–8.
72. Varadarajulu S, et al. The use of endoscopic ultrasound-guided gold markers in image-guided radiation therapy of pancreatic cancers: a case series. Endoscopy. 2010;42(5):423–5.
73. Farrell JJ, Sherrod A, Parekh D. EUS-guided fine-needle tattooing for preoperative localization of early pancreatic adenocarcinoma. Gastrointest Endosc. 2009;69(1):176–7.
74. Lennon AM, et al. EUS-guided tattooing before laparoscopic distal pancreatic resection (with video). Gastrointest Endosc. 2010;72(5):1089–94.
75. Larsen MH, Fristrup CW, Mortensen MB. Endoscopic ultrasound-guided fine-needle marking of a small pancreatic tumor. Endoscopy. 2009;41(Suppl 2):E175–6.
76. Hecht JR, et al. EUS or percutaneously guided intratumoral TNFerade biologic with 5-fluorouracil and radiotherapy for first-line treatment of locally advanced pancreatic cancer: a phase I/II study. Gastrointest Endosc. 2012;75(2):332–8.
77. Jurgensen C, et al. EUS-guided alcohol ablation of an insulinoma. Gastrointest Endosc. 2006;63(7):1059–62.
78. Levy MJ, et al. US-guided ethanol ablation of insulinomas: a new treatment option. Gastrointest Endosc. 2012;75(1):200–6.
79. Du YQ, Li ZS, Jin ZD. Endoscope-assisted brachytherapy for pancreatic cancer: from tumor killing to pain relief and drainage. J Interv Gastroenterol. 2011;1(1):23–7.
80. Jin Z, et al. Endoscopic ultrasonography-guided interstitial implantation of iodine 125-seeds combined with chemotherapy in the treatment of unresectable pancreatic carcinoma: a prospective pilot study. Endoscopy. 2008;40(4):314–20.
81. Poincloux L, et al. Endoscopic ultrasound-guided biliary drainage after failed ERCP: cumulative experience of 101 procedures at a single center. Endoscopy. 2015;47(9):794–801.
82. Weilert F. Prospective evaluation of simplified algorithm for EUS-guided intra-hepatic biliary access and anterograde interventions for failed ERCP. Surg Endosc. 2014;28(11):3193–9.
83. Oterdoom LH, van Weyenberg SJ, de Boer NK. Double-duct sign: do not forget the gallstones. J Gastrointestin Liver Dis. 2013;22(4):447–50.
84. Scheiman JM, et al. Can endoscopic ultrasound or magnetic resonance cholangiopancreatography replace ERCP in patients with suspected biliary disease? A prospective trial and cost analysis. Am J Gastroenterol. 2001;96(10):2900–4.
85. Jailwala J, et al. Triple-tissue sampling at ERCP in malignant biliary obstruction. Gastrointest Endosc. 2000;51(4 Pt 1):383–90.
86. Parsi MA, et al. Factors affecting the yield of brush cytology for the diagnosis of pancreatic and biliary cancers. Pancreas. 2011;40(1):52–4.
87. Parsi MA, et al. Diagnostic and therapeutic cholangiopancreatoscopy: performance of a new digital cholangioscope. Gastrointest Endosc. 2014;79(6):936–42.
88. Murakami M, et al. Bypass surgery or stent placement for biliary obstruction in patients with unresectable pancreatic cancer. Gan To Kagaku Ryoho. 2013;40(12):1705–7.
89. Yamamoto R, et al. Comparison of endoscopic stenting for malignant biliary obstruction: a single-center study. World J Gastrointest Endosc. 2015;7(9):889–94.
90. Kofokotsios A, et al. Palliation with endoscopic metal stents may be preferable to surgical intervention for patients with obstructive pancreatic head adenocarcinoma. Int Surg. 2015;100(6):1104–10.
91. Moss AC, et al. Do the benefits of metal stents justify the costs? A systematic review and meta-analysis of trials comparing endoscopic stents for malignant biliary obstruction. Eur J Gastroenterol Hepatol. 2007;19(12):1119–24.

92. Moss AC, Morris E, Mac Mathuna P. Palliative biliary stents for obstructing pancreatic carcinoma. Cochrane Database Syst Rev. 2006;1:CD004200.
93. Almadi MA, Barkun AN, Martel M. No benefit of covered vs uncovered self-expandable metal stents in patients with malignant distal biliary obstruction: a meta-analysis. Clin Gastroenterol Hepatol. 2013;11(1):27–37. e1
94. Saleem A, et al. Meta-analysis of randomized trials comparing the patency of covered and uncovered self-expandable metal stents for palliation of distal malignant bile duct obstruction. Gastrointest Endosc. 2011;74(2):321–7. e1-3
95. Cote GA, Sherman S. Endoscopic palliation of pancreatic cancer. Cancer J. 2012;18(6):584–90.
96. van der Gaag NA, et al. Preoperative biliary drainage for cancer of the head of the pancreas. N Engl J Med. 2010;362(2):129–37.
97. Fang Y, et al. Pre-operative biliary drainage for obstructive jaundice. Cochrane Database Syst Rev. 2012;9:CD005444.
98. Abrams RA, et al. Combined modality treatment of resectable and borderline resectable pancreas cancer: expert consensus statement. Ann Surg Oncol. 2009;16(7):1751–6.
99. Mullen JT, et al. Pancreaticoduodenectomy after placement of endobiliary metal stents. J Gastrointest Surg. 2005;9(8):1094–104. discussion 1104-5
100. Wasan SM, et al. Use of expandable metallic biliary stents in resectable pancreatic cancer. Am J Gastroenterol. 2005;100(9):2056–61.
101. Adler DG, Baron TH. Endoscopic palliation of malignant gastric outlet obstruction using self-expanding metal stents: experience in 36 patients. Am J Gastroenterol. 2002;97(1):72–8.
102. Espinel J, et al. Palliative treatment of malignant obstruction of gastric outlet using an endoscopically placed enteral Wallstent. Dig Dis Sci. 2001;46(11):2322–4.
103. Lopera JE, et al. Gastroduodenal stent placement: current status. Radiographics. 2004;24(6):1561–73.
104. Del Piano M, et al. Endoscopy or surgery for malignant GI outlet obstruction? Gastrointest Endosc. 2005;61(3):421–6.
105. Wong YT, et al. Gastric outlet obstruction secondary to pancreatic cancer: surgical vs endoscopic palliation. Surg Endosc. 2002;16(2):310–2.
106. Bessoud B, et al. Malignant gastroduodenal obstruction: palliation with self-expanding metallic stents. J Vasc Interv Radiol. 2005;16(2 Pt 1):247–53.
107. Brune IB, et al. Laparoscopic gastrojejunostomy and endoscopic biliary stent placement for palliation of incurable gastric outlet obstruction with cholestasis. Surg Endosc. 1997;11(8):834–7.
108. Holt AP, Patel M, Ahmed MM. Palliation of patients with malignant gastroduodenal obstruction with self-expanding metallic stents: the treatment of choice? Gastrointest Endosc. 2004;60(6):1010–7.
109. Kim JH, et al. Self-expanding coil stent with a long delivery system for palliation of unresectable malignant gastric outlet obstruction: a prospective study. Endoscopy. 2001;33(10):838–42.
110. Telford JJ, et al. Palliation of patients with malignant gastric outlet obstruction with the enteral Wallstent: outcomes from a multicenter study. Gastrointest Endosc. 2004;60(6):916–20.
111. Song HY, et al. A dual expandable nitinol stent: experience in 102 patients with malignant gastroduodenal strictures. J Vasc Interv Radiol. 2004;15(12):1443–9.
112. Jeurnink SM, et al. Surgical gastrojejunostomy or endoscopic stent placement for the palliation of malignant gastric outlet obstruction (SUSTENT study): a multicenter randomized trial. Gastrointest Endosc. 2010;71(3):490–9.
113. Tringali A, et al. Endoscopic treatment of malignant gastric and duodenal strictures: a prospective, multicenter study. Gastrointest Endosc. 2014;79(1):66–75.
114. Hosono S, et al. Endoscopic stenting versus surgical gastroenterostomy for palliation of malignant gastroduodenal obstruction: a meta-analysis. J Gastroenterol. 2007;42(4):283–90.

115. Jeurnink, S.M., et al., Stent versus gastrojejunostomy for the palliation of gastric outlet obstruction: a systematic review. J Gastroenterol. 2010;45(5):537–43.
116. Fiori E, et al. Palliative management of malignant antro-pyloric strictures. Gastroenterostomy vs. endoscopic stenting. A randomized prospective trial. Anticancer Res. 2004;24(1):269–71.
117. Mehta S, et al. Prospective randomized trial of laparoscopic gastrojejunostomy versus duodenal stenting for malignant gastric outflow obstruction. Surg Endosc. 2006;20(2):239–42.

Chapter 9
How to Treat Resectable Disease

Mary Dillhoff and Mark Bloomston

Introduction

Surgical resection is of critical importance in treatment if cure for pancreatic cancer is possible; however, a minority of patients have potentially resectable disease at presentation. Current guidelines suggest neoadjuvant therapy for resectable pancreatic cancer only in the context of a clinical trial; thus, proceeding to surgical resection is recommended if the mass is removable. However, most high-volume centers have trended toward neoadjuvant therapy even for resectable patients. Treatment of resectable disease will be defined and addressed, and surgical considerations will be addressed in this chapter.

Clinical Presentation

Patients presenting with painless jaundice, especially older patients, have concern for underlying malignancy. Approximately 70–80% of patients present with jaundice when the cancer is located in the head of the pancreas. Nearly 70% of pancreatic cancers are located in the head with the remaining in the body and tail [1]. Symptoms vary based on location; however, other concerning symptoms include weight loss, abdominal pain, and newly diagnosed diabetes [2, 3]. Left-sided lesions often present with abdominal and back pain, recent-onset diabetes, and nausea.

M. Dillhoff, M.D., M.S. (✉)
James Cancer Center and Solove Research Institute, Ohio State University,
390 W. 10th Avenue, Columbus, OH 43210, USA
e-mail: mary.dillhoff@osumc.edu

M. Bloomston, M.D.
21st Century Oncology, Fort Myers, FL, USA

T. Bekaii-Saab, B. El-Rayes (eds.), *Current and Emerging Therapies in Pancreatic Cancer*, DOI 10.1007/978-3-319-58256-6_9

Management of jaundice is an important part of the decision-making process prior to surgery. Preoperative biliary drainage was first suggested as a means to reduce operative complications as it was thought that jaundice increased postoperative complications [4]. In 2010 van der Gaag published a multicenter randomized controlled trial of preoperative biliary drainage vs. surgery alone. Patients with a bilirubin level of 2.3–14.6 mg per deciliter were randomized to preoperative plastic biliary stent placement followed by surgery 4–6 weeks later or surgery alone within 1 week of diagnosis. A significantly greater proportion of patients in the preoperative drainage group experienced serious complications compared to the early surgery group (74 vs. 39%). The largest increased risk in the biliary stent group was cholangitis in 26% of patients vs. 2% in non-stented patients. Perioperative outcomes were similar between the two groups [5]. In general, asymptomatic mild to moderate jaundice does not need to be corrected prior to surgery. However, in the presence of severe jaundice, cholangitis, severe pruritus, debilitated patient, or if neoadjuvant therapy is planned, biliary stenting should be considered.

Stent complications are a significant concern for patients undergoing these procedures. Metallic stents are considered superior to plastic stents in terms of stent-related complications. A meta-analysis of preoperative plastic vs. metal stents in resectable periampullary or pancreatic head tumors found that re-intervention rates were significantly reduced in the metal stent group (3.4%) vs. the plastic stent group (14.8% $p < 0.0001$) [6]. Costs have been shown to be slightly lower for plastic stents vs. metal stents $19,935 vs. $20,878 [7]. However, the difference in cost is a relatively small difference when taking into account the perceived cost to the patient if they have stent-related complications and require an additional intervention.

Diagnosis, Imaging, and Staging

For patients with painless jaundice or a newly diagnosed pancreas mass, cross-sectional imaging with intravenous contrast is mandatory for complete staging. Specific notation should be made of the relationship of the primary lesion to the mesenteric vasculature to allow classification of the lesion as resectable vs. borderline resectable or locally advanced (see determination of resectability below). This is best accomplished with imaging in both the arterial and venous phases. Perhaps the most important is the determination of metastatic disease in the lungs, liver, or elsewhere within the peritoneal cavity as pancreatectomy in the presence of distant disease does not provide a survival benefit. While computed tomography (CT) scanning typically provides the necessary information for determining resectability, both magnetic resonance imaging (MRI) and endoscopic ultrasound (EUS) are used as well in selected cases and will be discussed more thoroughly below. The relationship of the tumor to surrounding vasculature including the portal and superior mesenteric veins, celiac axis, superior mesenteric artery, and hepatic artery is critical to determine resectability of the disease (Figs. 9.1, 9.2, and 9.3). Multi-detector CT allows for high-resolution images as well as 3-D reconstruction. The so-called pancreas

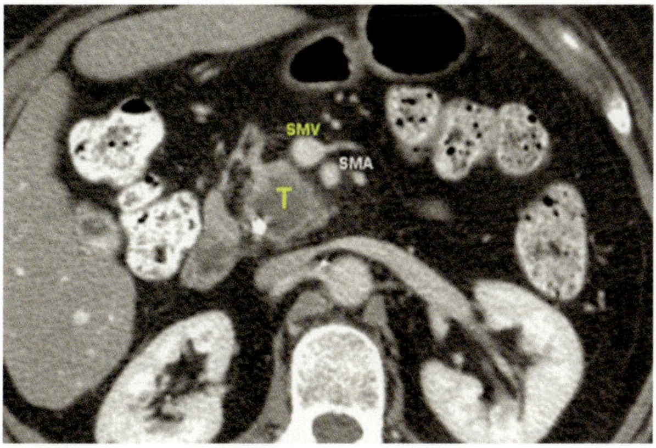

Fig. 9.1 Resectable pancreatic cancer with clear plane between tumor (T) and superior mesenteric vein (SMV) and superior mesenteric artery (SMA)

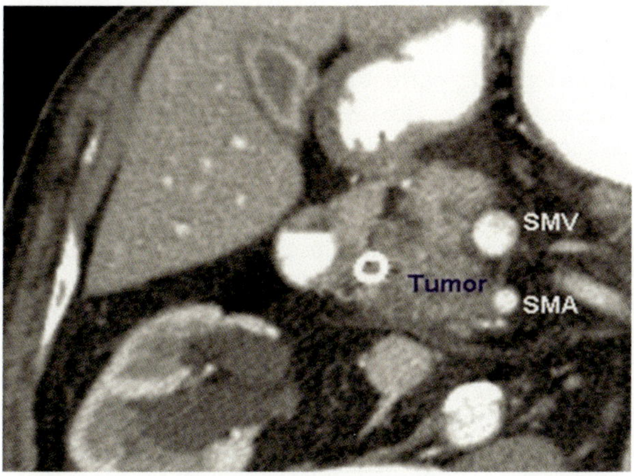

Fig. 9.2 Borderline resectable pancreatic cancer with less than 180° abutment of superior mesenteric artery (SMA) and plane between tumor and superior mesenteric vein (SMV)

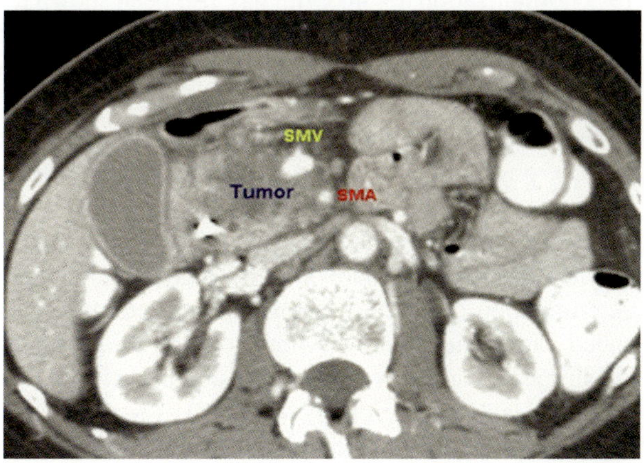

Fig. 9.3 Locally advanced unresectable pancreatic cancer with greater than 180° abutment of superior mesenteric vein (SMV) and encasement of the superior mesenteric artery (SMA)

protocol also adds the addition of fine cuts through the pancreas with both arterial and venous phases. MRI with contrast can be a useful addition in determining the relationship of local extension and is superior to CT in detecting small liver metastases. EUS is the most sensitive test for evaluating small pancreatic tumors, superior to both CT and MRI [8]. This is also the safest method to obtain tissue for pathologic confirmation. This is not recommended as a routine staging tool. EUS is essential if neoadjuvant therapy is to be undertaken for tissue confirmation prior to the start of therapy [9]. Decision-making and interpretation of the imaging studies and diagnostic evaluation are best undertaken by a multidisciplinary team that includes surgery, gastroenterology, medical oncology, radiation oncology, and pathology.

Endoscopic retrograde cholangiopancreatography (ERCP) combines endoscopy and fluoroscopic imaging for therapeutic intervention such as biliary decompression, when required. In addition, it may be used for duct brushing with cytology if a mass is not seen to biopsy by EUS.

The role of positron emission tomography (PET) scanning in pancreatic cancer continues to evolve. While inadequate as a sole modality for staging, it may improve detection of occult metastatic disease when used as an adjunct to standard CT [10]. However, in its current form, the addition of PET as part of the routine staging of pancreatic cancer does not greatly impact management and should be reserved for patients at highest risk for metastatic disease (e.g., borderline resectable/locally advanced, very elevated CA 19-9).

Serum CA 19-9 is best measured after biliary decompression as it may be falsely elevated. If elevated, it is useful in following patients for recurrence or to assess response to therapy. CA 19-9 is a sialylated Lewis A blood group antigen which is commonly expressed and shed in pancreatic diseases and many malignancies but is not specific to pancreatic cancer. CA 19-9 has a low positive predictive value, thus making it a poor screening biomarker [11]. CA 19-9 has been found to be prognostic in patients with resectable disease following surgery [12]. Berger and colleagues report median survival of patients undergoing resection, and a postoperative CA 19-9 level of <180 U/ml had a significantly prolonged median survival than those with CA 19-9 greater than 180 [13]. In patients receiving neoadjuvant therapy, CA 19-9 normalization to <40 U/ml has also been shown to be associated with improvement in overall survival (15 months vs. 11 months) for those not able to be resected and 38 months vs. 26 months for those undergoing resection [14]. Of note CA 19-9 may be undetectable in patients who are Lewis antigen negative [15].

In addition to imaging to determine that practicality of surgical resection, assessment of physiologic ability to undergo major operation is crucial. Standard preoperative assessment typically includes history and physical, assessment of functional status, laboratory evaluation, EKG, and possible cardiac work-up as indicated. While all of these measures provide a general assessment of a patient's well-being, determination of candidacy for pancreatectomy is best determined by an experienced pancreatic surgeon. After thorough initial staging, only 15–20% of patients are surgical candidates without consideration of neoadjuvant therapy.

Fine needle aspiration (FNA) by EUS is the safest method of obtaining pathologic confirmation of malignancy, preferable to the percutaneous approach. Pathologic confirmation is necessary prior to start of neoadjuvant chemotherapy; however, when proceeding directly to surgical resection, biopsy is not mandatory and should not delay surgery. The preference for EUS FNA is due to better yield, safety, and a theoretical decreased risk of seeding of the peritoneal cavity during percutaneous approaches. In addition, percutaneous approaches may have an increased risk of bleeding and infectious complications. If biopsy does not confirm malignancy consideration of one repeat, biopsy should be undertaken. It should be emphasized that biopsy is not mandatory prior to proceeding to resection if a high suspicion for pancreatic cancer exists. If biopsy does not confirm malignancy, alternative diagnosis such as autoimmune pancreatitis may be considered. Multidisciplinary teams are crucial to interpretation of these tests.

Determining Resectability

Determining if a tumor is able to be removed is based on the imaging studies described above and best determined by an experienced pancreatic surgeon, preferably as part of a multidisciplinary group. Essentially the imaging is used to estimate the ability to achieve complete (i.e., R0) resection at the relevant transection margins and vascular planes. R0 resection is a strong prognostic indicator for recurrence rates and overall survival [16–18]. The relationship of the tumor to mesenteric vasculature is the determinate of resectable vs. borderline and locally advanced pancreatic cancer (Figs. 9.1, 9.2, and 9.3). Preoperative imaging not only evaluates for distant metastatic disease but also the relationship of the mass to the superior mesenteric vein and portal vein, common hepatic artery, gastroduodenal artery, superior mesenteric artery, and celiac axis. The definitions of resectable, borderline, and locally advanced have been defined by many groups including the National Comprehensive Cancer Network (NCCN), Society of Surgical Oncology (SSO), Americas Hepato-Pancreato-Biliary Association (AHPBA), Society for Surgery of the Alimentary Tract (SSAT), and Alliance for Clinical Trials in Oncology. This has allowed the terminology to become more standard, although some differences remain between these groups' definitions (Table 9.1). Resectable pancreatic cancer is a tumor without contact of the celiac artery, hepatic artery, superior mesenteric

Table 9.1 Definitions of resectable/borderline/locally advanced disease

Surgical staging				
	Relationship to major vasculature			
Clinical stage	SMV/portal vein confluence	SMA	Celiac axis	Common hepatic artery
Resectable	No tumor contact or ≤180° contact without vein irregularity	No contact	No contact	No contact
Borderline	Contact >180° or ≤180° with compression or thrombosis and amenable to reconstruction	Contact ≤180°	≤180° (for body/tail tumors)	Contact without extension to celiac, short segment encasement
Locally advanced unresectable	Unreconstructible SMV/PV	Contact >180°	Contact	Long segment encasement

artery, or superior mesenteric vein. Some also include tumors that have limited involvement of the SMV/portal vein but are removable with R0 resection with vascular resection and reconstruction [19].

Role of Laparoscopy

Laparoscopy has long been used to evaluate for peritoneal disease not appreciated on cross-sectional imaging. The use varies greatly by institution and surgeon, ranging from routine to very selective use. This modality is most useful for patients with findings on imaging that are suspicious for metastatic disease but not obviously metastatic and/or not amenable to confirmatory biopsy. Those with peritoneal nodules or omental thickening, small indeterminate liver lesions, or ascites increase the clinical suspicion for underlying distant metastatic disease, thus increasing the utility for laparoscopy. Laparoscopy is not widely used for determining local resectability because evaluation of the mesenteric vasculature is not easily done with laparoscopy [20]. For patients with metastatic disease discovered by laparoscopy, an unnecessary laparotomy is avoided, thus shortening hospital length of stay and allowing chemotherapy to be initiated sooner [21, 22]. Most recently, a Cochrane review was published by Allen and colleagues evaluating the use of laparoscopy and again found that diagnostic laparoscopy decreases the rate of unnecessary laparotomy from 40% in those receiving work-up with CT alone to 18% for those receiving both CT and diagnostic laparoscopy [23]. Although rarely used in pancreatic malignancies, the addition of peritoneal washings for cytology may increase the sensitivity of diagnosing occult metastatic disease when used in conjunction with cross-sectional imaging and laparoscopy. Positive cytology occurs in up to 30% of potentially resectable pancreatic malignancies, and their survival is equivalent to those with distant metastatic disease. Thus, patients with positive cytology should be considered incurable and not eligible for resection [24].

Surgical Management and Considerations

For tumors in the head/uncinate of the pancreas, a pancreaticoduodenectomy or Whipple procedure is required. For tumors in the body/tail of the pancreas distal (subtotal), pancreatectomy is needed. Splenectomy is recommended as well for left-sided cancers. Many differences in surgical technique have been researched over many years including pylorus-preserving pancreaticoduodenectomy (PPPD), different anastomotic techniques, the use of drains, and the value of extended lymphadenectomy. No major difference in outcome has been shown with any of the above changes in technique.

Pylorus-preserving pancreaticoduodenectomy (PPPD) vs. standard pancreaticoduodenectomy has been evaluated in multiple randomized controlled trials. PPPD was introduced in an effort to prevent the long-term complications of dumping syndrome, bile reflux gastritis, and marginal ulcer. Trials have had conflicting results, but most have not found statistically significant differences in overall and disease-free survival, operating time, blood loss, length of stay, overall morbidity and mortality, resection margin status, quality of life, or delayed gastric emptying [25–27]. A Cochrane review evaluated PPPD vs. standard pancreaticoduodenectomy. Eight randomized controlled trials were included in the analysis with 512 patients. Postoperative morbidity, mortality, and long-term survival were not statistically different between groups. There was a statistical benefit of standard pancreaticoduodenectomy for delayed gastric emptying, but sensitivity analysis did not support this finding. There were some perioperative differences for PPPD with decreased blood loss, operative time, and red cell transfusion; however, none of these differences translated into lengthened survival or decreased length of stay. There was great heterogeneity within these studies; thus, these differences should be interpreted carefully [28]. Essentially, the use of pylorus preservation has been relegated to that of surgeon preference.

Given the morbidity associated with pancreatic fistula following pancreatectomy, the optimal management of the pancreatic duct has become the holy grail of pancreatic surgery. Many variations of anastomotic techniques have been attempted to reduce pancreatic fistula rates. Most commonly described and compared is pancreaticojejunostomy (PJ) vs. pancreaticogastrostomy (PG). Many trials have been performed addressing this question but evidence is still conflicting. There have been multiple meta-analyses published in the last several years again with some concluding that PG is associated with less postoperative pancreatic fistula (POPF) over PJ and others with no difference in the technique [29–33]. These results must be interpreted with caution as many surgeons feel the most reliable method of anastomosis is the technique that they use most commonly. Thus, changing technique may not result in lower POPF. Other techniques including occlusion of the pancreatic duct or binding technique have been described but are not routinely used in practice [34, 35]. Other techniques to create the pancreaticojejunostomy have been examined such as end to end, end to side, duct to mucosa, and invagination. All of these methods have been shown safe and are chosen based on surgeon's preference. Pancreatic duct stenting has been described for nearly a century; however, it has not been shown to decrease pancreatic fistula. A small randomized controlled trial confirmed that fistula rates and severity were similar between stent and no stent [36].

The addition of pharmaceuticals has also been evaluated to reduce the incidence of postoperative pancreatic fistulas (POPF). The somatostatin analog, octreotide, has been studied for many years with the premise that reduction of pancreatic secretions theoretically should reduce leak rates. The studies using octreotide have been mixed at best, and two prospective randomized controlled trials have not shown a decrease in fistula rates [37, 38]. A newer somatostatin analog with a longer half-life and broader binding profile than octreotide, pasireotide, was shown in a randomized controlled trial in 2014 to decrease the incidence of grade 3 or higher POPF from 21 to 9% [39]. The cost of this newer agent as prescribed in the trial and its off-label use, however, has thus far slowed its general adoption into practice at many institutions.

Lymph node status is an important predictor of survival in patients with pancreatic cancer. Lymph node involvement is estimated from 50 to 80%; thus extended lymphadenectomy has been proposed by some groups. However, several studies have shown that extended lymphadenectomy was associated with higher complication rates without improvement in quality of life or overall survival [40, 41]. The consensus meeting of the International Study Group on Pancreatic Surgery formulated a statement with regard to the recommended extent of lymphadenectomy. Lymphadenectomy should include the surrounding lymph nodes along the resection and not distant nodes (e.g., nodes to the left of the SMA, celiac, splenic artery, or left gastric). Several meta-analyses have also confirmed no improvement in survival with extended lymphadenectomies [42–44].

The routine use of operative drains continues to be a topic of discussion among pancreatic surgeons. Conlon and colleagues attempted to address the question in 2001 with a prospective randomized study of 179 patients undergoing pancreatectomy for peripancreatic tumors. The majority of patients (77%) underwent Whipple and the remainder distal pancreatectomy. The addition of drains did not reduce postoperative complications or death and increased the risk of intra-abdominal abscess, fluid collection, and pancreatic fistula [45]. A randomized multicenter trial was conducted more recently with 137 patients undergoing Whipple assigned to drain or no drain. The study was stopped early because of increased risk of death in the group not receiving drains (12 vs. 3%). Patients undergoing Whipple without drainage had an increased risk of complications and increased severity of complications including gastroparesis, intra-abdominal fluid collection, abscess, diarrhea, need for postoperative drain, and prolonged length of stay [46]. Cochrane review of 316 patients receiving drain vs. no drain done in 2015 was unable to conclude whether routine drainage affects mortality or surgical complications [47]. A multicenter randomized controlled trial evaluating drains in distal pancreatectomy has completed accrual and pending results. Given the data, routine drainage after pancreatic surgery to reduce mortality and surgical complications remains in question.

Vascular resections historically were abandoned during PD because of the high morbidity and mortality. However, venous resection has become widely acceptable. Rates of venous resection vary greatly by institution from 7 to 80% [48–50]. Perioperative morbidity and mortality are similar to standard resections. Venous resections vary depending on the tumor involvement with some requiring lateral venorrhaphy with primary closure, resection with vein patch, sleeve resection with primary anastomosis, or resection with interposition graft. The autologous graft of choice is most often the internal jugular vein or saphenous vein if adequate size. Prosthetic grafts are often debated because of the risk of infection when placed in a contaminated field. Primary anastomosis can often be performed even with a 5–7 cm gap after mobilization of the liver and right colon and ligation of the splenic vein [51].

Conclusion

Surgical resection remains the mainstay of therapy for long-term survival in patients with pancreatic cancer, although a minority are able to undergo resection with curative intent. The morbidity and mortality following resection have decreased dramatically since its inception a century ago, particularly in the last several decades.

Still, curative surgery remains underutilized by virtue of the perceived debilitating effects of pancreatectomy and the global nihilistic approach to pancreatic cancer. The reality is that mortality is now consistently below 5% at high-volume centers and patients (even elderly ones) can expect return to normal activities and good quality of life. Much progress on oncologic outcomes remains to be made. While current recommendations are for patients with resectable disease to undergo resection unless enrolled in a neoadjuvant therapy trial, most pancreatic surgeons will agree that once a tolerable, efficacious systemic therapy is identified, it is best administered prior to surgery. Until then, thoughtful consideration for resection utilizing high-quality cross-sectional imaging, sound surgical expertise, and a multidisciplinary team provides optimal outcomes.

References

1. Modolell I, Guarner L, Malagelada JR. Vagaries of clinical presentation of pancreatic and biliary tract cancer. Ann Oncol. 1999;10(4):82–4.
2. Kelsen DP, Portenoy R, Thaler H, Tao Y, Brennan M. Pain as a predictor of outcome in patients with operable pancreatic carcinoma. Surgery. 1997;122(1):53–9.
3. Chari ST, Leibson CL, Rabe KG, Timmons LJ, Ransom J, de Andrade M, et al. Pancreatic cancer-associated diabetes mellitus: prevalence and temporal association with diagnosis of cancer. Gastroenterology. 2008;134(1):95–101.
4. van der Gaag NA, Kloek JJ, de Castro SM, Busch OR, van Gulik TM, Gouma DJ. Preoperative biliary drainage in patients with obstructive jaundice: history and current status. J Gastrointest Surg. 2009;13(4):814–20.
5. van der Gaag NA, Rauws EA, van Eijck CH, Bruno MJ, van der Harst E, Kubben FJ, et al. Preoperative biliary drainage for cancer of the head of the pancreas. N Engl J Med. 2010;362(2):129–37.
6. Crippa S, Cirocchi R, Partelli S, Petrone MC, Muffatti F, Renzi C, et al. Systematic review and meta-analysis of metal versus plastic stents for preoperative biliary drainage in resectable periampullary or pancreatic head tumors. Eur J Surg Oncol. 2016;42(9):1278–85.
7. Chen VK, Arguedas MR, Baron TH. Expandable metal biliary stents before pancreaticoduodenectomy for pancreatic cancer: a Monte-Carlo decision analysis. Clin Gastroenterol Hepatol. 2005;3(12):1229–37.
8. Legmann P, Vignaux O, Dousset B, Baraza AJ, Palazzo L, Dumontier I, et al. Pancreatic tumors: comparison of dual-phase helical CT and endoscopic sonography. AJR Am J Roentgenol. 1998;170(5):1315–22.
9. Miura F, Takada T, Amano H, Yoshida M, Furui S, Takeshita K. Diagnosis of pancreatic cancer. HPB (Oxford). 2006;8(5):337–42.
10. Rijkers AP, Valkema R, Duivenvoorden HJ, van Eijck CH. Usefulness of F-18-fluorodeoxyglucose positron emission tomography to confirm suspected pancreatic cancer: a meta-analysis. Eur J Surg Oncol. 2014;40(7):794–804.
11. Ballehaninna UK, Chamberlain RS. The clinical utility of serum CA 19-9 in the diagnosis, prognosis and management of pancreatic adenocarcinoma: an evidence based appraisal. Journal of gastrointestinal oncology. 2012;3(2):105–19.
12. Kondo N, Murakami Y, Uemura K, Hayashidani Y, Sudo T, Hashimoto Y, et al. Prognostic impact of perioperative serum CA 19-9 levels in patients with resectable pancreatic cancer. Ann Surg Oncol. 2010;17(9):2321–9.
13. Berger AC, Garcia M Jr, Hoffman JP, Regine WF, Abrams RA, Safran H, et al. Postresection CA 19-9 predicts overall survival in patients with pancreatic cancer treated with adjuvant chemoradiation: a prospective validation by RTOG 9704. J Clin Oncol. 2008;26(36):5918–22.

14. Tzeng CW, Balachandran A, Ahmad M, Lee JE, Krishnan S, Wang H, et al. Serum carbohydrate antigen 19-9 represents a marker of response to neoadjuvant therapy in patients with borderline resectable pancreatic cancer. HPB. 2014;16(5):430–8.
15. Tempero MA, Uchida E, Takasaki H, Burnett DA, Steplewski Z, Pour PM. Relationship of carbohydrate antigen 19-9 and Lewis antigens in pancreatic cancer. Cancer Res. 1987;47(20):5501–3.
16. Sohn TA, Yeo CJ, Cameron JL, Koniaris L, Kaushal S, Abrams RA, et al. Resected adenocarcinoma of the pancreas-616 patients: results, outcomes, and prognostic indicators. J Gastrointest Surg. 2000;4(6):567–79.
17. Winter JM, Cameron JL, Campbell KA, Arnold MA, Chang DC, Coleman J, et al. 1423 pancreaticoduodenectomies for pancreatic cancer: a single-institution experience. J Gastrointest Surg. 2006;10(9):1199–210. discussion 210-1
18. Kuhlmann KF, de Castro SM, Wesseling JG, ten Kate FJ, Offerhaus GJ, Busch OR, et al. Surgical treatment of pancreatic adenocarcinoma; actual survival and prognostic factors in 343 patients. Eur J Cancer. 2004;40(4):549–58.
19. Varadhachary GR, Tamm EP, Abbruzzese JL, Xiong HQ, Crane CH, Wang H, et al. Borderline resectable pancreatic cancer: definitions, management, and role of preoperative therapy. Ann Surg Oncol. 2006;13(8):1035–46.
20. Hennig R, Tempia-Caliera AA, Hartel M, Buchler MW, Friess H. Staging laparoscopy and its indications in pancreatic cancer patients. Dig Surg. 2002;19(6):484–8.
21. Hashimoto D, Chikamoto A, Sakata K, Nakagawa S, Hayashi H, Ohmuraya M, et al. Staging laparoscopy leads to rapid induction of chemotherapy for unresectable pancreatobiliary cancers. Asian journal of endoscopic surgery. 2015;8(1):59–62.
22. Beenen E, van Roest MH, Sieders E, Peeters PM, Porte RJ, de Boer MT, et al. Staging laparoscopy in patients scheduled for pancreaticoduodenectomy minimizes hospitalization in the remaining life time when metastatic carcinoma is found. Eur J Surg Oncol. 2014;40(8):989–94.
23. Allen VB, Gurusamy KS, Takwoingi Y, Kalia A, Davidson BR. Diagnostic accuracy of laparoscopy following computed tomography (CT) scanning for assessing the resectability with curative intent in pancreatic and periampullary cancer. Cochrane Database Syst Rev. 2016;7:Cd009323.
24. Clark CJ, Traverso LW. Positive peritoneal lavage cytology is a predictor of worse survival in locally advanced pancreatic cancer. Am J Surg. 2010;199(5):657–62.
25. Tran KT, Smeenk HG, van Eijck CH, Kazemier G, Hop WC, Greve JW, et al. Pylorus preserving pancreaticoduodenectomy versus standard Whipple procedure: a prospective, randomized, multicenter analysis of 170 patients with pancreatic and periampullary tumors. Ann Surg. 2004;240(5):738–45.
26. Seiler CA, Wagner M, Bachmann T, Redaelli CA, Schmied B, Uhl W, et al. Randomized clinical trial of pylorus-preserving duodenopancreatectomy versus classical Whipple resection-long term results. Br J Surg. 2005;92(5):547–56.
27. Lin PW, Shan YS, Lin YJ, Hung CJ. Pancreaticoduodenectomy for pancreatic head cancer: PPPD versus Whipple procedure. Hepato-Gastroenterology. 2005;52(65):1601–4.
28. Huttner FJ, Fitzmaurice C, Schwarzer G, Seiler CM, Antes G, Buchler MW, et al. Pylorus-preserving pancreaticoduodenectomy (pp Whipple) versus pancreaticoduodenectomy (classic Whipple) for surgical treatment of periampullary and pancreatic carcinoma. Cochrane Database Syst Rev. 2016;2:Cd006053.
29. Xiong JJ, Tan CL, Szatmary P, Huang W, Ke NW, WM H, et al. Meta-analysis of pancreaticogastrostomy versus pancreaticojejunostomy after pancreaticoduodenectomy. Br J Surg. 2014;101(10):1196–208.
30. Crippa S, Cirocchi R, Randolph J, Partelli S, Belfiori G, Piccioli A, et al. Pancreaticojejunostomy is comparable to pancreaticogastrostomy after pancreaticoduodenectomy: an updated meta-analysis of randomized controlled trials. Langenbeck's archives of surgery / Deutsche Gesellschaft fur Chirurgie. 2016;401(4):427–37.

31. Guerrini GP, Soliani P, D'Amico G, Di Benedetto F, Negri M, Piccoli M, et al. Pancreaticojejunostomy versus Pancreaticogastrostomy after Pancreaticoduodenectomy: an up-to-date meta-analysis. Journal of investigative surgery. 2016;29(3):175–84.
32. Zhou Y, Yu J, Wu L, Li B. Meta-analysis of pancreaticogastrostomy versus pancreaticojejunostomy on occurrences of postoperative pancreatic fistula after pancreaticoduodenectomy. Asian journal of surgery. 2015;38(3):155–60.
33. Que W, Fang H, Yan B, Li J, Guo W, Zhai W, et al. Pancreaticogastrostomy versus pancreaticojejunostomy after pancreaticoduodenectomy: a meta-analysis of randomized controlled trials. Am J Surg. 2015;209(6):1074–82.
34. Tran K, Van Eijck C, Di Carlo V, Hop WC, Zerbi A, Balzano G, et al. Occlusion of the pancreatic duct versus pancreaticojejunostomy: a prospective randomized trial. Ann Surg. 2002;236(4):422–8; discussion 8.
35. Peng SY, Wang JW, Lau WY, Cai XJ, Mou YP, Liu YB, et al. Conventional versus binding pancreaticojejunostomy after pancreaticoduodenectomy: a prospective randomized trial. Ann Surg. 2007;245(5):692–8.
36. Winter JM, Cameron JL, Campbell KA, Chang DC, Riall TS, Schulick RD, et al. Does pancreatic duct stenting decrease the rate of pancreatic fistula following pancreaticoduodenectomy? Results of a prospective randomized trial. Journal of gastrointestinal surgery. 2006;10(9):1280–90; discussion 90.
37. Yeo CJ, Cameron JL, Lillemoe KD, Sauter PK, Coleman J, Sohn TA, et al. Does prophylactic octreotide decrease the rates of pancreatic fistula and other complications after pancreaticoduodenectomy? Results of a prospective randomized placebo-controlled trial. Ann Surg. 2000;232(3):419–29.
38. Lowy AM, Lee JE, Pisters PW, Davidson BS, Fenoglio CJ, Stanford P, et al. Prospective, randomized trial of octreotide to prevent pancreatic fistula after pancreaticoduodenectomy for malignant disease. Ann Surg. 1997;226(5):632–41.
39. Allen PJ, Gonen M, Brennan MF, Bucknor AA, Robinson LM, Pappas MM, et al. Pasireotide for postoperative pancreatic fistula. N Engl J Med. 2014;370(21):2014–22.
40. Yeo CJ, Cameron JL, Lillemoe KD, Sohn TA, Campbell KA, Sauter PK, et al. Pancreaticoduodenectomy with or without distal gastrectomy and extended retroperitoneal lymphadenectomy for periampullary adenocarcinoma, part 2: randomized controlled trial evaluating survival, morbidity, and mortality. Ann Surg. 2002;236(3):355–66. discussion 66-8
41. Riall TS, Cameron JL, Lillemoe KD, Campbell KA, Sauter PK, Coleman J, et al. Pancreaticoduodenectomy with or without distal gastrectomy and extended retroperitoneal lymphadenectomy for periampullary adenocarcinoma--part 3: update on 5-year survival. J Gastrointest Surg. 2005;9(9):1191–204. discussion 204-6
42. Michalski CW, Kleeff J, Wente MN, Diener MK, Buchler MW, Friess H. Systematic review and meta-analysis of standard and extended lymphadenectomy in pancreaticoduodenectomy for pancreatic cancer. Br J Surg. 2007;94(3):265–73.
43. Iqbal N, Lovegrove RE, Tilney HS, Abraham AT, Bhattacharya S, Tekkis PP, et al. A comparison of pancreaticoduodenectomy with extended pancreaticoduodenectomy: a meta-analysis of 1909 patients. European journal of surgical oncology. 2009;35(1):79–86.
44. Peparini N. Mesopancreas: a boundless structure, namely the rationale for dissection of the paraaortic area in pancreaticoduodenectomy for pancreatic head carcinoma. World J Gastroenterol. 2015;21(10):2865–70.
45. Conlon KC, Labow D, Leung D, Smith A, Jarnagin W, Coit DG, et al. Prospective randomized clinical trial of the value of intraperitoneal drainage after pancreatic resection. Ann Surg. 2001;234(4):487–93. discussion 93-4
46. Van Buren G, Bloomston M, Hughes SJ, Winter J, Behrman SW, Zyromski NJ, et al. A randomized prospective multicenter trial of pancreaticoduodenectomy with and without routine intraperitoneal drainage. Ann Surg. 2014;259(4):605–12.
47. Peng S, Cheng Y, Yang C, Lu J, Wu S, Zhou R, et al. Prophylactic abdominal drainage for pancreatic surgery. Cochrane Database Syst Rev. 2015;8:Cd010583.

48. Porembka MR, Hawkins WG, Linehan DC, Gao F, Ma C, Brunt EM, et al. Radiologic and intraoperative detection of need for mesenteric vein resection in patients with adenocarcinoma of the head of the pancreas. HPB. 2011;13(9):633–42.
49. Ramacciato G, Mercantini P, Petrucciani N, Giaccaglia V, Nigri G, Ravaioli M, et al. Does portal-superior mesenteric vein invasion still indicate irresectability for pancreatic carcinoma? Ann Surg Oncol. 2009;16(4):817–25.
50. Chua TC, Saxena A. Extended pancreaticoduodenectomy with vascular resection for pancreatic cancer: a systematic review. J gastrointest surg. 2010;14(9):1442–52.
51. Wang F, Arianayagam R, Gill A, Puttaswamy V, Neale M, Gananadha S, et al. Grafts for mesenterico-portal vein resections can be avoided during pancreatoduodenectomy. J Am Coll Surg. 2012;215(4):569–79.

Chapter 10
The Management of Locally Advanced Nonmetastatic Pancreas Cancer

Brent T. Xia, Young Kim, and Syed A. Ahmad

Abbreviations

AGEO	Association des Gastro-Entérologues Oncologues
AHPBA	Americas Hepato-Pancreato-Biliary Association
BR	Borderline resectable
CA	Celiac artery/axis
CI	Confidence interval
CRT	Chemoradiation therapy
CT	Computed tomography
DP	Distal pancreatectomy
DP-CAR	Distal pancreatectomy and splenectomy with celiac artery resection
ECOG	Eastern Cooperative Oncology Group
EGFR	Epidermal growth factor receptor
ERCP	Endoscopic retrograde cholangiopancreatography
EUS	Endoscopic ultrasound
FDG-PET/CT	Combined positron emission tomography/computed tomography using 18-fluorodeoxyglucose
FNA	Fine needle aspiration
FOLFIRINOX	Folinic acid, fluorouracil, irinotecan, and oxaliplatin
HA	Hepatic artery
LAPC	Locally advanced pancreatic cancer

B.T. Xia, M.D. • Y. Kim, M.D. • S.A. Ahmad, M.D. (✉)
Division of Surgical Oncology, Department of Surgery,
The University of Cincinnati Medical Center, 231 Albert Sabin Way,
ML 0558, SRU Room 1466, Cincinnati, OH 45267-0558, USA
e-mail: ahmadsy@uc.edu

T. Bekaii-Saab, B. El-Rayes (eds.), *Current and Emerging Therapies in Pancreatic Cancer*, DOI 10.1007/978-3-319-58256-6_10

MDACC	MD Anderson Cancer Center
MDCT	Multi-detector computed tomography
mFOLFIRINOX	Modified FOLFIRINOX
MRI	Magnetic resonance imaging
NCCN	National Comprehensive Cancer Network
NT	Neoadjuvant therapy
OR	Odds ratio
OS	Overall survival
PV	Portal vein
RECIST	Response Evaluation Criteria in Solid Tumors
SBRT	Stereotactic body radiation therapy
SEMS	Self-expanding metal stents
SMA	Superior mesenteric artery
SMV	Superior mesenteric vein
SSAT	Society for Surgery of the Alimentary Tract
SSO	Society of Surgical Oncology
TNM	Tumor-node-metastasis

Introduction

Pancreatic cancer is the fourth most common cause of cancer-related death in the United States, accounting for greater than 40,000 deaths in 2016 alone [1]. When compared to the 53,000 new diagnoses in the same year, this diagnosis/mortality ratio attests to the aggressive nature of pancreatic malignancy. Unfortunately, at the onset of symptoms and at the time of diagnosis, the majority (>50%) of pancreatic cancers have metastasized, resulting in less than 20% resectability rate [2]. The remaining 30–40% of patients present with borderline resectable (BR) and unresectable locally advanced pancreatic cancer (LAPC).

The 7th edition American Joint Committee on Cancer classifies pancreatic cancer based on tumor-node-metastasis (TNM) staging criteria [3]. Preoperative imaging is used to stratify patients based on primary tumor-vessel relationship to resectable, BR, unresectable, or metastatic disease. In patients with resectable disease, there is no tumor involvement of major blood vessels (T1–T3). Tumor growth into the celiac axis (CA) or superior mesenteric artery (SMA), factors that may preclude local curative resection, is T4 and stage three at minimum, with degree of vessel involvement differentiating between BR and LAPC.

This review will describe the definitions, clinical workup, and management of patients with borderline resectable pancreatic cancer (BRPC) and LAPC and discuss updates with regard to multimodality therapies for these subsets of patients.

Definitions

Borderline Resectable Pancreatic Cancer

Despite the simple concept of BR disease—disease burden that while technically resectable may result in an unfavorable rate of incomplete resection and locoregional recurrence—several groups have proffered criteria for expanding this definition with clinical criteria (Table 10.1) [4]. MD Anderson Cancer Center (MDACC) divides BR disease into three subtypes [4]. *Type A* disease encompasses the following criteria: ≤180° involvement of the SMA or CA, >180° involvement or encasement of the hepatic artery (HA), or short-segment occlusion of the superior mesenteric vein (SMV), portal vein (PV), or the SMV-PV confluence amenable to vascular resection and reconstruction. *Type B* disease is defined by tumor burden that may be technically resectable based on imaging but with high suspicion for extrapancreatic, metastatic disease. *Type C* disease reflects patient-level factors that contribute to marginal performance status.

In contrast, a consensus definition of the Americas Hepato-Pancreato-Biliary Association (AHPBA)/Society for Surgery of the Alimentary Tract (SSAT)/Society of Surgical Oncology (SSO) included any involvement—abutment or encasement—of the SMV-PV as BR disease [5]. The consensus definition was modified and adopted by the National Comprehensive Cancer Network (NCCN) in 2009. However, the NCCN definition did not differentiate well between BRPC and LAPC.

In an effort to remove ambiguity and promote multicenter cooperation, the Intergroup definition for BRPC was developed, taking into consideration prior retrospective reports of prognosis based on tumor-vessel interface (TVI) and in collaboration with investigators from the Alliance of Clinical Trials in Oncology, the Southwest Oncology Group, the Eastern Cooperative Oncology Group, and the Radiation Therapy Oncology Group [6–8]. Diagnosis is made using pancreas protocol computed tomography (CT) or magnetic resonance imaging (MRI) modalities and includes the following: (1) ≥180° TVI with the SMV or PV or short-segment occlusion amenable to resection and vascular reconstruction, (2) <180° TVI with the SMA, and (3) any TVI with the common HA, with normal proximal and distal vasculature amenable to resection and reconstruction.

Locally Advanced Pancreatic Cancer

Similar variations occur in the definition of LAPC between the MDACC, AHPBA/SSAT/SSO, and NCCN classification (Table 10.2). As in its definition of BRPC, the Intergroup definition uses objective descriptions of TVI instead of ambiguous terms such as "abutment" or "severely narrowed." Its classification of LAPC consists of the following: (1) unreconstructable occlusion of the SMV or PV, (2) ≥180° TVI

Table 10.1 Definitions of borderline resectable pancreatic cancer

Vessel	MD Anderson	AHPBA/SSAT/SSO	NCCN	Intergroup
SMV-PV	Short-segment occlusion	Abutment, encasement, or occlusion	Abutment with impingement or narrowing	TVI ≥ 180° and/or reconstructable occlusion
SMA	Abutment	Abutment	Abutment	TVI < 180°
CHA	Abutment or encasement	Abutment or encasement	Abutment or encasement	Reconstructable, short-segment TVI of any degree
CA	Abutment	No abutment or encasement	No abutment or encasement	TVI < 180°

AHPBA Americas Hepato-Pancreato-Biliary Association, *SSAT* Society for Surgery of the Alimentary Tract, *SSO* Society of Surgical Oncology, *NCCN* National Comprehensive Cancer Network, *SMV* superior mesenteric vein, *PV* portal vein, *SMA* superior mesenteric artery, *CHA* common hepatic artery, *CA* celiac artery, *TVI* tumor-vessel interface. Abutment, ≤ 180° involvement. Encasement, > 180° short-segment involvement. Reconstructable occlusion, normal vein or artery proximal and distal to the site of tumor-vessel involvement suitable for vascular reconstruction

Table 10.2 Definitions of locally advanced pancreatic cancer

Vessel	MD Anderson	AHPBA/SSAT/SSO	NCCN	Intergroup
SMV-PV	Unreconstructable tumor involvement	Unreconstructable tumor involvement	Unreconstructable tumor involvement or occlusion	Unreconstructable occlusion
SMA	Encasement	Encasement	Encasement or occlusion	TVI ≥ 180°
CHA	Long-segment encasement	Long-segment encasement	Unreconstructable tumor involvement	Unreconstructable TVI
CA	Encasement	Abutment	Abutment	TVI ≥ 180°

AHPBA Americas Hepato-Pancreato-Biliary Association, *SSAT* Society for Surgery of the Alimentary Tract, *SSO* Society of Surgical Oncology, *NCCN* National Comprehensive Cancer Network, *SMV* superior mesenteric vein, *PV* portal vein, *SMA* superior mesenteric artery, *CHA* common hepatic artery, *CA* celiac artery. Abutment, ≤ 180° involvement. Encasement, > 180° short-segment involvement

with the SMA, (3) unreconstructable TVI of the common HA, and (4) ≥180° TVI with the CA [7].

Clinical Workup

Imaging

Contrast-enhanced multi-detector computed tomography (MDCT) scan is the gold standard in diagnosing and staging pancreatic cancer. Acquisition of thin 2.5 mm slices of the pancreas during peak enhancement increases image resolution, with a reported sensitivity of 89–97% [9]. For tumors smaller than 1.5 cm, however, this rate decreases to 67% [10]. The characteristic appearance of pancreatic cancer on MDCT is an ill-defined mass that is hypodense in relation to the surrounding parenchyma, though a quarter of tumors are isodense and can be difficult to detect [11, 12].

For optimal detection of tumors, pancreas protocol CT scans are utilized to acquire images at two phases of peak contrast enhancement—the pancreatic phase and the hepatic phase [13]. Prior to the scan, water is given as a negative oral contrast agent to improve visualization of the periampullary region [14]. An arterial phase scan is performed approximately 20 s after injection of intravenous contrast. The *pancreatic phase* occurs after the arterial phase, approximately 40 s after injection of contrast, allowing enhancement and distinction of the pancreatic parenchyma from the neoplastic mass, as well as characterization of the mass in relationship to surrounding vasculature. Finally, the *hepatic phase* occurs approximately 1 min after injection of contrast and allows for venous enhancement of the liver to differentiate between normal hepatic parenchyma and hypovascular metastases, in addition to evaluation of the mesenteric and portal veins for vascular invasion. Isoattenuating tumors may be difficult to discriminate from normal parenchyma and require secondary signs such as ductal dilatation or mass effect to aid in detection [12].

Contrast-enhanced MRI is another modality that can be utilized to image the pancreas. A benefit of contrast-enhanced MRI is improved characterization of isoattenuating tumors that are difficult to see on MDCT [15]. Otherwise, it has been demonstrated to be equivalent to MDCT in detecting pancreatic cancer, with a sensitivity and specificity of 98% and 96%, respectively [16]. A major limitation of MRI is degradation of image quality with motion artifact [17].

In addition to contrast-enhanced MRI in characterizing subtle masses, combined positron emission tomography/computed tomography using 18-fluorodeoxyglucose (FDG-PET/CT) is an alternative option. In a single-center prospective study, FDG-PET/CT was reported to have a diagnostic accuracy of 89%, compared to 76% for MDCT for the detection of pancreatic cancer [18]. Furthermore, FDG-PET/CT plays an invaluable adjunctive role in cases of biliary strictures but lacking signs of malignancy on MDCT and MRI. In a quarter of study patients, clinical decision-making was altered due to FDG-PET/CT. Larger multicenter studies are needed to corroborate these promising findings before establishing FDG-PET/CT as a diagnostic and staging modality. In addition, its utility in staging BR and LAPC remains to be defined.

Endoscopic ultrasound (EUS) is another useful adjunct for detecting masses that are either indeterminate or not seen on CT despite a high clinical suspicion. Placement of the ultrasound probe in close proximity to the pancreas allows for high-resolution imaging in a focused location. The sensitivity and negative predictive value of EUS both approach 100% when the procedure is combined with fine needle aspiration (FNA) for tissue diagnosis [11]. The limitations of EUS are its invasive nature, dependency on operator skill, and inability to assess for metastatic disease. EUS can also be utilized for placement of fiducial markers, which are used as target points for stereotactic body radiation therapy (SBRT).

Tissue Diagnosis and Biliary Decompression

Prior to undergoing neoadjuvant therapy (NT), tissue confirmation of malignancy needs to be established. Currently, the need for surgical biopsy has been overtaken by FNA via percutaneous or endoscopic approaches, which is now considered the gold standard for obtaining tissue diagnosis [19]. Percutaneous and EUS-guided FNA have been demonstrated to be safe, cost-effective, accurate, and adequate in obtaining tissue cytology and histology [20]. Although there is a theoretical concern of seeding the needle tract or peritoneum with tumor, retrospective studies have neither demonstrated a recurrence-free nor overall survival disadvantage with the biopsy procedures [21, 22].

Another consideration for patients with head of the pancreatic tumors and obstructive jaundice is the need for biliary decompression, as many chemotherapy agents are cleared by the biliary system [23, 24]. This is typically performed by placement of a stent via endoscopic retrograde cholangiopancreatography (ERCP). Self-expanding metal stents (SEMS) are preferred over plastic stents due to longer patency and decreased complication rates [25, 26]. In a prospective study of resectable and borderline resectable patients who had SEMS placement prior to NT, stent-related complications—including stent occlusion (13%) and migration (2%)—did not interfere with technical aspects of surgical resection [27].

Neoadjuvant Regimens for Borderline Resectable Pancreatic Cancer

Although there are no randomized trials comparing NT to a surgery-first approach in patients with borderline resectable tumors, NT has become the treatment paradigm for this subset of patients in the United States. The primary purpose of NT is to downstage the tumor with the goal of achieving a margin-free, R0 resection. Additional benefits include early, well-tolerated systemic treatment of micrometastases and testing of tumor biology to select patients most likely to benefit from surgical intervention. Much of the data regarding neoadjuvant chemotherapy with or without chemoradiation therapy (CRT) comes from single-institution studies (Tables 10.3 and 10.4).

Gemcitabine Combination Therapies

One of the largest single-institution studies of BRPC comes from MDACC. Katz et al. reported 160 patients with BR tumors per the MDACC definition, of which 125 (78%) completed NT consisting of CRT ± gemcitabine-based chemotherapy prior to restaging [4]. Among patients restaged, 66 patients (41% of the original 160

Table 10.3 Prior studies of borderline resectable pancreatic cancer

Author [Ref], year	Period of inclusion	Staging definition	Neoadjuvant regimen	Number of patients	Type of study	Resected, *n* (% total)	R0 margins, n (% resected)	Median OS, months, all patients/resected patients
Mehta [71], 2001	Unknown	Other	5-FU-CRT	15	Retrospective single-center	9 (60%)	9 (100%)	12/30
Brown [72], 2008	2004–2007	–	CRT + CTX	13	Retrospective single-center	13 (100%)[a]	11 (85%)	–/–
McClaine [73], 2010	1990–2009	MDACC NCCN	Various	29	Retrospective single-center	12 (41%)	8 (67%)	–/23.3
Stokes [74], 2011	2005–2008	MDACC	Capecitabine-CRT	40	Retrospective single-center	16 (40%)	12 (75%)	12/23
Patel [75], 2011	2006–2009	Other	Gem/docetaxel/ capecitabine +5-FU-IMRT	18	Retrospective single-center	9 (50%)	8 (88%)	15.6/–
Chuong [76], 2011	2006–2010	Other	Gem/docetaxel/ capecitabine +5-FU-CRT	14	Retrospective single-center	14 (100%)	12 (86%)	–/–
Kang [28], 2012	2000–2010	NCCN	Gem-CRT	67	Retrospective single-center	32 (48%)	27 (84%)	–/26.3
Katz [54], 2012	2005–2010	MDACC AHPBA/SSAT/SSO	Gem-based CTX + Gem-CRT, or Gem-CRT alone	129	Retrospective single-center	85 (66%)	81 (95%)	22/33
Rose [77], 2014	2008–2012	AHPBA/SSAT/SSO	Gem/docetaxel	64	Retrospective single-center	31 (48%)	27 (87%)	23.6/not evaluable
Christians [31], 2014	2010–2012	Other	FOLFIRINOX + Gem or Capecitabine-CRT	18	Retrospective single-center	12 (66%)	12 (100%)	Not evaluable/not evaluable
Rashid [78], 2016	2006–2013	NCCN	Gem/docetaxel/ capecitabine + SBRT	101	Retrospective single-center	55 (54%)	53 (98%)	18/33
Katz [34], 2016	2013–2014	Intergroup	mFOLFIRINOX + capecitabine-CRT	22	Prospective, single-arm, multicenter	15 (68%)	14 (93%)	21.7/not evaluable

OS overall survival, *AHPBA* Americas Hepato-Pancreato-Biliary Association, *SSAT* Society for Surgery of the Alimentary Tract, *SSO* Society of Surgical Oncology, *NCCN* National Comprehensive Cancer Network, *5-FU* fluorouracil, *CRT* chemoradiation, *CTX* chemotherapy, *Gem* gemcitabine, *IMRT* intensity-modulated radiation therapy, *SBRT* stereotactic body radiation therapy

[a]Study reported resected a only patients

Table 10.4 Prior studies of borderline resectable and locally advanced pancreatic cancer

Author [Ref], year	Period of inclusion	Staging definition	Neoadjuvant regimen	Number of patients, BL/LAPC	Type of study	Resected, n (% total)	R0 margins, n (% resected)	Median OS, months, all patients/ resected patients
Pipas [79], 2005	2002–2004	Other	Gem/docetaxel + Gem-CRT	7/13	Retrospective single-center	13 (65%)	9 (69%)	14/–
Massucco [80], 2006	1999–2003	Other	Various	18/10	Retrospective single-center	8 (28%)	–	15.4/>21
Small [81], 2008	2002–2003	NCCN	Gem-CRT	9/14	Retrospective multicenter	4 (17%)	–	–/–
Turrini [82], 2009	1996–2006	MDACC	5-FU/ cisplatin-CRT	49/15	Retrospective single-center	9 (14%)	9 (100%)	14/24
Sahora [83], 2011	2001–2003	AHPBA/ SSAT/SSO	Gem/docetaxel	12/13	Prospective phase II, single-arm, single-center	8 (32%)	7 (87%)	13.5/16.3
Sahora [84], 2011	2003–2006	AHPBA/ SSAT/SSO	GEMOX	15/18	Prospective phase II, single-arm, single-center	13 (39%)	9 (69%)	16/22
Arvold [85], 2012	2005–2009	Other	Various	24/46	Retrospective single-center	14 (20%)	9 (64%)	14.2/19.4
Peddi [86], 2012	2009–2012	–	FOLFIRINOX	4/19	Retrospective multicenter	8 (35%)	–	–/–
Hosein [36], 2012	2008–2011	AHPBA/ SSAT/SSO	FOLFIRINOX	4/14	Retrospective single-center	9 (50%)	8 (88%)	–/–
Lee [87], 2012	2006–2008	NCCN	Gem/ capecitabine	18/25	Prospective, single-arm, single-center	17 (40%)	14 (82%)	16.6/23.1

Barugola [88], 2012	2001–2008	Other	Various	27/14	Retrospective single-center	41 (100%)[a]	29 (71%)	–/35
Mahaseth [44], 2013	2010–2012	–	FOLFIRINOX	4/24	Retrospective single-center	–	–	–/17.8
Boone [37], 2013	2011–2012	AHPBA/ SSAT/SSO	FOLFIRINOX	12/13	Retrospective single-center	9 (36%)	7 (77%)	–/–
Leone [49], 2013	2003–2009	Other	GEMOX + Gem-CRT	15/24	Prospective, single-arm, single-center	11 (28%)	9 (82%)	16.7/32
Moorcraft [89], 2014	2010–2013	–	FOLFIRINOX	9/13	Retrospective single-center	7 (32%)	4 (57%)	18.4/–
Ferrone [32], 2015	2011–2014	AHPBA/ SSAT/SSO	FOLFIRINOX	15/25	Retrospective single-center	40 (100%)[a]	35 (92%)	–/–
Addeo [90], 2015	2007–2012	MDACC		11/34	Retrospective single-center	45 (100%)	34 (76%)	17/–
Blazer [33], 2015	2011–2013	AHPBA/ SSAT/SSO	mFOLFIRINOX	18/25	Retrospective single-center	22 (51%)	19 (86%)	21.2–

BL borderline resectable, *LAPC* locally advanced pancreatic cancer, *OS* overall survival, *AHPBA* Americas Hepato-Pancreato-Biliary Association, *SSAT* Society for Surgery of the Alimentary Tract, *SSO* Society of Surgical Oncology, *NCCN* National Comprehensive Cancer Network, fluorouracil, *CRT* chemoradiation therapy, *CTX* chemotherapy, *Gem* gemcitabine, *GEMOX* gemcitabine and oxaliplatin, *FOLFIRINOX* folinic acid, fluorouracil, irinotecan, oxaliplatin, *mFOLFIRINOX* modified FOLFIRINOX

[a]Study reported resected only patients

patients) completed a resection of curative intent, with the majority achieving a R0 resection (62 patients, 94%). Patients who completed NT and resection had a significant survival advantage compared to patients who were not deemed surgical candidates (median overall survival [OS], 40 vs. 13 months, $P < 0.001$). This survival benefit remained when comparing the MDACC *Type A* borderline resectable patients due to vascular involvement who completed NT and surgery to those who did not (median OS, 40 vs. 15 months, $P < 0.001$).

Similar R0 resection rates were reported by Kang et al. in a retrospective observational study comparing 32 BRPC patients who were treated with neoadjuvant gemcitabine-based CRT to 104 patients with resectable disease who underwent upfront pancreatectomy [28]. In addition, there were no appreciable differences in the R0 rates (84% vs. 88%) and disease-specific survival (26.3 months vs. 30.4 months) between the two groups. Moreover, patients who received CRT had decreased T-staging and nodal involvement than the pancreatectomy-first patients ($P < 0.05$), suggesting that CRT not only has a local effect on the primary tumor but also a systemic effect on metastasis to the lymph nodes.

Favorable locoregional control was also observed in a prospective phase II trial conducted by Takahashi et al. in which 188 patients with resectable disease and 80 patients with BRPC both received gemcitabine-based CRT [29]. However, despite similar R0 resection and 5-year local recurrence rates between the two groups, patients with resectable disease had significantly higher 5-year survival rates (57% vs. 34%).

FOLFIRINOX

In the phase III ACCORD-11 trial, FOLFIRINOX (folinic acid, fluorouracil, irinotecan, and oxaliplatin) was demonstrated to have a significant response rate (31.6% vs. 9.4%, $P < 0.001$) and increased OS (11.1 vs. 6.8 months, $P < 0.001$) compared to single-agent gemcitabine among patients with metastatic pancreatic cancer [30]. The encouraging results of this study led to extrapolation of the FOLFIRINOX regimen to BRPC and LAPC. Christians et al. reported resection in 83% of patients and achieved a R0 resection in all patients [31]. Ferrone et al. reported similar results, with an 85% resection rate among 40 patients with BR and LAPC who underwent FOLFIRINOX prior to surgery and 92% obtaining a R0 resection [32]. In addition, compared to patients who were deemed resectable and underwent a surgery-first approach, BRPC patients treated with NT had significantly less lymph node involvement and increased OS.

Although response rates of patients treated with FOLFIRINOX in the ACCORD-11 trial were remarkable, there were significantly higher adverse events of grade 3–4 neutropenia, febrile neutropenia, thrombocytopenia, diarrhea, and neuropathy among patients in the FOLFIRINOX arm than the gemcitabine arm [30]. Due to these treatment toxicities, Blazer et al. utilized modified FOLFIRINOX (mFOLFIRINOX), which consisted of a lower dose of irinotecan and elimination of fluorouracil and leucovorin boluses, and reported a 61% resection rate and 82% RO resection rate among patients with BRPC [33]. Similarly, the Intergroup multicenter clinical trial demonstrated a pancreatectomy rate of 68% and R0 resection rate of 93% with mFOLFIRINOX in combination with capecitabine-based CRT [34].

A summary of studies on BRPC shown in Tables 10.3 and 10.4 displays the heterogeneity of staging definitions, treatment regimens, and therapeutic responses utilized. Thus, there is no universally accepted NT regimen, although induction therapy with gemcitabine combinations and mFOLFIRINOX has become attractive options. To address the lack of consistency in prior studies, the Intergroup trial—a prospective, multicenter single-arm trial—was conducted. This trial was designed to be a feasibility study to demonstrate multi-institutional cooperation in the management of this subset of patients. Thus, sample size in this study was limited to 22 patients. Among 22 patients who received mFOLFIRINOX, 15 (68%) underwent pancreatectomy, and the majority, 14 (93%), achieved an R0 resection [34]. In addition, one-third of patients developed a significant pathologic response of less than 5% residual viable tumor, despite only 27% of patients who had a radiologic partial or complete response after NT. The accrual goal of two patients per month was surpassed by an accrual rate of 2.6 patients per month among 14 institutions. Prior to and after completion of NT, all imaging was reviewed centrally to ensure trial compliance. Thus, not only has the Intergroup trial standardized the definition of BRPC, but it has also set the benchmark for how future clinical trials will be designed and conducted [7, 34].

Neoadjuvant Regimens for Locally Advanced Pancreatic Cancer

Neoadjuvant chemotherapy is the first-line treatment for patients with LAPC. As previously mentioned and depicted in Table 10.4, many retrospective and prospective studies examining NT regimens include patients with both BRPC and LAPC. Similar to the origin of BRPC treatments, neoadjuvant chemotherapy regimens for LAPC matured from the breakthroughs of randomized chemotherapy trials in patients with metastatic pancreatic cancer (Table 10.5).

FOLFIRINOX

As was the case with BRPC, the ACCORD-11 trial introduced FOLFIRINOX as a therapeutic opportunity to downstage tumors, achieve resectability, and attain long-term OS in LAPC cases [32]. Initially, reports from retrospective single-institution studies were limited by small patient populations, often comprised of both patients with BR and LAPC [32, 35–38]. One of the larger studies, the Association des Gastro-Entérologues Oncologues (AGEO) study, was a French multicenter observational cohort trial that prospectively enrolled 77 patients with LAPC to examine the efficacy and tolerability of FOLFIRINOX [39]. The AGEO group reported 6% ($n = 5$) of patients who stopped therapy due toxicities and a resection rate of 36% ($n = 28$) with 89% ($n = 25$) of resected patients achieving R0 margins.

Table 10.5 Prior studies of locally advanced pancreatic cancer (with more than 20 cases)

Author [Ref], year	Period of inclusion	Staging definition	Neoadjuvant regimen	Number of patients	Type of study	Resected, n (% total)	R0 margins, n (% resected)	Median OS, months, all patients / resected patients
Krishnan [91], 2007	1993–2005	Other	1. CRT 2. Chemo + CRT	323	Retrospective single-center	–	1. 7 (2.8%) 2. 2 (2.6%)	1. 8.5 2. 11.9
Chauffert [42], 2008	2000–2005	Other	1. CRT 2. Gem	119	Prospective randomized phase III multicenter	1. 2 (3.4%) 2. 3 (5%)	–	1. 8.6/– 2. 13/–
Wilkowski [92], 2009	2002–2005	Other	1. 5-FU-CRT 2. Gem-CRT 3. Gem-CRT + Gem	95	Prospective phase II, randomized, three-arm, multicenter	1. 4 (13%) 2. 8 (25%) 3. 6 (19%)	–	1. 9.6/– 2. 9.3/– 3. 7.3/–
Loehrer [93], 2011	2003–2005	Other	1. Gem 2. Gem + RT	74	Prospective, randomized, two-arm, single-center	–	-	1. 9.2/–- 2. 11.1/–
Habermehl [94], 2012	2001–2010	Other	Gem-CRT + Gem	215	Retrospective single-center	–(26%)	- (39%)	12.3/14.4
Faris [35], 2013	2010–2012	NCCN	FOLFIRINOX + CRT	22	Retrospective single-center	5 (23%)	5 (100%)	–/–
Marthey [39], 2015	2010–2012	Other	FOLFIRINOX	77	Observational multicenter	28 (36%)	25 (89%)	22/24.9
Sadot [40], 2015	2010–2013	NCCN	FOLFIRINOX ± CRT	101	Retrospective single-center	31 (31%)	16 (55%)	25/–
Nanda [45], 2015	2010–2013	NCCN	mFOLFIRINOX	29	Retrospective single-center	12 (41%)	10 (83%)	18.6/–
Hammel [52], 2016	2008–2011	Other	1. Gem ± CRT 2. Gem/ erlotinib ± CRT	223	Prospective phase III, randomized, two-arm, multicenter	18 (4%)	11 (2.5%)	12.8/30.9
Hackert [43], 2016	2001–2015	–	1. FOLFIRINOX 2. Gem + XRT	575	Retrospective single-center	1. 76 (61%) 2. 66 (52%)	1. 31 (41%) 2. 47 (31%)	1. 16/– 2. 16.5/–

OS overall survival, *AHPBA* Americas Hepato-Pancreato-Biliary Association, *SSAT* Society for Surgery of the Alimentary Tract, *SSO* Society of Surgical Oncology, *NCCN* National Comprehensive Cancer Network, *5-FU* fluorouracil, *CRT* chemoradiation therapy, *Gem* gemcitabine, *RT* radiation therapy, *FOLFIRINOX* folinic acid, fluorouracil, irinotecan, oxaliplatin, *mFOLFIRINOX* modified FOLFIRINOX

Similarly, Sadot et al. reviewed their experience of 101 LAPC cases from the Memorial Sloan Kettering Cancer Center and reported one-third of patients who were resected after induction with FOLFIRINOX, with 55% of patients achieving a R0 resection [40]. Compared to the AGEO group, Sadot et al.'s lower R0 margin rate, though still remarkable, may have been secondary to the variability with FOLFIRINOX treatment duration (1–20 cycles), a limitation given the retrospective nature of this study.

A meta-analysis by Suker et al. of 13 studies utilizing FOLFIRINOX in 355 LAPC cases yielded a resection rate of 25.9% and R0 resection of 78.4% among pooled proportion of cases [41]. The OS of FOLFIRINOX-treated patients was significantly longer than that of gemcitabine-treated patients (median OS, 24.2 vs. 14 months) [42]. Findings from a single-center review of 575 LAPC patients, reported by Hackert et al. after the meta-analysis was published, demonstrated a superior 60% resection rate for patients treated with FOLFIRINOX compared to 46% resection rate of patients treated with gemcitabine and radiation [43]. In addition, FOLFIRINOX treatment was independently associated with a favorable prognosis.

As previously mentioned, treatment toxicities associated with FOLFIRINOX are a significant factor in patient selection. In the meta-analysis, Suker et al. reported grade 3 and 4 adverse events comprising 60% of treatment toxicities or 60.4 adverse events per 100 patients [41]. In single-institution studies of LAPC, mFOLFIRINOX was demonstrated to reduce treatment toxicity without sacrificing efficacy [33, 44, 45]. Stein et al. validated these results in the first prospective study comparing mFOLFIRINOX to full-dose FOLFIRINOX in patients with metastasis and LAPC, reporting decreased adverse events and comparable efficacy with mFOLFIRINOX [46].

Gemcitabine and nab-Paclitaxel

The MPACT phase III randomized trial of patients with metastatic pancreatic cancer demonstrated improved response rate and 2 months longer OS with combination gemcitabine and albumin-bound paclitaxel (nab-paclitaxel) than single-agent gemcitabine [47]. As opposed to the ACCORD-11 trial, which excluded patients with an Eastern Cooperative Oncology Group (ECOG) score of two or more and demonstrated increased serious adverse events in patients treated with FOLFIRINOX, the MPACT trial did not demonstrate a difference in serious adverse events in the treatment groups [30, 47].

Although the use of gemcitabine and nab-paclitaxel for patients with LAPC is limited to a case report, the Locally Advanced Pancreatic Cancer Trial (LAPACT, NCT02301143) and Gemcitabine Abraxane Pancreas (GAP, NCT02043730) randomized trials are currently recruiting patients to compare efficacy of combination gemcitabine and nab-paclitaxel to single-agent gemcitabine [48].

Gemcitabine and Oxaliplatin

Another combination therapy, gemcitabine and oxaliplatin, has garnered interest as a therapeutic modality in treating LAPC. Leone et al. evaluated its use as induction therapy in 39 patients with BR and LAPC [49]. Eleven patients (9 BR, 2 LAPC) completed resection, with a median OS of 31.5 months compared to 12.3 months for unresected patients. Similar encouraging results were achieved in a multi-institutional phase II study of gemcitabine and oxaliplatin with radiation therapy in BRPC [50]. Among 68 patients from four institutions, 43 patients (63%) underwent resection, and the majority, 36 (84%), achieved a R0 resection.

Role of Radiation Therapy in LAPC

Chemotherapy is the first-line treatment for unresectable pancreas cancer, identified as a systemic disease. Theoretically, when followed by SBRT or CRT, which is used for local control, the opportunity to obtain an R0 resection is increased. A meta-analysis by Morganti et al. of 13 studies utilizing preoperative CRT in 510 LAPC cases yielded high median resection and R0 resection rates of 26.5% and 87.5%, respectively, and a median OS of 23.6 months among resected patients [51]. Although many retrospective studies and clinical trials have utilized SBRT and CRT following chemotherapy to treat patients with BR or unresectable disease, there is no agreement on an optimal regimen.

The LAP-07 phase III randomized trial sought to examine if the addition of CRT after 4 months of induction chemotherapy with gemcitabine ± erlotinib improved survival [52]. Among 442 patients randomized to either single-agent gemcitabine or in combination with erlotinib, patients with progression-free disease then underwent a second randomization—continue chemotherapy for an additional 2 months or CRT consisting of 54 Gy with capecitabine. Although patients treated with CRT post-chemotherapy had decreased local progression, there was no difference in the primary outcome of the study, median OS, when compared to chemotherapy alone (15.2 vs. 16.5 months, $P = 0.83$). However, these results do not close the door on CRT as an adjunct to chemotherapy, as the trial was designed in 2005, prior to studies reporting greater efficacy with FOLFIRINOX and combination gemcitabine and nab-paclitaxel in comparison with single-agent gemcitabine, historically, for treatment of LAPC.

Further trials are needed to evaluate the efficacy of CRT with these newer chemotherapy regimens. Trials are underway to examine the effect of SBRT and dose escalation after induction with FOLFIRINOX or combination gemcitabine and nab-paclitaxel. The Alliance Trial A021501 (NCT02839343), a prospective phase II study, will randomize BR patients to treatment with mFOLFIRINOX (seven courses) with the addition of hypofractionated SBRT (one course) or mFOLFIRINOX alone (eight courses), followed by resection for those deemed surgical candidates. The primary objective is to evaluate the 18-month OS with the longer course of chemotherapy. Secondary objectives are comparison of the two treatment arms in terms of regimen efficacy (R0 response rate, pathologic complete response rate, and event-free survival) and safety (incidence of adverse events).

Surgical Resection

Determining Resectability

The decision to proceed with resection post-NT has traditionally been determined by radiologic imaging, utilizing the Response Evaluation Criteria in Solid Tumors (RECIST) version 1.1 to evaluate for radiologic response post-NT [53]. However, the ability of CT imaging to distinguish between viable tumor and scarring in response to NT is questionable. A multi-institutional study conducted by Dholakia et al. reported no difference in the degree of tumor-vessel involvement between BR patients who underwent resection post-NT and those who remained unresectable [54]. In a MDACC review of 129 patients with BRPC, the majority of patients ($n = 85$) had stable disease, 12% had a partial response ($n = 15$), and only one patient had their tumor downstaged to resectable status after NT [54]. Yet, 66% ($n = 85$) of patients underwent resection and achieved a median OS of 33 months. The authors concluded that RECIST response was not an accurate predictor of resectability and that all patients should undergo an attempt at resection after NT, in the absence of systemic progression or local progression resulting in unresectability.

Vascular Resections

Due to limitations of current imaging modalities to accurately distinguish continued tumor involvement from downstaged desmoplastic reaction, en bloc vascular resections are frequently performed for patients with BR and LAPC patients who proceed to surgery. Prior reports have demonstrated feasibility of venous vascular resections, with similar morbidity and mortality compared to resections without vascular involvement [55, 56].

Yekebas et al. reviewed 585 LAPC cases and compared 449 patients who underwent pancreatectomy without a vascular resection to 136 patients who did receive a vascular resection [57]. The majority of vascular resections were performed due to involvement of the SMV-PV (94%, $n = 128$). The HA or SMA was resected in 10% ($n = 13$) of cases, and five patients underwent both venous and arterial reconstruction. In addition to similar in-hospital morbidity and mortality, there were no differences in median OS for patients with histopathologic proven vascular invasion who underwent vascular resection (15.2 months) and patients without vascular involvement (16 months).

In contrast to the abundance of literature on venous resections, there is a scarcity of reports examining arterial resections. In a retrospective analysis comparing 29 patients who underwent pancreatic resection with arterial en bloc resection to 449 patients who had a standard resection, higher morbidity (38% vs. 19.8%, $P = 0.031$) and mortality (14% vs. 4%, $P = 0.037$) rates, as well as a lower R0 resection rate (66% vs. 85.3%, $P = 0.027$), were reported in the arterial en bloc resection group [58]. Similarly, in a meta-analysis of 26 studies involving 366 patients who underwent arterial resection and 2243 patients who did not, Mollberg et al. reported increased mortality (odds ratio [OR], 5.04; 95% confidence interval [CI], 2.69–9.45; $P < 0.0001$) and decreased 1-year (OR, 0.49; 95% CI, 0.31–0.78; $P = 0.002$) and 3-year (OR, 0.39; 95% CI, 0.17–0.86; $P = 0.02$) survival among patients who underwent arterial resections compared to patients who did not [59]. Parallel outcome disparities are reported in patients who underwent arterial resections compared to patients who underwent venous resection. In a study of 184 BRPC patients treated with gemcitabine-based chemoradiation, Takahashi et al. reported worse survival outcomes among patients who underwent vascular resections for arterial involvement than for venous involvement [60]. Thus, unlike the feasibility and safety demonstrated with venous resections, arterial resections are associated with unfavorable surgical and prognostic outcomes.

Modified Appleby Procedure for Encasement of the Celiac Artery

The Appleby procedure was first described in 1953 as a total gastrectomy with resection of the CA for locally advanced gastric cancer [61]. Currently, the modified Appleby procedure involves a distal pancreatectomy (DP) and splenectomy with CA resection (DP-CAR) for locally advanced cancers of the body and tail of the pancreas [62]. Perfusion of the liver is achieved through retrograde flow of the preserved gastroduodenal artery.

Single-institution series report a 91% R0 resection rate and 5-year survival of 30–40% among patients who underwent DP-CAR [63–65]. In a matched 3:1 analysis of patients who underwent DP ($n = 51$) and DP-CAR ($n = 17$), Peters et al. reported similar R0 resection rates (DP-CAR vs. DP, 82.4% vs. 92.2%) and median OS (DP-CAR vs. DP, 19 vs. 20 months) [66]. The majority of patients who underwent DP-CAR received neoadjuvant FOLFIRINOX ($n = 15$), and only one patient (6.7%) had a R1 resection, compared to the surgery-first patients ($n = 2$) who had a 100% R1 resection. Furthermore, there were no differences in complication rates and mortality between the two procedures. However, these results may not be generalizable, as this study was conducted at high-volume, tertiary medical center and is not reflective of mortality rates as high as 18% from prior studies [65]. A matched analysis of the American College of Surgeons National Surgical Quality Improvement Program database comparing patients who underwent DP-CAR to DP reported higher 30-day mortality rates after DP-CAR (10% vs. 1%, $P < 0.03$) [67].

Future Directions

Despite the introduction of new neoadjuvant regimens and advancements in surgical technique and perioperative care, progress made by physicians and surgeons treating patients with pancreatic cancer continue to be outpaced by its rising incidence and mortality rate. Response and resection rates for BR and LAPC have improved over the past decade with the introduction of newer agents such as FOLFIRINOX and gemcitabine combinations, when compared historically to single-agent gemcitabine. As was the case with the ACCORD-11 and MPACT trials, future breakthroughs in the treatment of metastatic pancreatic cancer may carry over promising effective systemic therapies to downstage patients with advanced nonmetastatic disease [30, 47].

Targeted therapy, genomic profiling, and immunotherapy are prospective adjuncts to bridge the gap between modest advancements in medicine and the aggressive nature of pancreatic cancer. Mutations in proto-oncogene *KRAS*, which is directly downstream of epidermal growth factor receptor (*EGFR*) gene, have been reported in over 90% of pancreatic cancers and may be responsible for decreased efficacy of EGFR inhibitor erlotinib [68]. Silencing of *KRAS* expression has been demonstrated in increased erlotinib inhibition of EGFR in vitro [69].

Immunotherapy utilizing "checkpoint inhibitors," antibodies that target proteins expressed by cancer cells that allow it to hide from the body's immune system, has demonstrated promising response rates in other metastatic cancers. Although administration of single-agent ipilimumab (anti-CTLA-4) did not prolong survival in patients with metastatic pancreatic cancer, a delayed response occurred in one patient with progressive disease, suggestive of a potential immunotherapeutic influence [70]. Combination of immunotherapy with established treatment regimens may lead to a treatment breakthrough in patients with metastatic cancer, paving the way for more effective therapies to downstage patients with BR and LAPC.

References

1. Siegel RL, Miller KD, Jemal A. Cancer statistics, 2016. CA Cancer J Clin. 2016;66(1):7–30.
2. Sohn TA, Yeo CJ, Cameron JL, Koniaris L, Kaushal S, Abrams RA, et al. Resected adenocarcinoma of the pancreas-616 patients: results, outcomes, and prognostic indicators. J Gastrointest Surg. 2000;4(6):567–79.
3. Edge SB, Compton CC. The American joint committee on cancer: the 7th edition of the AJCC cancer staging manual and the future of TNM. Ann Surg Oncol. 2010;17(6):1471–4.
4. Katz MH, Pisters PW, Evans DB, Sun CC, Lee JE, Fleming JB, et al. Borderline resectable pancreatic cancer: the importance of this emerging stage of disease. J Am Coll Surg. 2008;206(5):833–46. discussion 46-8
5. Callery MP, Chang KJ, Fishman EK, Talamonti MS, William Traverso L, Linehan DC. Pretreatment assessment of resectable and borderline resectable pancreatic cancer: expert consensus statement. Ann Surg Oncol. 2009;16(7):1727–33.
6. Ishikawa O, Ohigashi H, Imaoka S, Furukawa H, Sasaki Y, Fujita M, et al. Preoperative indications for extended pancreatectomy for locally advanced pancreas cancer involving the portal vein. Ann Surg. 1992;215(3):231–6.

7. Katz MH, Marsh R, Herman JM, Shi Q, Collison E, Venook AP, et al. Borderline resectable pancreatic cancer: need for standardization and methods for optimal clinical trial design. Ann Surg Oncol. 2013;20(8):2787–95.
8. DS L, Reber HA, Krasny RM, Kadell BM, Sayre J. Local staging of pancreatic cancer: criteria for unresectability of major vessels as revealed by pancreatic-phase, thin-section helical CT. AJR Am J Roentgenol. 1997;168(6):1439–43.
9. Wong JC, Lu DS. Staging of pancreatic adenocarcinoma by imaging studies. Clin Gastroenterol Hepatol. 2008;6(12):1301–8.
10. Legmann P, Vignaux O, Dousset B, Baraza AJ, Palazzo L, Dumontier I, et al. Pancreatic tumors: comparison of dual-phase helical CT and endoscopic sonography. AJR Am J Roentgenol. 1998;170(5):1315–22.
11. Pietryga JA, Morgan DE. Imaging preoperatively for pancreatic adenocarcinoma. J Gastrointest Oncol. 2015;6(4):343–57.
12. Prokesch RW, Chow LC, Beaulieu CF, Bammer R, Jeffrey RB Jr. Isoattenuating pancreatic adenocarcinoma at multi-detector row CT: secondary signs. Radiology. 2002;224(3):764–8.
13. Xia BT, Ahmad SA. Clinical considerations for pancreatic cancer. Semin Roentgenol. 2016;51(2):74–81.
14. Makarawo TP, Negussie E, Malde S, Tilak J, Gayagoy J, Watson J, et al. Water as a contrast medium: a re-evaluation using the multidetector-row computed tomography. Am Surg. 2013;79(7):728–33.
15. Kim JH, Park SH, ES Y, Kim MH, Kim J, Byun JH, et al. Visually isoattenuating pancreatic adenocarcinoma at dynamic-enhanced CT: frequency, clinical and pathologic characteristics, and diagnosis at imaging examinations. Radiology. 2010;257(1):87–96.
16. Koelblinger C, Ba-Ssalamah A, Goetzinger P, Puchner S, Weber M, Sahora K, et al. Gadobenate dimeglumine-enhanced 3.0-T MR imaging versus multiphasic 64-detector row CT: prospective evaluation in patients suspected of having pancreatic cancer. Radiology. 2011;259(3):757–66.
17. Bipat S, Phoa SS, van Delden OM, Bossuyt PM, Gouma DJ, Lameris JS, et al. Ultrasonography, computed tomography and magnetic resonance imaging for diagnosis and determining resectability of pancreatic adenocarcinoma: a meta-analysis. J Comput Assist Tomogr. 2005;29(4):438–45.
18. Kauhanen SP, Komar G, Seppanen MP, Dean KI, Minn HR, Kajander SA, et al. A prospective diagnostic accuracy study of 18F-fluorodeoxyglucose positron emission tomography/computed tomography, multidetector row computed tomography, and magnetic resonance imaging in primary diagnosis and staging of pancreatic cancer. Ann Surg. 2009;250(6):957–63.
19. Roy A, Kim M, Hawes R, Varadarajulu S. Changing trends in tissue acquisition in malignant pancreatic neoplasms. J Gastroenterol Hepatol. 2016;31(2):501–5.
20. Matsuyama M, Ishii H, Kuraoka K, Yukisawa S, Kasuga A, Ozaka M, et al. Ultrasound-guided vs endoscopic ultrasound-guided fine-needle aspiration for pancreatic cancer diagnosis. World J Gastroenterol. 2013;19(15):2368–73.
21. Ikezawa K, Uehara H, Sakai A, Fukutake N, Imanaka K, Ohkawa K, et al. Risk of peritoneal carcinomatosis by endoscopic ultrasound-guided fine needle aspiration for pancreatic cancer. J Gastroenterol. 2013;48(8):966–72.
22. Ngamruengphong S, Swanson KM, Shah ND, Wallace MB. Preoperative endoscopic ultrasound-guided fine needle aspiration does not impair survival of patients with resected pancreatic cancer. Gut. 2015;64(7):1105–10.
23. Tempero MA, Arnoletti JP, Behrman SW, Ben-Josef E, Benson AB 3rd, Casper ES, et al. Pancreatic adenocarcinoma, version 2.2012: featured updates to the NCCN guidelines. J Natl Compr Cancer Netw. 2012;10(6):703–13.
24. Cooper AB, Tzeng CW, Katz MH. Treatment of borderline resectable pancreatic cancer. Curr Treat Options in Oncol. 2013;14(3):293–310.
25. Adams MA, Anderson MA, Myles JD, Khalatbari S, Scheiman JM. Self-expanding metal stents (SEMS) provide superior outcomes compared to plastic stents for pancreatic cancer patients undergoing neoadjuvant therapy. J Gastrointest Oncol. 2012;3(4):309–13.
26. Soderlund C, Linder S. Covered metal versus plastic stents for malignant common bile duct stenosis: a prospective, randomized, controlled trial. Gastrointest Endosc. 2006;63(7):986–95.

27. Aadam AA, Evans DB, Khan A, Oh Y, Dua K. Efficacy and safety of self-expandable metal stents for biliary decompression in patients receiving neoadjuvant therapy for pancreatic cancer: a prospective study. Gastrointest Endosc. 2012;76(1):67–75.
28. Kang CM, Chung YE, Park JY, Sung JS, Hwang HK, Choi HJ, et al. Potential contribution of preoperative neoadjuvant concurrent chemoradiation therapy on margin-negative resection in borderline resectable pancreatic cancer. J Gastrointest Surg. 2012;16(3):509–17.
29. Takahashi H, Ohigashi H, Gotoh K, Marubashi S, Yamada T, Murata M, et al. Preoperative gemcitabine-based chemoradiation therapy for resectable and borderline resectable pancreatic cancer. Ann Surg. 2013;258(6):1040–50.
30. Conroy T, Desseigne F, Ychou M, Bouche O, Guimbaud R, Becouarn Y, et al. FOLFIRINOX versus gemcitabine for metastatic pancreatic cancer. N Engl J Med. 2011;364(19):1817–25.
31. Christians KK, Tsai S, Mahmoud A, Ritch P, Thomas JP, Wiebe L, et al. Neoadjuvant FOLFIRINOX for borderline resectable pancreas cancer: a new treatment paradigm? Oncologist. 2014;19(3):266–74.
32. Ferrone CR, Marchegiani G, Hong TS, Ryan DP, Deshpande V, McDonnell EI, et al. Radiological and surgical implications of neoadjuvant treatment with FOLFIRINOX for locally advanced and borderline resectable pancreatic cancer. Ann Surg. 2015;261(1):12–7.
33. Blazer M, Wu C, Goldberg RM, Phillips G, Schmidt C, Muscarella P, et al. Neoadjuvant modified (m) FOLFIRINOX for locally advanced unresectable (LAPC) and borderline resectable (BRPC) adenocarcinoma of the pancreas. Ann Surg Oncol. 2015;22(4):1153–9.
34. Katz MH, Shi Q, Ahmad SA, Herman JM, Marsh RW, Collisson E, et al. Preoperative Modified FOLFIRINOX Treatment Followed by Capecitabine-Based Chemoradiation for Borderline Resectable Pancreatic Cancer: Alliance for Clinical Trials in Oncology Trial A021101. JAMA Surg. 2016;151(8):e161137.
35. Faris JE, Blaszkowsky LS, McDermott S, Guimaraes AR, Szymonifka J, Huynh MA, et al. FOLFIRINOX in locally advanced pancreatic cancer: the Massachusetts General Hospital cancer center experience. Oncologist. 2013;18(5):543–8.
36. Hosein PJ, Macintyre J, Kawamura C, Maldonado JC, Ernani V, Loaiza-Bonilla A, et al. A retrospective study of neoadjuvant FOLFIRINOX in unresectable or borderline-resectable locally advanced pancreatic adenocarcinoma. BMC Cancer. 2012;12:199.
37. Boone BA, Steve J, Krasinskas AM, Zureikat AH, Lembersky BC, Gibson MK, et al. Outcomes with FOLFIRINOX for borderline resectable and locally unresectable pancreatic cancer. J Surg Oncol. 2013;108(4):236–41.
38. Gunturu KS, Yao X, Cong X, Thumar JR, Hochster HS, Stein SM, et al. FOLFIRINOX for locally advanced and metastatic pancreatic cancer: single institution retrospective review of efficacy and toxicity. Med Oncol. 2013;30(1):361.
39. Marthey L, Sa-Cunha A, Blanc JF, Gauthier M, Cueff A, Francois E, et al. FOLFIRINOX for locally advanced pancreatic adenocarcinoma: results of an AGEO multicenter prospective observational cohort. Ann Surg Oncol. 2015;22(1):295–301.
40. Sadot E, Doussot A, O'Reilly EM, Lowery MA, Goodman KA, Do RK, et al. FOLFIRINOX induction therapy for stage 3 pancreatic adenocarcinoma. Ann Surg Oncol. 2015;22(11):3512–21.
41. Suker M, Beumer BR, Sadot E, Marthey L, Faris JE, Mellon EA, et al. FOLFIRINOX for locally advanced pancreatic cancer: a systematic review and patient-level meta-analysis. Lancet Oncol. 2016;17(6):801–10.
42. Chauffert B, Mornex F, Bonnetain F, Rougier P, Mariette C, Bouche O, et al. Phase III trial comparing intensive induction chemoradiotherapy (60 Gy, infusional 5-FU and intermittent cisplatin) followed by maintenance gemcitabine with gemcitabine alone for locally advanced unresectable pancreatic cancer. Definitive results of the 2000-01 FFCD/SFRO study. Ann Oncol. 2008;19(9):1592–9.
43. Hackert T, Sachsenmaier M, Hinz U, Schneider L, Michalski CW, Springfeld C, et al. Locally advanced pancreatic cancer: Neoadjuvant therapy with Folfirinox results in Resectability in 60% of the patients. Ann Surg. 2016;264(3):457–63.

44. Mahaseth H, Brutcher E, Kauh J, Hawk N, Kim S, Chen Z, et al. Modified FOLFIRINOX regimen with improved safety and maintained efficacy in pancreatic adenocarcinoma. Pancreas. 2013;42(8):1311–5.
45. Nanda RH, El-Rayes B, Maithel SK, Landry J. Neoadjuvant modified FOLFIRINOX and chemoradiation therapy for locally advanced pancreatic cancer improves resectability. J Surg Oncol. 2015;111(8):1028–34.
46. Stein SM, James ES, Deng Y, Cong X, Kortmansky JS, Li J, et al. Final analysis of a phase II study of modified FOLFIRINOX in locally advanced and metastatic pancreatic cancer. Br J Cancer. 2016;114(7):809–12.
47. Von Hoff DD, Ervin T, Arena FP, Chiorean EG, Infante J, Moore M, et al. Increased survival in pancreatic cancer with nab-paclitaxel plus gemcitabine. N Engl J Med. 2013;369(18):1691–703.
48. Olowokure O, Torregroza-Sanchez MP, Bedoya-Apraez ID. Gemcitabine plus nab-paclitaxel with chemoradiation in locally advanced pancreatic cancer (LAPC). J Gastrointest Oncol. 2013;4(2):E16–8.
49. Leone F, Gatti M, Massucco P, Colombi F, Sperti E, Campanella D, et al. Induction gemcitabine and oxaliplatin therapy followed by a twice-weekly infusion of gemcitabine and concurrent external-beam radiation for neoadjuvant treatment of locally advanced pancreatic cancer: a single institutional experience. Cancer. 2013;119(2):277–84.
50. Kim EJ, Ben-Josef E, Herman JM, Bekaii-Saab T, Dawson LA, Griffith KA, et al. A multi-institutional phase 2 study of neoadjuvant gemcitabine and oxaliplatin with radiation therapy in patients with pancreatic cancer. Cancer. 2013;119(15):2692–700.
51. Morganti AG, Massaccesi M, La Torre G, Caravatta L, Piscopo A, Tambaro R, et al. A systematic review of resectability and survival after concurrent chemoradiation in primarily unresectable pancreatic cancer. Ann Surg Oncol. 2010;17(1):194–205.
52. Hammel P, Huguet F, van Laethem JL, Goldstein D, Glimelius B, Artru P, et al. Effect of Chemoradiotherapy vs chemotherapy on survival in patients with locally advanced pancreatic cancer controlled after 4 months of gemcitabine with or without Erlotinib: the LAP07 randomized clinical trial. JAMA. 2016;315(17):1844–53.
53. Eisenhauer EA, Therasse P, Bogaerts J, Schwartz LH, Sargent D, Ford R, et al. New response evaluation criteria in solid tumours: revised RECIST guideline (version 1.1). Eur J Cancer. 2009;45(2):228–47.
54. Katz MH, Fleming JB, Bhosale P, Varadhachary G, Lee JE, Wolff R, et al. Response of borderline resectable pancreatic cancer to neoadjuvant therapy is not reflected by radiographic indicators. Cancer. 2012;118(23):5749–56.
55. Harrison LE, Klimstra DS, Brennan MF. Isolated portal vein involvement in pancreatic adenocarcinoma. A contraindication for resection? Ann Surg. 1996;224(3):342–7. discussion 7-9
56. Koniaris LG, Staveley-O'Carroll KF, Zeh HJ, Perez E, Jin XL, Maley WR, et al. Pancreaticoduodenectomy in the presence of superior mesenteric venous obstruction. J Gastrointest Surg. 2005;9(7):915–21.
57. Yekebas EF, Bogoevski D, Cataldegirmen G, Kunze C, Marx A, Vashist YK, et al. En bloc vascular resection for locally advanced pancreatic malignancies infiltrating major blood vessels: perioperative outcome and long-term survival in 136 patients. Ann Surg. 2008;247(2):300–9.
58. Bockhorn M, Burdelski C, Bogoevski D, Sgourakis G, Yekebas EF, Izbicki JR. Arterial en bloc resection for pancreatic carcinoma. Br J Surg. 2011;98(1):86–92.
59. Mollberg N, Rahbari NN, Koch M, Hartwig W, Hoeger Y, Buchler MW, et al. Arterial resection during pancreatectomy for pancreatic cancer: a systematic review and meta-analysis. Ann Surg. 2011;254(6):882–93.
60. Takahashi H, Akita H, Tomokuni A, Kobayashi S, Ohigashi H, Fijiwara Y, et al. Preoperative gemcitabine-based Chemoradiation therapy for borderline Resectable pancreatic cancer: impact of venous and arterial involvement status on surgical outcome and pattern of recurrence. Ann Surg. 2016;264(6):1091–7.
61. Appleby LH. The coeliac axis in the expansion of the operation for gastric carcinoma. Cancer. 1953;6(4):704–7.

62. Liu B. Modified Appleby operation in treatment of distal pancreatic cancer. Hepatobiliary Pancreat Dis Int. 2003;2(4):622–5.
63. Nakamura T, Hirano S, Noji T, Asano T, Okamura K, Tsuchikawa T, et al. Distal Pancreatectomy with en bloc celiac Axis resection (modified Appleby procedure) for locally advanced pancreatic body cancer: a single-center review of 80 consecutive patients. Ann Surg Oncol. 2016;23:969.
64. Hirano S, Kondo S, Hara T, Ambo Y, Tanaka E, Shichinohe T, et al. Distal pancreatectomy with en bloc celiac axis resection for locally advanced pancreatic body cancer: long-term results. Ann Surg. 2007;246(1):46–51.
65. Baumgartner JM, Krasinskas A, Daouadi M, Zureikat A, Marsh W, Lee K, et al. Distal pancreatectomy with en bloc celiac axis resection for locally advanced pancreatic adenocarcinoma following neoadjuvant therapy. J Gastrointest Surg. 2012;16(6):1152–9.
66. Peters NA, Javed AA, Cameron JL, Makary MA, Hirose K, Pawlik TM, et al. Modified Appleby procedure for pancreatic adenocarcinoma: does improved Neoadjuvant therapy warrant such an aggressive approach? Ann Surg Oncol. 2016;23:3757.
67. Beane JD, House MG, Pitt SC, Kilbane EM, Hall BL, Parmar AD, et al. Distal pancreatectomy with celiac axis resection: what are the added risks? HPB (Oxford). 2015;17(9):777–84.
68. Frank TS, Sun X, Zhang Y, Yang J, Fisher WE, Gingras MC, et al. Genomic profiling guides the choice of molecular targeted therapy of pancreatic cancer. Cancer Lett. 2015;363(1):1–6.
69. Diep CH, Munoz RM, Choudhary A, Von Hoff DD, Han H. Synergistic effect between erlotinib and MEK inhibitors in KRAS wild-type human pancreatic cancer cells. Clin Cancer Res. 2011;17(9):2744–56.
70. Royal RE, Levy C, Turner K, Mathur A, Hughes M, Kammula US, et al. Phase 2 trial of single agent Ipilimumab (anti-CTLA-4) for locally advanced or metastatic pancreatic adenocarcinoma. J Immunother. 2010;33(8):828–33.
71. Mehta VK, Fisher G, Ford JA, Poen JC, Vierra MA, Oberhelman H, et al. Preoperative chemoradiation for marginally resectable adenocarcinoma of the pancreas. J Gastrointest Surg. 2001;5(1):27–35.
72. Brown KM, Siripurapu V, Davidson M, Cohen SJ, Konski A, Watson JC, et al. Chemoradiation followed by chemotherapy before resection for borderline pancreatic adenocarcinoma. Am J Surg. 2008;195(3):318–21.
73. McClaine RJ, Lowy AM, Sussman JJ, Schmulewitz N, Grisell DL, Ahmad SA. Neoadjuvant therapy may lead to successful surgical resection and improved survival in patients with borderline resectable pancreatic cancer. HPB (Oxford). 2010;12(1):73–9.
74. Stokes JB, Nolan NJ, Stelow EB, Walters DM, Weiss GR, de Lange EE, et al. Preoperative capecitabine and concurrent radiation for borderline resectable pancreatic cancer. Ann Surg Oncol. 2011;18(3):619–27.
75. Patel M, Hoffe S, Malafa M, Hodul P, Klapman J, Centeno B, et al. Neoadjuvant GTX chemotherapy and IMRT-based chemoradiation for borderline resectable pancreatic cancer. J Surg Oncol. 2011;104(2):155–61.
76. Chuong MD, Hayman TJ, Patel MR, Russell MS, Malafa MP, Hodul PJ, et al. Comparison of 1-, 2-, and 3-dimensional tumor response assessment after Neoadjuvant GTX-RT in borderline-Resectable pancreatic cancer. Gastrointest Cancer Res. 2011;4(4):128–34.
77. Rose JB, Rocha FG, Alseidi A, Biehl T, Moonka R, Ryan JA, et al. Extended neoadjuvant chemotherapy for borderline resectable pancreatic cancer demonstrates promising postoperative outcomes and survival. Ann Surg Oncol. 2014;21(5):1530–7.
78. Rashid OM, Pimiento JM, Gamenthaler AW, Nguyen P, Ha TT, Hutchinson T, et al. Outcomes of a clinical pathway for borderline Resectable pancreatic cancer. Ann Surg Oncol. 2016;23(4):1371–9.
79. Pipas JM, Barth RJ Jr, Zaki B, Tsapakos MJ, Suriawinata AA, Bettmann MA, et al. Docetaxel/gemcitabine followed by gemcitabine and external beam radiotherapy in patients with pancreatic adenocarcinoma. Ann Surg Oncol. 2005;12(12):995–1004.
80. Massucco P, Capussotti L, Magnino A, Sperti E, Gatti M, Muratore A, et al. Pancreatic resections after chemoradiotherapy for locally advanced ductal adenocarcinoma: analysis of perioperative outcome and survival. Ann Surg Oncol. 2006;13(9):1201–8.

81. Small W Jr, Berlin J, Freedman GM, Lawrence T, Talamonti MS, Mulcahy MF, et al. Full-dose gemcitabine with concurrent radiation therapy in patients with nonmetastatic pancreatic cancer: a multicenter phase II trial. J Clin Oncol. 2008;26(6):942–7.
82. Turrini O, Viret F, Moureau-Zabotto L, Guiramand J, Moutardier V, Lelong B, et al. Neoadjuvant chemoradiation and pancreaticoduodenectomy for initially locally advanced head pancreatic adenocarcinoma. Eur J Surg Oncol. 2009;35(12):1306–11.
83. Sahora K, Kuehrer I, Schindl M, Koelblinger C, Goetzinger P, Gnant M. NeoGemTax: gemcitabine and docetaxel as neoadjuvant treatment for locally advanced nonmetastasized pancreatic cancer. World J Surg. 2011;35(7):1580–9.
84. Sahora K, Kuehrer I, Eisenhut A, Akan B, Koellblinger C, Goetzinger P, et al. NeoGemOx: gemcitabine and oxaliplatin as neoadjuvant treatment for locally advanced, nonmetastasized pancreatic cancer. Surgery. 2011;149(3):311–20.
85. Arvold ND, Ryan DP, Niemierko A, Blaszkowsky LS, Kwak EL, Wo JY, et al. Long-term outcomes of neoadjuvant chemotherapy before chemoradiation for locally advanced pancreatic cancer. Cancer. 2012;118(12):3026–35.
86. Peddi PF, Lubner S, McWilliams R, Tan BR, Picus J, Sorscher SM, et al. Multi-institutional experience with FOLFIRINOX in pancreatic adenocarcinoma. JOP. 2012;13(5):497–501.
87. Lee JL, Kim SC, Kim JH, Lee SS, Kim TW, Park DH, et al. Prospective efficacy and safety study of neoadjuvant gemcitabine with capecitabine combination chemotherapy for borderline-resectable or unresectable locally advanced pancreatic adenocarcinoma. Surgery. 2012;152(5):851–62.
88. Barugola G, Partelli S, Crippa S, Capelli P, D'Onofrio M, Pederzoli P, et al. Outcomes after resection of locally advanced or borderline resectable pancreatic cancer after neoadjuvant therapy. Am J Surg. 2012;203(2):132–9.
89. Moorcraft SY, Khan K, Peckitt C, Watkins D, Rao S, Cunningham D, et al. FOLFIRINOX for locally advanced or metastatic pancreatic ductal adenocarcinoma: the Royal Marsden experience. Clin Colorectal Cancer. 2014;13(4):232–8.
90. Addeo P, Rosso E, Fuchshuber P, Oussoultzoglou E, De Blasi V, Simone G, et al. Resection of borderline Resectable and locally advanced pancreatic adenocarcinomas after Neoadjuvant chemotherapy. Oncology. 2015;89(1):37–46.
91. Krishnan S, Rana V, Janjan NA, Varadhachary GR, Abbruzzese JL, Das P, et al. Induction chemotherapy selects patients with locally advanced, unresectable pancreatic cancer for optimal benefit from consolidative chemoradiation therapy. Cancer. 2007;110(1):47–55.
92. Wilkowski R, Boeck S, Ostermaier S, Sauer R, Herbst M, Fietkau R, et al. Chemoradiotherapy with concurrent gemcitabine and cisplatin with or without sequential chemotherapy with gemcitabine/cisplatin vs chemoradiotherapy with concurrent 5-fluorouracil in patients with locally advanced pancreatic cancer--a multi-centre randomised phase II study. Br J Cancer. 2009;101(11):1853–9.
93. Loehrer PJ Sr, Feng Y, Cardenes H, Wagner L, Brell JM, Cella D, et al. Gemcitabine alone versus gemcitabine plus radiotherapy in patients with locally advanced pancreatic cancer: an eastern cooperative Oncology group trial. J Clin Oncol. 2011;29(31):4105–12.
94. Habermehl D, Kessel K, Welzel T, Hof H, Abdollahi A, Bergmann F, et al. Neoadjuvant chemoradiation with gemcitabine for locally advanced pancreatic cancer. Radiat Oncol. 2012;7:28.

Chapter 11
Cytotoxic Therapy in Advanced Pancreatic Cancer: Where We Are and Where We Are Headed

Namrata Vijayvergia and Steven J. Cohen

Introduction

In 2016, pancreatic cancer will be the 12th most commonly diagnosed cancer and the fourth leading cause of cancer deaths in the United States. The incidence of pancreatic cancer has been slowly rising over the last decade. It is estimated that about 53,000 new cases will be diagnosed and 42,000 people will die from pancreatic cancer in 2016 [1]. The small difference between the incidence and death rate of pancreatic cancer reflects the early distant spread and inadequacy of current therapies. The 5-year survival rates for localized and advanced pancreatic cancer are 29% and less than 5%, respectively, which is lower than all other common cancers [2]. The majority of patients are diagnosed at an advanced stage and are not eligible for surgical resection [2]. Even those patients with early-stage disease undergoing curative surgery have a very high likelihood of relapse, making systemic therapy the mainstay of treatment for pancreatic cancer. The use of systemic cytotoxic chemotherapy in the treatment of metastatic pancreatic adenocarcinoma will thus be reviewed here.

N. Vijayvergia, M.D. (✉)
Fox Chase Cancer Center, Philadelphia, PA 19111, USA
e-mail: namrata.vijayvergia@fccc.edu

S.J. Cohen, M.D.
Abington Hospital-Jefferson Health, Abington, PA 19001, USA

T. Bekaii-Saab, B. El-Rayes (eds.), *Current and Emerging Therapies in Pancreatic Cancer*, DOI 10.1007/978-3-319-58256-6_11

First-Line Therapy

Single Agent

Before 1998, 5-fluorouracil (5-FU) was the only available therapy for advanced pancreatic cancer based upon superiority against best supportive care in small prospective studies and later a meta-analysis [3–5]. The low response rates ($\leq$7%) with single-agent 5-FU highlighted the need for further research [3]. In 1997, Burris et al. subsequently published a pivotal randomized trial that compared gemcitabine (1000 mg/m^2 weekly × 7 followed by 1 week break, then weekly × 3 every 4 weeks thereafter) to weekly bolus 5-fluorouracil (600 mg/m^2) as first-line therapy for 126 newly diagnosed patients with locally advanced or metastatic pancreatic cancer [6]. Patients were required to have no prior chemotherapy and a Karnofsky performance status greater than 50 to be eligible for the study. Although the objective response rate was poor in both arms (5.4% for gemcitabine arm and 0% for 5-FU arm), the gemcitabine group had a significantly better clinical benefit response, defined as improvement in pain, performance status, and/or weight (24% vs 5%). Median overall survival (5.6 months vs 4.4 months) and 1-year survival (18% vs 2%) were also modestly improved. Both gemcitabine and 5-FU were well tolerated with similar toxicities. On the basis of this trial, gemcitabine was approved for initial treatment of either locally advanced or metastatic pancreatic adenocarcinoma, and it became the standard of care. Several other classes of chemotherapeutic agents—anthracyclines, taxanes, camptothecins, and alkylating agents like streptozocin and ifosfamide—have been extensively studied in phase II trials for single-agent activity against pancreatic cancer [7–18]. They were all minimally active or inactive against pancreatic cancer. None of them had better response or survival rates than single-agent gemcitabine.

Combination Regimens

Once gemcitabine was established as a standard of care, clinical trials commonly evaluated combination regimens with a gemcitabine backbone, as summarized in Table 11.1 None of these studies found a combination regimen to be superior to gemcitabine alone. Two phase III studies evaluating the combination of gemcitabine with capecitabine versus gemcitabine alone found no significant improvement in median overall survival despite one of the trials demonstrating a higher response rate with the combination regimen [22, 28]. Phase III trials studying gemcitabine in combination with cisplatin or irinotecan also did not outperform gemcitabine alone [19, 29–31]. Similar outcomes were reported when gemcitabine was given with or without 5-FU [21, 32]. The combination of gemcitabine and oxaliplatin (GEMOX) was compared to gemcitabine alone in two large multicenter studies [20, 33]. In the GERCOR/GISCAD intergroup trial of 326 patients, GEMOX was associated with significant improvement in response rates (27% vs 17%) and median PFS (5.8 months vs 3.7 months) but with only a trend to improve OS (9 months vs 7.1 months, $p = 0.13$). On the other hand, the E6201 study, designed to compare

Table 11.1 Studies combining gemcitabine with different chemotherapeutic agents

Study Gem vs (Gem + X)	# patients	Overall survival control arm	Overall survival study arm
Cisplatin [19]	192	6.0 months	7.5 months
Oxaliplatin [20]	313	7.1 months	9.0 months
5-FU [21]	322	5.4 months	6.7 months
Capecitabine [22]	533	6.2 months	7.1 months
Pemetrexed [23]	565	6.3 months	6.2 months
Irinotecan [24]	360	6.6 months	6.3 months
Exatecan [25]	349	6.2 months	6.7 months
S-1 [26]	834	8.8 months	10.1 months
Nab-paclitaxel [27]	**861**	**6.7 months**	**8.5 months**

Gem = Gemcitabine
Combination with nab-paclitaxel resulted in a significant improvement in median overall survival

overall survival (OS) of standard weekly gemcitabine versus gemcitabine fixed-dose rate or GEMOX, showed no significant advantages for GEMOX. The median survival and 1-year survival were 4.9 months and 16% for gemcitabine and 5.7 months and 21% for GEMOX (HR, 0.88, p = 0.22) [33]. More recently, in the phase III GEST trial, S-1 (an oral fluoropyrimidine) was compared to gemcitabine monotherapy or a combination of gemcitabine + S-1 [26]. Although S-1 monotherapy was shown to be non-inferior to gemcitabine in OS (9.7 months vs 8.8 months for gemcitabine, $p < 0.001$), the combination of gemcitabine plus S-1 was not superior to gemcitabine monotherapy (OS 10.1 months vs 8.8 months, $p = 0.15$). Several older combination regimens containing 5-FU were studied in randomized trials in the 1980s and 1990s [34, 35]. None showed a survival benefit over single-agent 5-FU.

Given multiple combination therapy trials, ultimately a meta-analysis was performed to evaluate randomized trials comparing gemcitabine versus gemcitabine plus another cytotoxic drug [36]. The meta-analysis used 15 trials with 4465 patients. It revealed a significant survival benefit for combination therapy with a pooled hazard ratio of 0.91 (95% CI, 0.85–0.97, $p = 0.004$). Further analysis by type of combination showed a statistically significant benefit of combining gemcitabine with a platinum analog (n = 1248 from five studies; HR 0.85, p = 0.01) or a fluoropyrimidine (n = 1813 from six studies; HR 0.90, p = 0.036). Looking at patient characteristics, the only factor predictive of benefit from combination chemotherapy was patient performance status (ECOG 0–1/Karnofsky score 90–100) with a pooled HR of 0.76 and $p < 0.001$ (1108 patients from five studies).

Gemcitabine and Nab-Paclitaxel

Activity for the combination of gemcitabine and albumin-bound paclitaxel (nab-paclitaxel) was first reported in a phase I/II study involving 67 patients with previously untreated metastatic pancreatic cancer [37]. At the maximally tolerated dose, response rates of 48% and median survival of 12.2 months were observed. Guided by these encouraging results, Von Hoff et al. conducted a phase III study to evaluate the efficacy and safety of the combination of nab-paclitaxel and gemcitabine versus gemcitabine monotherapy in patients with metastatic pancreatic cancer (MPACT or Metastatic Pancreatic Adenocarcinoma Clinical Trial) [27]. This multicenter international study randomized 861 patients with a Karnofsky performance-status score of 70 or more to either nab-paclitaxel (125 mg/m^2) plus gemcitabine (1000 mg/m^2) on days 1, 8, and 15 every 4 weeks or gemcitabine alone (1000 mg/m^2 weekly × 7 followed by 1 week break, then weekly × 3 every 4 weeks thereafter) until disease progression. The primary endpoint was overall survival, and secondary endpoints were progression-free survival and overall response rate. Approximately 10% of the patients were older than 75 years of age, and 8% had a relatively poorer performance status (Karnofsky score = 70). Response rates (23% vs 7%), median progression-free survival (5.5 months vs 3.7 months), and median overall survival (8.5 months vs 6.7 months) were all significantly improved with the combination. The improved outcome from the combination came with the expected increase in toxicities compared to gemcitabine alone. The most commonly seen adverse events (grade 3 or higher) were neutropenia (38% vs 27%), fatigue (17% vs 7%), and neuropathy (17% vs 1%). Febrile neutropenia occurred in 3% of the patients treated with the combination regimen compared to 1% of those with single-agent therapy. Despite a higher incidence with gemcitabine + nab-paclitaxel, neuropathy of grade 3 or higher improved to grade 1 or lower in a median of 29 days. The use of subsequent anticancer therapy was similar between the two groups (38% in the nab-paclitaxel–gemcitabine group and 42% in the gemcitabine group). Stromal fibroblasts in pancreatic adenocarcinoma overexpress secreted protein acidic and rich in cysteine (SPARC), and its overexpression was previously found to be a marker of poor prognosis [38]. In the phase I/II trial of gemcitabine plus *nab*-paclitaxel [37], a significant improvement in overall survival was seen in patients with high SPARC expression compared to patients with low SPARC expression (17.8 vs 8.1 months, $p = 0.431$). Unfortunately, an analysis of SPARC expression in the MPACT study did not demonstrate an association with survival and thus not a predictive marker for nab-paclitaxel (HR 1.019, $p = 0.903$) [39].

FOLFIRINOX

Prior to presentation of the MPACT trial, researchers in France were studying the combination of 5-FU, oxaliplatin, and irinotecan (FOLFIRINOX) in advanced pancreatic cancer. Conroy et al. in 2005 reported results from a phase II study using this regimen. Forty-six patients with advanced pancreatic cancer, the majority with metastatic disease, received this regimen for a median of eight cycles. Time to disease progression was 8.2 months and median overall survival was 10.2 months [40]. FOLFIRINOX was then studied in a phase II randomized study conducted in 176 treatment-naïve patients with metastatic pancreatic cancer [41]. Objective response rates were significantly higher with the combination regimen (39% vs 11% with gemcitabine alone). This study was expanded to the phase III ACCORD 11/PRODIGE study, conducted at

48 centers in France. In this study, 342 patients with newly diagnosed metastatic pancreatic cancer were randomly assigned to receive FOLFIRINOX (oxaliplatin 85 mg/m^2, irinotecan 180 mg/m^2, leucovorin 400 mg/m^2, and 5-FU 400 mg/m^2 bolus followed by 2400 mg/m^2 over 46 h as continuous infusion every 2 weeks) or gemcitabine alone (1000 mg/m^2 weekly for 7 of 8 weeks and then weekly for 3 of 4 weeks) within 1 week of enrollment. Patients had to be ≤75 years of age, have a performance status of ECOG 0–1, and be treatment naïve for metastatic disease. Duration of therapy goal was set at 6 months. The patient-selection criteria of this study were very rigorous (ECOG 0–1, age less than 76). Only 38% of the patients had carcinoma of the pancreatic head, likely related to the exclusion of patients with a high bilirubin level, resulting in a lower proportion of enrolled patients with biliary stents (14.3%).

The primary endpoint was overall survival, and secondary endpoints were progression-free survival, tumor response, safety, and quality of life (QoL). The multidrug combination was found to be significantly more efficacious than gemcitabine. At the preplanned interim analysis, the primary endpoint had been met and enrollment was stopped at 250 patients. The objective response rate was 31.6% vs 9.4% ($p < 0.001$), and median PFS was 6.4 months versus 3.3 months ($p < 0.001$) favoring the combination. With a median follow-up of 26.6 months, the median overall survival was better in the FOLFIRINOX group as compared with the gemcitabine group (11.1 months vs 6.8 months ($p < 0.001$)), and landmark overall survival rates at 6, 12, and 18 months were 75.9%, 48.4%, and 18.6%, respectively, in the FOLFIRINOX group as compared with 57.6%, 20.6%, and 6.0%, respectively, in the gemcitabine group. However, FOLFIRINOX was significantly more toxic than gemcitabine, as shown in Table 11.2 Incidences of grade 3 or 4 neutropenia, febrile neutropenia, thrombocytopenia, diarrhea, and sensory neuropathy were significantly higher in the FOLFIRINOX group, whereas the incidence of grade 3 or 4 transaminitis was significantly higher in the gemcitabine group. Second-line therapy was administered in 47% of patients in the FOLFIRINOX group and in 50% in the gemcitabine group. QoL was assessed using the European Organisation for Research and Treatment of Cancer Quality of Life Questionnaire C30 every 2 weeks. The time until definitive deterioration ≥20 points on this scale was significantly longer for FOLFIRINOX compared with gemcitabine for global health score; physical, role, cognitive, and social functioning; and six symptom domains (fatigue, nausea/vomiting, pain, dyspnea, anorexia, and constipation) [43]. Thus, despite its toxicities, FOLFIRINOX significantly reduced QoL impairment compared with gemcitabine.

Dose modifications

In the MPACT study, only 71% of the nab-paclitaxel doses and 63% of the gemcitabine doses remained at full dose due to protocol-driven reductions secondary to toxicities. In the clinic, administering three weekly doses out of four at full dose is quite challenging. Thus, there has been significant interest in developing and testing alternative doses and schedules of gemcitabine and nab-paclitaxel. A recent retrospective analysis of a prospectively established database of patients who received a modified regimen combining gemcitabine at 1000 mg/m^2 and nab-paclitaxel at

Table 11.2 Comparing MPACT and ACCORD11/PRODIGE studies

	MPACT trial [27]		ACCORD 11/PRODIGE [42]	
	Gemcitabine + nab-paclitaxel	Gemcitabine	FOLFIRINOX	Gemcitabine
ORR	23%*	7%*	31.6%*	9.4%*
PFS	5.5 m*	3.7 m*	6.4 m*	3.3 m*
OS	8.5 m*	6.7 m*	11.1 m*	6.8 m*
OS at 1 year	35%*	22%*	48.6%*	20.6%*
Grade 3/4 neutropenia	38%	27%	45.7%*	21%*
Febrile neutropenia	3%	1%	5.4%*	1.2%*
Diarrhea	6%	1%	12.8%*	1.8%*
Neuropathy	17%	1%	9%*	0%*
Fatigue	17%	1%	23.6%	17.8%

*Statistically significant difference
ORR overall response rate, *PFS* progression-free survival, *OS* overall survival

125 mg/m^2 every 2 weeks for first-line therapy was reported at GI-ASCO 2015 [44]. Sixty-three patients were evaluable for toxicity, and 47 were evaluable for response. Patients on the modified regimen had a median progression-free survival of 4.8 months (95% confidence interval [CI] = 2.6–7.4) and median overall survival of 11.1 months (95% CI = 5.3–not reached). With the modified regimen, 27% of patients experienced neurotoxicity of any grade, with the rate of grade 3 or 4 toxicity less than 2%. In clinical practice, a modified dose (nab-paclitaxel at 100 mg/m^2) or schedule (two out of three weeks or every other week treatments) of this regimen is routinely used to improve tolerability.

Similarly, the side effect profile of FOLFIRINOX has prompted various modifications to improve its tolerability. A Brazilian retrospective study of 19 patients with metastatic pancreatic adenocarcinoma who were treated with a modified dose FOLFIRINOX (no bolus 5-FU and reduced dose of at least one agent since the first cycle) was presented at ASCO 2013 [45]. Prophylactic G-CSF was given to 14 (73%) patients. Grade 3/4 toxicities were reported in 10 patients (52.6%): nausea/vomiting 1 (5.2%), diarrhea 1 (5.2%), fatigue 3 (15.7%), neutropenia 4 (21%), thrombocytopenia 1 (5.2%), and febrile neutropenia 3 (15.6%). Elevations in AST and ALT above the upper limit of normality were identified in 5 (26.31%). No deaths were reported due to toxicity. At 4.5 months follow-up, median overall or progression-free survival was not reached. Similar results have been published from other small series using modified FOLFIRINOX (omitting 5-FU bolus, 25% dose reduction in irinotecan and prophylactic growth factor support) in this disease [46]. A recent phase II using modified FOLFIRINOX (25% dose reductions of irinotecan and bolus 5-FU, prophylactic pegfilgrastim) suggested a similar response rate and improved tolerability compared to full dose FOLFIRINOX in advanced pancreatic cancer. Grade 3/4 toxicities were vomiting, peripheral sensory neuropathy (3.2%), febrile neutropenia (4.8%), anemia (6.4%), neutropenia (16.2%), fatigue (12.9%), and thrombocytopenia (11.3%). Neutropenia ($p < 0.0001$) and vomiting ($p = 0.006$) were significantly decreased. Response rate in 29 evaluable pts was 31.4% and similar to historical data (31.6%, $p = 0.82$) [47]. Given the above experiences, the current NCI national group standard is to administer FOLFIRINOX without the 5-FU bolus and with growth factor support. Dose reduction of irinotecan to 150 mg/m^2 is increasingly considered as well.

Thus, there are currently two appropriate frontline combination regimens (gem/nab-paclitaxel and FOLFIRINOX) for patients with metastatic pancreatic cancer. Both have demonstrated superiority to the historical standard gemcitabine in prospective randomized studies. The two regimens have never been compared head to head in a prospective study, but Table 11.2 illustrates their comparative efficacy and adverse event profile. A lack of predictive biomarkers guiding selection of FOLFIRINOX versus gem/nab-paclitaxel necessitates individualization of therapy based on patient's age, performance status, and preferences. Other chemotherapy options including gemcitabine plus erlotinib [48] or even gemcitabine monotherapy may be considered in patients with poor or compromised performance status.

Second-Line Therapy

The choice of second-line therapy is largely dictated by the previous treatment regimen, side effects, and patients' performance status. Supportive data for second-line therapy initially came from the CONKO-003 study which was a multicenter, randomized trial that studied a folinic acid and fluorouracil/oxaliplatin combination referred to as OFF (oxaliplatin 85 mg/m^2 on days 8 and 22 plus short-term infusional FU (2000 mg/m^2 over 24 h) and leucovorin (200 mg/m^2 over 30 min), both given on days 1, 8, 15, and 22) versus folinic acid and fluorouracil (FF) in 168 gemcitabine refractory metastatic pancreatic cancer patients [49]. After a median follow-up of 54.1 months, the median overall survival in the OFF arm was significantly better compared to the FF arm (5.9 months and 3.3 months, respectively, hazard ratio 0.66; 95% CI, 0.48–0.91; $p = 0.010$). Time to progression with OFF (2.9 months; 95% CI, 2.4–3.2) versus FF (2.0 months; 95% CI, 1.6–2.3) was significantly extended as well (HR, 0.68; 95% CI, 0.50–0.94; log-rank $p = 0.019$). Toxicities were similar between the treatment arms, with the exception of grade 1–2 neurotoxicity (38.2% vs 7.1%, $p < 0.001$). In contrast, the PANCREOX study failed to demonstrate a benefit of adding oxaliplatin to infusional 5-FU/leucovorin in the second-line setting [50]. This was a smaller, second-line, phase III, randomized study of 108 patients with advanced pancreatic cancer who had previously received gemcitabine. Patients were randomly assigned to mFOLFOX6 or infusional 5-FU/leucovorin. There was no observed difference in progression-free survival between the two arms (median 3.1 vs 2.9 months, $p = 0.99$), and overall survival was inferior in patients assigned to the combination arm (median 6.1 vs 9.9 months, $p = 0.02$). Increased toxicity was observed with the addition of oxaliplatin in this setting with grade 3/4 adverse events occurring in 63% of mFOLFOX6 patients and 11% of

5-FU/leucovorin patients. Based on the results of CONKO-003 study and the efficacy of FOLFIRINOX in the first line, FOLFOX is generally considered an active regimen in the second-line setting for advanced pancreatic cancer. The activity of single-agent irinotecan in pancreatic cancer has been investigated in several small studies, with little evidence of efficacy [51–53]. Nanoliposomal irinotecan is designed to improve the time in circulation and the intratumoral levels of irinotecan and its active metabolite SN-38 [54]. Promising results were seen in a phase II study of 40 patients with previously treated metastatic pancreatic cancer who received nanoliposomal irinotecan at 120 mg/m^2 every 3 weeks. The median overall survival was 5.2 months with a 1-year survival rate of 25% and acceptable toxicity profile [55]. This led to the larger phase III NAPOLI-I study that included metastatic pancreatic cancer patients with previous exposure to gemcitabine-based therapy. Four hundred and seventeen patients were randomly assigned to either nanoliposomal irinotecan plus fluorouracil and folinic acid ($n = 117$), single-agent nanoliposomal irinotecan ($n = 151$), or 5-FU and folinic acid ($n = 149$) [56]. Primary endpoint was overall survival. The median survival was longer with combination therapy compared to the 5-FU arm (median 6.1 vs 4.2 months, hazard ratio 0.67, 95% CI 0.49–0.92), as was progression-free survival (3.1 vs 1.5 months with control). Median overall survival was not significantly different in the single-agent nanoliposomal irinotecan and fluorouracil groups (4.9 months vs 4.2 months; hazard ratio 0.99, 0.77–1.28, $p = 0.94$). Grade 3 or higher adverse events occurring most frequently in the combination arm were neutropenia (27%), diarrhea (13%), vomiting (11%), and fatigue (14%). Based upon these results, nanoliposomal irinotecan was approved, in combination with 5-FU and leucovorin, for patients with metastatic pancreatic cancer who have previously received gemcitabine-based regimen.

Gemcitabine-based second-line regimens for patients receiving FOLFIRINOX in first line have not been as well studied. A multicenter prospective study evaluated the safety and efficacy of gemcitabine and nab-paclitaxel after FOLFIRINOX therapy in 57 patients. The disease control rate was 58%, with a 17.5% objective response rate. Median overall survival was 8.8 months (95% CI, 6.2–9.7), and median progression-free survival was 5.1 months (95% CI, 3.2–6.2). Since the start of first-line chemotherapy, median survival was 18 months (95% CI, 16–21). Incidence of grade 3 or higher toxicities was 40%, consisting of neutropenia (12.5%), neurotoxicity (12.5%), asthenia (9%), and thrombocytopenia (6.5%). On balance, NCCN guidelines recommend second-line fluoropyrimidine-based chemotherapy for those previously treated with gemcitabine-based regimen and second-line gemcitabine-based therapy for those previously treated with fluoropyrimidine-based treatment [57]. This also reflects the common treatment pattern in clinical practice.

Other Novel Chemotherapeutic Agents

Evofosfamide (formerly TH-302) is a prodrug that converts into a DNA-alkylating agent in the hypoxic tumor microenvironment. A phase I/II clinical study (NCT00743379) of solid tumors investigating evofosfamide doses of 240–575 mg/m^2

on days 1, 8, and 15 of a 28-day cycle established the recommended phase II dose of the combination with gemcitabine at 340 mg/m^2. A subsequent randomized phase II study combining it with gemcitabine suggested improvement in progression-free survival compared to gemcitabine alone (5.6 months vs 3.6 months, $p = 0.005$) and a nonsignificant trend toward better overall survival (9.2 months vs 6.9 months, $p = 0.8$) [58]. This led to the phase III MAESTRO study of gemcitabine ± evofosfamide [59] that enrolled 693 patients with newly diagnosed advanced pancreatic cancer. There was no significant difference in overall survival (median OS 8.7 m with combination vs 7.6 m with gemcitabine alone, HR = 0.84 (95% CI, 0.71–1.01, $p = 0.059$)). Median progression-free survival was 5.5 months with evofosfamide + gemcitabine compared to 3.7 months with gemcitabine + placebo (HR = 0.77 (95% CI, 0.65–0.92, $p = 0.004$)).

A nucleoside transporter protein, human equilibrative nucleoside transporter 1 (hENT1), promotes transport of gemcitabine into malignant cells and was evaluated as a predictive marker of gemcitabine therapy in pancreatic cancer. CO-101 is a novel gemcitabine analog which is not dependent on the nucleoside transport mechanism. The Low hENT1 and Adenocarcinoma of the Pancreas (LEAP) study randomized metastatic pancreatic cancer patients to either gemcitabine or CO-101. The cohort was divided into high and low hENT1 expression groups, and the primary endpoint was overall survival in the low hENT1 tumor expression subgroup. There was no difference in survival between treatments in the low hENT1 subgroup or overall population (HR of 0.994 and 1.072, respectively). Similarly, low versus high hENT1 expression did not affect survival in patients treated with gemcitabine [60].

Lurbinectedin (PM01183) binds covalently to tumor DNA, forming adducts that are capable of inducing double-stranded breaks and interfering with the transcriptional machinery [61]. A phase I study in solid tumors demonstrated an activity signal in metastatic pancreatic cancer among others with reversible myelosuppression as its main dose-limiting toxicity [61]. Synergy in combination with fluoropyrimidines was also reported [62]. In the subsequent phase I study of the combination of lurbinectedin and capecitabine (NCT02210364), four patients with metastatic pancreatic cancer were enrolled, but only two had stable disease as their best response [63]. No other studies are currently evaluating its role in pancreatic cancer.

Conclusion

Although the treatment of advanced pancreatic cancer has improved significantly in the last decade, prognosis remains poor with median survival less than a year. Despite the promise of molecularly targeted and "personalized" medicine, the major advances in pancreatic cancer over the last few years have involved traditional or bioengineered cytotoxic agents. Further development of cytotoxic agents based on promising preclinical data should be continued.

References

1. Siegel RL, Miller KD, Jemal A. Cancer statistics, 2016. CA Cancer J Clin. 2016;66:7–30.
2. SEER Stat Fact Sheets: Pancreas cancer. Available from URL: http://seer.cancer.gov/statfacts/html/pancreas.html. Accessed 22 Feb 2016.
3. DeCaprio JA, Mayer RJ, Gonin R, Arbuck SG. Fluorouracil and high-dose leucovorin in previously untreated patients with advanced adenocarcinoma of the pancreas: results of a phase II trial. J Clin Oncol. 1991;9:2128–33.
4. Palmer KR, Kerr M, Knowles G, Cull A, Carter DC, Leonard RCF. Chemotherapy prolongs survival in inoperable pancreatic carcinoma. Br J Surg. 1994;81:882–5.
5. Fung MC, Takayama S, Ishiguro H, Sakata T, Adachi S, Morizane T. Chemotherapy for advanced or metastatic pancreatic cancer: analysis of 43 randomized trials in 3 decades (1974-2002). Gan To Kagaku Ryoho. 2003;30:1101–11.
6. Burris HA 3rd, Moore MJ, Andersen J, et al. Improvements in survival and clinical benefit with gemcitabine as first-line therapy for patients with advanced pancreas cancer: a randomized trial. J Clin Oncol. 1997;15:2403–13.
7. Schein PS, Lavin PT, Moertel CG, et al. Randomized phase II clinical trial of adriamycin, methotrexate, and actinomycin-D in advanced measurable pancreatic carcinoma: a gastrointestinal tumor study group report. Cancer. 1978;42:19–22.
8. Wils J, Bleiberg H, Blijham G, et al. Phase II study of epirubicin in advanced adenocarcinoma of the pancreas. Eur J Cancer Clin Oncol. 1985;21:191–4.
9. Carter SK, Comis RL. The integration of chemotherapy into a combined modality approach for cancer treatment. VI. Pancreatic adenocarcinoma. Cancer Treat Rev. 1975;2:193–214.
10. Ajani JA, Abbruzzese JL, Goudeau P, et al. Ifosfamide and mesna: marginally active in patients with advanced carcinoma of the pancreas. J Clin Oncol. 1988;6:1703–7.
11. The Gastrointestinal Tumor Study Group. Ifosfamide is an inactive substance in the treatment of pancreatic carcinoma. Cancer. 1989;64:2010–3.
12. Androulakis N, Kourousis C, Dimopoulos MA, et al. Treatment of pancreatic cancer with docetaxel and granulocyte colony-stimulating factor: a multicenter phase II study. J Clin Oncol. 1999;17:1779–85.
13. Rougier P, Adenis A, Ducreux M, et al. A phase II study: docetaxel as first-line chemotherapy for advanced pancreatic adenocarcinoma. Eur J Cancer. 2000;36:1016–25.
14. Lenzi R, Yalcin S, Evans DB, Abbruzzese JL. Phase II study of docetaxel in patients with pancreatic cancer previously untreated with cytotoxic chemotherapy. Cancer Invest. 2002;20:464–72.
15. Okada S, Sakata Y, Matsuno S, et al. Phase II study of docetaxel in patients with metastatic pancreatic cancer: a Japanese cooperative study. Cooperative group of docetaxel for pancreatic cancer in Japan. Br J Cancer. 1999;80:438–43.
16. Whitehead RP, Jacobson J, Brown TD, Taylor SA, Weiss GR, Macdonald JS. Phase II trial of paclitaxel and granulocyte colony-stimulating factor in patients with pancreatic carcinoma: a southwest oncology group study. J Clin Oncol. 1997;15:2414–9.
17. Wagener DJ, Verdonk HE, Dirix LY, et al. Phase II trial of CPT-11 in patients with advanced pancreatic cancer, an EORTC early clinical trials group study. Ann Oncol. 1995;6:129–32.
18. O'Reilly S, Donehower RC, Rowinsky EK, Ord S, Grochow LB. A phase II trial of topotecan in patients with previously untreated pancreatic cancer. Anticancer Drugs. 1996;7:410–4.
19. Heinemann V, Quietzsch D, Gieseler F, et al. Randomized phase III trial of gemcitabine plus cisplatin compared with gemcitabine alone in advanced pancreatic cancer. J Clin Oncol. 2006;24:3946–52.
20. Louvet C, Labianca R, Hammel P, et al. Gemcitabine in combination with oxaliplatin compared with gemcitabine alone in locally advanced or metastatic pancreatic cancer: results of a GERCOR and GISCAD phase III trial. J Clin Oncol. 2005;23:3509–16.
21. Berlin JD, Catalano P, Thomas JP, Kugler JW, Haller DG, Benson AB 3rd. Phase III study of gemcitabine in combination with fluorouracil versus gemcitabine alone in patients with advanced pancreatic carcinoma: eastern cooperative oncology group trial E2297. J Clin Oncol. 2002;20:3270–5.

22. Cunningham D, Chau I, Stocken DD, et al. Phase III randomized comparison of gemcitabine versus gemcitabine plus capecitabine in patients with advanced pancreatic cancer. J Clin Oncol. 2009;27:5513–8.
23. Oettle H, Richards D, Ramanathan RK, et al. A phase III trial of pemetrexed plus gemcitabine versus gemcitabine in patients with unresectable or metastatic pancreatic cancer. Ann Oncol. 2005;16:1639–45.
24. Rocha Lima CM, Green MR, Rotche R, et al. Irinotecan plus gemcitabine results in no survival advantage compared with gemcitabine monotherapy in patients with locally advanced or metastatic pancreatic cancer despite increased tumor response rate. J Clin Oncol. 2004;22:3776–83.
25. Abou-Alfa GK, Letourneau R, Harker G, et al. Randomized phase III study of exatecan and gemcitabine compared with gemcitabine alone in untreated advanced pancreatic cancer. J Clin Oncol. 2006;24:4441–7.
26. Ueno H, Ioka T, Ikeda M, et al. Randomized phase III study of gemcitabine plus S-1, S-1 alone, or gemcitabine alone in patients with locally advanced and metastatic pancreatic cancer in Japan and Taiwan: GEST study. J Clin Oncol. 2013;31:1640–8.
27. Von Hoff DD, Ervin T, Arena FP, et al. Increased survival in pancreatic cancer with nab-paclitaxel plus gemcitabine. N Engl J Med. 2013;369:1691–703.
28. Herrmann R, Bodoky G, Ruhstaller T, et al. Gemcitabine plus capecitabine compared with gemcitabine alone in advanced pancreatic cancer: a randomized, multicenter, phase III trial of the Swiss group for clinical cancer research and the central European cooperative oncology group. J Clin Oncol. 2007;25:2212–7.
29. Colucci G, Labianca R, Di Costanzo F, et al. Randomized phase III trial of gemcitabine plus cisplatin compared with single-agent gemcitabine as first-line treatment of patients with advanced pancreatic cancer: the GIP-1 study. J Clin Oncol. 2010;28:1645–51.
30. Wang X, Ni Q, Jin M, et al. Gemcitabine or gemcitabine plus cisplatin for in 42 patients with locally advanced or metastatic pancreatic cancer. Zhonghua Zhong Liu Za Zhi. 2002;24:404–7.
31. Stathopoulos GP, Syrigos K, Aravantinos G, et al. A multicenter phase III trial comparing irinotecan-gemcitabine (IG) with gemcitabine (G) monotherapy as first-line treatment in patients with locally advanced or metastatic pancreatic cancer. Br J Cancer. 2006;95: 587–92.
32. Di Costanzo F, Carlini P, Doni L, et al. Gemcitabine with or without continuous infusion 5-FU in advanced pancreatic cancer: a randomised phase II trial of the Italian oncology group for clinical research (GOIRC). Br J Cancer. 2005;93:185–9.
33. Poplin E, Feng Y, Berlin J, et al. Phase III, randomized study of gemcitabine and oxaliplatin versus gemcitabine (fixed-dose rate infusion) compared with gemcitabine (30-minute infusion) in patients with pancreatic carcinoma E6201: a trial of the eastern cooperative oncology group. J Clin Oncol. 2009;27:3778–85.
34. Cullinan SA, Moertel CG, Fleming TR, et al. A comparison of three chemotherapeutic regimens in the treatment of advanced pancreatic and gastric carcinoma. Fluorouracil vs fluorouracil and doxorubicin vs fluorouracil, doxorubicin, and mitomycin. JAMA. 1985;253:2061–7.
35. Cullinan S, Moertel CG, Wieand HS, et al. A phase III trial on the therapy of advanced pancreatic carcinoma. Evaluations of the Mallinson regimen and combined 5-fluorouracil, doxorubicin, and cisplatin. Cancer. 1990;65:2207–12.
36. Heinemann V, Boeck S, Hinke A, Labianca R, Louvet C. Meta-analysis of randomized trials: evaluation of benefit from gemcitabine-based combination chemotherapy applied in advanced pancreatic cancer. BMC Cancer. 2008;8:1.
37. Von Hoff DD, Ramanathan RK, Borad MJ, et al. Gemcitabine plus nab-paclitaxel is an active regimen in patients with advanced pancreatic cancer: a phase I/II trial. J Clin Oncol. 2011;29:4548–54.
38. Infante JR, Matsubayashi H, Sato N, et al. Peritumoral fibroblast SPARC expression and patient outcome with resectable pancreatic adenocarcinoma. J Clin Oncol. 2007;25:319–25.
39. Hidalgo M, Plaza C, Illei P, et al. SPARC analysis in the phase III MPACT trial of nab-paclitaxel (NAB-P) plus gemcitabine (GEM) vs GEM alone for patients with metastatic pancreatic cancer (PC). Ann Oncol. 2014;25:ii106.

40. Conroy T, Paillot B, Francois E, et al. Irinotecan plus oxaliplatin and leucovorin-modulated fluorouracil in advanced pancreatic cancer–a groupe tumeurs digestives of the federation nationale des centres de Lutte Contre le cancer study. J Clin Oncol. 2005;23:1228–36.
41. Ychou MDF, Guimbaud R. Randomized phase II trial comparing folfirinox (5FU/leucovorin [LV], irinotecan [I] and oxaliplatin [O]) vs gemcitabine (G) as first-line treatment for metastatic pancreatic adenocarcinoma (MPA). First results of the ACCORD 11 trial (abstract 4516). J Clin Oncol. 2007;25(18):4516.
42. Conroy T, Desseigne F, Ychou M, et al. FOLFIRINOX versus gemcitabine for metastatic pancreatic cancer. N Engl J Med. 2011;364:1817–25.
43. Gourgou-Bourgade S, Bascoul-Mollevi C, Desseigne F, et al. Impact of FOLFIRINOX compared with gemcitabine on quality of life in patients with metastatic pancreatic cancer: results from the PRODIGE 4/ACCORD 11 randomized trial. J Clin Oncol. 2013;31:23–9.
44. Bekaii-Saab KKTS. Modified gemcitabine and nab-paclitaxel in patients with metastatic pancreatic cancer (MPC): a single-institution experience. J Clin Oncol. 2015;33(3):366.
45. Safety and efficacy of modified dose-attenuated FOLFIRINOX chemotherapy in patients over 65 years with advanced pancreatic adenocarcinoma. ASCO. Chicago: J Clin Oncol. 2015;33(3_suppl):468. DOI: 10.1200/jco.2015.33.3_suppl.468
46. Mahaseth H, Brutcher E, Kauh J, et al. Modified FOLFIRINOX regimen with improved safety and maintained efficacy in pancreatic adenocarcinoma. Pancreas. 2013;42:1311–5.
47. James ES, Yao X, Cong X, et al. Interim analysis of a phase II study of dose-modified FOLFIRINOX (mFOLFIRINOX) in locally advanced (LAPC) and metastatic pancreatic cancer (MPC). J Clin Oncol. 2014;32:e15226. (Meeting Abstracts)
48. Moore MJ, Goldstein D, Hamm J, et al. Erlotinib plus gemcitabine compared with gemcitabine alone in patients with advanced pancreatic cancer: a phase III trial of the national cancer institute of Canada clinical trials group. J Clin Oncol. 2007;25:1960–6.
49. Oettle H, Riess H, Stieler JM, et al. Second-line oxaliplatin, folinic acid, and fluorouracil versus folinic acid and fluorouracil alone for gemcitabine-refractory pancreatic cancer: outcomes from the CONKO-003 trial. J Clin Oncol. 2014;32:2423–9.
50. Gill S, Ko Y-J, Cripps MC, et al. PANCREOX: a randomized phase 3 study of 5FU/LV with or without oxaliplatin for second-line advanced pancreatic cancer (APC) in patients (pts) who have received gemcitabine (GEM)-based chemotherapy (CT). ASCO Annual Meeting Proceedings, 2014: 4022.
51. Yi SY, Park YS, Kim HS, et al. Irinotecan monotherapy as second-line treatment in advanced pancreatic cancer. Cancer Chemother Pharmacol. 2009;63:1141–5.
52. Gebbia V, Maiello E, Giuliani F, Borsellino N, Arcara C, Colucci G. Irinotecan plus bolus/infusional 5-fluorouracil and leucovorin in patients with pretreated advanced pancreatic carcinoma: a multicenter experience of the Gruppo Oncologico Italia Meridionale. Am J Clin Oncol. 2010;33:461–4.
53. Zaniboni A, Aitini E, Barni S, et al. FOLFIRI as second-line chemotherapy for advanced pancreatic cancer: a GISCAD multicenter phase II study. Cancer Chemother Pharmacol. 2012;69:1641–5.
54. Kalra AV, Kim J, Klinz SG, et al. Preclinical activity of nanoliposomal irinotecan is governed by tumor deposition and intratumor prodrug conversion. Cancer Res. 2014;74:7003–13.
55. Ko AH, Tempero MA, Shan YS, et al. A multinational phase 2 study of nanoliposomal irinotecan sucrosofate (PEP02, MM-398) for patients with gemcitabine-refractory metastatic pancreatic cancer. Br J Cancer. 2013;109:920–5.
56. Wang-Gillam A, Li C-P, Bodoky G, et al. Nanoliposomal irinotecan with fluorouracil and folinic acid in metastatic pancreatic cancer after previous gemcitabine-based therapy (NAPOLI-1): a global, randomised, open-label, phase 3 trial. Lancet. 2016;387:545–57.
57. NCCN Clinical practice guidelines in oncology: pancreatic cancer version 2. 2015. Available from URL: http://www.nccn.org/professionals/physician_gls/pdf/pancreatic.pdf.

58. Borad MJ, Reddy SG, Bahary N, et al. Randomized phase II trial of gemcitabine plus TH-302 versus gemcitabine in patients with advanced pancreatic cancer. J Clin Oncol. 2015;33:1475–81.
59. Van Cutsem E, Lenz H-J, Furuse J, et al. Evofosfamide (TH-302) in combination with gemcitabine in previously untreated patients with metastatic or locally advanced unresectable pancreatic ductal adenocarcinoma: primary analysis of the randomized, double-blind phase III MAESTRO study. ASCO Annual Meeting Proceedings. 2016;34(4S):193.
60. Poplin E, Wasan H, Rolfe L, et al. Randomized, multicenter, phase II study of CO-101 versus gemcitabine in patients with metastatic pancreatic ductal adenocarcinoma: including a prospective evaluation of the role of hENT1 in gemcitabine or CO-101 sensitivity. J Clin Oncol. 2013;31(35):4453–61.
61. Elez ME, Tabernero J, Geary D, et al. First-in-human phase I study of Lurbinectedin (PM01183) in patients with advanced solid tumors. Clin Cancer Res. 2014;20:2205–14.
62. Aviles P, Guillen MJ, Galmarini C, et al. Synergism of lurbinectedin (PM01183) combined with 5-fluorouracil (5-FU): in vitro and in vivo studies. Cancer Res. 2013;73:5498.
63. Sauri T, Aftimos P, Szyldergemajn S, et al. 482plurbinectedin (PM01183) on days (D) 1 & 8 in combination with capecitabine (XEL) in patients (PTS) with metastatic breast (MBC), colorectal (CRC) or pancreatic (PAC) cancer. Ann Oncol. 2014;25:iv161.

Chapter 12
Molecularly Targeted Therapies in Pancreatic Cancer

Walid L. Shaib and Bassel F. El-Rayes

Introduction

Molecularly targeted therapies are designed to inhibit specific cellular signaling pathways involved in cancer growth, resistance, and metastasis. Potential advantages of targeted therapies over conventional cytotoxic therapies are improved safety due to selective inhibition of cancer-related pathways and enhanced activity. Furthermore, targeted therapies are the cornerstone for "personalized" or "precision" medicine, where the molecular profile of the tumor rather than histologic features drives the treatment decision. The early success of agents like imatinib in chronic myelogenous leukemia and gastrointestinal stromal tumors catapulted molecularly targeted therapies to the forefront of cancer management. In pancreatic ductal adenocarcinoma (PDAC), several classes of targeted therapies have been evaluated in large randomized clinical trials. Although these clinical trials were supported by promising preclinical data, the results have been largely disappointing. Currently, the clinical standard of care for PDAC remains heavily dependent on conventional cytotoxic drugs and radiation therapy. Ongoing trials are evaluating novel targeted therapies including agents targeting the microenvironment (discussed in Chap. 13), DNA repair (discussed in Chap. 14), and cancer stem cells.

The most commonly mutated signaling pathways in PDAC are Ras-MAPK, p16/CDKN2A, TP53, SMAD4, and TGF-beta. These signaling pathways are key regulators of carcinogenesis and progression of PDAC. The most common genetic alterations in PDAC cells are telomere abnormalities and chromosomal instabilities. Other less common genetic mutations include BRCA2, PALB2, FANCC, FANCG, FBXW7, BAX, RB1, and many others that involve amplifications, chromosomal deletions, and DNA mismatch repair genes [1, 2]. Table 12.1 summarizes the clinical trials that evaluated targeted agents used in the treatment of pancreatic cancer discussed in this chapter.

W.L. Shaib, M.D. • B.F. El-Rayes, M.D. (✉)
Department of Hematology and Oncology, Winship Cancer Institute, Emory University, 1365C Clifton Rd., Atlanta, GA 30322, USA
e-mail: bassel.el-rayes@emoryhealthcare.org

T. Bekaii-Saab, B. El-Rayes (eds.), *Current and Emerging Therapies in Pancreatic Cancer*, DOI 10.1007/978-3-319-58256-6_12

Table 12.1 A summary of the clinical trials that evaluated targeted agents used in the treatment of pancreatic cancer

Author	Target	Study drug	Phase	OS	PFS	P-value
Van Cutsem et al. [10]	KRAS farnesyl transferase	Tipifarnib/gem vs gem/placebo	III	6.4 vs 6.1	3.7 vs 3.6	0.75
Moore et al. [15] NCIC CTGPA.3	EGFR	Erlotinib/gem vs gem	III	6.2 vs 5.9		0.038
Philip et al. [18] SWOG S0205	EGFR	Cetuximab/gem vs gem	III	6.3 vs 5.9		0.23
Santos et al. [20] AIO-PK0104	EGFR	Erlotinib/gem vs capecitabine/gem	III	6.2 vs 6.9		0.9
Kindler et al. [29] **CALGB80303**	**VEGF**	**Bevacizumab/gem vs gem/placebo**	**III**	**5.8 vs 5.9**		**0.95**
Van Cutsem et al. [30] **AViTA**	**VEGF/EGFR**	**Erlotinib/bevacizumab/gem vs gem/ erlotinib/placebo**	**III**	**7.1 vs 6.0**		**0.21**
Kindler et al. [32]	**VEGFR**	**Axitinib/gem vs gem/placebo**	**III**	**8.5 vs 8.3**		**0.54**
Harder et al. [40]	Her2/neu	Trastuzumab/capecitabine	II single arm ($n = 17$)	6.9	23.5% at 3 months	
Infante et al. [58]	**MEK**	**Trametinib/gem vs gem/placebo**	**II**	**8.4 vs 6.7**		**0.45**
Van Cutsem et al. [59]	**MEK**	**Pimasertib/gem vs gem**	**II**		**3.7 vs 2.8**	**0.61**
Bodoky et al. [60]	MAPK	Selumetinib vs capecitabine (second line)	II	5.4 vs 5.0		0.92
Wolpin et al. [62]	**mTOR**	**Everolimus (second line)**	**II**	**4.5**	**1.8**	
Hurwitz et al. [48] RECAP	JAK 1/2	Ruxolitinib/capecitabine vs capecitabine/ placebo **(second line)**	II	4.5 vs 4.3		0.25
Hofland et al. [55]	**MUC1**	**^{90}Y clivatuzumab tetraxetan vs best supportive care (third-line interim analysis)**		**4.0 vs 2.8**		**0.021**

Farnesylation

KRAS mutation is present in >80% of PDAC tumors. An essential step in *KRAS* posttranscriptional activation is farnesylation, which is key in the transport of the *RAS* protein to the cell membrane [3]. Selective inhibitors of farnesyl transferases (e.g., tipifarnib) have been used to inhibit processing and activation of *KRAS*. Preclinical data using tipifarnib in PDAC models demonstrated significant clinical activity [4]. Phase I studies of farnesyl transferase inhibitors as monotherapy or in combination with other chemotherapeutic agents like capecitabine [5] and irinotecan [6] were promising [7–9]. Based on the promising preclinical data and the safety profile, a phase III double-blind, placebo-controlled study randomized 688 patients with previously untreated stage IV pancreatic cancer to gemcitabine with or without tipifarnib. Primary endpoint was survival. This trial did not demonstrate any benefit for adding tipifarnib to standard chemotherapy [10].

Matrix Metalloproteinases (MMPs)

The matrix metalloproteinases are a family of zinc-containing proteolytic enzymes that degrade proteins in the extracellular matrix. Four main subgroups have been defined: the collagenases, the gelatinases, the stromelysins, and the membrane-bound MMPs. MMPs regulate cytokines, growth factors, and growth factor receptors which affect cell migration, apoptosis, and proliferation as well as growth factor sequestration. Loss of the tight control of MMP activity in cancer contributes to excessive destruction of the extracellular matrix, neovascularization, tumor spread, and metastases [11]. A phase III clinical trial randomized patients between gemcitabine alone and an MMP inhibitor, BAY 12-9566 (tanomastat), in the first-line treatment setting with a primary endpoint being overall survival (OS). The trial accrued 277 patients. It was closed to accrual after the second interim analysis due to worsening survival in the study arm. The median OS on the BAY 12-9566 arm and the gemcitabine arm was 3.7 months and 6.6 months, respectively ($P < 0.001$) [12].

Another phase III trial using the same design randomized 414 patients in first-line treatment to gemcitabine alone and marimastat at three dose levels, and the OS was the primary endpoint. The degree of significance was not reached at all the dose levels (5, 10, or 25 mg of marimastat and gemcitabine; 3.7, 3.5, 4.2, and 5.6 months, respectively, $P = 0.19$) [13]. The same group reported a phase III double-blind, placebo-controlled, randomized trial of 239 patients in the first-line treatment of unresectable PDAC comparing gemcitabine and marimastat to gemcitabine and placebo. The OS was the primary endpoint. There was no significant difference in survival between the groups (OS 5.5 and 5.4 months, $P = 0.95$) [14].

Epidermal Growth Factor Receptor

Epidermal growth factor receptor (EGFR) is a member of the erbB/human epidermal growth factor receptor family of tyrosine kinases, which includes erbB2/HER2, erbB3/HER3, and erbB4/HER4. Members of the EGFR family possess intrinsic tyrosine kinase activity. Activation of EGFR by a ligand leads to autophosphorylation in tyrosine residues located on the intracellular domains of the receptor. The activated tyrosine kinase in turn phosphorylates and activates intracellular signaling pathways including PI3K/Akt and Ras-MPK. These pathways are critical in cancer growth and metastasis. The inhibition of this tyrosine phosphorylation results in the inhibition of angiogenesis and proliferation of cancer cells. In preclinical models, EGFR promotes pancreatic tumorigenesis. Two independent groups showed that EGFR deletion or treatment with erlotinib diminished pancreatic intraepithelial neoplasia (PanIN) lesion formation and impaired its progression to PDAC.

Erlotinib is a selective competitive inhibitor of the tyrosine kinase domain of the EGFR. In a phase III study, patients with previously untreated stage IV pancreatic cancer were randomized to gemcitabine with or without erlotinib (NCIC CTG PA.3) [15]. The OS benefit was 0.3 months (6.2 vs 5.9 months, $P = 0.038$). Given this marginal benefit, erlotinib is not widely used in clinical practice [16]. EGFR inhibition was evaluated in another phase III that randomized patients with newly diagnosed pancreatic cancer to a monoclonal antibody against EGFR (cetuximab) in combination with gemcitabine versus gemcitabine alone. Cetuximab, a monoclonal antibody, binds to the extracellular ligand-binding domain of EGFR, suppressing EGFR-dependent signaling through inhibition of ligand-dependent activation and receptor dimerization and induction of antibody-dependent cell-mediated cytotoxicity [17]. A total of 745 patients were enrolled with locally advanced/metastatic PDAC. The median survival time, which was the primary endpoint, was reported at 6.3 months for the gemcitabine plus cetuximab arm compared to 5.9 months for the gemcitabine-alone arm ($P = 0.23$). This difference was not statistically significant [18]. Both these trials used EGFR inhibitors (erlotinib and cetuximab) and were evaluated in molecularly unselected patients [19]. The two molecules differ in that the erlotinib is an EGFR tyrosine kinase inhibitor that binds to the intracellular tyrosine kinase domain and the cetuximab is an anti-EGFR monoclonal antibody that binds to the extracellular ligand-binding domain. This could be one explanation to the difference in survival outcomes. In the effort of finding predictive biomarkers for EGFR inhibitors, *KRAS* and *EGFR* gene copy numbers were evaluated in 117 patients enrolled on the trial. The results did not demonstrate a predictive value for either *KRAS* mutational status or EGFR copy number [20].

AIO-PK0104 study is a multicenter trial comparing gemcitabine/erlotinib followed by capecitabine with capecitabine/erlotinib followed by gemcitabine in advanced PDAC. The study demonstrated that both treatment strategies are feasible and of comparable efficacy (OS of 6.2 vs 6.9, $P = 0.90$). *KRAS* wild-type status was associated with improved survival (HR 1.68, $P = 0.005$) for erlotinib-treated patients [21]. Another post hoc analysis of the AIO-PK0104 study found that *KRAS* codon

12 mutations constituted 70% of the patients and showed no association for response ($P = 0.40$). *KRAS* wild-type patients had an improved survival (HR 1.68, $P = 0.005$), and this trend was also observed during non-erlotinib-containing second-line chemotherapy. Based on the data, the authors concluded that *KRAS* is more likely a prognostic rather than predictive biomarker [22].

Angiogenesis

Vascular endothelial growth factors (VEGFs) through interaction with VEGF receptors (VEGFR) have a central role in controlling angiogenesis and lymphangiogenesis, both of which are important in PDAC pathogenesis, progression, and metastasis [23, 24]. VEGF is expressed in all PDAC tumors [23]. VEGF-A/VEGFR-2 signaling plays an important role in inducing invasion and migration of PDAC cells. VEGFR-2 and phosphorylated VEGFR-2 (pVEGFR-2) were expressed in 69% and 50% of 107 PDAC, respectively, suggesting that these receptors are important targets in PDAC treatment [25, 26]. Bevacizumab, a monoclonal antibody against VEGF-A, has shown activity against a vast number of tumors including colorectal [27] and lung cancers [28]. CALGB initiated a phase III trial comparing gemcitabine and bevacizumab (10 mg/kg) combination to gemcitabine alone in patients with advanced-stage pancreatic cancer (CALGB 80303). The trial randomized 602 patients. The primary endpoint was OS. The results of the trial did not show any significant difference ($P = 0.95$) or in any of the secondary endpoints [29]. The addition of bevacizumab to gemcitabine/erlotinib combination was evaluated in a phase II trial. The AViTA (addition of bevacizumab to gemcitabine and erlotinib) enrolled 605 patients to gemcitabine/erlotinib/bevacizumab or gemcitabine/erlotinib/placebo combinations. The primary endpoint was OS, and this was not met (7.1 vs 6.0 months, $P = 0.21$) [30].

Axitinib is a tyrosine kinase inhibitor of VEGFR and has shown clinical activity in renal cell cancer [31]. The combination of gemcitabine and axitinib was compared to gemcitabine alone in patients with treatment-naïve advanced-stage pancreatic cancer in a phase III trial enrolling 632 patients. Primary endpoint was OS. No difference in OS was observed (8.5 vs 8.3 months, $P = 0.54$) [32]. A shared flaw in the design of these trials is lack of a biomarker to select patients who may benefit from anti-angiogenic therapy. Currently there are no validated predictive biomarkers [33]. Pant et al. evaluated baseline serum albumin as a predictive biomarker in a pooled analysis from seven prospective clinical trials evaluating gemcitabine-based therapy with or without bevacizumab. The authors reviewed data from 264 patients. Normal baseline albumin was associated with significantly improved OS (10.2 vs 4.1 months, $P = 0.0001$) for patients receiving bevacizumab. Albumin level of >3.4 g/dL was proposed to be a prognostic factor in advanced-stage bevacizumab-treated PDAC patients in a pooled prospective analysis [34].

Ramucirumab is a monoclonal antibody against VEGFR-1 and VEGFR-2. In clinical trials, it has shown activity in colorectal [35] and gastric cancer [36, 37]. An ongoing phase II randomized, placebo-controlled trial combining FOLFIRINOX with ramucirumab is currently accrual (NCT02581215) [38]. The rationale behind this combination is that the fluoropyrimidine backbone, and contrary to gemcitabine treatment, increases bone marrow-derived circulating endothelial progenitor cells and pro-angiogenic growth factors, making these suitable targets to VEGFR inhibition.

Her2/neu

Her2/neu amplification estimate was reported at 2% in an analysis of 490 tumors from patients with pancreatic cancer [39]. Targeting Her2/neu in patients with pancreatic cancer who had overexpression of the Her2/neu by immunohistochemistry staining 3+ pattern was evaluated in a phase II multicenter single-arm trial combining trastuzumab and capecitabine. Her2/neu 3+ expression on immunohistochemistry (IHC) was 11% of 212 patients. Trastuzumab and capecitabine resulted in a progression-free survival at 12 weeks (primary endpoint) of only 23.5% and an OS of 6.9 months [40]. Trastuzumab was also studied in combination with gemcitabine in a phase II trial. Her2/neu 2+/3+ by IHC staining was seen in 16% of 269 patients. Treatment with gemcitabine/trastuzumab combination resulted in an OS of 7 months and the 1-year survival of 19% that was comparable to gemcitabine single-agent treatment [41]. The results of these trials are disappointing for targeting Her2/neu overexpression in pancreatic cancer.

Janus Kinase Inhibition (JAK 1/2)

The Janus kinase (JAK)-activated STAT (signal transducer and activator of transcription) pathway contributes to pancreatic cancer cellular proliferation and survival [42]. The JAK pathway is commonly activated by inflammatory cytokines such as IL-6. Multiple clinical studies have demonstrated a negative prognostic value for elevated markers of systemic inflammation in PDAC patients [43, 44]. CRP and hypoalbuminemia are markers of inflammation and are known to be negative prognostic factors in pancreatic cancer [45]. In preclinical PDAC models, the JAK/STAT and related inflammatory pathways play a crucial role in cancer progression. Initially ruxolitinib was approved for myelofibrosis with the specific target mutation of JAK 2 V617F mutation [46]. In a series of 26 patients with PDAC, this mutation was not identified [47]. In RECAP, patients who progressed on gemcitabine were randomized to either capecitabine alone or combination of capecitabine and ruxolitinib, a JAK 1/2 inhibitor [48]. A total of 127 patients were randomized. No difference in survival outcomes was observed (4.5 vs 4.3, respectively, $P = 0.25$). In the prespecified subgroup of patients with systemic inflammation as measured by elevated serum C-reactive protein (CRP > 13 mg/L), survival significantly favored the ruxolitinib/capecitabine combination (3- and 6-month survivals of 48% and

42% vs 29% and 11%, respectively, $P = 0.01$). Based on these results, JANUS 1 and JANUS 2 phase III trials restricted enrollment to patients with elevated CRP (NCT02117479). Both studies were closed after a planned interim analysis demonstrated no added benefit of ruxolitinib to capecitabine [49]. Trials combining gemcitabine with ruxolitinib or gemcitabine and nab-paclitaxel with ruxolitinib are ongoing (NCT01822756). Ruxolitinib in combination with gemcitabine/nab-paclitaxel is in phase I/II clinical trial [50].

MUC1

Human mucin 1 (MUC1) is a protein secreted by over 85% of PDAC and absent in normal pancreas [51]. Patients with metastatic PDAC and MUC1 expressing circulating tumor cells had inferior survival outcomes [52]. Clivatuzumab tetraxetan (PAM4) is a monoclonal antibody that specifically targets pancreatic MUC1. The antibody part, clivatuzumab (targeted at MUC1), is conjugated with tetraxetan and has a chelator for yttrium-90. Initial phase I trial that evaluated single-agent PAM4 demonstrated promising responses to treatment in small set of patients with pancreatic cancer [53]. A second phase I study of repeated cycles of the same drug in combination with low-dose gemcitabine demonstrated an encouraging response rate of 16% and a disease control rate of 42% and a median survival of 7.7 months (including 11.8 months for those who received repeated cycles) [54]. Major toxicities were related to myelosuppression. Encouraged by the results of these early trials, a phase III study was conducted comparing best supportive care to low-dose gemcitabine with ^{90}Y clivatuzumab in the third-line setting (NCT01956812), following a planned interim analysis on OS, after more than 50% of the required 371 deaths had occurred. The interim analysis showed that the treatment arm of ^{90}Y clivatuzumab tetraxetan combined with low-dose gemcitabine and best supportive care did not demonstrate a sufficient improvement in OS and the study was terminated for futility [55].

MEK/MAPK

The MEK/MAPK and PI3K/Akt/mTOR pathways are downstream pathways to *KRAS*. Efforts to target these downstream effectors of *KRAS* activation are in study [56], although results have been disappointing. The difficulty in targeting *KRAS* mutation led to the hypothesis that targeting downstream targets such as MEK could lead to same results as the direct target of the *KRAS*. Trametinib, a mitogen/extracellular signal-related kinase (MEK) 1/2 inhibitor, was approved in treatment of unresectable or metastatic BRAF V600E/K-mutated melanoma [57]. A randomized double-blind phase II study was designed to determine OS in patients with pancreatic cancer treated with trametinib and gemcitabine versus gemcitabine alone. The trial enrolled 160 chemo-naïve PDAC patients. There was no significant difference in OS (8.4 vs 6.7 months, $P = 0.45$) [58]. Another selective, noncompetitive MEK 1/2 inhibitor, pimasertib, was studied in a randomized phase II trial in combination with gemcitabine in chemo-naïve PDAC patients. A total of 88 patients were randomized, and the primary endpoint, which was progression-free survival, was not met (3.7 vs 2.8 months, respectively, $P = 0.61$) [59]. Selumetinib, a mitogen-activated protein kinase (MAPK) inhibitor, demonstrated similar efficacy as capecitabine in a phase II study randomizing 77 PDAC patients in the second-line treatment setting after failure to gemcitabine. The OS was the primary endpoint and was not met (5.4 vs 5.0 months, $P = 0.92$) [60]. Similarly, targeting mTOR, using everolimus, has failed to show activity in previously treated metastatic pancreatic cancer. The trial was a phase II single arm that enrolled 33 patients. The median progression-free survival and overall survival were 1.8 and 4.5 months, respectively [61, 62]. Patients with pancreatic cancer in the setting of Peutz–Jeghers syndrome harbor an alteration in the STK11 tumor suppressor gene. STK11 encodes an mTOR1 inhibitor, and hence cancers with this mutation are dependent on mTOR activity. A remarkable response to mTOR inhibition was reported in a patient with pancreatic cancer with STK11 mutation highlighting the importance of selecting patients with appropriate mutation profile for testing molecularly targeted agents [63].

Activating RAS mutations may signal through multiple pathways. Inhibition of MEK may upregulate the activation of the PI3K/Akt pathway, necessitating a strategy to target multiple pathways simultaneously. Ah et al. tested this hypothesis by combining selumetinib with erlotinib in patients with metastatic pancreatic cancer who have progressed on one prior therapy [64]. Although no partial responses were observed, median OS was about 7.5 months with 51% disease control rate. A combination of selumetinib and MK-2206 (Akt inhibitor) did not improve OS in patients progressing after gemcitabine-based chemotherapy when compared to FOLFOX in a randomized phase II study [65]. Based on the current evidence, targeting the signaling pathways downstream from *RAS* has, at best, yielded modest activity. The design of these trials and lack of molecular selection of patients may have contributed to the observed negative results.

Targeting RAS

Several strategies targeting *RAS* are being evaluated in pancreatic cancer. These pathways include viral-mediated targeting of *RAS*-mutated cells (Reolysin®), dislodging RAS from cell membrane, and inhibiting *RAS* transcription. Salirasib inhibits *RAS*-dependent cell growth by dislodging all RAS isoforms from the plasma membrane with activity demonstrated in PDAC cell lines and xenograft models [66]. A phase I study combining salirasib with gemcitabine in advanced PDAC demonstrated a median OS of 6.2 months and a 1-year survival of 37 % [67]. Posttranscriptional inhibition of RAS expression through small interfering RNA (siRNA) is a promising approach for therapy in pancreatic cancer. Using pancreatic tumor xenografts, Rejiba et al. demonstrated suppression of mutant *KRAS* expression using specific siRNA leading to tumor growth inhibition [68]. A major challenge of using siRNA clinically has been developing a drug delivery strategy. A biodegradable polymeric matrix encompassing siRNA such as anti-KRAS^{G12D} siRNA (known as local drug eluter; siG12D LODER) is designed to provide slow and stable local drug release within a tumor over a period of a few months. This method of drug delivery can suppress *KRAS* expression, in vitro and in vivo, resulting in antitumor activity and improved survival in mouse models [69]. This was studied in a phase I/II first-line treatment trial followed by gemcitabine treatment in locally advanced pancreatic cancer. A total of 15 patients were enrolled. Stable disease was defined in 12 patients. Median OS was 15.1 months. The combination was well tolerated [70].

Hedgehog Pathway

Inhibition of the hedgehog pathway decreases the growth of various types of tumors, including PDAC [71, 72]. Cancer-associated stromal fibroblasts overexpress the hedgehog receptor smoothened (SMO), leading to activation of the sonic hedgehog pathway [73]. In preclinical study, the SMO receptor inhibitor saridegib with gemcitabine in gemcitabine-resistant mice resulted in increased tumor vasculature and extended survival [74]. However, a phase IB/II study comparing gemcitabine ± the hedgehog inhibitor vismodegib in PDAC did not translate to any benefit [75]. Another mutation that has been identified is the TCH1 that encodes genes for the hedgehog receptor. These mutations have not been reported in PDAC.

STAT3

The interaction and crossroad effect of the JAK and STAT pathways have always been linked to each other. STAT3 is aberrantly activated in human PDAC and has also been shown to be critically important for PDAC precursor lesion formation [76, 77]. Increase in STAT3 phosphorylation predicts poor outcome in PDAC following resection with curative intent [78]. Furthermore, it has been shown that inhibition of STAT3 results in increased sensitivity to gemcitabine chemotherapy as well as reduction in tumor burden and delay of tumor progression in PDAC [79]. β-Catenin expression has been correlated with resistance of pancreatic cancer cells to chemotherapy [80]. Blockade of the STAT3 and β-catenin pathways, therefore, offers a novel and potentially highly effective strategy to target cancer stem cells and resistance to existing chemotherapy. STAT3 increases the expression of the stemness-associated genes Sox2, c-Myc, Nanog, and β-catenin.

BBI608, a STAT3 inhibitor, has demonstrated potent anticancer stem cell effects in a broad spectrum of cancer types while sparing normal hematopoietic stem cells. BBI608 has also demonstrated inhibitory activity against a broad spectrum of heterogeneous (bulk or non-stem) cancer cells. BBI608 has demonstrated potent antitumor activity as monotherapy in vivo in a variety of murine xenograft models of human cancer including colorectal, pancreatic, head and neck, breast, prostate, gastric, and liver cancers. In an open-label, multicenter study, 31 patients received BBI608 in combination with gemcitabine and nab-paclitaxel. This combination was well tolerated. The median progression-free survival was encouraging at 7.8 months [81] (NCT02231723). A phase III trial is planned comparing gemcitabine/nab-paclitaxel with BBI608 to gemcitabine and nab-paclitaxel.

Conclusion

Molecularly targeted therapies have had no impact on the treatment of pancreatic cancer. Multiple randomized trials evaluating agents targeting intracellular signaling pathways, angiogenesis, tumor stroma, and tumor antigens have failed to identify any active agents. With the exception of erlotinib, the management of pancreatic cancer remains heavily dependent on cytotoxic chemotherapy regimens. Many mechanisms have been proposed to explain this lack of activity of targeted agents in pancreatic cancer. First, trials have not selected patients based on molecular profile. The success of targeted agents in other disease types has heavily depended on selecting patients with certain molecular profiles such as ALK activation in non-small cell lung cancer (NSCLC) [82]. Identifying predictive biomarkers is an essential step prior to initiating large randomized trials. The development of PARP inhibitors in patients with impaired DNA repair is an example of the change in drug development strategies in pancreatic cancer. A second challenge in the treatment of pancreatic cancer has been the lack of an active chemotherapy backbone regimen to combine with targeted agents. The success of anti-angiogenic agents in colorectal cancer, for example, was enhanced by the activity of 5FU-based therapy. In pancreatic cancer, anti-angiogenic agents were developed using a single-agent gemcitabine backbone regimen that has modest activity. The new generations of trials are evaluating novel agents in the setting of more active combination chemotherapy regimens. A third challenge has been the lack of predicative preclinical models that can guide drug development. Newer models including organoids, patient-derived xenografts, and genetically engineered mouse models hold promise for better preclinical prediction of activity of targeted agents. Finally, novel targeted therapies currently in clinical trials have encouraging preliminary activity and could provide a valuable addition to the more active chemotherapy combinations.

References

1. Hruban RH, Petersen GM, Goggins M, et al. Familial pancreatic cancer. Ann Oncol. 1999;10(Suppl 4):69–73.
2. Bardeesy N, Sinha M, Hezel AF, et al. Loss of the Lkb1 tumour suppressor provokes intestinal polyposis but resistance to transformation. Nature. Sep 12 2002;419(6903):162–7.

3. Jančík S, Drábek J, Radzioch D, Hajdúch M. Clinical relevance of KRAS in human cancers. Biomed Res Int. 2010;2010:150960.
4. Siegel-Lakhai WS, Crul M, Zhang S, et al. Phase I and pharmacological study of the farnesyltransferase inhibitor tipifarnib (Zarnestra, R115777) in combination with gemcitabine and cisplatin in patients with advanced solid tumours. Br J Cancer. Nov 28 2005;93(11):1222–9.
5. Gore L, Holden SN, Cohen RB, et al. A phase I safety, pharmacological and biological study of the farnesyl protein transferase inhibitor, tipifarnib and capecitabine in advanced solid tumors. Ann Oncol. Nov 2006;17(11):1709–17.
6. Sparreboom A, Kehrer DF, Mathijssen RH, et al. Phase I and pharmacokinetic study of irinotecan in combination with R115777, a farnesyl protein transferase inhibitor. Br J Cancer. Apr 19 2004;90(8):1508–15.
7. Zujewski J, Horak ID, Bol CJ, et al. Phase I and pharmacokinetic study of farnesyl protein transferase inhibitor R115777 in advanced cancer. J Clin Oncol Off J Am Soc Clin Oncol. Feb 2000;18(4):927–41.
8. Cohen SJ, Gallo J, Lewis NL, et al. Phase I and pharmacokinetic study of the farnesyltransferase inhibitor R115777 in combination with irinotecan in patients with advanced cancer. Cancer Chemother Pharmacol. Jun 2004;53(6):513–8.
9. Patnaik A, Eckhardt SG, Izbicka E, et al. A Phase I, Pharmacokinetic, and Biological Study of the Farnesyltransferase Inhibitor Tipifarnib in Combination with Gemcitabine in Patients with Advanced Malignancies. Clinical Cancer Res. Oct 15 2003;9:4761–71.
10. Van Cutsem E, van de Velde H, Karasek P, et al. Phase III trial of gemcitabine plus tipifarnib compared with gemcitabine plus placebo in advanced pancreatic cancer. J Clin Oncol Off J Am Soc Clin Oncol. Apr 15 2004;22(8):1430–8.
11. Jones LE, Humphreys MJ, Campbell F, Neoptolemos JP, Boyd MT. Comprehensive analysis of matrix metalloproteinase and tissue inhibitor expression in pancreatic cancer: increased expression of matrix metalloproteinase-7 predicts poor survival. Clin Cancer Res. Apr 15 2004;10(8):2832–45.
12. Moore MJ, Hamm J, Dancey J, et al. Comparison of gemcitabine versus the matrix metalloproteinase inhibitor BAY 12-9566 in patients with advanced or metastatic adenocarcinoma of the pancreas: a phase III trial of the national cancer institute of Canada clinical trials group. J Clin Oncol Off J Am Soc Clin Oncol. Sep 1 2003;21(17):3296–302.
13. Bramhall SR, Rosemurgy A, Brown PD, Bowry C, Buckels JA, Marimastat Pancreatic Cancer Study G. Marimastat as first-line therapy for patients with unresectable pancreatic cancer: a randomized trial. J Clin Oncol Off J Am Soc Clin Oncol. Aug 1 2001;19(15):3447–55.
14. Bramhall SR, Schulz J, Nemunaitis J, Brown PD, Baillet M, Buckels JA. A double-blind placebo-controlled, randomised study comparing gemcitabine and marimastat with gemcitabine and placebo as first line therapy in patients with advanced pancreatic cancer. Br J Cancer. Jul 15 2002;87(2):161–7.
15. Moore MJ, Goldstein D, Hamm J, et al. Erlotinib plus gemcitabine compared with gemcitabine alone in patients with advanced pancreatic cancer: a phase III trial of the national cancer institute of Canada clinical trials group. J Clin Oncol. May 20 2007;25(15):1960–6.
16. Miksad RA, Schnipper L, Goldstein M. Does a statistically significant survival benefit of erlotinib plus gemcitabine for advanced pancreatic cancer translate into clinical significance and value? J Clin Oncol Off J Am Soc Clin Oncol. 2007;25(28):4506–7. author reply 4508
17. Baselga J. Why the epidermal growth factor receptor? The rationale for cancer therapy. Oncologist. 2002;7(Suppl 4):2–8.
18. Philip PA, Benedetti J, Corless CL, et al. Phase III study comparing gemcitabine plus cetuximab versus gemcitabine in patients with advanced pancreatic adenocarcinoma: southwest oncology group-directed intergroup trial S0205. J Clin Oncol Off J Am Soc Clin Oncol. Aug 1 2010;28(22):3605–10.
19. https://http://www.ncbi.nlm.nih.gov/pubmed/20606093–comments.
20. da Cunha Santos G, Dhani N, Tu D, et al. Molecular predictors of outcome in a phase 3 study of gemcitabine and erlotinib therapy in patients with advanced pancreatic cancer: national cancer institute of Canada clinical trials group study PA.3. Cancer. Dec 15 2010;116(24):5599–607.

21. Boeck S, Jung A, Laubender RP, et al. EGFR pathway biomarkers in erlotinib-treated patients with advanced pancreatic cancer: translational results from the randomised, crossover phase 3 trial AIO-PK0104. Br J Cancer. Feb 5 2013;108(2):469–76.
22. Boeck S, Jung A, Laubender RP, et al. KRAS mutation status is not predictive for objective response to anti-EGFR treatment with erlotinib in patients with advanced pancreatic cancer. J Gastroenterol. Apr 2013;48(4):544–8.
23. Ellis LM, Takahashi Y, Fenoglio CJ, Cleary KR, Bucana CD, Evans DB. Vessel counts and vascular endothelial growth factor expression in pancreatic adenocarcinoma. Eur J Cancer. Feb 1998;34(3):337–40.
24. Doi Y, Yashiro M, Yamada N, Amano R, Noda S, Hirakawa K. VEGF-A/VEGFR-2 signaling plays an important role for the motility of pancreas cancer cells. Ann Surg Oncol. Aug 2012;19(8):2733–43.
25. Higgins KJ, Abdelrahim M, Liu S, Yoon K, Safe S. Regulation of vascular endothelial growth factor receptor-2 expression in pancreatic cancer cells by Sp proteins. Biochem Biophys Res Commun. Jun 23 2006;345(1):292–301.
26. Doi Y, Yashiro M, Yamada N, et al. Significance of phospho-vascular endothelial growth factor receptor-2 expression in pancreatic cancer. Cancer Sci. Jun 2010;101(6):1529–35.
27. Bennouna J, Sastre J, Arnold D, et al. Continuation of bevacizumab after first progression in metastatic colorectal cancer (ML18147): a randomised phase 3 trial. Lancet Oncol. Jan 2013;14(1):29–37.
28. Zinner RG, Obasaju CK, Spigel DR, et al. PRONOUNCE: randomized, open-label, phase III study of first-line pemetrexed + carboplatin followed by maintenance pemetrexed versus paclitaxel + carboplatin + bevacizumab followed by maintenance bevacizumab in patients ith advanced nonsquamous non-small-cell lung cancer. J Thorac Oncol. Jan 2015;10(1):134–42.
29. Kindler HL, Niedzwiecki D, Hollis D, et al. Gemcitabine plus bevacizumab compared with gemcitabine plus placebo in patients with advanced pancreatic cancer: phase III trial of the cancer and leukemia group B (CALGB 80303). J Clin Oncol Off J Am Soc Clin Oncol. Aug 1 2010;28(22):3617–22.
30. Van Cutsem E, Vervenne WL, Bennouna J, et al. Phase III trial of bevacizumab in combination with gemcitabine and erlotinib in patients with metastatic pancreatic cancer. J Clin Oncol Off J Am Soc Clin Oncol. May 1 2009;27(13):2231–7.
31. European Medicines Agency. Inlyta®film-coated tablets: summary of product characteristics (online).http://www.emea.eu/docs/en_GB/document_library/EPAR_-_Product_Information/human/002406//WC500132188.pdf.
32. Kindler HL, Ioka T, Richel DJ, et al. Axitinib plus gemcitabine versus placebo plus gemcitabine in patients with advanced pancreatic adenocarcinoma: a double-blind randomised phase 3 study. Lancet Oncol. Mar 2011;12(3):256–62.
33. Duda DG, Ancukiewicz M, Jain RK. Biomarkers of antiangiogenic therapy: how do we move from candidate biomarkers to valid biomarkers? J Clin Oncol Off J Am Soc Clin Oncol. Jan 10 2010;28(2):183–5.
34. Pant S, Martin LK, Geyer S, et al. Baseline serum albumin is a predictive biomarker for patients with advanced pancreatic cancer treated with bevacizumab: a pooled analysis of 7 prospective trials of gemcitabine-based therapy with or without bevacizumab. Cancer. Jun 15 2014;120(12):1780–6.
35. Tabernero J, Yoshino T, Cohn AL, et al. Ramucirumab versus placebo in combination with second-line FOLFIRI in patients with metastatic colorectal carcinoma that progressed during or after first-line therapy with bevacizumab, oxaliplatin, and a fluoropyrimidine (RAISE): a randomised, double-blind, multicentre, phase 3 study. Lancet Oncol. May 2015;16(5):499–508.
36. Wilke H, Muro K, Van Cutsem E, et al. Ramucirumab plus paclitaxel versus placebo plus paclitaxel in patients with previously treated advanced gastric or gastro-oesophageal junction adenocarcinoma (RAINBOW): a double-blind, randomised phase 3 trial. Lancet Oncol. Oct 2014;15(11):1224–35.
37. Fuchs CS, Tomasek J, Yong CJ, et al. Ramucirumab monotherapy for previously treated advanced gastric or gastro-oesophageal junction adenocarcinoma (REGARD): an international, randomised, multicentre, placebo-controlled, phase 3 trial. Lancet. Jan 4 2014;383(9911):31–9.

38. clinicaltrial.gov.
39. Chou A, Waddell N, Cowley MJ, et al. Clinical and molecular characterization of HER2 amplified-pancreatic cancer. Genome Med. 2013;5(8):78.
40. Harder J, Ihorst G, Heinemann V, et al. Multicentre phase II trial of trastuzumab and capecitabine in patients with HER2 overexpressing metastatic pancreatic cancer. Br J Cancer. Mar 13 2012;106(6):1033–8.
41. Safran H, Iannitti D, Ramanathan R, et al. Herceptin and gemcitabine for metastatic pancreatic cancers that overexpress HER-2/neu. Cancer Investig. 2004;22(5):706–12.
42. Quintas-Cardama A, Verstovsek S. Molecular pathways: Jak/STAT pathway: mutations, inhibitors, and resistance. Clin Cancer Res. Apr 15 2013;19(8):1933–40.
43. Nixon AB, Pang H, Starr MD, et al. Prognostic and predictive blood-based biomarkers in patients with advanced pancreatic cancer: results from CALGB80303 (alliance). Clin Cancer Res. Dec 15 2013;19(24):6957–66.
44. Nakachi K, Furuse J, Ishii H, Suzuki E, Yoshino M. Prognostic factors in patients with gemcitabine-refractory pancreatic cancer. Jpn J Clin Oncol. Feb 2007;37(2):114–20.
45. McMillan DC, Elahi MM, Sattar N, Angerson WJ, Johnstone J, McArdle CS. Measurement of the systemic inflammatory response predicts cancer-specific and non-cancer survival in patients with cancer. Nutr Cancer. 2001;41(1–2):64–9.
46. Mascarenhas J, Hoffman R. Ruxolitinib: the first FDA approved therapy for the treatment of myelofibrosis. Clin Cancer Res. Jun 1 2012;18(11):3008–14.
47. Chou DH, Vetere A, Choudhary A, et al. Kinase-independent small-molecule inhibition of JAK-STAT signaling. J Am Chem Soc. Jun 24 2015;137(24):7929–34.
48. Hurwitz HI, Uppal N, Wagner SA, et al. Randomized, double-blind, phase II study of ruxolitinib or placebo in combination with capecitabine in patients with metastatic pancreatic cancer for whom therapy with gemcitabine has failed. J Clin Oncol. 2015;33(34):4039–47.
49. Incyte press release JANUS 1. 2016; http://www.businesswire.com/news/home/20160211005321/en/Incyte-Announces-Decision-Discontinue-JANUS-Studies-Ruxolitinib. Accessed 12 Apr 2016.
50. US National Library of Medicine. ClinicalTrials.gov [online], https://clinicaltrials.gov/ct2/show/NCT02119663. 2015.
51. CF Q, Li Y, Song YJ, et al. MUC1 expression in primary and metastatic pancreatic cancer cells for in vitro treatment by (213)Bi-C595 radioimmunoconjugate. Br J Cancer. Dec 13 2004;91(12):2086–93.
52. Dotan E, Alpaugh RK, Ruth K, et al. Prognostic significance of MUC-1 in circulating tumor cells in patients with metastatic pancreatic adenocarcinoma. Pancreas. 2016;45(8):1131–5.
53. Gulec SA, Cohen SJ, Pennington KL, et al. Treatment of advanced pancreatic carcinoma with 90Y-Clivatuzumab Tetraxetan: a phase I single-dose escalation trial. Clin Cancer Res. Jun 15 2011;17(12):4091–100.
54. Ocean AJ, Pennington KL, Guarino MJ, et al. Fractionated radioimmunotherapy with (90) Y-clivatuzumab tetraxetan and low-dose gemcitabine is active in advanced pancreatic cancer: a phase 1 trial. Cancer. Nov 15 2012;118(22):5497–506.
55. Immunomedics provides update on phase 3 PANCRIT-1 trial of clivatuzumab tetraxetan in patients with advanced pancreatic cancer. 2016; https://globenewswire.com/news-release/2016/03/14/819641/0/en/Immunomedics-Provides-Update-on-Phase-3-PANCRIT-1-Trial-of-Clivatuzumab-Tetraxetan-in-Patients-With-Advanced-Pancreatic-Cancer.html. Accessed 12 Apr 2016.
56. Paulson AS, Tran Cao HS, Tempero MA, Lowy AM. Therapeutic advances in pancreatic cancer. Gastroenterology. Jun 2013;144(6):1316–26.
57. Flaherty KT, Infante JR, Daud A, et al. Combined BRAF and MEK inhibition in melanoma with BRAF V600 mutations. N Engl J Med. Nov 2012;367(18):1694–703.
58. JR I. A randomized, double-blind, placebo-controlled trial of trametinib, a MEK inhibitor, in combination with gemcitabine for patients with untreated metastatic adenocarcinoma of the pancreas [abstract]. J Clin Oncol. 2013;31(Suppl. 4):a291.
59. Eric VC. Phase II randomized trial of MEK inhibitor pimasertib or placebo combined with gemcitabine in the first-line treatment of metastatic pancreatic cancer [abstract]. J Clin Oncol. 2015;33(Suppl. 3):a344.

60. Bodoky G, Timcheva C, Spigel DR, et al. A phase II open-label randomized study to assess the efficacy and safety of selumetinib (AZD6244 [ARRY-142886]) versus capecitabine in patients with advanced or metastatic pancreatic cancer who have failed first-line gemcitabine therapy. Investig New Drugs. Jun 2012;30(3):1216–23.
61. Garrido-Laguna I, Tan AC, Uson M, et al. Integrated preclinical and clinical development of mTOR inhibitors in pancreatic cancer. Br J Cancer. Aug 24 2010;103(5):649–55.
62. Wolpin BM, Hezel AF, Abrams T, et al. Oral mTOR inhibitor everolimus in patients with gemcitabine-refractory metastatic pancreatic cancer. J Clin Oncol Off J Am Soc Clin Oncol. Jan 10 2009;27(2):193–8.
63. Klumpen HJ, Queiroz KC, Spek CA, et al. mTOR inhibitor treatment of pancreatic cancer in a patient with Peutz-Jeghers syndrome. J Clin Oncol Off J Am Soc Clin Oncol. Feb 20 2011;29(6):e150–3.
64. Ko AH, Tempero MA, Bekaii-Saab TB, et al. Dual MEK/EGFR inhibition for advanced, chemotherapy-refractory pancreatic cancer: A multicenter phase II trial of selumetinib (AZD6244; ARRY-142886) plus erlotinib. Paper presented at: ASCO Annual Meeting Proceedings. 2013.
65. Chung VM, McDonough SL, Philip PA, et al. SWOG S1115: Randomized phase II trial of selumetinib (AZD6244; ARRY 142886) hydrogen sulfate (NSC-748727) and MK-2206 (NSC-749607) vs. mFOLFOX in pretreated patients (Pts) with metastatic pancreatic cancer. Paper presented at: ASCO Annual Meeting Proceedings. 2015.
66. Weisz B, Giehl K, Gana-Weisz M, et al. A new functional Ras antagonist inhibits human pancreatic tumor growth in nude mice. Oncogene. Apr 22 1999;18(16):2579–88.
67. Laheru D, Shah P, Rajeshkumar NV, et al. Integrated preclinical and clinical development of S-trans, trans-farnesylthiosalicylic acid (FTS, Salirasib) in pancreatic cancer. Investig New Drugs. 2012;30(6):2391–9.
68. Réjiba S, Wack S, Aprahamian M, Hajri A. K-ras oncogene silencing strategy reduces tumor growth and enhances gemcitabine chemotherapy efficacy for pancreatic cancer treatment. Cancer Sci. 2007;98(7):1128–36.
69. Khvalevsky EZ, Gabai R, Rachmut IH, et al. Mutant KRAS is a druggable target for pancreatic cancer. Proc Natl Acad Sci. 2013;110(51):20723–8.
70. Golan T, Khvalevsky EZ, Hubert A, et al. RNAi therapy targeting KRAS in combination with chemotherapy for locally advanced pancreatic cancer patients. Oncotarget. Sep 15 2015;6(27):24560–70.
71. Feldmann G, Habbe N, Dhara S, et al. Hedgehog inhibition prolongs survival in a genetically engineered mouse model of pancreatic cancer. Gut. Oct 2008;57(10):1420–30.
72. Kelleher FC. Hedgehog signaling and therapeutics in pancreatic cancer. Carcinogenesis. Apr 2011;32(4):445–51.
73. Walter K, Omura N, Hong SM, et al. Overexpression of smoothened activates the sonic hedgehog signaling pathway in pancreatic cancer-associated fibroblasts. Clin Cancer Res. Mar 15 2010;16(6):1781–9.
74. Olive KP, Jacobetz MA, Davidson CJ, et al. Inhibition of hedgehog signaling enhances delivery of chemotherapy in a mouse model of pancreatic cancer. Science (New York, NY). Jun 12 2009;324(5933):1457–61.
75. Catenacci DVT, Bahary N, Nattam SR, et al. Final analysis of a phase IB/randomized phase II study of gemcitabine (G) plus placebo (P) or vismodegib (V), a hedgehog (Hh) pathway inhibitor, in patients (pts) with metastatic pancreatic cancer (PC): a university of Chicago phase II consortium study. J Clin Oncol. 2013;31(15_suppl):4012. (Meeting Abstracts). May 20, 2013
76. Scholz A, Heinze S, Detjen KM, et al. Activated signal transducer and activator of transcription 3 (STAT3) supports the malignant phenotype of human pancreatic cancer. Gastroenterology. Sep 2003;125(3):891–905.
77. Fukuda A, Wang SC, JPt M, et al. Stat3 and MMP7 contribute to pancreatic ductal adenocarcinoma initiation and progression. Cancer Cell. Apr 12 2011;19(4):441–55.

78. Denley SM, Jamieson NB, McCall P, et al. Activation of the IL-6R/Jak/stat pathway is associated with a poor outcome in resected pancreatic ductal adenocarcinoma. J Gastrointest Surg. May 2013;17(5):887–98.
79. Venkatasubbarao K, Peterson L, Zhao S, et al. Inhibiting signal transducer and activator of transcription-3 increases response to gemcitabine and delays progression of pancreatic cancer. Mol Cancer. 2013;12(1):104.
80. Singh A, Settleman J. EMT, cancer stem cells and drug resistance: an emerging axis of evil in the war on cancer. Oncogene. Aug 26 2010;29(34):4741–51.
81. Safi Shahda BFE-R, O'Neil BH, Starodub A, Hanna WT, Borodyansky L, Oh C, Li C, Bekaii-Saab TS. A phase Ib study of cancer stem cell (CSC) pathway inhibitor BBI-608 in combination with gemcitabine and nab-paclitaxel (nab-PTX) in patients (pts) with metastatic pancreatic ductal adenocarcinoma (mPDAC). J Clin Oncol. 2016;34(suppl 4S):284. 2016 Gastrointestinal Cancers Symposium
82. Solomon BJ, Mok T, Kim DW, et al. First-line crizotinib versus chemotherapy in ALK-positive lung cancer. N Engl J Med. Dec 4 2014;371(23):2167–77.

Chapter 13
Targeting the Tumor Microenvironment

Julia Carnevale and Andrew H. Ko

Introduction and Overview

Pancreatic cancer is a stroma-rich malignancy, characterized by a dense desmoplastic reaction at the primary pancreatic site that may comprise more than half of the tumor volume [1]. However, rather than merely representing some sort of inert fibrotic scaffolding, evidence has accumulated over the years that this stromal compartment, also often referred to as the tumor microenvironment (TME), is a dynamic entity that evolves and changes during the course of pancreatic tumorigenesis, impacting the biology of pancreatic cancer in a myriad of ways. This includes playing critical roles in tumor growth, invasiveness, metastatic spread, stemness, resistance to therapy, and immune escape.

The accumulation of these discoveries has led researchers to focus on identifying pharmacologic approaches to target the stroma in order to inhibit the malignant potential of pancreatic cancer and improve drug delivery. However, studies using a variety of different genetically engineered mouse models have also suggested that the tumor stroma may function to *restrain* pancreatic cancer growth in some contexts, serving in a protective capacity—thus highlighting both the multiplicity and diversity of functions of the stromal compartment and our need to proceed with caution as we seek to manipulate the TME for therapeutic benefit. Herein we will review many of the research efforts underway that seek to modulate different aspects of the TME to attenuate tumor growth and improve delivery of potent treatments for patients with pancreatic cancer.

J. Carnevale, M.D. • A.H. Ko, M.D. (✉)
Helen Diller Family Comprehensive Cancer Center, University of California San Francisco, 550 16th Street, Box 3211, San Francisco, CA 94143, USA
e-mail: andrew.ko@ucsf.edu

T. Bekaii-Saab, B. El-Rayes (eds.), *Current and Emerging Therapies in Pancreatic Cancer*, DOI 10.1007/978-3-319-58256-6_13

The Starring Role of Pancreatic Stellate Cells

In addition to a rich extracellular matrix comprised of multiple collagens, glycoproteins, and growth factors, the TME features a variety of cell types including mesenchymal cells (most notably fibroblasts of various types, including pancreatic stellate cells), inflammatory cells, and vascular endothelium (*see* Table 13.1).

Pancreatic cancer-associated fibroblasts comprise a large percentage of the cellular compartment of the TME. There is considerable heterogeneity in these fibroblasts [2, 3], distinguished by differential expression of specific protein markers, with many of the cells likely derived from the bone marrow rather than originating from within the pancreas itself [4–7]. The most well-studied subset of fibroblasts that play a central role in tumor–stromal interactions and the development and maintenance of desmoplasia are termed *pancreatic stellate cells* (*PSCs*), so-called because of their star-shaped morphology, cytoplasmic storage of vitamin A in the form of lipid droplets, and similarity in behavior to hepatic stellate cells, the primary mediators of fibrosis in the liver [8, 9]. Analogously, PSCs represent the primary cells responsible for the production of fibrosis in response to pancreatic injury, pancreatitis, and cancer [10–13]. In healthy pancreas tissue, PSCs, which are typically found in a periacinar location, remain in a quiescent state; however, under inflammatory conditions, these cells are activated, becoming highly proliferative and differentiating into myofibroblasts, where they deposit extracellular matrix, including

Table 13.1 Components of the pancreatic cancer microenvironment

Component	Examples
Mesenchymal cells	Cancer-associated fibroblasts Pancreatic stellate cells (PSCs) (aka myofibroblasts)
Immune cells	Mast cells Myeloid-derived suppressor cells (MDSCs) Neutrophils Tumor-associated macrophages (TAM) T lymphocytes (primarily regulatory)
Extracellular matrix proteins	Collagens I, III, IV Fibroblast-associated protein Fibronectin Growth factors Hyaluronic acid Laminin Matrix metalloproteinase 2 (MMP-2), MMP-9, MMP-11 SPARC/osteonectin Thrombospondin-1/2
Vasculature	Endothelial cells Pericytes

Abbreviations: MMP, matrix metalloproteinase; SPARC, secreted protein acidic and rich in cysteine

A.H. Ko, Progress in the Treatment of Metastatic Pancreatic Cancer and the Search for Next Opportunities. *J Clin Oncol,* 33(16), 2015: 1781.

collagens I and III, fibronectin, and matrix metalloproteinases that remodel the matrix [12, 14]. PSCs can be distinguished from non-stellate pancreatic fibroblasts (PFBs) based on surface protein expression, most notably α-smooth muscle actin (SMA), which is not usually expressed in PFBs [10]. Specific to cancer, pancreatic tumor cells activate PSCs via various secreted factors, including transforming growth factor (TGF)-β1, fibroblast growth factor (FGF)-2, and platelet-derived growth factor (PDGF), as well as Sonic Hedgehog (SHH) [11, 15–18]. (The role of SHH will be discussed in greater detail in a later section in this chapter.) The reverse also holds true: PSCs play a critical role in influencing multiple aspects of pancreatic tumor biology and signaling, with the concentration of PSCs within pancreatic tumors providing potentially useful prognostic information. In one analysis performed by Erkan and colleagues of 233 patients who underwent surgery for their pancreatic cancer, those whose tumors contained the highest ratio of α-smooth muscle actin (as a proxy for PSC activity) relative to collagen deposition—which the investigators referred to as an "activated stromal index"—had the lowest median survival rate [19]. Fujita et al. similarly showed in a retrospective analysis of 109 patients undergoing pancreatectomy at their institution that higher intratumoral levels of α-SMA mRNA expression were associated with shorter survival [20].

The potentially agonistic role for PSCs in pancreatic cancer tumor growth, survival, and metastasis has been demonstrated in a series of *in vitro* and *in vivo* co-culture experiments, in which tumor cells were either exposed to media from PSCs or co-cultured with PSCs themselves, and metrics of the malignant phenotype measured. In one such study, following isolation of PSCs obtained from patients undergoing pancreatic cancer resection, Hwang et al. showed that pancreatic cancer cell lines grown in media taken from these cultured PSCs (both immortalized and non-immortalized) resulted in increased proliferation, invasion, and colony formation on soft agar [21]. Co-injection of pancreatic cancer cell lines with immortalized PSCs also led to increased tumor progression and metastasis in an *in vivo* orthotopic mouse model. Mouse experiments performed by Vonlaufen et al. produced similar findings; athymic mice receiving intrapancreatic injection of a MIA PaCa-2 cell line together with PSCs, compared to the pancreatic cancer cell line alone, demonstrated larger tumors, more fibrotic bands containing activated PSCs within tumors, and an increased number of regional and distant metastases [22].

It is believed that the increased metastatic potential of tumor cells is mediated in large part by various secreted factors by PSCs, including matrix metalloproteinases and SPARC (secreted protein acidic and rich in cysteine), which are known to promote and increase tumor cell invasion. (SPARC, which has been the subject of considerable interest for its putative role in mediating tumoral uptake of the chemotherapy drug nanoparticle-bound (nab)-paclitaxel, will be discussed in greater detail later in this chapter.) In addition, Xu and colleagues performed a sex mismatch study (injecting fluorescently labeled male human PSCs plus female pancreatic cancer cells into the pancreas of female mice) to track PSCs and further evaluate their role in metastases [23]. Indeed, they found that PSCs exhibit transendothelial migration (i.e., can intravasate/extravasate to and from blood vessels), thus actually being able to accompany cancer cells to distant sites of metastasis.

Adding to their multiplicity of roles, PSCs may also be important in tumor angiogenesis, as they do secrete proangiogenic molecules, including vascular endothelial growth factor (VEGF), especially under hypoxic conditions [24]. PSCs have been demonstrated in mouse studies to increase the concentration of CD31+ (endothelial) cells in primary pancreatic tumors when injected locally [23]. Conversely, at the same time, they may help sustain the hypovascular, hypoxic microenvironment that characterizes pancreatic tumors via their role in stromal deposition [25, 26].

Several groups have demonstrated that PSCs also help mediate the immunosuppressive microenvironment of pancreatic tumors. Ene-Obong and colleagues showed in a series of studies on both human pancreatic cancer samples and a well-validated genetically engineered murine model of pancreatic cancer expressing both oncogenic Kras and mutant p53 in pancreatic cells (*Kras*$^{LSL\text{-}G12D/+}$, *Trp53*$^{LSL\text{-}R172H/+}$, *Pdx-1-Cre*; herein referred to as the KPC mouse) [27] that activated PSCs reduce migration of CD8(+) T cells to the juxtatumoral stromal compartment, suggesting that PSCs also play a role in preventing an effective antitumor immune response [26]. PSCs have further been demonstrated by Mace et al. to promote the differentiation of myeloid-derived suppressor cells (MDSCs) [28].

Finally, multiple lines of evidence support the hypothesis that PSCs may contribute to the therapeutic resistance that notoriously characterizes pancreatic cancer. As noted, PSCs are responsible for laying down much of the ECM that may represent a physical barrier hampering adequate drug delivery and acquisition of resistance to chemotherapy. Lonardo et al. reported that PSCs also form a niche for cancer stem cells within pancreatic tumors by secreting embryonic morphogen nodal/activin at the tumor/stroma interface, promoting *in vitro* sphere formation and invasiveness of pancreatic cancer stem cells [29], the compartment of pancreatic tumors known to be particularly resistant to standard therapies. Mantoni and colleagues performed a series of both co-culture assays and *in vivo* experiments to demonstrate that PSCs also radioprotect pancreatic cancer cells and that this radioprotection occurs in a β1-integrin-dependent manner [1].

Taken as a whole, these data implicate pancreatic stellate cells as an intriguing candidate for potential therapeutic intervention when considering stromal-targeting strategies. As such, a variety of clinical approaches have been taken that focused specifically on therapeutically targeting PSCs. One such broad approach leverages the fact that PSCs express high levels of the vitamin D receptor (VDR), as shown by Sherman et al. [30]. These investigators found that VDR acts as a master transcriptional regulator of PSCs to push them from an activated to a quiescent state. Consequently, administration of a potent vitamin D analogue, calcitriol, in KPC mice led to stromal remodeling, increased intratumoral uptake of gemcitabine, reduced tumor volume, and a 57% increase in survival compared to mice treated with chemotherapy alone [30]. A number of clinical trials are ongoing to test vitamin D analogues, such as paricalcitol and calcitriol, in combination with standard chemotherapies in the neoadjuvant and advanced settings (http://clinicaltrials.gov; NCT02030860, NCT02754726, NCT00238199).

It has additionally been observed that vitamin A (retinol) can also restore PSC quiescence. Froeling et al. administered all-trans-retinoic acid (ATRA) to KPC mice which induced quiescence and reduced motility of PSCs, leading to reduced proliferation and increased apoptosis of surrounding pancreatic cancer cells [31]. Based on this research, there is now a phase I clinical trial open testing ATRA in combination with chemotherapy in patients with metastatic pancreatic cancer (the STAR-PAC trial).

However, we need to proceed with caution when targeting the fibroblast compartment of pancreatic tumors given the potential protective role these cells may play in this disease, as highlighted by a set of experiments performed by Ozdemir and colleagues [32]. These investigators generated transgenic mice in which α-SMA-positive myofibroblasts could be selectively targeted in their pancreatic tumors; the result of depleting these myofibroblast cells (presumably derived from PSCs) was the development of pancreatic cancers that not only showed significant remodeling of the extracellular matrix but also were highly undifferentiated and hypovascular. In total, these tumors behaved in a biologically more aggressive fashion and resulted in significant reduction in animal survival. (Similar findings were also observed in an analysis of resected human pancreatic cancer specimens, in which lower numbers of myofibroblasts correlated with worse survival.) Notably, these myofibroblast-depleted tumors exhibited a decrease in T-effector cells and an increase in suppressive T regulatory cells, associated with increased CTLA-4 expression. Administration of an anti-CTLA-4 antibody in this setting resulted in a rescue of the phenotype of myofibroblast-depleted tumors, with a reduction in undifferentiated cancer cells, and attenuated PDAC progression, which was associated with a significant extension in overall survival in these mice [32]. This observation suggests a possible clinical strategy that could be explored in which immunotherapy is combined with stromal-depleting agents.

Another distinct fibroblast subtype, the carcinoma-associated fibroblast (CAF) (identified by expression of the membrane protein fibroblast activation protein-α (FAP)), also appears to play a unique immunosuppressive role in pancreatic tumor biology [33]. Depleting these cells in mouse models of pancreatic cancer, which has been shown to sensitize tumors to immunotherapy, may represent an additional therapeutic approach that can potentially be tested in clinic in the future.

Immune Cells: Key Constituents of the Microenvironment

Studies of well-established genetically engineered mouse models, including the KPC mouse, have shown that from the very earliest stages of pancreatic cancer development, there is a rich and progressive infiltration of leukocytes [34]. This leukocyte infiltrate is dominated by immunosuppressive cells, such as tumor-associated macrophages (TAMs), myeloid-derived suppressor cells (MDSCs), and regulatory T cells (Tregs). Tregs, characterized by a CD4+ CD25+ FoxP3+ phenotype, are primary mediators of immune evasion in cancer [35], most notably by suppression of conventional T-helper cells, and have been shown in some studies to correlate with poorer prognosis in patients with pancreatic cancer [36]. MDSCs, which are elevated in both the circulation and the TME of patients with pancreatic cancer, also represent key players in suppressing host immunity via inhibition of T cell activation and migration, as well as promoting expansion of the population of Treg cells [35, 37]. TAMs, meanwhile, play a myriad of roles, including contributing to tumor angiogenesis, growth, and stromal remodeling [35, 38, 39]. Other immune cell types, including neutrophils and mast cells, can also be found in variable concentrations within the TME.

Conversely, there generally appears to be a striking paucity of activated cytotoxic (effector) CD8+ T cells or NK cells to counter this dense immunosuppressive infiltrate [40–42]. This imbalance between anti- and pro-inflammatory cell types in the TME of pancreatic cancer reflects its uniquely immunosuppressive milieu and why this malignancy is commonly referred to as non-immunogenic [42]. Efforts are ongoing both to more precisely characterize the immune cell composition in human pancreatic tumor specimens and especially to develop novel therapeutic strategies to prime the host immune system and induce a more robust cytotoxic T cell response against pancreatic cancer.

Given the remarkable transformative impact that immunotherapy has had in other solid tumor types, notably melanoma, lung cancer, genitourinary malignancies, and head and neck tumors, it is not surprising that there have been and continue to be intensive clinical efforts trying to exploit and unleash the host immune system to similar effect in pancreatic cancer, albeit with limited efficacy to date. These strategies include, but are not limited to, genetically modified cellular and attenuated live bacterial-based vaccines, immune checkpoint inhibitors (antibodies against PD-1, PD-L1, CTLA-4, IDO inhibitors, and others), and various other agents designed to inhibit any specific one or more of the immunosuppressive cell types noted above. While Chap. 15 of this book provides a more in-depth look at these different immunotherapeutic strategies in pancreatic cancer, this section offers one representative example to illustrate how our understanding of one specific immune cell type, the *tumor-associated macrophage (TAM)*, has informed a diverse array of approaches in which these particular cells are being targeted.

Targeting TAMs. Of the many elements comprising the pancreatic cancer TME that contribute to immunosuppression, the predominance and negative prognostic value of TAMs (particularly M2-polarized, or anti-inflammatory, TAMs) [43–45] have made these cells a particularly intriguing candidate for therapeutic targeting. TAMs are derived from inflammatory monocytes which are recruited from the bone marrow, extravasate into tumor tissues, and differentiate into macrophages that inhibit T cell response. In addition to playing a leading role in creating this immunosuppressive milieu within the TME, TAMs also have versatile functions in promoting cancer cell proliferation, stimulating tumor angiogenesis and extracellular matrix breakdown, and enhancing tumor invasion and metastasis [46].

Sanford and colleagues reported that inflammatory monocytes were increased in the peripheral blood of patients with pancreatic cancer compared with healthy controls and that increased levels correlated inversely with survival in patients following pancreatic cancer surgery [47]. Moreover, these same investigators determined that mobilization of these cells from the bone marrow into the circulation, as well as recruitment of these cells to sites of inflammation where they develop into (tumor-associated) macrophages, is dependent on the chemokine CCL2 and its receptor CCR2. The potential therapeutic implications of this finding were realized by treating tumor-bearing wild-type mice with a CCR2 antagonist (PF-04136309), in whom a marked decrease in TAMs was found with a corresponding increase in effector T cells, suggesting enhanced antitumor adaptive immunity. Importantly, these treated mice showed a significant reduction in tumor growth as well as a significant decrease in liver metastases compared to vehicle-treated mice. Furthermore, combination of the CCR2 antagonist with gemcitabine proved to be additive in inhibiting tumor growth and dramatically reducing rates of liver metastases [47].

Based on these encouraging preclinical data, an open-label, dose-finding, non-randomized phase Ib study was conducted in treatment-naive patients with borderline resectable or locally advanced pancreatic adenocarcinoma who were treated with six cycles of either FOLFIRINOX ($n = 8$) or FOLFIRINOX plus PF-04136309 ($n = 39$) [48]. Forty-nine percent of patients receiving the CCR2 inhibitor achieved an objective tumor response, and the combination therapy did not confer significantly added toxicity when compared to chemotherapy alone. Importantly, the authors confirmed the on-target effects of the experimental agent, with (1) a significant decline in peripheral CCR2-positive monocytes when compared to baseline, (2) a reduction in levels of TAMs in tumor biopsy specimen posttreatment and (3) a rise in intratumoral CD8- and CD4-positive T cells with a relative decline in regulatory T cells in posttreatment compared to baseline samples. These findings suggested a reversal of immunosuppression and restored antitumor immunity. Based on these promising results, successor studies are in development or currently underway evaluating this strategy for different stages of pancreatic cancer and/or in combination with other chemotherapy regimens (NCT02732938).

An alternative strategy for targeting TAMs entails "reprogramming" these cells for antitumor activity. CD40 agonists may represent one such approach [49, 50]. CD40, a member of the tumor necrosis factor receptor (TNFR) superfamily, plays an important role in induction of tumor apoptosis and regulation of immune activation, especially in cross talk between T cells and antigen-presenting cells [51–55]. However, in the context of pancreatic adenocarcinoma, Beatty and colleagues found that CD40 agonists mediate their antitumor activity independent of T cells, but rather by activating macrophages to infiltrate tumors, become tumoricidal, and facilitate the depletion of stroma [49]. Specifically, these investigators observed that treatment of genetically engineered KPC mice with the CD40 agonist antibody FGK45 could induce tumor regressions with associated stromal degradation and that this drug effect was lost when the mice were depleted of macrophages (but not CD4- or CD8-positive T cells).

The clinical impact of CD40 activation has been explored in a phase I clinical trial of the agonist CD40 antibody (CP-870,893) in combination with gemcitabine for treatment-naive patients with advanced pancreatic cancer [50]. The overall objective response rate (ORR) in this small (21 patients) study was 19%, with a median progression-free survival (PFS) of 5.2 months and median overall survival (OS) of 8.4 months. The most common adverse event observed was grade 1–2 cytokine release syndrome, reflecting systemic immune activation, and a rapid (albeit transient) decrease in peripheral monocyte levels following CP-870,893 infusion. While on-treatment biopsies were not mandated for this study, serial FDG-PET/CT scans were performed, with somewhat heterogeneous metabolic responses noted. Other trials either ongoing (NCT02588443) or in development are seeking to further elucidate the activity of CD40 agonists in pancreatic cancer, not only to assess their clinical activity but also to look for the pharmacodynamic and immunologic effects of this class of agents.

A third and final example in this category of TAM-targeting agents involves blockade of colony-stimulating factor-1 (CSF-1) and/or its receptor (CSF-1R), a signaling axis involved in the infiltration and activation of macrophages within tumors. A number of preclinical studies in different tumor models have shown that inhibition of CSF-1/CSF-1R signaling can block tumor progression and metastasis [56–60]. Mitchem et al. specifically studied this approach in orthotopic pancreatic cancer models and found that inhibitors of CSF-1R depleted mature TAMs, resulting in improved efficacy of chemotherapy, fewer metastases, and increased antitumor T cell immunity [58]. Zhu and colleagues showed that CSF-1R blockade upregulates T cell checkpoints such as PD-L1 and CTLA-4, and combining CSF-1R and immune checkpoint inhibitors could potently elicit tumor regressions in preclinical models [61], offering a promising therapeutic strategy to explore in the clinical arena.

The therapeutic agents targeting CSF-1/CSF-1R that are furthest along in clinical development include PLX3397, a selective CSF-1R inhibitor, and emactuzumab, an anti-CSF-1R monoclonal antibody. These agents have shown particularly promising clinical activity in a rare tumor type, tenosynovial giant-cell tumor, that is characterized by overexpression of CSF-1 which binds to and recruits CSF-1R-expressing cells of the mononuclear phagocyte lineage [62, 63]. Specific to pancreatic cancer, there currently are numerous active clinical trials testing CSF-1/CSF-1R blockade in a variety of different capacities (NCT02777710, NCT02452424, NCT02718911, NCT01316822, NCT01346358, NCT02526017, NCT02829723).

Blood Vessels and the TME

Pancreatic adenocarcinoma in general is a hypovascular, poorly perfused tumor, with fewer large-diameter vessels compared to adjacent normal human pancreas [30, 64, 65]. This is due in large part to the dense desmoplastic stroma associated with pancreatic tumors that compresses and distorts blood vessels [64, 66]. As will be discussed in subsequent sections in this chapter, various stromal-depleting strategies, such as recombinant hyaluronidase and inhibitors of Hedgehog signaling, have been shown, at least in preclinical models, to increase tumor vascular density and patency, resulting in improved drug delivery [64, 67].

The hypovascular nature of pancreatic cancer raises important questions regarding the extent to which angiogenesis is important and plays a role in this malignancy. Multiple groups have reported on the frequency of overexpression of the proangiogenic molecule VEGF-A (vascular endothelial growth factor-A) in human pancreatic cancer, with some but not all reports finding a correlation between VEGF-A levels and poorer clinical outcomes in patients, including shorter survival [65, 68–70]. Experiments in subcutaneous or orthotopic nude mouse models of human pancreatic cancer in which VEGF signaling was targeted (e.g., via antisense RNA, a diphtheria toxin–VEGF fusion protein, or an adenoviral vector encoding the soluble form of the decoy receptor VEGFR-1) have demonstrated evidence of reduced tumor growth [71–73], lending some rationale to studying antiangiogenic strategies in pancreatic cancer clinical trials.

To date, however, clinical trials focused on blocking VEGF signaling in pancreatic cancer have been disappointing, with no survival benefit observed in two large phase III clinical trials with the addition of the anti-VEGF antibody bevacizumab to standard therapy (gemcitabine or gemcitabine plus erlotinib) in the first-line metastatic setting [74, 75]. Small-molecule inhibitors of VEGFR, such as axitinib and sunitinib, have likewise not demonstrated any benefit when tested in either the first- or second-line settings in this disease [76, 77]. An alternative strategy directly targeting existing tumor vasculature consists of paclitaxel embedded within a cationic liposome membrane (EndoTAG-1), which selectively binds to negatively charged tumor endothelial cells [78]. A randomized controlled phase II study suggested some improvement in clinical outcomes with the addition of this novel agent to gemcitabine in patients with advanced pancreatic cancer [78], but further testing in a larger phase III trial has not been forthcoming.

Despite these less than overwhelming results, interest remains in how best to employ antiangiogenic strategies in pancreatic cancer. This may include evaluating other angiogenic pathways beyond VEGF, as well as studying combination strategies in which antiangiogenic therapies are administered together with other stromal-depleting/remodeling agents or immunotherapies [65]. In general, mechanistic arguments could be made to justify why therapeutic approaches that either impair *or* increase tumor perfusion might be beneficial, highlighting the conundrum and ongoing uncertainty regarding targeting tumor vasculature in this disease [66].

Hedgehog Signaling: Lessons Learned in Targeting the Tumor Stroma

Hedgehog signaling represents an important developmental pathway in normal mammalian embryogenesis, including normal pancreatic formation [79, 80]. Aberrant expression of Sonic Hedgehog (SHH), the most common Hedgehog ligand, as well as its associated signaling components Patched (PTCH1, the cognate receptor for Hedgehog ligands) and Smoothened (SMO, a co-receptor), is also frequently seen in pancreatic cancer, with increasing activity as tumors progress from early precursor (PanIN) lesions to invasive adenocarcinoma [81–88]. Studies involving global sequencing analysis have identified this pathway as one of the central elements undergoing transformation in nearly all pancreatic cancers [82].

Yauch et al. used xenograft mouse models of pancreatic and colon cancer to show that ligand-dependent activation of the Hedgehog pathway occurs in the tumor microenvironment, as opposed to within the epithelium [89]. Specifically, these investigators found that while Hedgehog ligands are produced by tumor cells, the signal is then transduced in the stromal compartment of tumors, where stromal cells express the SHH receptor PTCH1. Upon ligand binding, this leads to activation of SMO and subsequent downstream activation of the GLI family of transcription factors, which represent useful expression markers of Hedgehog signaling activity [90]. Administration of a Hedgehog pathway antagonist in these mice resulted in inhibition of tumor growth via downregulation of Hedgehog target genes in the stromal microenvironment, but not within the tumor epithelium. In sum, these findings suggested a paracrine requirement for Hedgehog signaling (between tumor and stroma) in the tumorigenesis of Hedgehog-expressing malignancies.

Subsequent studies specific to pancreatic cancer confirmed this paracrine model of Hedgehog-mediated tumorigenesis. Tian and colleagues expressed an oncogenic allele of SMO in mouse pancreas that activated Hedgehog signaling in a cell-autonomous manner, showing that the signaling is restricted principally to α-SMA-expressing spindle cells adjacent to tumor epithelium, rather than in the epithelial cells themselves [91]. These researchers then microdissected human and mouse pancreatic specimens to confirm that Hedgehog target gene expression (GLI1) was significantly higher (40- to 120-fold in human samples) in the stromal compartment compared to tumor epithelium. Bailey et al. demonstrated that Hedgehog signaling contributes to the development of the desmoplastic stroma in pancreatic tumors, in part, by promoting the differentiation and proliferation of PSCs [18]. Administration of a blocking antibody to SHH to mice with orthotopically implanted pancreatic tumors significantly decreased the degree of desmoplasia observed.

The therapeutic implications of Hedgehog inhibition were most clearly suggested by a series of experiments conducted by Olive et al., who used the KPC mouse model to highlight how the desmoplastic stroma associated with pancreatic cancer represents a poorly perfused, poorly vascularized physical barrier that impairs effective drug delivery to the tumor [67]. Recognizing the role that Hedgehog signaling plays in promoting this desmoplasia, these investigators studied the effects of IPI-926, a semisynthetic derivative of cyclopamine that blocks Hedgehog signaling by potently inhibiting Smoothened (SMO), on these mice. When given alone or in combination with gemcitabine, IPI-926 was shown to deplete the desmoplastic stroma and increase intratumoral vascularity. Mice treated with the combination showed increased intratumoral concentration of gemcitabine metabolites, indicating improved drug delivery. An intervention–survival study on these mice, which included monitoring of tumor volumes, showed that mice treated with the gemcitabine/IPI-926 exhibited more frequent tumor shrinkage (albeit transient), had fewer metastases to the liver, and had prolonged survival, when compared to vehicle-treated controls, whereas no significant differences were observed with gemcitabine or IPI-926 alone.

Based on these preclinical findings with promising mechanistic rationale, several clinical trials were initiated evaluating IPI-926 and other Hedgehog signaling inhibitors in combination with chemotherapy in advanced pancreatic cancer. However, surprising results were reported from the largest of these studies, a randomized phase II trial of gemcitabine plus either IPI-926 or placebo as first-line treatment of metastatic pancreatic cancer. Specifically, this study found that patients receiving IPI-926 had *higher* rates of progressive disease and correspondingly *shorter* overall survival, when compared to the control group [92]. Another randomized phase II study evaluating a different SMO inhibitor (vismodegib) in combination with gemcitabine as first-line therapy in patients with metastatic pancreatic cancer showed no detrimental effect, but no significant improvement in overall survival, compared to gemcitabine plus placebo [93]. Other smaller single-arm studies reported somewhat more promising efficacy results with this general strategy [94, 95] but overall were too small to interpret.

Following the disappointing results from these clinical trials, several preclinical studies were published in succession that helped shed some light on why manipulation of the tumor stroma, via Hedgehog inhibition or other means, could potentially produce detrimental effects. Rhim et al. developed KPC mice in which SHH was conditionally deleted and found that while the SHH-deleted tumors had significantly reduced stromal content, as predicted, these tumors were also more aggressive and exhibited an undifferentiated phenotype, increased vascularity, and heightened proliferation [96]. They further showed that *long-term* administration of IPI-926 (as opposed to the short course of treatment of this drug in the experiments by Olive et al.) mimicked SHH deletion, with tumors that were more highly proliferative, vascular, and poorly differentiated than those arising in control mice treated with vehicle or gemcitabine alone. These findings suggested that the short-term, beneficial effects of increased drug delivery conferred by Hedgehog inhibition may eventually be overcome by the deleterious effects of long-term inhibition of this pathway. In addition to inducing dramatic changes in tumor histology and biology, loss of SHH also produced tumors that were more sensitive to VEGF inhibition, suggesting a genetic subset of pancreatic cancers in whom antiangiogenic strategies may be appropriate to revisit.

Similar results were reported by Lee et al. in a series of experiments performed on three separate genetically engineered mouse models of pancreatic cancer, in which either genetic or pharmacologic reduction of Hedgehog signaling decreased survival and accelerated tumor progression [97]. Conversely, administration of an oral small molecule (SAG21k) that activates Hedgehog signaling mediated hyperplasia of stromal cells (particularly those with a myofibroblast-like phenotype, likely PSCs) and expression of collagen I, as well as decreased proliferation and progenitor-like character in the epithelial compartment. Intriguingly, these authors suggest that on the basis of these results, there may be a role for Hedgehog pathway *activation* in clinical trials of pancreatic cancer, although certainly this would have to be balanced against the increased desmoplasia that would result—again, highlighting the need to understand both the pros and cons of therapeutically targeting tumor stroma.

Directly Targeting the Extracellular Matrix

The extracellular matrix (ECM) of pancreatic cancer is composed predominantly of collagen and a complex mixture of proteoglycans and glycosaminoglycans. Of these, one glycosaminoglycan of particular interest in pancreatic cancer is hyaluronic acid (HA), a negatively charged polymer consisting of disaccharide repeats (alternating *N*-acetylglucosamine and glucuronic acid units) that represents a major component of the ECM [64]. In addition to regulating multiple biological processes via signaling through receptors CD44 and RHAMM (receptor for HA-mediated motility), including angiogenesis, epithelial–mesenchymal transition, proliferation, and migration [98, 99], HA also contributes to the viscoelasticity of the ECM via sequestering mobile cations and solvating water [99]. High levels of HA in the ECM lead to elevated interstitial fluid pressure, which in turn compresses tumor vasculature and hampers the ability of small-molecule cytotoxic therapies to reach tumor cells [67, 100–102]. Expression of HA has been associated with lower overall survival rates in a number of malignancies, including pancreatic cancer [103].

Enzymes that degrade hyaluronidases exist naturally [104] and can be isolated and modified for use as cancer therapeutics. The one furthest along in clinical development is PEGPH20, a recombinant form of human hyaluronidase that has been pegylated to prolong its half-life in circulation to over 20 h. PEGPH20 has been tested in xenograft models of pancreatic cancer where it has been shown to inhibit tumor growth [105, 106]. Provenzano et al. further tested PEGPH20 treatment in the KPC mouse model, in which pancreatic tumors develop that faithfully recapitulate the high intratumoral hyaluronic acid content of human pancreatic cancer [64]. In this model, administration of PEGPH20 plus gemcitabine resulted in dramatically lower intratumoral interstitial fluid pressure, increased patent vasculature, and consequently improved tumor drug delivery. Mice treated with the combination of PEGPH20 plus gemcitabine showed prolonged survival compared to gemcitabine alone [64]. Jacobetz et al. independently reported similar results with the combinations of PEGPH20 plus intraperitoneal gemcitabine and with PEGPH20 plus intravenous doxorubicin [99].

The mechanistic rationale and provocative preclinical findings have prompted PEGPH20 to be studied in the clinical arena as a potential cancer therapeutic agent. A phase Ib study examined the combination of PEGPH20 at escalating doses in combination with standard gemcitabine in 28 patients with advanced pancreatic cancer [107]. The most common PEGPH20-related adverse events were musculoskeletal and extremity pain, peripheral edema, and fatigue, although none of these adverse events were serious or necessitated PEGPH20 discontinuation. Thromboembolic events were also observed in 29% of patients. Median progression-free survival (PFS) and overall survival (OS) rates were 5.0 and 6.6 months, respectively. Notably, in the subset of patients whose tumors showed high levels of HA expression, median PFS and OS were 7.2 and 13.0 months ($n = 6$), compared to 3.5 and 5.7 months for patients with HA-low tumors ($n = 11$).

Subsequently, a randomized phase II trial was undertaken looking at the combination of gemcitabine and nab-paclitaxel with or without PEGPH20 in patients with previously untreated metastatic pancreatic cancer. Importantly, for this study, a companion diagnostic assay was developed to be able to determine HA expression within tumors as a potential predictive biomarker for this treatment approach. Final analysis of stage 1 data from this study was presented at the American Society of Clinical Oncology (ASCO) Annual Meeting in 2016, at which point a total of 135 patients had been treated [108]. In the subset of patients with HA-high tumors (comprising approximately a third of study subjects), the addition of PEGPH20 to chemotherapy led to a clinically meaningful improvement in median progression-free survival compared to chemotherapy alone (9.2 vs 6.3 months, respectively; HR 0.48), whereas this difference was less striking in patients with HA-low tumors (median PFS 5.3 vs 4.3 months; HR 0.69). Response rate was also higher in the PEGPH20-containing treatment arm compared to the control arm in patients with HA-high tumors (55% vs 33%). Of note, due to high rates of thromboembolic events observed early on the study, the trial was amended to mandate enoxaparin (LMWH) prophylaxis for patients on both treatment arms, which appeared to mitigate this risk.

Given the promising efficacy results of this trial, with incorporation of a potentially useful biomarker, a global phase III randomized controlled trial of similar design as the phase II (gemcitabine/nab-paclitaxel with or without PEGPH20) was initiated in 2016 (NCT02715804). However, this study is limited exclusively to patients with HA-high tumors to try and enrich for the subgroup of pancreatic cancers most likely to benefit from this stromal-targeting strategy.

Aside from HA, other efforts to target the extracellular matrix have involved inhibiting growth factors that stimulate extracellular matrix (ECM) formation. Connective tissue growth factor (CTGF), for example, is a glycoprotein overexpressed in human pancreatic adenocarcinomas and some pancreatic cancer cell lines [109] that plays multiple roles in tumor biology, including modulating deposition of ECM and angiogenesis [110]. Several investigators have shown that administration of FG-3019, a neutralizing CTGF-specific monoclonal antibody, confers antitumor activity in pancreatic cancer both *in vitro* and *in vivo* [109, 110], although unlike other stromal-targeting agents, it does not appear to enhance delivery of concurrently administered chemotherapy agents like gemcitabine [111]. On the basis of this preclinical work, this "antifibrotic" agent has been and is being tested in pancreatic cancer clinical trials in combination with standard chemotherapy in the metastatic and locally advanced settings [112, 113].

CTGF itself is a downstream modulator of TGF-β, a key signal transduction molecule which, as noted earlier in this chapter, is involved in the activation of PSCs that leads to desmoplasia. Due to both the tumor-suppressing and tumor-promoting effects of TGF-β signaling, blocking this pathway has been met with some trepidation in the past. Whatcott and colleagues assessed the effects of LY2157299, a TGF-βR1 inhibitor, in combination with gemcitabine on KPC mice, and found a marked reduction in overall stromal content, including collagen I deposition [98]. This same agent has since been evaluated in a randomized, double-blind phase II trial in combination with chemotherapy in patients with advanced pancreatic cancer. As reported at the 2016 ASCO Annual Meeting, addition of LY2157299 (also known as galunisertib) to gemcitabine conferred modest improvements in overall and progression-free survival compared to gemcitabine plus placebo (median OS 9.1 vs 7.6 months [HR 0.89]; median PFS 3.6 vs 2.8 months [HR 0.80], respectively), with greater benefit observed in patients with lower baseline TGF-β1 levels [114]. An alternative strategy that has been explored in pancreatic cancer is an antisense oligonucleotide targeting TGF-β2 called trabedersen, which showed antitumor activity in pancreatic cancer cell culture and in orthotopic mouse model [115]. This agent was subsequently evaluated in a phase I/II trial in which one long-term responder with metastatic pancreatic cancer was reported [116], but further clinical development has not been reported.

Do Chemotherapy Agents Remodel the TME?

In addition to the investigational therapeutic approaches described elsewhere in this chapter, there is also preclinical and clinical evidence that one of the standard chemotherapeutic agents approved for use in pancreatic cancer, albumin-bound paclitaxel (nab-paclitaxel), exerts some effects on the TME. In the original phase I/II report of gemcitabine plus nab-paclitaxel that led to the pivotal phase III MPACT trial, von Hoff et al. performed parallel experiments using patient-derived xenograft models of pancreatic cancer to demonstrate that exposure to nab-paclitaxel depleted the desmoplastic stroma [117]. The reduction in tumor stroma and the accompanying increase in vascularization facilitated the delivery of gemcitabine and consequently increased intratumoral levels of gemcitabine. Furthermore, the authors hypothesized that a key albumin-binding protein called SPARC (secreted protein acidic and rich in cysteine) expressed by stromal fibroblasts may represent an important mediator facilitating the uptake of nab-paclitaxel in the TME that contributes to stromal depletion. Indeed, early clinical data suggested that stromal expression of SPARC may serve as a useful predictor of sensitivity to treatment with nab-paclitaxel [117], in addition to representing a poor prognostic factor overall [118]. However, subsequent analysis performed on archival tumor specimens as well as plasma samples from the MPACT trial failed to corroborate any predictive utility for SPARC in patients receiving either gemcitabine plus nab-paclitaxel or gemcitabine alone [119].

In a separate small but intriguing study, Alvarez et al. reported that patients with resectable or borderline resectable pancreatic cancer who received two cycles of gemcitabine plus nab-paclitaxel prior to surgical resection showed decreased tumor stiffness (as measured by endoscopic ultrasound elastography) [120]. Histological evaluation of these patients' surgical specimens revealed tumors with a less abundant and less organized network of type I collagen fibers compared to a denser, well-organized collagen fiber network seen in the samples from patients who were either untreated or received conventional (non-nab-paclitaxel-containing) chemoradiation.

Furthermore, patients treated with nab-paclitaxel plus gemcitabine had fewer cancer-associated fibroblasts (CAFs) in their tumor specimens. Parallel experiments performed on genetically engineered mice suggested that these stromal altering effects were likely attributable to the nab-paclitaxel rather than the gemcitabine [120].

Conclusion

Pancreatic cancer retains its title as one of the most aggressive and lethal of all malignancies, characterized by aggressive biology, an early propensity to metastasize, chemoresistance, and poor immunogenicity. The uniquely complex tumor microenvironment associated with this disease helps explain many of these adverse features. Both laboratory and clinical exploration has deepened our understanding of the role that the varied cellular and acellular components of the TME play and how we may be able to therapeutically exploit each of them to improve the outlook for patients diagnosed with pancreatic cancer. Clinical trials of novel therapies designed to target elements of the TME have met with mixed success to date, and history teaches us that we must proceed with caution when manipulating the stromal compartment. Nonetheless, it is likely that such approaches will find their place alongside, or in combination with, cytotoxic therapies, immunotherapies, and other molecularly targeted strategies in changing the paradigm in how we treat this challenging disease in the future.

References

1. Mantoni TS, Lunardi S, Al-Assar O, Masamune A, Brunner TB. Pancreatic stellate cells radioprotect pancreatic cancer cells through beta1-integrin signaling. Cancer Res. 2011;71(10):3453–8.
2. Iacobuzio-Donahue CA, Ryu B, Hruban RH, Kern SE. Exploring the host desmoplastic response to pancreatic carcinoma: gene expression of stromal and neoplastic cells at the site of primary invasion. Am J Pathol. 2002;160(1):91–9.
3. Sugimoto H, Mundel TM, Kieran MW, Kalluri R. Identification of fibroblast heterogeneity in the tumor microenvironment. Cancer Biol Ther. 2006;5(12):1640–6.
4. Direkze NC, Hodivala-Dilke K, Jeffery R, Hunt T, Poulsom R, Oukrif D, et al. Bone marrow contribution to tumor-associated myofibroblasts and fibroblasts. Cancer Res. 2004;64(23):8492–5.
5. Ishii G, Sangai T, Oda T, Aoyagi Y, Hasebe T, Kanomata N, et al. Bone-marrow-derived myofibroblasts contribute to the cancer-induced stromal reaction. Biochem Biophys Res Commun. 2003;309(1):232–40.
6. Watanabe T, Masamune A, Kikuta K, Hirota M, Kume K, Satoh K, et al. Bone marrow contributes to the population of pancreatic stellate cells in mice. Am J Physiol Gastrointest Liver Physiol. 2009;297(6):G1138–46.
7. Scarlett CJ, Colvin EK, Pinese M, Chang DK, Morey AL, Musgrove EA, et al. Recruitment and activation of pancreatic stellate cells from the bone marrow in pancreatic cancer: a model of tumor-host interaction. PLoS One. 2011;6(10):e26088.

8. Blomhoff R, Wake K. Perisinusoidal stellate cells of the liver: important roles in retinol metabolism and fibrosis. FASEB J. 1991;5(3):271–7.
9. Apte MV, Haber PS, Applegate TL, Norton ID, McCaughan GW, Korsten MA, et al. Periacinar stellate shaped cells in rat pancreas: identification, isolation, and culture. Gut. 1998;43(1):128–33.
10. Erkan M, Adler G, Apte MV, Bachem MG, Buchholz M, Detlefsen S, et al. StellaTUM: current consensus and discussion on pancreatic stellate cell research. Gut. 2012;61(2):172–8.
11. Apte MV, Park S, Phillips PA, Santucci N, Goldstein D, Kumar RK, et al. Desmoplastic reaction in pancreatic cancer: role of pancreatic stellate cells. Pancreas. 2004;29(3):179–87.
12. Apte MV, Haber PS, Darby SJ, Rodgers SC, McCaughan GW, Korsten MA, et al. Pancreatic stellate cells are activated by proinflammatory cytokines: implications for pancreatic fibrogenesis. Gut. 1999;44(4):534–41.
13. Haber PS, Keogh GW, Apte MV, Moran CS, Stewart NL, Crawford DH, et al. Activation of pancreatic stellate cells in human and experimental pancreatic fibrosis. Am J Pathol. 1999;155(4):1087–95.
14. Omary MB, Lugea A, Lowe AW, Pandol SJ. The pancreatic stellate cell: a star on the rise in pancreatic diseases. J Clin Invest. 2007;117(1):50–9.
15. Bachem MG, Schunemann M, Ramadani M, Siech M, Beger H, Buck A, et al. Pancreatic carcinoma cells induce fibrosis by stimulating proliferation and matrix synthesis of stellate cells. Gastroenterology. 2005;128(4):907–21.
16. Lohr M, Schmidt C, Ringel J, Kluth M, Muller P, Nizze H, et al. Transforming growth factor-beta1 induces desmoplasia in an experimental model of human pancreatic carcinoma. Cancer Res. 2001;61(2):550–5.
17. Duner S, Lopatko Lindman J, Ansari D, Gundewar C, Andersson R. Pancreatic cancer: the role of pancreatic stellate cells in tumor progression. Pancreatology. 2010;10(6):673–81.
18. Bailey JM, Swanson BJ, Hamada T, Eggers JP, Singh PK, Caffery T, et al. Sonic hedgehog promotes desmoplasia in pancreatic cancer. Clin Cancer Res. 2008;14(19):5995–6004.
19. Erkan M, Michalski CW, Rieder S, Reiser-Erkan C, Abiatari I, Kolb A, et al. The activated stroma index is a novel and independent prognostic marker in pancreatic ductal adenocarcinoma. Clin Gastroenterol Hepatol. 2008;6(10):1155–61.
20. Fujita H, Ohuchida K, Mizumoto K, Nakata K, Yu J, Kayashima T, et al. Alpha-smooth muscle actin expressing stroma promotes an aggressive tumor biology in pancreatic ductal adenocarcinoma. Pancreas. 2010;39(8):1254–62.
21. Hwang RF, Moore T, Arumugam T, Ramachandran V, Amos KD, Rivera A, et al. Cancer-associated stromal fibroblasts promote pancreatic tumor progression. Cancer Res. 2008;68(3):918–26.
22. Vonlaufen A, Joshi S, Qu C, Phillips PA, Xu Z, Parker NR, et al. Pancreatic stellate cells: partners in crime with pancreatic cancer cells. Cancer Res. 2008;68(7):2085–93.
23. Xu Z, Vonlaufen A, Phillips PA, Fiala-Beer E, Zhang X, Yang L, et al. Role of pancreatic stellate cells in pancreatic cancer metastasis. Am J Pathol. 2010;177(5):2585–96.
24. Masamune A, Kikuta K, Watanabe T, Satoh K, Hirota M, Shimosegawa T. Hypoxia stimulates pancreatic stellate cells to induce fibrosis and angiogenesis in pancreatic cancer. Am J Physiol Gastrointest Liver Physiol. 2008;295(4):G709–17.
25. Erkan M, Kleeff J, Gorbachevski A, Reiser C, Mitkus T, Esposito I, et al. Periostin creates a tumor-supportive microenvironment in the pancreas by sustaining fibrogenic stellate cell activity. Gastroenterology. 2007;132(4):1447–64.
26. Lunardi S, Muschel RJ, Brunner TB. The stromal compartments in pancreatic cancer: are there any therapeutic targets? Cancer Lett. 2014;343(2):147–55.
27. Hingorani SR, Petricoin EF, Maitra A, Rajapakse V, King C, Jacobetz MA, et al. Preinvasive and invasive ductal pancreatic cancer and its early detection in the mouse. Cancer Cell. 2003;4(6):437–50.
28. Mace TA, Ameen Z, Collins A, Wojcik S, Mair M, Young GS, et al. Pancreatic cancer-associated stellate cells promote differentiation of myeloid-derived suppressor cells in a STAT3-dependent manner. Cancer Res. 2013;73(10):3007–18.

29. Lonardo E, Frias-Aldeguer J, Hermann PC, Heeschen C. Pancreatic stellate cells form a niche for cancer stem cells and promote their self-renewal and invasiveness. Cell Cycle. 2012;11(7):1282–90.
30. Sherman MH, Yu RT, Engle DD, Ding N, Atkins AR, Tiriac H, et al. Vitamin D receptor-mediated stromal reprogramming suppresses pancreatitis and enhances pancreatic cancer therapy. Cell. 2014;159(1):80–93.
31. Froeling FE, Feig C, Chelala C, Dobson R, Mein CE, Tuveson DA, et al. Retinoic acid-induced pancreatic stellate cell quiescence reduces paracrine Wnt-beta-catenin signaling to slow tumor progression. Gastroenterology. 2011;141(4):1486–97. 1497 e1-14
32. Ozdemir BC, Pentcheva-Hoang T, Carstens JL, Zheng X, Wu CC, Simpson TR, et al. Depletion of carcinoma-associated fibroblasts and fibrosis induces immunosuppression and accelerates pancreas cancer with reduced survival. Cancer Cell. 2014;25(6):719–34.
33. Kraman M, Bambrough PJ, Arnold JN, Roberts EW, Magiera L, Jones JO, et al. Suppression of antitumor immunity by stromal cells expressing fibroblast activation protein-alpha. Science (New York, NY). 2010;330(6005):827–30.
34. Clark CE, Beatty GL, Vonderheide RH. Immunosurveillance of pancreatic adenocarcinoma: insights from genetically engineered mouse models of cancer. Cancer Lett. 2009;279(1):1–7.
35. Evans A, Costello E. The role of inflammatory cells in fostering pancreatic cancer cell growth and invasion. Front Physiol. 2012;3:270.
36. Hiraoka N, Onozato K, Kosuge T, Hirohashi S. Prevalence of FOXP3+ regulatory T cells increases during the progression of pancreatic ductal adenocarcinoma and its premalignant lesions. Clin Cancer Res. 2006;12(18):5423–34.
37. Gabitass RF, Annels NE, Stocken DD, Pandha HA, Middleton GW. Elevated myeloid-derived suppressor cells in pancreatic, esophageal and gastric cancer are an independent prognostic factor and are associated with significant elevation of the Th2 cytokine interleukin-13. Cancer Immunol Immunother. 2011;60(10):1419–30.
38. Ostrand-Rosenberg S, Sinha P, Beury DW, Clements VK. Cross-talk between myeloid-derived suppressor cells (MDSC), macrophages, and dendritic cells enhances tumor-induced immune suppression. Semin Cancer Biol. 2012;22(4):275–81.
39. Ruffell B, Affara NI, Coussens LM. Differential macrophage programming in the tumor microenvironment. Trends Immunol. 2012;33(3):119–26.
40. Clark CE, Hingorani SR, Mick R, Combs C, Tuveson DA, Vonderheide RH. Dynamics of the immune reaction to pancreatic cancer from inception to invasion. Cancer Res. 2007;67(19):9518–27.
41. von Bernstorff W, Voss M, Freichel S, Schmid A, Vogel I, Johnk C, et al. Systemic and local immunosuppression in pancreatic cancer patients. Clin Cancer Res. 2001;7(3 Suppl):925s–32s.
42. Lutz ER, Wu AA, Bigelow E, Sharma R, Mo G, Soares K, et al. Immunotherapy converts nonimmunogenic pancreatic tumors into immunogenic foci of immune regulation. Cancer Immunol Res. 2014;2(7):616–31.
43. Chen SJ, Zhang QB, Zeng LJ, Lian GD, Li JJ, Qian CC, et al. Distribution and clinical significance of tumour-associated macrophages in pancreatic ductal adenocarcinoma: a retrospective analysis in China. Curr Oncol. 2015;22(1):e11–9.
44. Cui R, Yue W, Lattime EC, Stein MN, Xu Q, Tan XL. Targeting tumor-associated macrophages to combat pancreatic cancer. Oncotarget. 2016;7(31):50735–54.
45. Kurahara H, Shinchi H, Mataki Y, Maemura K, Noma H, Kubo F, et al. Significance of M2-polarized tumor-associated macrophage in pancreatic cancer. J Surg Res. 2011;167(2):e211–9.
46. Qian BZ, Pollard JW. Macrophage diversity enhances tumor progression and metastasis. Cell. 2010;141(1):39–51.
47. Sanford DE, Belt BA, Panni RZ, Mayer A, Deshpande AD, Carpenter D, et al. Inflammatory monocyte mobilization decreases patient survival in pancreatic cancer: a role for targeting the CCL2/CCR2 axis. Clin Cancer Res. 2013;19(13):3404–15.

48. Nywening TM, Wang-Gillam A, Sanford DE, Belt BA, Panni RZ, Cusworth BM, et al. Targeting tumour-associated macrophages with CCR2 inhibition in combination with FOLFIRINOX in patients with borderline resectable and locally advanced pancreatic cancer: a single-centre, open-label, dose-finding, non-randomised, phase 1b trial. Lancet Oncol. 2016;17(5):651–62.
49. Beatty GL, Chiorean EG, Fishman MP, Saboury B, Teitelbaum UR, Sun W, et al. CD40 agonists alter tumor stroma and show efficacy against pancreatic carcinoma in mice and humans. Science (New York, NY). 2011;331(6024):1612–6.
50. Beatty GL, Torigian DA, Chiorean EG, Saboury B, Brothers A, Alavi A, et al. A phase I study of an agonist CD40 monoclonal antibody (CP-870,893) in combination with gemcitabine in patients with advanced pancreatic ductal adenocarcinoma. Clin Cancer Res. 2013;19(22):6286–95.
51. Bennett SR, Carbone FR, Karamalis F, Flavell RA, Miller JF, Heath WR. Help for cytotoxic-T-cell responses is mediated by CD40 signalling. Nature. 1998;393(6684):478–80.
52. French RR, Chan HT, Tutt AL, Glennie MJ. CD40 antibody evokes a cytotoxic T-cell response that eradicates lymphoma and bypasses T-cell help. Nat Med. 1999;5(5):548–53.
53. Ridge JP, Di Rosa F, Matzinger P. A conditioned dendritic cell can be a temporal bridge between a CD4+ T-helper and a T-killer cell. Nature. 1998;393(6684):474–8.
54. Schoenberger SP, Toes RE, van der Voort EI, Offringa R, Melief CJ. T-cell help for cytotoxic T lymphocytes is mediated by CD40-CD40L interactions. Nature. 1998;393(6684):480–3.
55. Aggarwal BB. Signalling pathways of the TNF superfamily: a double-edged sword. Nat Rev Immunol. 2003;3(9):745–56.
56. DeNardo DG, Brennan DJ, Rexhepaj E, Ruffell B, Shiao SL, Madden SF, et al. Leukocyte complexity predicts breast cancer survival and functionally regulates response to chemotherapy. Cancer Discov. 2011;1(1):54–67.
57. Lin EY, Nguyen AV, Russell RG, Pollard JW. Colony-stimulating factor 1 promotes progression of mammary tumors to malignancy. J Exp Med. 2001;193(6):727–40.
58. Mitchem JB, Brennan DJ, Knolhoff BL, Belt BA, Zhu Y, Sanford DE, et al. Targeting tumor-infiltrating macrophages decreases tumor-initiating cells, relieves immunosuppression, and improves chemotherapeutic responses. Cancer Res. 2013;73(3):1128–41.
59. Pyonteck SM, Akkari L, Schuhmacher AJ, Bowman RL, Sevenich L, Quail DF, et al. CSF-1R inhibition alters macrophage polarization and blocks glioma progression. Nat Med. 2013;19(10):1264–72.
60. Strachan DC, Ruffell B, Oei Y, Bissell MJ, Coussens LM, Pryer N, et al. CSF1R inhibition delays cervical and mammary tumor growth in murine models by attenuating the turnover of tumor-associated macrophages and enhancing infiltration by CD8+ T cells. Oncoimmunology. 2013;2(12):e26968.
61. Zhu Y, Knolhoff BL, Meyer MA, Nywening TM, West BL, Luo J, et al. CSF1/CSF1R blockade reprograms tumor-infiltrating macrophages and improves response to T-cell checkpoint immunotherapy in pancreatic cancer models. Cancer Res. 2014;74(18):5057–69.
62. Cassier PA, Italiano A, Gomez-Roca CA, Le Tourneau C, Toulmonde M, Cannarile MA, et al. CSF1R inhibition with emactuzumab in locally advanced diffuse-type tenosynovial giant cell tumours of the soft tissue: a dose-escalation and dose-expansion phase 1 study. Lancet Oncol. 2015;16(8):949–56.
63. Tap WD, Wainberg ZA, Anthony SP, Ibrahim PN, Zhang C, Healey JH, et al. Structure-guided blockade of CSF1R kinase in Tenosynovial Giant-cell tumor. N Engl J Med. 2015;373(5):428–37.
64. Provenzano PP, Cuevas C, Chang AE, Goel VK, Von Hoff DD, Hingorani SR. Enzymatic targeting of the stroma ablates physical barriers to treatment of pancreatic ductal adenocarcinoma. Cancer Cell. 2012;21(3):418–29.
65. Craven KE, Gore J, Korc M. Overview of pre-clinical and clinical studies targeting angiogenesis in pancreatic ductal adenocarcinoma. Cancer Lett. 2016;381(1):201–10.

66. Feig C, Gopinathan A, Neesse A, Chan DS, Cook N, Tuveson DA. The pancreas cancer microenvironment. Clin Cancer Res. 2012;18(16):4266–76.
67. Olive KP, Jacobetz MA, Davidson CJ, Gopinathan A, McIntyre D, Honess D, et al. Inhibition of Hedgehog signaling enhances delivery of chemotherapy in a mouse model of pancreatic cancer. Science (New York, NY). 2009;324(5933):1457–61.
68. Seo Y, Baba H, Fukuda T, Takashima M, Sugimachi K. High expression of vascular endothelial growth factor is associated with liver metastasis and a poor prognosis for patients with ductal pancreatic adenocarcinoma. Cancer. 2000;88(10):2239–45.
69. Itakura J, Ishiwata T, Friess H, Fujii H, Matsumoto Y, Buchler MW, et al. Enhanced expression of vascular endothelial growth factor in human pancreatic cancer correlates with local disease progression. Clin Cancer Res. 1997;3(8):1309–16.
70. Ellis LM, Takahashi Y, Fenoglio CJ, Cleary KR, Bucana CD, Evans DB. Vessel counts and vascular endothelial growth factor expression in pancreatic adenocarcinoma. Eur J Cancer. 1998;34(3):337–40.
71. Luo J, Guo P, Matsuda K, Truong N, Lee A, Chun C, et al. Pancreatic cancer cell-derived vascular endothelial growth factor is biologically active in vitro and enhances tumorigenicity in vivo. Int J Cancer. 2001;92(3):361–9.
72. Hotz HG, Gill PS, Masood R, Hotz B, Buhr HJ, Foitzik T, et al. Specific targeting of tumor vasculature by diphtheria toxin-vascular endothelial growth factor fusion protein reduces angiogenesis and growth of pancreatic cancer. J Gastrointest Surg. 2002;6(2):159–66. discussion 66
73. Hoshida T, Sunamura M, Duda DG, Egawa S, Miyazaki S, Shineha R, et al. Gene therapy for pancreatic cancer using an adenovirus vector encoding soluble flt-1 vascular endothelial growth factor receptor. Pancreas. 2002;25(2):111–21.
74. Kindler HL, Niedzwiecki D, Hollis D, Sutherland S, Schrag D, Hurwitz H, et al. Gemcitabine plus bevacizumab compared with gemcitabine plus placebo in patients with advanced pancreatic cancer: phase III trial of the cancer and leukemia group B (CALGB 80303). J Clin Oncol. 2010;28(22):3617–22.
75. Van Cutsem E, Vervenne WL, Bennouna J, Humblet Y, Gill S, Van Laethem JL, et al. Phase III trial of bevacizumab in combination with gemcitabine and erlotinib in patients with metastatic pancreatic cancer. J Clin Oncol. 2009;27(13):2231–7.
76. Kindler HL, Ioka T, Richel DJ, Bennouna J, Letourneau R, Okusaka T, et al. Axitinib plus gemcitabine versus placebo plus gemcitabine in patients with advanced pancreatic adenocarcinoma: a double-blind randomised phase 3 study. Lancet Oncol. 2011;12(3):256–62.
77. O'Reilly EM, Niedzwiecki D, Hall M, Hollis D, Bekaii-Saab T, Pluard T, et al. A cancer and leukemia group B phase II study of sunitinib malate in patients with previously treated metastatic pancreatic adenocarcinoma (CALGB 80603). Oncologist. 2010;15(12):1310–9.
78. Lohr JM, Haas SL, Bechstein WO, Bodoky G, Cwiertka K, Fischbach W, et al. Cationic liposomal paclitaxel plus gemcitabine or gemcitabine alone in patients with advanced pancreatic cancer: a randomized controlled phase II trial. Ann Oncol. 2012;23(5):1214–22.
79. Ingham PW, McMahon AP. Hedgehog signaling in animal development: paradigms and principles. Genes Dev. 2001;15(23):3059–87.
80. Hebrok M, Kim SK, St Jacques B, McMahon AP, Melton DA. Regulation of pancreas development by hedgehog signaling. Development (Cambridge, England). 2000;127(22):4905–13.
81. Berman DM, Karhadkar SS, Maitra A, Montes De Oca R, Gerstenblith MR, Briggs K, et al. Widespread requirement for Hedgehog ligand stimulation in growth of digestive tract tumours. Nature. 2003;425(6960):846–51.
82. Jones S, Zhang X, Parsons DW, Lin JC, Leary RJ, Angenendt P, et al. Core signaling pathways in human pancreatic cancers revealed by global genomic analyses. Science (New York, NY). 2008;321(5897):1801–6.

83. Liu MS, Yang PY, Yeh TS. Sonic hedgehog signaling pathway in pancreatic cystic neoplasms and ductal adenocarcinoma. Pancreas. 2007;34(3):340–6.
84. Morton JP, Lewis BC. Shh signaling and pancreatic cancer: implications for therapy? Cell Cycle. 2007;6(13):1553–7.
85. Morton JP, Mongeau ME, Klimstra DS, Morris JP, Lee YC, Kawaguchi Y, et al. Sonic hedgehog acts at multiple stages during pancreatic tumorigenesis. Proc Natl Acad Sci U S A. 2007;104(12):5103–8.
86. Quint K, Stintzing S, Alinger B, Hauser-Kronberger C, Dietze O, Gahr S, et al. The expression pattern of PDX-1, SHH, patched and Gli-1 is associated with pathological and clinical features in human pancreatic cancer. Pancreatology. 2009;9(1–2):116–26.
87. Steg A, Vickers SM, Eloubeidi M, Wang W, Eltoum IA, Grizzle WE, et al. Hedgehog pathway expression in heterogeneous pancreatic adenocarcinoma: implications for the molecular analysis of clinically available biopsies. Diagn Mol Pathol. 2007;16(4):229–37.
88. Thayer SP, di Magliano MP, Heiser PW, Nielsen CM, Roberts DJ, Lauwers GY, et al. Hedgehog is an early and late mediator of pancreatic cancer tumorigenesis. Nature. 2003;425(6960):851–6.
89. Yauch RL, Gould SE, Scales SJ, Tang T, Tian H, Ahn CP, et al. A paracrine requirement for hedgehog signalling in cancer. Nature. 2008;455(7211):406–10.
90. Rubin LL, de Sauvage FJ. Targeting the hedgehog pathway in cancer. Nat Rev Drug Discov. 2006;5(12):1026–33.
91. Tian H, Callahan CA, DuPree KJ, Darbonne WC, Ahn CP, Scales SJ, et al. Hedgehog signaling is restricted to the stromal compartment during pancreatic carcinogenesis. Proc Natl Acad Sci U S A. 2009;106(11):4254–9.
92. Update from Phase 2 study of saridegib plus gemcitabine in patients with metastatic pancreatic cancer. Infinity Pharmaceuticals. 2012. http://phx.corporate-ir.net/phoenix.zhtml?c=121941&p=irol-newsArticle&ID=1653550.
93. Catenacci DVT, Junttila MR, Karrison T, Bahary N, Horiba MN, Nattam SR, et al. Randomized phase Ib/II study of gemcitabine plus placebo or vismodegib, a hedgehog pathway inhibitor, in patients with metastatic pancreatic cancer. J Clin Oncol. 2015;33(36):4284–92.
94. De Jesus-Acosta A, O'Dwyer, PJ, Ramanathan, RK, Von Hoff, DD, Maitra, A, Rasheed, Z, Zheng, L, Rajeshkumar, NV, Le, DT, Hoering, A, Bolejack, V, Yabuuchi, S, Laheru, DA. A phase II study of vismodegib, a hedgehog (Hh) pathway inhibitor, combined with gemcitabine and nab-paclitaxel (nab-P) in patients (pts) with untreated metastatic pancreatic ductal adenocarcinoma (PDA). J Clin Oncol. 2014;32(suppl 3; abstr 257). 2014 Gastrointestinal Cancers Symposium.
95. Ko AH, LoConte N, Tempero MA, Walker EJ, Kate Kelley R, Lewis S, et al. A phase I study of FOLFIRINOX plus IPI-926, a hedgehog pathway inhibitor, for advanced pancreatic adenocarcinoma. Pancreas. 2016;45(3):370–5.
96. Rhim AD, Oberstein PE, Thomas DH, Mirek ET, Palermo CF, Sastra SA, et al. Stromal elements act to restrain, rather than support, pancreatic ductal adenocarcinoma. Cancer Cell. 2014;25(6):735–47.
97. Lee JJ, Perera RM, Wang H, DC W, Liu XS, Han S, et al. Stromal response to hedgehog signaling restrains pancreatic cancer progression. Proc Natl Acad Sci U S A. 2014;111(30):E3091–100.
98. Whatcott CJ, Han H, Von Hoff DD. Orchestrating the tumor microenvironment to improve survival for patients with pancreatic cancer: normalization, not destruction. Cancer J (Sudbury, Mass). 2015;21(4):299–306.
99. Jacobetz MA, Chan DS, Neesse A, Bapiro TE, Cook N, Frese KK, et al. Hyaluronan impairs vascular function and drug delivery in a mouse model of pancreatic cancer. Gut. 2013;62(1):112–20.
100. Provenzano PP, Hingorani SR. Hyaluronan, fluid pressure, and stromal resistance in pancreas cancer. Br J Cancer. 2013;108(1):1–8.

101. DuFort CC, DelGiorno KE, Carlson MA, Osgood RJ, Zhao C, Huang Z, et al. Interstitial pressure in pancreatic ductal adenocarcinoma is dominated by a gel-fluid phase. Biophys J. 2016;110(9):2106–19.
102. Singha NC, Nekoroski T, Zhao C, Symons R, Jiang P, Frost GI, et al. Tumor-associated hyaluronan limits efficacy of monoclonal antibody therapy. Mol Cancer Ther. 2015;14(2):523–32.
103. Whatcott CJ, Diep CH, Jiang P, Watanabe A, LoBello J, Sima C, et al. Desmoplasia in primary tumors and metastatic lesions of pancreatic cancer. Clin Cancer Res. 2015;21(15):3561–8.
104. McLeskey SB, Dowds C, Carballada R, White RR, Saling PM. Molecules involved in mammalian sperm-egg interaction. Int Rev Cytol. 1998;177:57–113.
105. Jiang P, Li X, Thompson CB, Huang Z, Araiza F, Osgood R, et al. Effective targeting of the tumor microenvironment for cancer therapy. Anticancer Res. 2012;32(4):1203–12.
106. Thompson CB, Shepard HM, O'Connor PM, Kadhim S, Jiang P, Osgood RJ, et al. Enzymatic depletion of tumor hyaluronan induces antitumor responses in preclinical animal models. Mol Cancer Ther. 2010;9(11):3052–64.
107. Hingorani SR, Harris WP, Beck JT, Berdov BA, Wagner SA, Pshevlotsky EM, et al. Phase Ib study of PEGylated recombinant human hyaluronidase and gemcitabine in patients with advanced pancreatic cancer. Clin Cancer Res. 2016;22(12):2848–54.
108. Bullock A, Hingorani SR, Wu XW, Jiang P, Chondros D, Khelifa S, Aldrich C, Pu J, Eugene AE. Final analysis of stage 1 data from a randomized phase II study of PEGPH20 plus nab-paclitaxel/gemcitabine in stage IV previously untreated pancreatic cancer patients (pts), utilizing Ventana companion diagnostic assay. J Clin Oncol. 2016;34(suppl; abstr 4104):2016.
109. Dornhofer N, Spong S, Bennewith K, Salim A, Klaus S, Kambham N, et al. Connective tissue growth factor-specific monoclonal antibody therapy inhibits pancreatic tumor growth and metastasis. Cancer Res. 2006;66(11):5816–27.
110. Aikawa T, Gunn J, Spong SM, Klaus SJ, Korc M. Connective tissue growth factor-specific antibody attenuates tumor growth, metastasis, and angiogenesis in an orthotopic mouse model of pancreatic cancer. Mol Cancer Ther. 2006;5(5):1108–16.
111. Neesse A, Frese KK, Bapiro TE, Nakagawa T, Sternlicht MD, Seeley TW, et al. CTGF antagonism with mAb FG-3019 enhances chemotherapy response without increasing drug delivery in murine ductal pancreas cancer. Proc Natl Acad Sci U S A. 2013;110(30):12325–30.
112. Vincent J, Picozzi V, Pipas J, Koong A, Giaccia A. FG-3019, a human monoclonal antibody to connective tissue growth factor (CTGF), with gemcitabine/erlotinib in patients with locally advanced or metastatic pancreatic ductal adenocarcinoma (abstract). J Clin Oncol. 2014;32(suppl)(5s):4138.
113. Picozzi V, Rocha F, Helton S, Mody K. Randomized, open-label trial of gemcitabine/nab-paclitaxel (G/NP) ±FG-3019 as neoadjuvant chemotherapy in locally advanced, unresectable pancreatic cancer (abstract). J Clin Oncol. 2016;34(suppl):457.
114. Melisi D, Garcia-Carbonero R, Macarulla T, Pezet DA. Phase II, double-blind study of galunisertib+gemcitabine vs gemcitabine+placebo in patients with unresectable pancreatic cancer (abstract). J Clin Oncol. 2016;34(suppl):4019.
115. Schlingensiepen KH, Jaschinski F, Lang SA, Moser C, Geissler EK, Schlitt HJ, et al. Transforming growth factor-beta 2 gene silencing with trabedersen (AP 12009) in pancreatic cancer. Cancer Sci. 2011;102(6):1193–200.
116. Oettle H, Seufferlein T, Luger T, Schmid R. Final results of a phase I/II study in patients with pancreatic cancer, malignant melanoma, and colorectal carcinoma with trabedersen (abstract). J Clin Oncol. 2012;34(suppl):4034.
117. Von Hoff DD, Ramanathan RK, Borad MJ, Laheru DA, Smith LS, Wood TE, et al. Gemcitabine plus nab-paclitaxel is an active regimen in patients with advanced pancreatic cancer: a phase I/II trial. J Clin Oncol. 2011;29(34):4548–54.

118. Infante JR, Matsubayashi H, Sato N, Tonascia J, Klein AP, Riall TA, et al. Peritumoral fibroblast SPARC expression and patient outcome with resectable pancreatic adenocarcinoma. J Clin Oncol. 2007;25(3):319–25.
119. Hidalgo M, Plaza C, Musteanu M, Illei P, Brachmann CB, Heise C, et al. SPARC expression did not predict efficacy of nab-paclitaxel plus gemcitabine or gemcitabine alone for metastatic pancreatic cancer in an exploratory analysis of the phase III MPACT trial. Clin Cancer Res. 2015;21(21):4811–8.
120. Alvarez R, Musteanu M, Garcia-Garcia E, Lopez-Casas PP, Megias D, Guerra C, et al. Stromal disrupting effects of nab-paclitaxel in pancreatic cancer. Br J Cancer. 2013;109(4):926–33.

Chapter 14
Synthetic Lethality: Achilles Heel in Select Patient Subpopulations

Min Yuen Teo and Eileen M. O'Reilly

What Is Synthetic Lethality?

Synthetic lethality is a principle first described in the early twentieth century when it was observed that certain nonallelic genes were lethal in fruit flies only in combination, even when the homozygous parents were perfectly viable [1, 2]. In modern biological context, it is defined as a type of genetic interaction where the "co-occurrence of two genetic events results in organismal or cellular death" [2–4].

There has been numerous well-documented examples of synthetic lethality in cancer described in the scientific literature, including the dependence of WEE1 in the setting of *SET domain-containing 2* (SETD2) deficiency [5] and reliance on *enhancer of zeste 2 polycomb repressive complex 2 subunit* (EZH2) activity in the setting of SWI/SNF mutation [6]; the latter has in fact led to current clinical development of EZH2 inhibitors in tumors lacking components of SWI/SNF complex. However, the concept of synthetic lethality has been best studied to date in the setting of BRCA1/2 tumors.

BRCA1 and BRCA2 are crucial components of a tightly modulated pathway which responds predominantly to double-strand breaks. Double-strand breaks are by far the most lethal of DNA damages and are repaired by either the homologous recombination or nonhomologous end-joining pathways. Homologous recombination is the preferred repair mechanism due to high-fidelity DNA repair and lower error rates [7]. Cells with defective double-strand repair show a high degree of

M.Y. Teo
Department of Medicine, Memorial Sloan Kettering Cancer Center, 300 East 66h Street, Office 1021, New York, NY 10065, USA

E.M. O'Reilly (✉)
Department of Medicine, Memorial Sloan Kettering Cancer Center, 300 East 66h Street, Office 1021, New York, NY 10065, USA

Weill Cornell Medical College, New York, NY, USA
e-mail: oreillye@mskcc.org

T. Bekaii-Saab, B. El-Rayes (eds.), *Current and Emerging Therapies in Pancreatic Cancer*, DOI 10.1007/978-3-319-58256-6_14

chromosomal instability, including chromosome breaks and radial chromosomes, which may lead to acquired mutations with consequential oncogenesis [8–10].

Due to both endogenous and environmental stressors [7], DNA damage can occur in the form of base modification, single-strand breaks, double-stand breaks, and intra-strand and inter-strand cross-links [11]. Destruction is first detected by checkpoint kinases *ataxia telangiectasia mutated* (ATM) and *ataxia telangiectasia and Rad3-related protein* (ATR), which lead to downstream activation of the Fanconi anemia complex. Once activated, the Fanconi anemia complex proceeds to recruit other component proteins of the homologous recombination mechanism including the BRCA1 and BRCA2 genes which encode for proteins which play a central role in homologous recombination pathway [12, 13]. Clinically significant mutations in these genes are frequently frameshift insertions or deletions which are translated into functionally impaired proteins [14], thereby contributing to defective homologous recombination mechanism. The impaired mechanism leads to accumulation of mutations and chromosomal defects which increase the risk of carcinogenesis and, conversely, increased sensitivity to cross-linking properties of cytotoxic agents [15–17].

In the absence of effective double-strand breakage repair, alternative DNA repair mechanisms are frequently hobbled. PAR-1 is a nuclear protein which localizes to the site of DNA damage and contributes to the majority of PARP activity. PARP is a critical component of the base excision repair pathway, an important pathway in repair of single-strand breakage. Conversely, loss of PARP-1 increases the formation of DNA lesions that might be repaired by components of homologous recombination. In cells with loss of function of BRCA1/2, PARP inhibition further interrupts alternative DNA repair pathways, leading to accumulation of large numbers of chromatid aberrations and subsequent cell cycle arrest and cell death and therefore demonstration of synthetic lethality [16].

The Clinical Application of Synthetic Lethality Across Different Cancer Types

While the principle and mechanistic evidence of synthetic lethality have been well recognized in preclinical studies, the clinical application has only arisen relatively recently with the development of PARP inhibitors.

Ovarian cancer and breast cancer are the two diseases at the forefront of efforts to capitalize on the concept of synthetic lethality for therapeutic vulnerability, largely driven by the recognition of BRCA1/2-related cancers as part of hereditary breast-ovarian cancer syndrome. Olaparib is one of the first small molecule PARP inhibitors which has entered clinical evaluation and, more importantly, to demonstrate clinical evidence of synthetic lethality. In its phase 1 study, a total of 60 patients with various cancer types were enrolled, 23 of which were confirmed BRCA1/2 mutation carriers. Two patients were not evaluable for antitumor activity, while two other patients had cancers not commonly associated with BRCA1/2 mutation, and their disease progressed rapidly despite therapy. Of the remaining 19 patients with ovarian, breast, and prostate cancer, 12 patients derived clinical benefit with radiologic or tumor marker responses or meaningful disease stabilization of over 4 months. Olaparib has since been extensively investigated in ovarian cancer and has demonstrated improvement in progression-free survival in combination with chemotherapy and as maintenance treatment in the first-line setting [18] and durable response in relapsed disease [19] most notably among patients with germline BRCA1/2 mutations, culminating in FDA approval for olaparib in this disease.

Development of PARP inhibition in breast cancer was transiently stalled due to the negative phase III study of carboplatin plus gemcitabine in combination with iniparib [20], but it was later identified that iniparib was found to harbor very low PARP inhibitory activity [21]. More recently, the large adaptive I-SPY 2 trial successfully demonstrated clinical activity of veliparib in combination with carboplatin with enhanced pathologic complete response rates among triple negative breast cancer patients undergoing neoadjuvant therapy and is therefore selected to undergo phase III evaluation [22].

Beyond breast and ovarian cancer, a recently reported phase II study demonstrated the clinical activity of olaparib in a cohort of heavily pretreated patients with metastatic castration prostate cancer, with a response rate of 33%. Interestingly, 88% of responders were found to harbor either somatic or germline mutations in BRCA1/2 and other DNA damage repair genes [23], further proving the validity of synthetic lethality as a clinical target. In fact, it was more recently shown that up to 11.8% of men with metastatic castration-resistant prostate cancer harbor germline deleterious mutations in DNA damage repair genes. Up to three quarters of these mutations were represented by *BRCA2* (44%), *ATM* (13%), *CHEK2* (12%), and *BRCA1* (7%) (PMID 27433846). Interestingly, the noted prevalence was significantly higher than men with localized disease (4.6%) and general population with no known cancer diagnosis (2.7%) [24].

BRCA1/2 Mutations and Alterations in Homologous Recombination Genes Are More Prevalent in Pancreatic Adenocarcinoma than Previously Thought

It is estimated that 5–15% of pancreatic adenocarcinoma has an inheritable component and is linked to various inherited cancer susceptibility syndromes [25] such as hereditary breast and ovarian cancer syndrome [25], Lynch syndrome, Peutz-Jeghers, familial atypical multiple mole melanoma syndrome, and hereditary pancreatitis [26]. Many of these have well-studied and characterized genomic etiologies related to single gene defects.

Hereditary breast and ovarian cancer syndrome is by far the most studied and encompasses a significant proportion of inheritable pancreatic adenocarcinoma, estimated to be between 4 and 7% of all pancreatic adenocarcinomas [27, 28]. Correlation between pancreatic cancer and hereditary breast and ovarian cancer syndrome was first gleaned from large population-based studies on hereditary breast and ovarian cancer syndromes. The large Hereditary Breast Cancer study enrolled over 5000 female carriers of BRCA1/2 mutations. With an average follow-up time of 2 years, eight cases of pancreatic cancers were diagnosed. Although low by absolute numbers, this observation represented a significantly higher standardized incidence rate compared to the general population, with a standardized incidence radio of 2.55 for *BRCA1* carriers and 2.13 for *BRCA2* carriers [29]. Similarly, the Breast Cancer Linkage Consortium study which enrolled over 3728 women with germline *BRCA2* mutation observed 3.51 times increased risk for development of pancreatic cancer [30].

While the two studies described above were mainly designed to study women with BRCA1/2-mutated breast cancers, other investigators have sought to answer a similar question with slightly different methodologies. Studies examining pancreatic cancer patients with strong family histories provided additional supporting evidence by demonstrating enrichment of related genetic variants.

In one of the earliest studies of 29 patients with pancreatic cancer and highly significant family history from the National Familial Pancreatic Tumor Registry (NFPTR), germline DNA analysis found BRCA2 mutation 17.2% of the patients, while no germline mutations in the other three genes tested for the study were observed (*MP2K4*, *MADH4*, and *ACVR1B*) [31]. Similarly, Lucas and colleagues identified germline BRCA1/2 mutations in 21.9% of 32 patients with pancreatic cancer and 18.9% in patients without a cancer diagnosis currently enrolled in their high-risk pancreatic cancer prevention and genetics program [32].

In one of the largest published series to date, 175 patients with pancreatic cancer treated in Memorial Sloan Kettering Cancer Center (MSKCC) underwent clinical genetic counseling and germline DNA analysis. Patients were enrolled based on suspicious personal or family history. Among all enrolled patients, 56.0% had Ashkenazi Jewish ancestry, 26.3% had personal history of prior malignancies, and 30–50% had family history of malignancies in first-degree relatives. In this study, pathogenic mutations were identified in 15.1% of patients, including 13 patients with *BRCA2* mutation, four patients with BRCA1 mutations, p16 mutations in two further patients, *PALB2* in one patient, and four patients with germline mutations in mismatch repair genes [28]. Patients with Ashkenazi Jewish ancestry were more likely to be tested positive for BRCA1/2 genes (13.7%) compared to those with non-Ashkenazi Jewish ancestry (7.1%).

While these studies, including the Hereditary Breast Cancer and Breast Cancer Linkage Consortium studies, have convincingly demonstrated the link between risk of pancreatic carcinogenesis and germline BRCA1/2 mutations, these studies enrolled specifically high-risk patients, enriched for strong personal or family history for pancreatic cancers or other BRCA-related malignancies, or known carrier status. The inherent selection bias therefore precludes any meaningful estimation of the magnitude or incidence of the correlation. However, a recent Canadian study sought to address this particular question: In an unselected cohort of patients with pancreatic adenocarcinoma, 11 of 306 patients (3.6%) were found to harbor pathogenic BRCA2 mutations and another three patients (1.0%) with BRCA1 mutations [27]. A high rate of Ashkenazi ancestry was noted in the study cohort at 10.8%. When analyzed separately, BRCA1/2 mutations were observed in four of 13 (12.1%) Ashkenazi Jewish patients and in 10 of 273 (3.7%) non-Ashkenazi Jewish patients ($p = 0.05$), which reflects the relatively similar observation from the MSKCC series described previously.

As discussed above, the DNA response and repair mechanism, including that of homologous recombination, consist of a complex network of many enzymes and proteins, and therefore it is conceivable that alterations in other members of the mechanism might demonstrate similar phenotypic consequences. Recent works by different groups have implicated germline mutations in other components of homologous recombination beyond BRCA1/2.

In a series of an unselected cohort of 96 pancreatic cancer patients from the Mayo Clinic Pancreatic Cancer patient registry, 14 pathogenic mutations in 13 patients were identified in eight genes, namely, *ATM*, *BRCA2*, checkpoint kinase 2 (*CHEK2*), MutS homolog 6 (*MSH6*), BRCA1-associated RING domain 1 (*BARD1*), *BRCA1*, Fanconi anemia complementation group M (*FANCM*), and Nibrin (*NBN*), majority of which are components of the homologous recombination pathway [33]. Similar observations were noted in a significantly larger sample set of 638 patients with familial pancreatic cancer without known germline mutations. Whole genome sequencing identified truncating mutations in a wide range of DNA damage repair genes at low frequencies, including *ATM*, polymerase (DNA directed) Nu (*POLN*), polymerase (DNA directed) theta (*POLQ*), Fanconi anemia complementation group C (*FANCC*), Fanconi anemia complementation group M (*FANCM*), etc. [34]. The Ontario Pancreas Cancer Study investigated the prevalence of germline mutations in a limited panel of genes—including *ATM*, *BRCA1*, *BRCA2*, *APC*, *CDKN2A*, and various mismatch repair genes. Among 290 probands, 11 pathogenic mutations were identified, of which 3 were alterations in the *ATM* gene [35]. In another study of the Mayo Clinic Pancreatic Cancer Cohort, four pathogenic mutations in ATM were noted out of 14 pathogenic mutations in 13/96 patients [33], while another regional pancreatic database observed four mutations in ATM out of 11 mutations seen in 10/70 patients [36], therefore conferring a prevalence of 1.0–5.7% among high-risk patients with pancreatic cancers.

Other groups, on the other hand, focused on incidence of selected genes. *Partner and localizer of BRCA2* (PALB2) has attracted particular attention. The PALB2 protein recruits BRCA2 to sites of DNA damage [37], forms a complex with both BRCA1 and BRCA2 in homologous recombination repair [38], and contributes to formation of rad51 nucleofilaments [39]. However, the incidence of germline PALB2 mutations appears to be relatively low. Zhen and colleagues observed a deleterious mutation in the PALB2 gene in 0.6% of patients with familial pancreatic cancer [40], and no PALB2 mutations were detected at all in a Dutch series of 28 non-BRCA1/2 familial pancreatic cancer families and 28 non-BRCA1/2 familial breast cancer families with at least one confirmed case of pancreatic cancer [41]. However, another series of 39 cases with a confirmed family history of pancreatic cancer revealed three cases of *PALB2* mutation (7.7%) [42]. In a large Italian series of non-BRCA1/2 familial breast cancer families, frequency of germline *PALB2* mutation was estimated to be 2.1% [42]. Collectively, these studies suggested that the true incidence of a germline *PALB2* mutation in pancreatic cancer patients with family history might be in the range of 1.5–2.1%.

Van der Heijden and colleagues observed mutations in *FANCC* and Fanconi anemia complementation group G (*FANCG*) genes in a small subset of patients with early-onset pancreatic adenocarcinoma [43]. In a large screening study of 421 patients with pancreatic cancers, two truncating mutations in *FANCC* were observed, but none were observed for *FANCG* although they were not associated with family history [44]. Rogers and colleagues examined genomic DNA from 38 patients with familial pancreatic cancer for mutations in *FANCC* and *FANCG* genes. Several polymorphisms of indeterminate functional significance were reported. The authors observed that these genes did not appear to contribute to the clustering of pancreatic cancers seen in the setting in familial pancreatic cancer and concluded that these genes were uncommon causes of inherited pancreatic cancers [45].

Taken together, these studies indicated that familial pancreatic adenocarcinoma patients harbor germline mutations in other components of the DNA damage response or homologous recombination mechanism. However, the prevalence of individual mutations is low, comparable to observations in other cancer types [46–48]. Besides Roger and colleagues' work on *FANCC* and *FANCG* genes [5], the low prevalence of these mutations and the lack of large pancreatic germline cohorts to date render it challenging to evaluate the penetrance strength of these mutations or their absolute risk in pancreatic carcinogenesis.

Early Signals of Potential Synthetic Lethality: BRCA1/2-Mutated Pancreatic Adenocarcinoma and Platinum or DNA-Targeting Cytotoxic Chemotherapy

FOLFIRINOX (5-Fluorouracil, oxaliplatin, irinotecan, leucovorin) and gemcitabine plus nab-paclitaxel are the current standards of care for advanced pancreatic adenocarcinoma based on superior survival data from the French PRODIGE4/ACORD11 trial [49] and the MPACT study [50], respectively, compared to single agent gemcitabine. Details of the studies are discussed elsewhere in this issue. Nevertheless, overall survival for these cancers remains poor, with medians in the range of 6–11 months and a small number of patients living beyond 2 years.

It is postulated that, for a subset of pancreatic cancers with BRCA1/2 or related mutations, their inability to repair DNA damage and inherent genomic susceptibility can enhance sensitivity to platinum-based chemotherapy or other DNA-targeting agents. This was indeed the observation gleaned from other cancer types [51]. With pancreatic adenocarcinoma, there are preclinical models which have also supported the hypothesis. This is best illustrated in a recent pancreatic xenograft study. BRCA-mutant xenografts were significantly more sensitive to cisplatin than BRCA wild-type xenografts [52].

Nevertheless, this observation has only been supported by case reports and small series for pancreatic adenocarcinoma [53–56]. Sonnenblick and colleagues reported a case of a 60-year-old patient with pancreatic cancer and BRCA2 germline mutation. The patient was treated with gemcitabine with progressive disease as best response. Cisplatin was added to gemcitabine, which led to a dramatic radiographic and biochemical complete response [53]. Chalasani and colleagues presented the case of a 49-year-old woman with germline BRCA2 mutation and metastatic pancreatic adenocarcinoma who achieved substantial partial response with third-line chemotherapy with capecitabine and mitomycin C, a cross-linking agent with identical mode of action as cisplatin [54]. Another case reported a 71-year-old BRCA2 carrier with dual diagnosis of prostate and pancreatic adenocarcinomas, who achieved disease control with second-line irinotecan for over 27 cycles of treatment [55].

In a small series of ten patients with pancreatic adenocarcinoma and known germline BRCA2 mutations [57], six patients achieved a mean duration of response of 4.8 months, ranging from 2 to 8 months, with platinum-based combination chemotherapy. Seven patients were treated with topoisomerase-I inhibitors alone or in combination with other agents, and these patients experienced a mean duration of disease response of 8.3 months. Two patients who were exposed to mitomycin C responded for 2.3 and 3 months, respectively. In another small series of 15 patients, six patients received platinum-based chemotherapy as first-line therapy, five of those experienced partial radiographic response, including one complete response with FOLFIRINOX [58]. Golan and colleagues reported superior overall survival in platinum-treated patients with either stage III disease (48 months versus 10 months) or stage IV disease (15 months versus 7 months) [59]. Although these are small series with highly selected patients, the data to date collectively suggest that superior disease control might be attainable in patients with BRCA1/2 mutations.

Synthetic Lethality and PARP Inhibition in Pancreatic Adenocarcinoma

As described previously, the discovery of synthetic lethality as a biological concept and observable phenomenon in vitro [16] has led to effective use of PARP inhibitors in other BRCA-related cancers [18, 23, 60]. In pancreatic cancer, preclinical studies have reaffirmed comparable observations. In pancreatic cancer xenografts, increased sensitivity to cisplatin but not gemcitabine was observed in BRCA1/2-mutated tumors [52]. In murine models, the addition of PARP inhibitor to cisplatin could increase time to cancer and overall survival [61].

Early clinical data have been promising. In a small retrospective series of 15 patients with pancreatic cancer and confirmed germline BRCA mutations (4 with BRCA1 and 11 with BRCA2), two patients were treated with PARP inhibitors either alone or in combination with chemotherapy in the first-line non-curative setting and enjoyed partial response lasting 2 and 6 months, respectively. Of two patients who were treated with PARP inhibitors in the second-line setting, one sustained stable disease for 6 months [58]. While the clinical responses were not uniformly positive, it has nonetheless spurned sufficiently interest to develop the concept further in pancreatic cancer which has a severe unmet need for effective therapies. This led to several PARP inhibitors in various stages of clinical evaluation and development, including olaparib, veliparib, and rucaparib.

In a large phase II study, patients with advanced solid tumor cancers and confirmed germline BRCA1/2 mutations were treated with single-agent olaparib at 200 mg BID. There were 23 patients with gemcitabine-refractory metastatic pancreatic cancer among the study cohorts. Objective responses were observed in 21.7% of patients, while 34.8% of patients demonstrated stable disease of at least 8 weeks' duration. Median progression-free and overall survivals were 4.6 and 9.8 months, respectively [62]. In a phase I study of gemcitabine and olaparib, the recommended phase 2 dose was determined to be gemcitabine 600 m/mg2 and olaparib 100 mg BID. The study included a dose expansion cohort where patients with treatment-naïve locally advanced or metastatic pancreatic cancer were randomized to olaparib plus gemcitabine at the maximum tolerated dose as determined or standard dose gemcitabine. The combination did not appear to confer improvement in disease control or survival rates; however, patients were not routinely genotyped in this study [63]. Although no further development was planned for the combination, olaparib is currently being investigated in various other clinical settings for pancreatic cancer, including in a phase 1 study of olaparib in combination with irinotecan, cisplatin, and mitomycin C (NCT01296763) and in the phase III POLO trial (NCT02184195). The trial aims to accrue approximately 145 patients with confirmed deleterious germline BRCA1/2 mutations who achieve at least disease stabilization following 16 weeks or more of platinum-based chemotherapy. Patients will be randomized in a 3:2 ratio to olaparib as maintenance therapy or placebo. The primary endpoint is a progression-free survival. As of January 2016, over 635 patients have been screened, and results were available for 590 patients, of which 46 patients (7.8%) showed germline BRCA mutations. Thirty-six of these patients (6.2%) had newly found to harbor germline BRCA mutations as a result of study screening process [64]. Table 14.1 summarizes ongoing trials.

Veliparib is also currently undergoing extensive drug development in pancreatic cancer. Some single-agent clinical activity has previously been observed. Some clinical activity for single-agent veliparib was also observed in a study of 16 patients with confirmed BRCA1/2 or *PALB2* mutation. Five had BRCA1 mutation while 11 had *BRCA2* mutations. Only one partial response was noted which progressed at 6 months, while four patients achieved stable disease, and ten had progressive disease as best response [65]. Veliparib was also examined in combination with cisplatin and gemcitabine in a phase IB dose-finding study [66]. A total of 17 patients were enrolled, and the randomized phase II dose of veliparib was determined to be 80 mg PO BID days 1–12 combined with cisplatin 25 mg/m^2 and gemcitabine 600 mg/m^2 IV days 3 and 10, every 21 days. Nine patients had BRCA1/2 mutation, while the remaining patients were BRCA wild type and enrolled based on strong personal or family history of malignancy. No significant activity was noted in the

Table 14.1 Ongoing clinical trials

Treatment	Clinical trials identifier	Phase	Patient population	Selected eligibility requirements	Primary endpoint
Olaparib	NCT02677038	II	At least one prior chemotherapy in the metastatic setting	Germline BRCA1/2 negative. Previously identified genetic aberrations associated with HRD will be eligible, e.g., somatic BRCA mutation, FA gene, or RAD51 mutations	Response rate
Olaparib versus placebo	NCT02184195	III	Nonprogression after at least 12 weeks of platinum-based chemotherapy	Germline BRCA1/2 mutation	Progression-free survival
Cediranib + olaparib	NCT02498613	II	At least one prior chemotherapy in the metastatic setting	Mixed disease cohort, BRCA mutation excluded	Response rate
Olaparib	NCT02511223	II	At least one prior chemotherapy in the metastatic setting	Tested negative for germline BRCA1/2; previously identified loss of ATM by IHC or family history of BRCA-associated cancers; previously identified genetic aberrations associated with HRD will be eligible, e.g., somatic BRCA mutation, FA gene, or RAD51 mutations	Response rate

(continued)

Table 14.1 (continued)

Treatment	Clinical trials identifier	Phase	Patient population	Selected eligibility requirements	Primary endpoint
Gemcitabine + veliparib + IMRT	NCT01908478	I	Unresectable disease	Unselected	Dose finding
Gemcitabine + cisplatin ± veliparib	NCT01585805	II	Part 1: first-line metastatic setting; part 2: single agent in previously treated disease	Confirmed BRCA1/2 or PALB2 mutation	Response rate
mFOLFOX6 + veliparib	NCT01489865	I/II	First line	Confirmed BRCA1/2, PALB2 of FA gene mutations	Dose finding

latter group, but for the BRCA-mutated subgroup, six out of nine patients experienced partial response, while the remaining patients had stable disease as best response. In another dose-finding study, veliparib was tested in combination with FOLFIRI. Among the 96 patients enrolled, partial responses were noted in 2 out of 14 patients who had a diagnosis of pancreatic cancer [67].

Other ongoing studies involving veliparib includes a randomized phase II study of cisplatin, gemcitabine, plus veliparib versus cisplatin and gemcitabine (NCT01585805), a phase 1 study of veliparib in combination with gemcitabine and intensity-modulated radiation therapy in patients with locally advanced disease (NCT01908478), and a phase I/II study of veliparib in combination with FOLFOX in metastatic pancreatic adenocarcinoma (NCT01489865).

Rucaparib is another PARP inhibitor in a much earlier stage of development. A phase II trial enrolled patients with metastatic pancreatic adenocarcinoma with known somatic or germline BRCA1/2 mutation and at least one prior line of systemic therapy. Nineteen patients were treated before the study was closed due to lack of responses in the first 15 patients. However, partial responses were subsequently noted in two patients and complete response in one patient. All responders only had one prior line of treatment and were platinum sensitive [68].

Conclusion

Pancreatic adenocarcinoma remains a difficult disease to treat with challenging outcomes. At a molecular level, it is characterized by diverse underlying mechanisms of disease progression and treatment resistance, including genomic instability [69]. The recognition of BRCA-related pancreatic adenocarcinoma as a clinically relevant subtype offers new opportunities for biology-driven drug development and biomarker-directed therapeutics. To date, preclinical optimism has not been translated into a high level of preliminary clinical signals based on early readouts. These observations are consistent with observations in breast, ovarian, and prostate cancers. Nevertheless, numerous studies are still ongoing, evaluating PARP inhibitors in combination with different systemic cytotoxic agents. New agents targeting different components of DNA damage response and repair mechanism, such as ATM and ATR inhibitors, are currently under phase 1 evaluation, and their role in yielding insight regarding disease-related synthetic lethality remains to be seen.

References

1. Dobzhansky T. Genetics of natural populations. Xiii. Recombination and variability in populations of *Drosophila pseudoobscura*. Genetics. 1946;31:269–90.
2. Nijman SM. Synthetic lethality: general principles, utility and detection using genetic screens in human cells. FEBS Lett. 2011;585:1–6.

3. Boone C, Bussey H, Andrews BJ. Exploring genetic interactions and networks with yeast. Nat Rev Genet. 2007;8:437–49.
4. JLt H, Garvik B, Hartwell L. Principles for the buffering of genetic variation. Science. 2001;291:1001–4.
5. Pfister SX, Markkanen E, Jiang Y, et al. Inhibiting WEE1 selectively kills histone H3K36me3-deficient cancers by dNTP starvation. Cancer Cell. 2015;28:557–68.
6. Kim KH, Kim W, Howard TP, et al. SWI/SNF-mutant cancers depend on catalytic and non-catalytic activity of EZH2. Nat Med. 2015;21:1491–6.
7. Houtgraaf JH, Versmissen J, van der Giessen WJ. A concise review of DNA damage checkpoints and repair in mammalian cells. Cardiovasc Revasc Med. 2006;7:165–72.
8. Zhu C, Mills KD, Ferguson DO, et al. Unrepaired DNA breaks in p53-deficient cells lead to oncogenic gene amplification subsequent to translocations. Cell. 2002;109:811–21.
9. Chapman JR, Taylor MR, Boulton SJ. Playing the end game: DNA double-strand break repair pathway choice. Mol Cell. 2012;47:497–510.
10. Jackson SP, Bartek J. The DNA-damage response in human biology and disease. Nature. 2009;461:1071–8.
11. Hoeijmakers JH. Genome maintenance mechanisms for preventing cancer. Nature. 2001;411:366–74.
12. Moynahan ME, Pierce AJ, Jasin M. BRCA2 is required for homology-directed repair of chromosomal breaks. Mol Cell. 2001;7:263–72.
13. Moynahan ME, Chiu JW, Koller BH, Jasin M. Brca1 controls homology-directed DNA repair. Mol Cell. 1999;4:511–8.
14. Konstantinopoulos PA, Ceccaldi R, Shapiro GI, D'Andrea AD. Homologous recombination deficiency: exploiting the fundamental vulnerability of ovarian cancer. Cancer Discov. 2015;5:1137–54.
15. Turner N, Tutt A, Ashworth A. Hallmarks of 'BRCAness' in sporadic cancers. Nat Rev Cancer. 2004;4:814–9.
16. Ashworth A. A synthetic lethal therapeutic approach: poly(ADP) ribose polymerase inhibitors for the treatment of cancers deficient in DNA double-strand break repair. J Clin Oncol Off J Am Soc Clin Oncol. 2008;26:3785–90.
17. Keim R, Ferguson DJ. Contralateral recurrence and prognostic factors in familial non-BRCA1/2-associated breast cancer (Br J Surg 2006; 93: 961–968). Br J Surg. 2007;94:121. author reply –2
18. Oza AM, Cibula D, Benzaquen AO, et al. Olaparib combined with chemotherapy for recurrent platinum-sensitive ovarian cancer: a randomised phase 2 trial. Lancet Oncol. 2015;16:87–97.
19. Matulonis UA, Penson RT, Domchek SM, et al. Olaparib monotherapy in patients with advanced relapsed ovarian cancer and a germline BRCA1/2 mutation: a multistudy analysis of response rates and safety. Ann Oncol. 2016;27:1013–9.
20. O'Shaughnessy J, Schwartzberg L, Danso MA, et al. Phase III study of iniparib plus gemcitabine and carboplatin versus gemcitabine and carboplatin in patients with metastatic triple-negative breast cancer. J Clin Oncol Off J Am Soc Clin Oncol. 2014;32:3840–7.
21. Sinha G. Downfall of iniparib: a PARP inhibitor that doesn't inhibit PARP after all. J Natl Cancer Inst. 2014;106:djt447.
22. Rugo HS, Olopade OI, DeMichele A, et al. Adaptive randomization of Veliparib-carboplatin treatment in breast cancer. N Engl J Med. 2016;375:23–34.
23. Mateo J, Carreira S, Sandhu S, et al. DNA-repair defects and Olaparib in metastatic prostate cancer. N Engl J Med. 2015;373:1697–708.
24. Pritchard CC, Mateo J, Walsh MF, et al. Inherited DNA-repair Gene mutations in men with metastatic prostate cancer. N Engl J Med. 2016;375:443–53.
25. Mersch J, Jackson MA, Park M, et al. Cancers associated with BRCA1 and BRCA2 mutations other than breast and ovarian. Cancer. 2015;121:269–75.
26. Connor AA, Gallinger S. Hereditary pancreatic cancer syndromes. Surg Oncol Clin N Am. 2015;24:733–64.

27. Holter S, Borgida A, Dodd A, et al. Germline BRCA mutations in a large clinic-based cohort of patients with pancreatic adenocarcinoma. J Clin Oncol Off J Am Soc Clin Oncol. 2015;33:3124–9.
28. Salo-Mullen EE, O'Reilly EM, Kelsen DP, et al. Identification of germline genetic mutations in patients with pancreatic cancer. Cancer. 2015;121:4382–8.
29. Iqbal J, Ragone A, Lubinski J, et al. The incidence of pancreatic cancer in BRCA1 and BRCA2 mutation carriers. Br J Cancer. 2012;107:2005–9.
30. Breast Cancer Linkage C. Cancer risks in BRCA2 mutation carriers. J Natl Cancer Inst. 1999;91:1310–6.
31. Murphy KM, Brune KA, Griffin C, et al. Evaluation of candidate genes MAP2K4, MADH4, ACVR1B, and BRCA2 in familial pancreatic cancer: deleterious BRCA2 mutations in 17%. Cancer Res. 2002;62:3789–93.
32. Lucas AL, Frado LE, Hwang C, et al. BRCA1 and BRCA2 germline mutations are frequently demonstrated in both high-risk pancreatic cancer screening and pancreatic cancer cohorts. Cancer. 2014;120:1960–7.
33. Hu C, Hart SN, Bamlet WR, et al. Prevalence of pathogenic mutations in cancer predisposition genes among pancreatic cancer patients. Cancer Epidemiol Biomarkers Prev. 2016;25:207–11.
34. Roberts NJ, Norris AL, Petersen GM, et al. Whole genome sequencing defines the genetic heterogeneity of familial pancreatic cancer. Cancer Discov. 2016;6:166–75.
35. Grant RC, Selander I, Connor AA, et al. Prevalence of germline mutations in cancer predisposition genes in patients with pancreatic cancer. Gastroenterology. 2015;148:556–64.
36. Geurts J, Evans DB, Tsai S. Genetic screening for patients with pancreatic cancer: frequency of high-risk mutations. ASCO Meeting Abstracts. 2015;33:e12526.
37. Park JY, Zhang F, Andreassen PR. PALB2: the hub of a network of tumor suppressors involved in DNA damage responses. Biochim Biophys Acta. 2014;1846:263–75.
38. Sy SM, Huen MS, Chen J. PALB2 is an integral component of the BRCA complex required for homologous recombination repair. Proc Natl Acad Sci U S A. 2009;106:7155–60.
39. Ahlskog JK, Larsen BD, Achanta K, Sorensen CS. ATM/ATR-mediated phosphorylation of PALB2 promotes RAD51 function. EMBO Rep. 2016;17:671–81.
40. Zhen DB, Rabe KG, Gallinger S, et al. BRCA1, BRCA2, PALB2, and CDKN2A mutations in familial pancreatic cancer: a PACGENE study. Genetics in medicine: official journal of the American College of Medical. Genetics. 2015;17:569–77.
41. Harinck F, Kluijt I, van Mil SE, et al. Routine testing for PALB2 mutations in familial pancreatic cancer families and breast cancer families with pancreatic cancer is not indicated. Eur J Hum Genet. 2012;20:577–9.
42. Peterlongo P, Catucci I, Pasquini G, et al. PALB2 germline mutations in familial breast cancer cases with personal and family history of pancreatic cancer. Breast Cancer Res Treat. 2011;126:825–8.
43. van der Heijden MS, Yeo CJ, Hruban RH, Kern SE. Fanconi anemia gene mutations in young-onset pancreatic cancer. Cancer Res. 2003;63:2585–8.
44. Couch FJ, Johnson MR, Rabe K, et al. Germ line Fanconi anemia complementation group C mutations and pancreatic cancer. Cancer Res. 2005;65:383–6.
45. Rogers CD, van der Heijden MS, Brune K, et al. The genetics of FANCC and FANCG in familial pancreatic cancer. Cancer Biol Ther. 2004;3:167–9.
46. Tung N, Battelli C, Allen B, et al. Frequency of mutations in individuals with breast cancer referred for BRCA1 and BRCA2 testing using next-generation sequencing with a 25-gene panel. Cancer. 2015;121:25–33.
47. Kurian AW, Hare EE, Mills MA, et al. Clinical evaluation of a multiple-gene sequencing panel for hereditary cancer risk assessment. J Clin Oncol Off J Am Soc Clin Oncol. 2014;32:2001–9.
48. Maxwell KN, Wubbenhorst B, D'Andrea K, et al. Prevalence of mutations in a panel of breast cancer susceptibility genes in BRCA1/2-negative patients with early-onset breast cancer. Genetics in medicine: official journal of the American College of Medical. Genetics. 2015;17:630–8.

49. Conroy T, Desseigne F, Ychou M, et al. FOLFIRINOX versus gemcitabine for metastatic pancreatic cancer. N Engl J Med. 2011;364:1817–25.
50. Von Hoff DD, Ervin T, Arena FP, et al. Increased survival in pancreatic cancer with nab-paclitaxel plus gemcitabine. N Engl J Med. 2013;369:1691–703.
51. Silver DP, Richardson AL, Eklund AC, et al. Efficacy of neoadjuvant Cisplatin in triple-negative breast cancer. J Clin Oncol Off J Am Soc Clin Oncol. 2010;28:1145–53.
52. Lohse I, Borgida A, Cao P, et al. BRCA1 and BRCA2 mutations sensitize to chemotherapy in patient-derived pancreatic cancer xenografts. Br J Cancer. 2015;113:425–32.
53. Sonnenblick A, Kadouri L, Appelbaum L, et al. Complete remission, in BRCA2 mutation carrier with metastatic pancreatic adenocarcinoma, treated with cisplatin based therapy. Cancer Biol Ther. 2011;12:165–8.
54. Chalasani P, Kurtin S, Dragovich T. Response to a third-line mitomycin C (MMC)-based chemotherapy in a patient with metastatic pancreatic adenocarcinoma carrying germline BRCA2 mutation. JOP. 2008;9:305–8.
55. James E, Waldron-Lynch MG, Saif MW. Prolonged survival in a patient with BRCA2 associated metastatic pancreatic cancer after exposure to camptothecin: a case report and review of literature. Anticancer Drugs. 2009;20:634–8.
56. Lowery M, Shah MA, Smyth E, et al. A 67-year-old woman with BRCA 1 mutation associated with pancreatic adenocarcinoma. J Gastrointest Cancer. 2011;42:160–4.
57. Vyas O, Leung K, Ledbetter L, et al. Clinical outcomes in pancreatic adenocarcinoma associated with BRCA-2 mutation. Anticancer Drugs. 2015;26:224–6.
58. Lowery MA, Kelsen DP, Stadler ZK, et al. An emerging entity: pancreatic adenocarcinoma associated with a known BRCA mutation: clinical descriptors, treatment implications, and future directions. Oncologist. 2011;16:1397–402.
59. Golan T, Kanji ZS, Epelbaum R, et al. Overall survival and clinical characteristics of pancreatic cancer in BRCA mutation carriers. Br J Cancer. 2014;111:1132–8.
60. Lee JM, Hays JL, Annunziata CM, et al. Phase I/Ib study of olaparib and carboplatin in BRCA1 or BRCA2 mutation-associated breast or ovarian cancer with biomarker analyses. J Natl Cancer Inst. 2014;106:dju089.
61. Lowery MA, Lee A, Tobias E, et al. Evaluation of PARP inhibition as a platinum sparing strategy in Brca2-deficient pancreatic tumors. ASCO Meeting Abstracts. 2014;32:e15237.
62. Kaufman B, Shapira-Frommer R, Schmutzler RK, et al. Olaparib monotherapy in patients with advanced cancer and a germline BRCA1/2 mutation. J Clin Oncol. 2015;33:244–50.
63. Bendell J, O'Reilly EM, Middleton MR, et al. Phase I study of olaparib plus gemcitabine in patients with advanced solid tumours and comparison with gemcitabine alone in patients with locally advanced/metastatic pancreatic cancer. Ann Oncol. 2015;26:804–11.
64. Golan T, Oh D-Y, Reni M, et al. POLO: a randomized phase III trial of olaparib maintenance monotherapy in patients (pts) with metastatic pancreatic cancer (mPC) who have a germline BRCA1/2 mutation (gBRCAm). ASCO Meeting Abstracts. 2016;34:TPS4152.
65. Lowery MA, Kelsen DP, Smith SC, et al. Phase II trial of veliparib (V) in patients (pts) with previously treated BRCA or PALB2-mutated (mut) pancreas adenocarcinoma (PC). ASCO Meeting Abstracts. 2015;33:358.
66. O'Reilly EM, Lowery MA, Segal MF, et al. Phase IB trial of cisplatin (C), gemcitabine (G), and veliparib (V) in patients with known or potential BRCA or PALB2-mutated pancreas adenocarcinoma (PC). ASCO Meeting Abstracts. 2014;32:4023.
67. Berlin J, Ramanathan RK, Strickler JH, et al. A phase 1 dose-escalation study of veliparib with bimonthly FOLFIRI in patients with advanced solid tumors. ASCO Meeting Abstracts. 2574;2014:32.
68. Domchek SM, Hendifar AE, McWilliams RR, et al. RUCAPANC: an open-label, phase 2 trial of the PARP inhibitor rucaparib in patients (pts) with pancreatic cancer (PC) and a known deleterious germline or somatic BRCA mutation. ASCO Meeting Abstracts. 2016;34:4110.
69. Knudsen ES, O'Reilly EM, Brody JR, Witkiewicz AK. Genetic diversity of pancreatic ductal adenocarcinoma and opportunities for precision medicine. Gastroenterology. 2016;150:48–63.

Chapter 15
Immunotherapies in Pancreatic Cancer

Mohamad Bassam Sonbol and Mitesh J. Borad

Pancreatic cancer is the fourth leading cause of cancer-related deaths in the United States. Most of the new cases of pancreatic cancers (approximately 53,070 cases annually) are diagnosed in advanced stages with 5-year survival of 2% [17]. The mainstay of treatment in pancreatic cancer had been with gemcitabine until a recent study showed the superiority of the nab-paclitaxel addition to gemcitabine compared to the monotherapy. In addition, FOLFIRINOX (fluorouracil, leucovorin, oxaliplatin, and irinotecan) is another regimen that has been shown to be effective and has been added to the "arsenal" of treatment approaches against this lethal cancer. However, even with the addition of the latter, the median overall survival has only improved to 11.1 months [18]. Hence, there remains an unmet need for new therapeutic agents. With a better understanding of the pancreatic microenvironment, there has been a great focus on the use of immunotherapies in pancreatic cancer in an attempt to attain a further survival benefit.

Pancreatic Cancer Microenvironment

The complex tumor microenvironment in pancreatic cancer plays a crucial role in this cancer resistance to therapeutic agents and its poor prognosis. Effector T-cells, which play an important role in antitumor activity via antigen-presenting cells (APC) activation, are decreased in numbers in pancreatic microenvironment

M.B. Sonbol, M.D. • M.J. Borad, M.D. (✉)
Department of Hematology/Medical Oncology, Mayo Clinic, Phoenix, AZ, USA
e-mail: Borad.Mitesh@mayo.edu

T. Bekaii-Saab, B. El-Rayes (eds.), *Current and Emerging Therapies in Pancreatic Cancer*, DOI 10.1007/978-3-319-58256-6_15

[1–3].On the other hand, immunosuppressive cells, such as T-regulatory cells (T-regs) and myeloid-derived suppressor cells (MDSCs), are found to be increased in number [2]. These immunosuppressive cells play an important role in hindering host immune response and accelerating angiogenesis, thus leading to tumor growth and extension. In addition to the abovementioned cellular activity, multiple inhibitory receptors and enzymes have been described in the pancreatic microenvironment and lead to worse prognosis. For example, indoleamine 2,3-dioxygenase (IDO) is one of the enzymes that when increased, as seen in pancreatic cancer, attracts T-regs into the microenvironment and leads to increase in the number of effector T-cells [3, 4]. The prognostic value of these cellular changes has been described previously. The number of T-regs and MDSCs is inversely related to survival, whereas effector $CD4^+$ T-cells correlate with better prognosis [2]. CD40 is another co-stimulatory molecule that is expressed on T-cells, and when binding to its ligand CD40 on APCs within pancreatic tumor stroma, it leads to upregulation of the surface expression of MHC which results in T-cell activation.

A better understanding of the microenvironment in pancreatic cancer has led to identifying multiple immunological targets that are currently under investigation.

In this chapter, we describe some of the immunotherapies that are being investigated in pancreatic cancer with a focus on checkpoint inhibitors. Virotherapy and vaccines are covered in depth in accompanying chapters.

Immune Checkpoint Inhibitors

As described previously, multiple receptors work as co-stimulatory or co-inhibitory signals affecting the host reaction to tumor growth. Program death (PD-1) and its ligand (PD-L1), along with cytotoxic T-lymphocyte-associated protein-4 (CTLA-4), have received recent attention with FDA approval of multiple PD-1/PD-L1 immunotherapy agents in melanoma and bladder, lung, kidney, and head and neck cancers.

PD-1 is a co-inhibitory molecule that is expressed in multiple cells including CD4+ and CD8+ T-cells, T-regs, and natural killer cells (NK). PD-L1 is mainly expressed in several solid tumors and tumor-infiltrating lymphocytes (TILs). The interaction between PD-1 and its ligand PD-L1 leads to decreased T-cell proliferation, cytokine release, and cytolytic activity of PD-1+ T-cells.

Several phase I/II trials have incorporated the use of immune checkpoint inhibitors as monotherapies, or in combination with other agents such as chemotherapy, vaccines, or a combination of checkpoint inhibitors (Table 15.1).

Table 15.1 Summary of completed phase I/II clinical trials investigating checkpoin inhibitors in pancreatic cancer

Study	Checkpoint inhibitor	Phase	Primary endpoint	Median PFS*	Median OS*	Comments	Ref
Brahmer et al.	BMS-936559	I	Safety, efficacy	N/A	N/A	Study on advanced solid tumors. No objective response in pancreatic cancer patients	Mulvihill et al. [5] ; Brahmer et al. [6] #179}
Segal et al.	Durvalumab (MEDI4736)	I/II	Safety, efficacy	N/A	N/A	Phase II study evaluating the durvalumab in combination with tremelimumab has been initiated (ALPS study)	{Segal, 2014 #190}
Royal et al.	Ipilimumab	II	Efficacy	N/A	N/A	Generally ineffective except for one patient with delayed response	Noonan et al. [7]; {Royal et al. [8] #180}
Kaylan et al.	Ipilimumab/gem	Ib	MTD	2.5 months	8.5 months	43% response rate with PR and SD of 2/16 and 5/16, respectively	{Kaylan, 2016 #191}
Beatty et al.	CP-870,893	I	MTD, safety, and efficacy	N/A	7.4 months	Cytokine release syndrome was most common AE. PR and SD were 4/21 and 11/21, respectively	Nakao et al.[9] ; Beatty, et al. [10] #181}

(continued)

Table 15.1 (continued)

Study	Checkpoint inhibitor	Phase	Primary endpoint	Median PFS*	Median OS*	Comments	Ref
Le et al.	Ipilimumab/GVAX	Ib	Safety, efficacy	N/A	5.7 months	Two-arm study: Ipilimumab vs. Ipilimumab with GVAX. Although statistically nonsignificant, OS favored the combination arm (5.7 vs. 3.6 months, *P* 0.072)	{Le, 2013 #194}

PFS-progression-free survival; OS-overall survival; MTD-maximal tolerable dosage; SD-stable disease; PR-partial response; AE-adverse event

Checkpoint Inhibitors as Monotherapies and Dual Checkpoint Inhibitors

BMS-936559, a PD-L1-specific, IgG4 monoclonal antibody, was studied in a phase I clinical trial of advanced solid tumors. There was no objective response in patients with pancreatic cancer that were included in the efficacy population of the study [6]. MEDI4736, durvalumab, is another PD-L1-specific monoclonal antibody that has been studied in a phase I expansion study in multiple tumor types including 32 patients with pancreatic adenocarcinoma. Grade 3/4 toxicity was reported in 13% of patients with adverse events leading to discontinuation of treatment in one patient due to grade 3 elevated liver function tests. Tumor shrinkage was detectable in a subset of patients, including pancreatic cancer. Upon a median follow-up of 6 weeks, objective response rate was seen in 7% (2/29) of patients, and disease control was achieved in 21% (6/29) [19]. A phase 2 study evaluating the efficacy of the combination of durvalumab with the CTLA-4 inhibitor tremelimumab is currently underway (ALPS study: NCT02558894).

Ipilimumab, an anti-CTLA-4 agent, has been shown to be relatively ineffective in 27 patients with locally advanced/metastatic pancreatic cancer with only one patient having delayed response after initial progressive disease [8]. In another phase Ib study, ipilimumab was combined with gemcitabine in 16 patients with advanced pancreatic cancer. Response (partial response + stable disease) was seen in 43% of patients with 2 out of 16 having partial response and 5 having stable disease. Median PFS was 2.5 months with OS of 8.5 months. The combination was generally tolerable [20]. Another phase1/2 randomized clinical trial is currently underway and comparing ipilimumab combined with the PD-1 inhibitor nivolumab vs. nivolumab monotherapy (NCT01928394).

Pembrolizumab, a PD-1 inhibitor that has been FDA approved and shown to be effective in multiple other solid tumors, is currently under investigation in multiple clinical trials in pancreatic cancer as single agent (NCT02331251, NCT02054806), in combination with hypofractionated radiotherapy (NCT02303990), and in combination with chemoradiation (CRT) in neoadjuvant settings (NCT02305186). Results of these trials are yet to be published.

In a study utilizing CD40 pathway, CP-870,893, a humanized CD40 agonist, was given in combination with gemcitabine to 21 previously untreated advance pancreatic cancer patients. Four patients had partial response and 11 with stable disease. Median OS was 7.4 months [10].

A single agent therapeutic approach focusing on overcoming T-cell immunologic endpoints with PD-1/PD-L1 and anti-CTLA-4-directed agents in pancreatic cancer has been so far discouraging. This minimal-response pancreatic cancer compared to the promising results with other types of solid tumors can be explained by the unique microenvironment. Besides the paucity of the effector T-cells in the pancreatic microenvironment, the dense pancreatic cancer stroma restricts immune cell migration and comprises a barrier in front of the cancer antigen recognition. Hence, an important concept in potentiating the checkpoint inhibitors is by finding ways to invite more lymphocytes into the tumor stroma in an attempt to expose this "fortress." Multiple strategies are currently under development to help in exposing the microenvironment by either inducing an "immunogenic blast" with introducing cancer antigens to the immune system with chemotherapy or radiation or by further sensitizing the immune system using vaccines and viruses.

Checkpoint Inhibitors Combined with Vaccines

The main principle behind vaccine immunotherapy is to mount an immune response against the tumor by administering a tumor-specific antigen. In general, vaccine immunotherapy can be divided into whole-cell vaccines (GVAX and algenpantucel-L) and synthetic vaccines (using whole protein or peptide). This will be covered in more detail in another chapter.

GVAX is an allogeneic-irradiated whole-cell pancreatic tumor vaccine. It consists of two allogeneic pancreatic tumor cell lines that have been modified with plasmid vector encoding the cDNA for human GM-CSF. GM-CSF activates and recruits the APCs, which mounts an immune response by engaging with the tumor antigen expressed by the vaccine {Jaffee, 2001 #192; Kleponis, 2015 #193}.

In a preclinical study, it was found that PD-L1 is weakly expressed at a low frequency in untreated human and murine pancreatic ductal adenocarcinomas, but treatment with a GVAX significantly upregulated PD-L1 expression after treatment of tumor-bearing mice. Furthermore, anti-PD-1/PD-L1 antibodies enhanced antitumor activities of the GVAX and improved murine survival compared with PD-1 antibody monotherapy or GVAX therapy alone [11]. Based on the abovementioned preclinical data and looking at the combination of nivolumab with GVAX in metastatic pancreatic cancer patients (NCT02243371) and in the adjuvant settings in patients with surgically resectable pancreatic cancer (NCT02451982), two clinical trials have been initiated. On the other hand, the combination of the anti-CTLA-4 ipilimumab with GVAX has been shown to be potentially effective. In a study of 30 patients with previously treated advanced pancreatic cancer, ipilimumab was combined with GVAX in one arm compared to ipilimumab monotherapy in the other arm. Stable disease was seen in two patients in the monotherapy arm compared to three in the combination arm. The OS was favoring the combination arm compared to the ipilimumab monotherapy arm (5.7 vs. 3.6 months, respectively, $P = 0.072$). Immune-related adverse events were seen in 73% of patients in monotherapy arm compared to 80% in the combination arm. Twenty percent of patients in both arms experience grades 3–4 IRAEs (colitis, Guillain-Barré syndrome, nephritis, and pneumonitis) [21]. A preliminary announcement of negative results of a follow-up study has been made, and the final results are awaiting presentation/publication.

Other Potential Targets

Bruton's tyrosine kinase (BTK) has been identified as a potential target in the treatment of pancreatic cancer. Both murine and human pancreas ductal adenocarcinomas (PDACs) exhibit increased BTK activation in tumor CD20+, CD11b+cells.

Inhibition of BTK in a preclinical study, as shown by Gunderson et al., led to slowed progression of orthotopic tumors in a T-cell-dependent manner [12]. In addition, this was accompanied by an increase in effector and memory CD8+ T-cells which could potentiate the efficacy of immune checkpoint inhibitors when combined with ibrutinib. The combination of ibrutinib with durvalumab, MEDI4736, is currently being studied in a phase Ib/II clinical trial (NCT02403271, recruiting). On the other hand, NCT02436668, RESOLVE trial, is a phase II/III clinical trial that is studying the combination of ibrutinib vs. placebo, in combination with nab-paclitaxel and gemcitabine in the first-line treatment of patients with metastatic pancreatic adenocarcinoma (recruiting).

There has been emerging evidence that inflammation plays an important role in the tumorigenesis process in pancreatic cancer. Recently, specific inflammatory signaling pathways such as STAT3/IL-6, NF-kB, and CXCR2 have been implicated in PDAC progression. CXCR2 is a receptor for multiple human chemokines and was found to regulate the migration of MDSCs. In a preclinical study, the inhibition of CXCR2 reduced metastasis and improved response to gemcitabine and anti-PD-1 by allowing T-cell infiltration [13]. The combination of ulocuplumab, a fully human IgG4 anti-CXCR4 antibody, with nivolumab is currently being studied in a phase I/II study (NCT02472977) in solid tumors including patients with pancreatic cancer.

On the other hand, the importance of IL-6 in pancreatic cancer has been shown before, and several studies have demonstrated that elevated IL-6 levels are associated with increased tumor size and poor prognosis. IL-6 binds to its membrane receptor complexes containing the common signal-transducing receptor chain glycoprotein 130 (GP130), which subsequently leads to series of signaling events that include the JAK/STAT, MAPK, and PI3K pathways. The activation of IL-6/STAT3 pathway can modulate the pancreatic cancer microenvironment with increasing the amount of immunosuppressive cells such as MDSCs and T-regs [14]. Therefore, targeting IL-6 as monotherapy or combined with other therapeutic methods is currently being studied. In a preclinical study on pancreatic cancer cells, the administration of bazedoxifene, an IL6-GP130 inhibitor, led to apoptosis and suppressed tumor growth in pancreatic cancer cells via STAT3 phosphorylation and STAT3 DNA binding. In addition, a synergistic effect was seen when bazedoxifene was combined with paclitaxel or gemcitabine, leading to further inhibition of cell viability and cell migration in pancreatic cancer cells [15]. In another more recently published study, combining IL-6 with PD-L1 blockade in mice with pancreatic cancer limited the tumor progression and enhanced the overall survival. The authors also showed that this dual inhibition was accompanied by a change at the level of the microenvironment with increased number of infiltrating effector T-cells in the tumor [14].

Another potential target is the focal adhesion kinase (FAK) which is an intracellular, nonreceptor kinase encoded by *PTK2*. FAK is overexpressed and activated in a variety of cancer including pancreatic cancer where it serves as a scaffolding protein and its overexpression is correlated with tumor size. Moreover, FAK overexpression is correlated with increased fibrosis and poor T-cell infiltration. Therefore, multiple FAK inhibitors have been developed and currently being studied in different malignancies in preclinical and early phase I studies. In a recent preclinical study on mouse model of human PDAC, the VS-4718 FAK inhibitor led to suppression of tumor progression and increased survival [16]. In addition, FAK inhibition promoted the responsiveness to PD-1 antagonist. Therefore, the combination of VS-4718 (defactinib) with checkpoint immunotherapy is currently being tested in a phase I clinical trial (NCT02546531).

Conclusion

The treatment of pancreatic cancer remains very challenging. As the effect of cytotoxic agents has plateaued, immunotherapeutic interventions could be the way to improve survival in this deadly disease. However, the use of immune agents as monotherapies has not been promising, and combining such agents together or with other targeted therapies might be needed to alter the microenvironment in order to make the cancer more susceptible to immunotherapies. In addition, further studies are needed to identify which patient populations might be more susceptible to immunotherapies (such as mismatch repair deficient tumors).

References

1. Fridman WH, Pages F, Sautes-Fridman C, Galon J. The immune contexture in human tumours: impact on clinical outcome. Nat Rev Cancer. 2012;12(4):298–306.
2. Ino Y, Yamazaki-Itoh R, Shimada K, Iwasaki M, Kosuge T, Kanai Y, Hiraoka N. Immune cell infiltration as an indicator of the immune microenvironment of pancreatic cancer. Br J Cancer. 2013;108(4):914–23.
3. Kunk PR, Bauer TW, Slingluff CL, Rahma OE. From bench to bedside a comprehensive review of pancreatic cancer immunotherapy. J Immunother Cancer. 2016;4:14.
4. Witkiewicz A, Williams TK, Cozzitorto J, Durkan B, Showalter SL, Yeo CJ, Brody JR. Expression of indoleamine 2,3-dioxygenase in metastatic pancreatic ductal adenocarcinoma recruits regulatory T cells to avoid immune detection. J Am Coll Surg. 2008;206(5):849–54. discussion 854-846
5. Mulvihill S, Warren R, Venook A, Adler A, Randlev B, Heise C, Kirn D. Safety and feasibility of injection with an E1B-55 kDa gene-deleted, replication-selective adenovirus (ONYX-015) into primary carcinomas of the pancreas: a phase I trial. Gene Ther. 2001;8(4):308–15.
6. Brahmer JR, Tykodi SS, Chow LQ, Hwu WJ, Topalian SL, Hwu P, Drake CG, Camacho LH, Kauh J, Odunsi K, Pitot HC, Hamid O, Bhatia S, Martins R, Eaton K, Chen S, Salay TM, Alaparthy S, Grosso JF, Korman AJ, Parker SM, Agrawal S, Goldberg SM, Pardoll DM, Gupta A, Wigginton JM. Safety and activity of anti-PD-L1 antibody in patients with advanced cancer. N Engl J Med. 2012;366(26):2455–65.
7. Noonan AM, Farren MR, Geyer SM, Huang Y, Tahiri S, Ahn D, Mikhail S, Ciombor KK, Pant S, Aparo S, Sexton J, Marshall JL, Mace TA, Wu CS, El-Rayes B, Timmers CD, Zwiebel J, Lesinski GB, Villalona-Calero MA, Bekaii-Saab TS. Randomized phase 2 trial of the Oncolytic virus Pelareorep (Reolysin) in upfront treatment of metastatic pancreatic adenocarcinoma. Mol Ther. 2016;24(6):1150–8.

8. Royal RE, Levy C, Turner K, Mathur A, Hughes M, Kammula US, Sherry RM, Topalian SL, Yang JC, Lowy I, Rosenberg SA. Phase 2 trial of single agent Ipilimumab (anti-CTLA-4) for locally advanced or metastatic pancreatic adenocarcinoma. J Immunother. 2010;33(8):828–33.
9. Nakao A, Kasuya H, Sahin TT, Nomura N, Kanzaki A, Misawa M, Shirota T, Yamada S, Fujii T, Sugimoto H, Shikano T, Nomoto S, Takeda S, Kodera Y, Nishiyama Y. A phase I dose-escalation clinical trial of intraoperative direct intratumoral injection of HF10 oncolytic virus in non-resectable patients with advanced pancreatic cancer. Cancer Gene Ther. 2011;18(3):167–75.
10. Beatty GL, Chiorean EG, Fishman MP, Saboury B, Teitelbaum UR, Sun W, Huhn RD, Song W, Li D, Sharp LL, Torigian DA, O'Dwyer PJ, Vonderheide RH. CD40 agonists alter tumor stroma and show efficacy against pancreatic carcinoma in mice and humans. Science. 2011;331(6024):1612–6.
11. Soares KC, Rucki AA, Wu AA, Olino K, Xiao Q, Chai Y, Wamwea A, Bigelow E, Lutz E, Liu L, Yao S, Anders RA, Laheru D, Wolfgang CL, Edil BH, Schulick RD, Jaffee EM, Zheng L. PD-1/PD-L1 blockade together with vaccine therapy facilitates effector T-cell infiltration into pancreatic tumors. J Immunother. 2015;38(1):1–11.
12. Gunderson AJ, Kaneda MM, Tsujikawa T, Nguyen AV, Affara NI, Ruffell B, Gorjestani S, Liudahl SM, Truitt M, Olson P, Kim G, Hanahan D, Tempero MA, Sheppard B, Irving B, Chang BY, Varner JA, Coussens LM. Bruton tyrosine kinase-dependent immune cell cross-talk drives pancreas cancer. Cancer Discov. 2016;6(3):270–85.
13. Steele CW, Karim SA, Leach JD, Bailey P, Upstill-Goddard R, Rishi L, Foth M, Bryson S, McDaid K, Wilson Z, Eberlein C, Candido JB, Clarke M, Nixon C, Connelly J, Jamieson N, Carter CR, Balkwill F, Chang DK, Evans TR, Strathdee D, Biankin AV, Nibbs RJ, Barry ST, Sansom OJ, Morton JP. CXCR2 inhibition profoundly suppresses metastases and augments immunotherapy in pancreatic ductal adenocarcinoma. Cancer Cell. 2016;29(6):832–45.
14. Mace TA, Shakya R, Pitarresi JR, Swanson B, McQuinn CW, Loftus S, Nordquist E, Cruz-Monserrate Z, Yu L, Young G, Zhong X, Zimmers TA, Ostrowski MC, Ludwig T, Bloomston M, Bekaii-Saab T, Lesinski GB. IL-6 and PD-L1 antibody blockade combination therapy reduces tumour progression in murine models of pancreatic cancer. Gut. 2016; doi:10.1136/gutjnl-2016-311585.
15. Wu X, Cao Y, Xiao H, Li C, Lin J. Bazedoxifene as a novel GP130 inhibitor for pancreatic cancer therapy. Mol Cancer Ther. 2016;15(11):2609–19.
16. Jiang H, Hegde S, Knolhoff BL, Zhu Y, Herndon JM, Meyer MA, Nywening TM, Hawkins WG, Shapiro IM, Weaver DT, Pachter JA, Wang-Gillam A, DeNardo DG. Targeting focal adhesion kinase renders pancreatic cancers responsive to checkpoint immunotherapy. Nat Med. 2016;22(8):851–60.
17. Siegel RL, Miller KD, Jemal A. Cancer statistics, CA Cancer J Clin. 2016;66(1): p. 7–30.
18. Conroy T, Desseigne F, Ychou M, Bouché O, Guimbaud R, Bécouarn Y, Adenis A, Raoul JL, Gourgou-Bourgade S, de la Fouchardière C, Bennouna J, Bachet JB, Khemissa-Akouz F, Péré-Vergé D, Delbaldo C, Assenat E, Chauffert B, Michel P, Montoto-Grillot C, Ducreux M. FOLFIRINOX versus Gemcitabine for Metastatic Pancreatic Cancer. N Engl J Med. 2011;364(19):1817–1825.
19. Segal NH, Hamid O, Hwu W, Massard C, Butler M, Antonia S, Blake-Haskins A, Robbins PB, Li X, Vasselli J, Khleif S. 1058PDA phase I multi-arm dose-expansion study of the anti-programmed cell death-ligand-1 (PD-L1) antibody MEDI4736: preliminary data. Ann Oncol. 2014;25 (suppl_4):iv365–iv365.
20. Kalyan A, et al. Ipilimumab and gemcitabine for advanced pancreas cancer: A phase Ib study. J Clin Oncol. 2016;34(15_suppl): p. e15747–e15747.
21. Le DT, Lutz E, Uram JN, Sugar EA, Onners B, Solt S, Zheng L, Diaz LA, Donehower RC, Jaffee EM, Laheru DA, Evaluation of ipilimumab in combination with allogeneic pancreatic tumor cells transfected with a GM-CSF gene in previously treated pancreatic cancer. J Immunother. 36 (7):382-389.

Chapter 16
Vaccine Therapy in Pancreatic Cancer

Benjamin A. Weinberg and Michael J. Pishvaian

Introduction

Pancreatic ductal adenocarcinoma (PDA) is a devastating illness, with only 7.7% of patients alive 5 years after their initial diagnosis [1]. Even in the most optimal circumstance, in which patients with resectable disease who undergo resection and complete adjuvant therapy, median overall survival (mOS) is only 28.0 months [2]. Improvement is desperately needed for patients with metastatic disease (mPDA), with meager mOS estimates ranging from 8.5 months with gemcitabine and nab-paclitaxel to 11.1 months with FOLFIRINOX (oxaliplatin, irinotecan, leucovorin, and fluorouracil) [3, 4]. Thus, researchers have been actively exploring alternatives to conventional cytotoxic chemotherapy, and one of the most exciting avenues involves training the immune system to attack the cancer directly. Unfortunately, PDA is frequently thought of as poorly immunogenic with no objective responses to single-agent checkpoint inhibitors (anti-programmed death 1 (anti-PD-1) or anti-programmed death ligand 1 (anti-PD-L1)) [5]. However, studies demonstrate that by appropriately priming PDA cells using vaccines, one can induce them to become immunogenic and susceptible to checkpoint inhibitors and other immunotherapy approaches [6]. In this chapter we review the rationale for using vaccines to fight PDA, the targets unique to PDA that have been previously utilized, methods to augment the immune response to PDA vaccines, and key prior and ongoing trials of PDA vaccines in the clinic.

B.A. Weinberg, M.D. • M.J. Pishvaian, M.D., Ph.D. (✉)
Division of Hematology and Oncology, Lombardi Comprehensive Cancer Center, Georgetown University, Washington, DC, USA
e-mail: pishvaim@georgetown.edu

T. Bekaii-Saab, B. El-Rayes (eds.), *Current and Emerging Therapies in Pancreatic Cancer*, DOI 10.1007/978-3-319-58256-6_16

Vaccine Background

The immune system has long been recognized as a potential partner in attacking cancer cells. Early successes, such as high-dose interleukin-2 (IL-2) in melanoma [7, 8] and renal cell carcinoma [9, 10] and bacillus Calmette-Guérin (BCG) in early stage bladder cancer [11], focused on ways to amplify a nonspecific immune response using preexisting immune effector cells that already recognized tumor antigens. These findings further stimulated interest in developing cancer vaccines that could induce clonal expansion of B and T cells that recognize specific tumor antigens. This method has the added benefit of generating memory B and T cell populations that can engage in active surveillance and mount a response upon repeat recognition of tumor cells.

Active-specific immunotherapy using cancer vaccines can induce the development of antibodies directed against tumor antigens. Anti-idiotype antibodies (AIAs) against tumor-associated antigens (TAAs) destroy cancer cells via antibody-dependent cytotoxicity (ADCC) [12]. These AIAs are formulated by first administering a TAA, resulting in the production of an anti-TAA antibody (Ab1) which then itself generates antibodies against itself (Ab2, the AIA), a mirror image of Ab1, and a mimic of the original TAA, which then can again stimulate antibody production against the original TAA (Ab3, the anti-AIA) [13]. The end result is an antibody that targets the TAA without requiring the presence of the foreign TAA protein. The AIA is processed, presented to antigen-presenting cells (APCs), and then presented to the major histocompatibility complex (MHC) of T cells, inducing targeted CD4- and CD8-driven immune responses [14].

Other cancer vaccines use different modalities to stimulate an immune response. Whole cell vaccines are destroyed tumor cells whose contents are taken up by APCs causing activation of B and T cells. These vaccines can be autologous, as used in adjuvant studies derived from resected tumor specimens, or allogeneic, derived from preexisting tumor cell lines [15].

Recombinant viral DNA vaccines use a preexisting viral coat to infect cells and house a reengineered viral genome that expresses a specific TAA. Once inside the cell, viral DNA encoding for the TAA protein is transcribed to mRNA and ultimately translated in the cytoplasm, leading to intracellular production and processing of the TAA, its presentation to the cell surface via MHC class I or II, and recognition by $CD8^+$ or $CD4^+$ T cells, respectively [16, 17].

While peptide vaccines are the most simple and easy to use cancer vaccines, they have numerous disadvantages in PDA: many peptides cannot be presented by MHCs, $CD8^+$ cytotoxic T lymphocytes (CTLs) may be ineffective at killing PDA cells, TAAs and MHCs are often downregulated, and dendritic cell (DC) function may be decreased in patients with advanced PDA [18–21].

In contrast, DC vaccines more effectively stimulate specific CTL responses [22]. DCs are more effective at presenting antigens compared with activated macrophages and B cells as they have higher numbers of MHC, costimulatory, and adhesion molecules, and they migrate to lymph nodes where they can interact and stimulate T cells [23]. DCs are normally found within the tumor microenvironment but are frequently suppressed by tumor production of cytokines (interleukin-6 (IL-6), IL-10, and vascular endothelial growth factor (VEGF)) [22, 24, 25] and condition T cells to become suppressive (FOXP3[+] and IL-13-producing CD4[+] T and natural killer (NK) cells) [26, 27]. However, if this local suppression can be overcome, dendritic cells are effective killers of cancer cells because they can recognize multiple tumor antigens and expand multiple lineages (NK cells and CTLs) targeting different antigens [22]. There are two methods of producing DC vaccines: (1) generating DCs ex vivo by bombarding them with TAAs and reinjecting them into patients where they travel via lymphatics, interact with T cells, and induce an immune response and (2) using TAAs within monoclonal antibodies directed against receptors on DCs in order to deliver a large amount of antigen to DCs within lymphatics [22].

Vaccines have been studied in multiple oncology settings, including for use in adjuvant treatment and in advanced and metastatic disease. In the adjuvant setting, vaccine therapy is designed to create a surveillance mechanism by which residual tumor cells could be recognized by the immune system. In the advanced setting, vaccines may be used to stimulate a CTL response with the goal of disease control.

Vaccine Targets

Numerous TAAs and pathway targets for PDA vaccines have been studied, and in this section, we review the reasoning as to why these targets are important in PDA cells and the early phase clinical trials performed to study these agents.

CEA

Carcinoembryonic antigen (CEA) is a 180-kDa glycoprotein that is expressed on over 90% of PDA tumors [28, 29]. It is a member of the immunoglobulin superfamily encoded on chromosome 19 [30]. CEA is normally expressed during fetal development and is implicated in intercellular adhesion [31, 32]. CTLs are able to recognize CEA epitopes that bind MHCs A2, A3, and A24, but otherwise CEA is considered poorly immunogenic because of exposure during fetal development and immune tolerance [29]. One method to augment its immunogenicity is to modify the human leukocyte antigen (HLA)-A2 CEA CAP-1 epitope to CAP1-6D, increasing CTL recognition by 100–1000-fold [33]. This technique was used to make CEAVac, a vaccine comprised of the CEA peptide CAP1-6D, montanide (incomplete Freund's adjuvant, IFA), and granulocyte-macrophage colony-stimulating factor (GM-CSF) [34]. In a phase I trial, Geynisman and colleagues randomized 19 patients with previously treated PDA expressing HLA-A2 and CEA to one of three dose levels of CEAVac (10 μg, 100 μg, or 1000 μg) given every 2 weeks until disease progression [34]. Seventy-four percent of the patients had metastatic PDA. Of the 14 patients who received at least 3 doses of CEAVac, 1 patient with locally advanced PDA at dose level 1000 μg had a complete response (CR) and was alive at 71 months, and another patient at dose level 100 μg had stable disease (SD) for 11 months and was alive at 39 months. Both patients had strong CTL responses measured by Enzyme-Linked ImmunoSpot (ELISpot) assay and indeed mean CTL response correlated with dose level (248 spots per 10^4 $CD8^+$ cells at dose level 1000 μg vs 37 spots at dose level 10 μg, $P = 0.037$). Treatment was well tolerated with no grade 3 or 4 toxicities. While CEAVac monotherapy at dose level 1000 μg elicited a CTL response, these results did not translate into significant clinical efficacy.

Another CEA vaccine studied in CEA-expressing adenocarcinoma is ALVAC, a reengineered canarypox virus encoding CEA. A phase I study using a recombinant vaccinia-CEA virus vaccine failed to show any antineoplastic effect in humans but was shown to be safe and able to elicit CTL responses [35]. The canarypox virus has several advantages over vaccinia because it is an avian virus that does not replicate in mammals, humans are unlikely to have been previously exposed to it, and it induces strong CTL responses [36, 37]. In a phase I study, ALVAC-CEA was administered to 20 patients, including 2 patients with pancreatic cancer, at three different dose levels (2.5×10^5, 2.5×10^6, and 2.5×10^7 plaque-forming units) [38]. Of the 15 patients with measurable disease, no patients had an objective response to treatment, although 7 of 9 HLA-A2-positive patients had an increase in CEA-specific CTL precursors (based on limiting dilution assays of peripheral blood mononuclear cells, PBMCs). Higher dose levels did not result in higher rates of CTL responses, and no grade 3 or 4 toxicities occurred.

Building on this trial, a pilot study of ALVAC-CEA plus the T cell costimulatory molecule B7.1 was performed in 39 patients with CEA-expressing tumors [39]. B7.1, also known as CD80, works by binding to CD28 on T cells which leads to the production of cytokines including IL-2 and interferon (IFN) γ, forming a costimulatory signal that prevents an anergic response by the T cell to the antigen [40]. Again, 3 dose levels were used, 2.5×10^7, 1.0×10^8, and 4.5×10^8 plaque-forming units, and 3 patients enrolled had PDA. Thirty patients who received at least 4 injections of the vaccine were evaluable, 8 patients had SD, and no patients had CRs or partial responses (PRs). Twelve of 15 HLA-A2-positive patients had a significant increase in CEA-specific T cell precursor frequency by ELISpot assay.

Another phase I trial of ALVAC-CEA-B7.1 of 18 patients with metastatic CEA-expressing tumors only had 1 patient with PDA, but again this study showed that the vaccine can produce CEA-specific T cell responses and was well tolerated [37]. Three patients had SD which correlated with their CTL response. Thus, the addition of B7.1 may have augmented the immunogenicity of the ALVAC-CEA as evidenced by increase of specific CTL responses and possible clinical efficacy based on stabilization of disease. The second stage of this study used GM-CSF as an adjuvant to enhance antigen processing and presentation to DCs [41]. Thirty patients received the vaccine alone and another 30 received the vaccine plus GM-CSF. While more patients who received GM-CSF had SD compared to those who received vaccine alone (44% vs 27%, $P = 0.1213$), this clinical benefit did not correlate with CEA-specific T cell precursors as there was a statistically significant increase in patients who received vaccine alone but not on those patients who received GM-CSF [41].

MUC-1

Mucin 1 (MUC-1) is a MHC-independent TAA and highly glycosylated transmembrane protein in epithelial cells that may be involved in metastasis due to its anti-adhesion properties and promotion of invasion [42]. MUC-1 expression on circulating tumor cells (CTCs) in mPDA is a negative prognostic biomarker [43]. In a phase I trial, 63 patients (including 24 patients with PDA) received a synthetic mucin peptide combined with BCG [44]. No patients had an objective response, but 3 patients (including 1 with PDA) had SD. Out of 22 tested patients, only 7 had an at least twofold increase in mucin-specific CTLs after vaccination. Patients did have adverse reactions to vaccination including skin breakdown (98%), fever (64%), chills (48%), anorexia (40%), hypoalbuminemia (40%), and rigors (16%), and higher levels of IL-6 were associated with the development of constitutional symptoms ($P = 0.001$).

A synthetic MUC-1 peptide (GVTSAPDTRPAPGSTAPPAH$_5$-CONH$_2$) loaded autologous DC vaccine was studied in 10 patients with resected PDA and 2 patients with resected biliary cancer in an adjuvant phase I/II study [45]. The vaccine was tolerated well without any adverse events, although no specific CTL responses were seen. mOS was 26 months, and 4 of the 12 patients were alive after more than 4 years of follow-up and without recurrent disease. This MUC-1 peptide with DC construct has not been further explored in published clinical trials.

Kaufman and colleagues conducted a phase I trial of a poxvirus vaccine and a fowlpox virus vaccine targeting both CEA and MUC-1 in 10 patients with advanced pancreatic cancer using 3 costimulatory molecules (B7.1, ICAM-1, and LFA-3, or TRIad of COstimulatory molecules (TRICOM)) [46]. As discussed previously, activation of a T cell by an APC requires both an interaction between the peptide/MHC complex and T cell receptor (TCR) and a second interaction using a costimulatory molecule. Each costimulatory molecule has distinct T cell ligands (B7.1 binds to CD28/cytotoxic T-lymphocyte-associated protein 4 (CTLA-4), ICAM-1 binds to CD11a/CD18, and LFA-3 binds to CD2), and the 3 checkpoint interactions work synergistically to lower the threshold of T cell activation in animal models [47]. In the phase I trial, patients received a recombinant vaccinia viral vaccine with CEA, MUC-1, and TRICOM (PANVAC-V) followed by 3 vaccines of the same construct using a fowlpox virus (PANVAC-F) every 2 weeks. All vaccinations were followed by 4 daily doses of GM-CSF. Patients could continue monthly booster vaccines for up to 12 months if they did not have progressive disease (PD). The 2 different viral rectors were used in a prime-boost sequence that had been shown to generate superior T cell responses in studies of malaria using *Plasmodium falciparum* circumsporozoite antigen (PfCSF) and in prostate cancer using prostate-specific antigen (PSA) [48, 49].

In the phase I trial of PANVAC, 5 of 8 evaluable patients had antigen-specific CTL responses by ELISpot assay, and patients who developed anti-CEA or anti-MUC-1 immune responses had improved mOS compared to those patients without immune responses (15.1 vs 3.9 months, $P = 0.002$) [46]. The only adverse events were minor injection site reactions, and there were no grade 3 or 4 adverse events. Thus, PANVAC demonstrated both potential clinical efficacy and safety in this small study of PDA patients. We have proposed a clinical trial of PANVAC with the anti-PD-L1 antibody durvalumab (see section on ongoing vaccine clinical trials below) to further augment this immune response.

RAS

The RAS superfamily contains over 150 small GTPase proteins that regulate a variety of cellular functions by serving as molecular switches that bind GTP ("on" state) and hydrolyze it to GDP ("off" state) [50]. Within this family, humans have three *RAS* genes (*HRAS*, *KRAS*, and *NRAS*), and mutated *RAS* genes are oncogenes that play crucial roles in the development of many types of malignancies [51]. *RAS* mutation status carries vital prognostic and predictive information for patients with metastatic colorectal cancer (mCRC) as anti-epidermal growth factor receptor (anti-EGFR)-directed therapies are not as effective in *RAS*-mutated tumors, and patients with *RAS*-mutated tumors have inferior overall survival compared with patients with *RAS* wild-type tumors [52–54]. In PDA, more than 90% of tumors harbor *KRAS* mutations in codons 12, 13, or 61, and the vast majority of mutations occur in codon 12 (most commonly G12V, G12D, and G12R) [55]. *KRAS* mutations are thought to play in early role in oncogenesis as they are present in precursor PDA lesions (pancreatic intraepithelial neoplasia, PanIN) [56, 57]. Activated KRAS mediates multiple downstream signal transduction cascades including the mitogen-activated protein kinase (MAPK) and phosphatidylinositol-3-kinase (PI3K)/AKT pathways [58]. Thus, this pathway is an important potential therapeutic target, although no targeted therapies have been developed despite over 30 years of studying RAS [59]. This is still a burgeoning field of research, and recent advances include targeting the active site of RAS, using siRNA, and co-targeting other critical pathways such as YAP1 and c-Myc [60].

Given its near ubiquity in PDA, there has been a strong interest in targeting *KRAS* mutations by using vaccines. Gjertsen and colleagues first demonstrated that a synthetic peptide vaccine comprised of residues 5–21 of p21 *RAS* (KLVVVGAXGVGKSALTI where X is the mutated amino acid, G to V, D, or R) could elicit a T cell response by extracting PBMCs from a PDA patient, loading them with a vaccine targeting their tumor's specific *RAS* mutation and reinfusing them back to the patient [61]. In this phase I/II study, 5 patients with advanced PDA received the vaccine, and 2 patients developed a proliferative T cell response in PBMCs and had SD at 2 months [62]. Further analysis of 1 patient with a G12V mutation showed the development of specific $CD4^+$ and $CD8^+$ T cell responses [63].

To augment the immune response, another phase I/II study combined the synthetic *RAS* peptide with GM-CSF in 10 patients with resected PDA and 38 patients with advanced PDA [64]. Resected patients received a vaccine matched to their specific *RAS* mutation, while those with advanced disease received a mixture of four peptide vaccines (containing the G12V, G12R, G12D, and G12C substitutions). Fifty-eight percent of patients developed an immune response as measured by delayed-type hypersensitivity (DTH) reaction or T cell response. Tumor biopsies in 1 of 4 patients with advanced disease revealed tumor infiltrating lymphocytes (TILs) reactive against the patient's G12R mutation. Overall, immune responders with advanced PDA had improved mOS compared to nonresponders with advanced PDA (148 vs 61 days, $P = 0.0002$) [64]. In a long-term follow-up of patients who received the vaccine in the adjuvant setting, mOS was 27.5 months and was 28 months among immune responders, and 4 of 20 evaluable patients were alive at 10 years [65]. No further clinical data using this vaccine have been published.

Another mutant *RAS* peptide vaccine (using residues 5–17 with G12C, G12V, or G12D mutations corresponding to *RAS* mutation of the patient's tumor) using Detox™ PC adjuvant (composed of the cell wall skeleton of *Mycobacterium phlei* and monophosphoryl lipid A from *Salmonella*) was first studied in a pilot adjuvant trial in 5 PDA and 7 colorectal cancer patients [66]. Five of 11 evaluable patients had a positive immune response as measured by IFN γ gene expression, and the mOS of the PDA patients was more than 44.4 months. The same vaccine and Detox™ PC adjuvant were further evaluated in a trial of 53 patients with advanced cancer (including 11 with PDA) plus either IL-2, GM-CSF, or both IL-2 and GM-CSF [67]. IL-2 promotes the growth of tumor-specific lymphocytes and clonal TILs [68–70]. Fifty-four percent of patients had an immune response by ELISpot testing, 31% with vaccine plus IL-2, 92% with vaccine plus GM-CSF, and 36% with vaccine plus IL-2 and GM-CSF ($P = 0.003$), and there was no correlation between immune response and OS ($P = 0.086$) [67]. IL-2 may have negatively impacted the formation of an immune response due to the expansion of T regulatory cells (Tregs), but this finding was not directly assessed as few samples were tested for Tregs in this study. There have been no other published clinical data using this vaccine.

Another pilot adjuvant trial by Abou-Alfa and colleagues examined a different 21-mer synthetic *RAS* peptide in 24 patients with resected PDA [71]. Again, the vaccine matched the *RAS* mutation of the patient's tumor (G12R, G12 V, G12D, or wild-type *RAS*) and used GM-CSF as an adjuvant. However, only 9 patients were evaluable for an immune response, only 1 patient had a specific DTH response to their *RAS* mutation, 3 patients had nonspecific DTH responses, and mOS was 20.3 months [71]. This vaccine has also not been studied further due to its poor immunogenicity.

Carbone and colleagues studied custom 17-mer *KRAS*- or *TP53*-derived peptides loaded into PBMCs of 39 patients including 9 patients with PDA (all of whom received *KRAS*-targeting vaccines) [72]. Only one patient had an immune response by CTL activity and IFNγ response. This vaccine construct has also not been further evaluated.

Palmer and colleagues reported a phase I/II trial of TG01, a mixture of seven RAS peptides, with GM-CSF and gemcitabine as adjuvant therapy in 18 patients with resected PDA [73]. About 87.5% of patients had an immune response by DTH persisting after gemcitabine, and the vaccine was well tolerated except for allergic reactions in 4 patients including 2 cases of anaphylaxis. This trial is still ongoing.

Finally, another vaccine targeting KRAS in PDA is GI-4000. GI-4000 is comprised of 4 strains of heat-inactivated recombinant yeast (*Saccharomyces cerevisiae*) that each express a modified RAS protein. Each strain has a different combination of 3 modified RAS proteins of the 7 most common *RAS* mutations (GI-4014: Q61L, G12V, and Q61R; GI-4015: Q61L, G12C, and Q61R; GI-4016: Q61L, G12D, and Q61R; GI-4020: Q61L, G12R, and Q61H) [74]. In a phase I study, Cohn and colleagues enrolled 32 patients with advanced colorectal cancer, non-small cell lung cancer, or pancreatic cancer who failed at least 1 line of therapy [75]. Only 9 patients had *RAS* mutations of whom 7 had mutations contained within vaccine strains, and 6 patients received GI-4014, GI-4015, and GI-4016. There were no serious adverse events reported. Two of 3 evaluable patients had evidence of a mutation-specific CTL response by proliferation and cytokine secretion assays (final results of the study were not published). A phase II study presented by Muscarella and colleagues randomized 176 patients with resected *RAS*-mutated PDA 1:1 to receive GI-4000 or placebo in 3 weekly injections followed by 6 cycles of adjuvant gemcitabine (stratified by R0 or R1 resection status) [76]. Patients continued monthly GI-4000 or placebo monthly during off weeks from gemcitabine and monthly until intolerance, disease progression, or death. In an unplanned analysis of 39 patients with R1 resections, the GI-4000 arm had a significantly higher rate of mutation-specific CTL response by ELISpot (47% vs 8%, $P = 0.032$), and there was improved mOS in immune responders compared to those who received placebo (596 vs 444 days, P not reported). mOS was slightly longer in the GI-4000 arm compared to placebo (524 vs 444 days, P not reported). There were no significant adverse events associated with GI-4000. The final results of this completed study have not yet been published.

TP53

Like *KRAS*, *TP53* is frequently mutated in PDA, present in approximately 50% of tumors [55]. *TP53* mutations correlate with a poor prognosis and increased metastatic potential [77, 78]. *TP53* normally encodes the p53 protein that negatively regulates cell growth and is activated in the setting of cellular stress or damage, functioning as a tumor suppressor gene [79]. Thus, *TP53* is an excellent therapeutic target in PDA.

In a phase II study, Chai and colleagues treated 36 patients with mPDA with a DC vaccine (16 patients) or a DC vaccine combined with recombinant adenovirus-p53 gene therapy [80]. There were no serious adverse events reported. DC vaccine alone had a disease control rate (DCR: CR, PR, or SD) of 37.5% and mOS of 5.5 months, compared to a DCR of 45% and mOS 6.8 months for those patients treated with the combination. This vaccine construct has not been further studied.

β-hCG

β-human chorionic gonadotropin (β-hCG) is a hormone used as a marker for pregnancy that is also expressed by a variety of malignancies [81]. In 1 study, 56% of PDA tumors stained positive by immunohistochemistry (IHC) using a monoclonal antibody directed against β-hCG [82]. Iversen and colleagues reported results of a phase II trial of CTP37-DT, a synthetic peptide of the terminal peptide of β-hCG conjugated to diphtheria toxoid (DT), with gemcitabine vs vaccine alone in 55 patients with untreated mPDA [83]. There was improved mOS in the combination group (6.6 vs 4.7 months with vaccine alone). This vaccine has not been further explored in PDA.

Survivin

Survivin regulates cell cycle progression by blocking caspase activation and inhibiting programmed cell death [84]. Given its antiapoptotic properties, overexpression of survivin is associated with PDA carcinogenesis [85]. It is an ideal TAA as it is expressed in fetal tissue and tumors but not in normal fully differentiated cells [86]. In a phase I study of HLA-A*2402-positive patients and survivin-positive advanced PDA, Kameshima and colleagues explored the use of an HLA-A24-restricted survivin-derived peptide vaccine (survivin-2B80-88, AYACNTSTL) with IFA and IFNα adjuvants (based on a prior study in advanced colorectal cancer) [87, 88]. IFNα stimulates DC proliferation and activation and is thought to augment the immune response [89]. In the study, 6 patients were vaccinated and 4 had SD. All 4 patients with SD had an over 200% increase tetramer staining for peptide-specific CTLs postvaccination and positive response by ELISpot testing [88]. Further studies of this peptide have not been published.

Gastrin

Gastrin is a growth peptide, and its expression is upregulated in PDA [90]. G17DT contains a synthetic gastrin peptide linked to DT, and antigastrin antibodies induced by G17DT can inhibit the growth of PDA cells [91]. In a phase II trial, 30 patients with advanced PDA received 3 doses of G17DT at 100 or 250 μg [92]. Twenty of the 30 (67%) patients developed antigastrin antibodies, including 14 of 17 patients

(82%) in the 250 μg group ($P = 0.018$). Three patients with an antibody response did have grade 3 local injection site reactions (defined as abscess, ulceration, or necrosis). mOS from day of injection was 217 days for responders vs 121 days for nonresponders ($P = 0.0023$). G17DT was well tolerated, induced an antibody response in most patients at the 250 μg dose, and did improve mOS in responders compared to nonresponders.

This study led to the larger phase III trial of 154 patients with untreated advanced PDA unsuitable or unwilling to take chemotherapy who were randomized 1:1 to receive G17DT (250 μg on weeks 0, 1, 3, 24, and 52) or placebo [93]. Seventy-nine patients received G17DT and 74 received placebo. Injection site reactions occurred in 18% of patients who received G17DT. In the intention-to-treat (IIT) population, 64.5% of patients treated with G17DT developed an anti-G17DT antibody response, and their mOS was superior to nonresponders and to those who received placebo (176 vs 63 vs 83 days, respectively, $P = 0.003$ by log-rank analysis) [93]. However, the overall HR for mortality of 0.75 (95% CI 0.51–1.10, $P = 0.138$), comparing G17DT treatment to placebo, was not statistically significant. Therefore, further trials of G17DT in advanced PDA have not been performed.

Telomerase

Telomerase is an enzyme that preserves telomere length at the end of chromosomes, supporting cellular immortalization and carcinogenesis in malignancy [94]. The human catalytic unit of telomerase (hTERT) is overexpressed on PDA cells but not benign pancreatic tissue [95]. GV1001 is a synthetic peptide of hTERT (611–626: EARPALLTSRLRFIPK) and is well recognized by $CD4^+$ T cells via MHC class I. Bernhardt and colleagues used the vaccine in 48 patients with untreated advanced PDA at 1 of 3 dose levels (112 μg, 560 μg, or 1.87 mg) plus GM-CSF [96]. The vaccine was well tolerated and generated an immune response in 24 of 38 patients by DTH test or specific T cell response, including 75% of those patients at the 560 μg dose level. Immune responders had improved mOS compared to nonresponders (216 vs 88 days, $P = 0.0001$), and the 560 μg group had improved mOS (260 days) compared to 112 μg (119 days, $P = 0.006$) and 1.87 mg (153 days, $P = 0.05$).

Building on this early work with GV1001, Middleton and colleagues performed a phase III open-label trial of 6 cycles of gemcitabine (1000 mg/m^2 IV days 1, 8, and 15) and capecitabine (830 mg/m^2 PO twice daily 21 out of every 28 days) plus GM-CSF and GV1001 (560 μg days 1, 3, 5, once weekly weeks 2–4, then monthly starting week 6) [97]. In this trial, 1062 patients with untreated advanced PDA were randomized 1:1:1 to received chemotherapy alone, chemotherapy followed by GV1001, or concurrent chemoimmunotherapy. Unfortunately, it was a negative trial as GV1001 did not improve mOS: 7.9 months with chemotherapy alone (95% CI 7.1–8.8), 6.9 months with sequential therapy (95% CI 6.4–7.6, HR 1.2, 98.25% CI 1.0–1.5, $P = 0.0466$), and 8.4 months with concurrent therapy (95% CI 7.3–9.7, HR

1.05, 98.25% CI 0.8–1.3, $P = 0.6378$) [97]. Another study of GV1001 monotherapy compared to gemcitabine was terminated prematurely due to lack of efficacy [98]. Further studies of GV1001 in PDA have not yet been published. A phase I study of radiation, tadalafil, sargramostim, gemcitabine, and GV1001 in locally advanced PDA is currently ongoing (NCT01342224).

WT1

Wilms tumor gene (*WT1*) protein is expressed on a variety of cancers (including 65% of PDA), plays a role in carcinogenesis, and naturally induces an immune response [99–102]. In a phase I study, 9 patients with advanced PDA and 16 patients with advanced biliary cancer and appropriate HLA type (HLA-A*0201, HLA-A*0206, and/or HLA-A*2404 positive) received gemcitabine and a WT1 vaccine (HLA-A02-restricted 126–134 peptide, RMFPNAPYL or a HLA-A24-restricted 235–243 peptide, CYTWNQMNL) [103]. The vaccine was administered with montanide (IFA). Two vaccine dose levels were evaluated (1 and 3 mg), and the higher dose level was well tolerated with no reported dose-limiting toxicities (DLTs). The vaccine generated WT1-specific PMBCs in 13 of 20 evaluable patients, and mOS of the PDA patients was 259 days. There is evidence that gemcitabine works synergistically with the WT1 vaccine by shifting the WT1 protein from the nucleus to the cytoplasm, promoting its antigen presentation and generation of a WT1-specific CTL response [104].

Following this study, a large phase I trial of 32 HLA-A*2402-positive patients with advanced PDA used the 3 mg vaccine dose with montanide adjuvant every 2 weeks plus gemcitabine [105]. There was only 1 DLT (cerebrovascular ischemia) reported. Eighteen of 31 evaluable patients had an immune response by positive DTH test. mOS in all patients was 8.1 months and was statistically better in responders vs nonresponders (10.9 vs 3.9 months, $P = 0.003$) [105].

Further studies of WT1 utilized DC vaccines pulsed with WT1. In a phase I trial, Koido and colleagues treated 10 patients with mPDA and 1 patient with cholangiocarcinoma who possessed the appropriate HLA types with concurrent gemcitabine and mature DCs pulsed with MHC-restricted WT1 peptides [106]. The treatment was well tolerated, although 1 patient with rapidly progressing PDA died of a cerebral infarction. Only 4 of 10 evaluable patients had an immune response by DTH, although immune responders did have improved mOS than nonresponders, and 3 patients with PDA and strong DTH reactions had a mOS of 717 days. An analysis of markers for response in the PDA patients revealed increased posttreatment neutrophil to lymphocyte ratio, HLA-DR, and CD83 as potential positive prognostic biomarkers [107].

Finally, another phase I study by Mayanagi and colleagues looked at the same regimen (WT1 DC vaccine plus gemcitabine) as first-line therapy in 10 HLA-A*2402-positive advanced PDA patients [108]. Adverse effects were consistent with prior studies including gemcitabine. Sixty percent of patients had an immune response by DTH, and there was a significant increase in WT1-specific T cells after DC vaccination (compared to pre-vaccination, $P = 0.036$). While there were no objective responses, 60% of patients had SD, and mOS was 243 days. Given the lack of significant response, further studies of WT1 vaccines have not been reported.

VEGFR2

Vascular endothelial growth factor 2 (VEGFR2) promotes tumor growth via neovascularization and plays a role in PDA development and metastasis, and its overexpression represents a poor prognosis in patients with PDA [109–111]. Elpamotide is an epitope peptide of VEGFR2-169 (RFVPDGNRI), HLA restricted to HLA-A*2402. In a phase I study, Miyazawa and colleagues enrolled 21 HLA-A*2402-positive patients with advanced PDA to received gemcitabine, IFA, and 3 escalating doses of elpamotide (0.5, 1, or 2 mg on days 1, 8, 15, and 22 every 28 days) [112]. Of the 18 patients who received at least 4 doses of vaccine, no grade 4 adverse events were reported, CTL responses by ELISpot were seen in 61% of patients, and mOS was 7.7 months.

Given these findings, a larger phase II/III trial by Yamaue and colleagues randomized 153 patients with untreated advanced PDA and the HLA-A*2402 genotype 2:1 to receive elpamotide plus gemcitabine or placebo plus gemcitabine [113]. Patients in the elpamotide arm had slightly higher rates of fever (31% vs 20.8%, $P = 0.01$) and aspartate aminotransferase (AST) elevation (36% vs 20.8%, $P = 0.015$) compared to the placebo arm. mOS was the same in both groups (8.36 months with elpamotide vs 8.54 months with placebo, HR 0.87, $P = 0.897$), although patients who received elpamotide who developed a severe infusion site reaction had improved mOS compared to those who did not develop a severe reaction (15.67 months vs 8.28 months, HR 0.8, 95% CI 0.39–1.64, *P* value not reported). Thus, while the addition of the vaccine to gemcitabine did not improve mOS, there was a trend toward improved mOS in immune responders. Further studies of using elpamotide in PDA have not been reported in the literature.

VXM01 is an oral DNA vaccine that contains a plasmid encoding VEGFR2 and uses the vector *Salmonella typhi* Ty21a as a live-attenuated bacterial carrier (the oral vaccine against typhoid fever) [114]. In a phase I trial, Schmitz-Winnenthal and colleagues randomized 45 patients with advanced PDA (previously treated with gemcitabine) 2:1 to receive escalating doses of VXM01 (30 patients) or placebo (15 patients). No DLTs occurred so the maximum tolerated dose was not reached [115]. There was no difference in CTL responses or objective responses between the 2 groups, although there was indirect evidence of antiangiogenic vaccination effect by increase in serum VEGF-A, collagen IV, and blood pressure [116, 117]. This trial was extended to add monthly booster vaccinations to maintain a specific CTL response (prime-boost vaccination). In this extended phase I trial, 12 of 18 vaccinated patients had a CTL response, and mOS was 9.3 months compared to 8.4 months in 8 patients who received placebo, and those vaccinated with a CTL response had improved mOS compared to nonresponders (10.3 vs 5.4 months, *P* value not reported) [118]. No further studies of VXM01 in PDA have been published.

KIF20A

Kinesin family member 20A (KIF20A, also known as RAB6KIFL) is an intracellular trafficking protein that promotes movement of organelles, helps form the mitotic spindle, and plays a role in PDA carcinogenesis [119]. Inhibiting KIF20A decreases invasion and proliferation of PDA cells [120]. The KIF20A peptide is also an effective TAA as it can generate specific HLA-A2-restricted CTLs and is not overexpressed in normal adult tissues [121]. Asahara and colleagues conducted a phase I/II trial of 31 patients with advanced PDA and HLA-A*2402 positivity [122]. Twenty-nine patients received at least 4 doses of the KIF20A-66 peptide (KVYLRVRPLL, 1 mg or 3 mg dose on days 1, 8, 15, and 22 every 28 days) with IFA. The 3 mg dose was well tolerated, and a CTL response was detected in 70% of patients overall. mOS was 142 days which was improved compared to historical controls (9 patients with unmatched HLA, mOS 83 days, $P = 0.0468$).

Another phase I trial evaluated adding gemcitabine to the KIF20A peptide with IFA (administered at 3 dose levels, 0.5, 1, or 3 mg on days 1, 8, 15, and 22 every 28 days) in 9 patients with advanced PDA and positive for HLA-A*2402 [123]. There were no grade 3–4 adverse events related to KIF20A. Specific CTL responses determined by ELISpot were generated in 8 of 9 patients, and mOS was 173 days.

A phase II trial of the adjuvant cocktail OCV-C01 (containing KIF20A, VEGFR1, and VEGFR2 peptides) with gemcitabine in 30 patients with resected PDA showed a median disease-free survival (DFS) of 15.8 months, and mOS was not yet reached [124]. Another phase II study of OCV-C01 with IFA and gemcitabine in 68 patients with untreated PDA and unknown HLA status showed a mOS of 9.2 months [125]. These studies are still ongoing in Japan.

HSP

Heat shock proteins (HSPs) and their related heat shock response pathways play vital roles in pancreatic oncogenesis by chaperoning and stabilizing multiple oncoproteins [126]. Maki and colleagues conducted a phase I study of an autologous HSP vaccine (HSPPC-96) produced from tumor tissue in 10 patients with resected PDA [127]. Patients did not receive other adjuvant therapy and mOS was 2.2 years, but there was no correlation between development of an immune response and survival. No further studies of HSP vaccine in PDA have been reported.

Whole Tumor Cell Vaccines

Algenpantucel-L

Algenpantucel-L is a whole cell allogeneic vaccine which contains 2 irradiated human PCA cell lines (HAPa-1 and HAPa-2) genetically engineered to express the murine α [1, 3]-galactosyltransferase (αGT) gene [128]. Anti-αGT antibodies can stimulate NK cells via ADCC as well as the complement system and in theory can cause hyperacute rejection of PDA cells analogous to rejection of allogeneic solid organ transplants [129, 130]. Hardacre and colleagues enrolled 73 patients in an adjuvant phase II trial of algenpantucel-L followed by gemcitabine plus algenpantucel-L, chemoradiation with 5-FU plus algenpantucel-L, and finally more gemcitabine plus algenpantucel-L [128]. Two dose levels were studied (100 million cells–300 million cells per dose). The primary objective was DFS at 1 year which was seen in 62% of patients. mOS was not reached, and OS at 1 year was 86%. DFS at 1 year was significantly higher in patients who received the higher treatment dose compared to the lower dose (81% vs 51%, $P = 0.02$), and there was trend toward higher OS at 1 year (96% vs 79%, $P = 0.053$) [128]. Unfortunately, a phase III trial of adjuvant gemcitabine (with or without 5-FU chemoradiation) plus algenpantucel-L or chemotherapy/chemoradiation alone was a negative trial, results not formally published yet (NCT01072981). Another ongoing phase III study is using FOLFIRINOX or gemcitabine plus nab-paclitaxel with or without algenpantucel-L in borderline resectable or locally advanced unresectable PDA (PILLAR trial, NCT01836432).

GM-CSF (GVAX)

GVAX is a vaccine comprised of 2 allogeneic, lethally irradiated PDA cell lines reengineered with a plasmid vector to express GM-CSF [131, 132]. In early mouse studies, GM-CSF proved to be an important cytokine in generating an immune response in poorly immunogenic tumors by attracting APCs [133, 134]. In a phase I dose-escalation study of GVAX in PDA, 14 patients with resected PDA (stages I–III) received 1 dose of GVAX followed by chemoradiation with 5-FU then 3 monthly doses of GVAX [135]. There were no DLTs and DTH responses seen in 3 patients. DFS was 13 months, and 3 patients were still without disease at over 25 months [135]. Given these results, 60 patients with resected PDA were given the highest dose level (5×10^8 cells) and chemoradiation per the phase I schedule with the addition of a potential booster dose 6 months after the fourth GVAX dose [136]. In this phase II study, the treatment was again well tolerated, and no DLTs were reported. mDFS was 17.3 months (95% CI 14.6–22.8), and mOS was 24.8 months (95% CI 21.2–31.6). GVAX generated a mesothelin-specific CTL response in 88% of patients who were HLA-A0101 or HLA-A0201 positive (mesothelin-binding epitopes), and this response correlated with improved DFS [136]. Thus, the adjuvant GVAX plus chemoradiation regimen was safe and produced survival estimates on par with historical controls.

To augment the immunogenicity of GVAX, Laheru and colleagues added pre-vaccination cyclophosphamide (Cy) to deplete Tregs that normally suppress the immune response [137]. In a nonrandomized open-label pilot study, 30 patients with advanced PDA received GVAX (5×10^8 cells per dose) every 3 weeks for 6 doses, and an additional 20 patients received 250 mg/m^2 Cy IV 1 day prior to each GVAX dose. In both groups the treatment was well tolerated with few grade 3–4 adverse events: dehydration (2%), asthenia (4%), and fatigue (4%). mOS in the GVAX alone group was 2.3–4.3 months in the group who received Cy (cohorts were unmatched and not directly compared) [137]. In terms of mesothelin-specific CD8$^+$ T cell responses, 9 of 10 evaluable patients who received Cy had evidence of a response, while only 4 of 8 patients who received GVAX alone had a response. These results indicate that Cy administered prior to GVAX can augment the CTL response.

Another method to increase the immunogenicity of GVAX is to add a checkpoint inhibitor that blocks CTLA-4. Immune responses can be downregulated by the binding of CTLA-4 on the activated T cell surface with B7 antigens on APCs, resulting in apoptosis of the T cell. In a phase II study, Royal and colleagues first evaluated the use of ipilimumab (a fully humanized anti-CTLA-4 antibody that blocks the CTLA-4/B7 interaction) as a single agent in 27 patients with advanced PDA [138]. Ipilimumab was given as 3 mg/kg IV every 3 weeks, 4 doses per course with maximum 2 courses. Unfortunately, the treatment was not effective as there were no objective responses by RECIST criteria, and there were 3 reported immune-related grade 3–4 adverse events (colitis, hypophysitis, and encephalitis in 1 patient each) [138]. Prior preclinical work demonstrated potential synergy between CTLA-4 blockade and GM-CSF-based vaccines [139]. In a phase Ib trial, Le and colleagues randomized 30 patients with previously treated advanced PDA 1:1 to receive ipilimumab alone or ipilimumab plus GVAX. Ipilimumab was administered at 10 mg/kg IV based on successful studies in advanced melanoma, given every 3 weeks for 4 doses followed by maintenance dosing every 12 weeks (GVAX was administered prior to ipilimumab infusions in the combination arm) [140–142]. mOS was longer in the combination arm, although not statistically significant (5.7 vs 3.6 months, HR 0.51, 95% CI 0.23–1.08, $P = 0.072$) [142]. Among 19 analyzable patients who were either HLA-A1 or HLA-A2 positive, 14 patients had mesothelin-specific CTL responses by ELISpot. Patients with OS greater than 4.3 months had significant increases in specific CTL responses relative to baseline ($P = 0.014$), suggesting that CTL response correlates with improved survival. There were several grade 3–4 immune-related adverse events (rash, colitis (2), Guillain-Barre syndrome, pneumonitis, and nephritis) [142]. This study showed that addition of a checkpoint inhibitor could augment the immune response and potentially improve survival.

Finally, Le and colleagues studied GVAX and Cy with the addition of a live-attenuated *Listeria monocytogenes* vaccine reengineered to secrete mesothelin (CRS-207) [143–145]. CRS-207 stimulates both the innate and adaptive immune system by turning on T cells and NK cells [145]. The combination of GVAX and CRS-207 uses a heterologous prime-boost strategy to increase the immune response. Ninety patients with previously treated mPDA were randomized 2:1 to receive 2 doses of GVAX and Cy followed by 4 doses of CRS-207 or to receive 6 doses of

GVAX and Cy every 3 weeks. In patients who received at least 3 doses of vaccine, mOS was significantly longer in the CRS-207 arm (9.7 vs 4.6 months, HR 0.53, 95% CI 0.29–0.96, $P = 0.02$). Notable adverse events in the CRS-207 arm included lymphopenia (8%), increased AST (5%), fatigue (5%), and pyrexia (5%). An increase in mesothelin-specific CTL response in HLA-A1-, HLA-A2-, or HLA-A3-positive patients was seen only in the CRS-207 arm (compared to baseline CTL levels, $P = 0.042$). Generation of a mesothelin-specific CTL response again correlated with improved survival [143]. An ongoing trial of GVAX, Cy, CRS-207, and nivolumab is ongoing (NCT02243371, see section on ongoing vaccine clinical trials below).

Ongoing Vaccine Clinical Trials

Randomized Phase II Study of the Efficacy and Immune Response of GVAX Pancreas (with Cyclophosphamide) and CRS-207 with or Without Nivolumab in Patients with Previously Treated Metastatic Pancreatic Adenocarcinoma (STELLAR, NCT02243371)

Given the prior experiences of combining GVAX with checkpoint inhibition (anti-CTLA-4), there is ongoing interest in combining GVAX with other checkpoint inhibitors such as nivolumab, a fully humanized IgG4 anti-PD-1 monoclonal antibody. Interestingly, patients with PDA tumors with high PD-L1 expression have fewer TILs and a significantly worse prognosis than patients with low PD-L1 PDA tumors [146]. However, prior studies of single-agent checkpoint inhibitors (anti-CTLA-4 and anti-PD-L1 antibodies) have not shown clinical efficacy in PDA [5, 138]. PDA tumors exposed to GVAX have increased TILs and an upregulated immunosuppressive microenvironment including increased PD-L1 expression [6, 147]. Thus, it may be possible to transform a previously "non-immunogenic" PDA tumor to one that is susceptible to the immune system.

Building on this foundation with the prime-boost vaccination protocol of GVAX followed by CRS-207, Le and colleagues plan to enroll 108 patients with mPDA who have failed only 1 line of prior therapy for metastatic disease in phase II study [148]. Patients are randomized 1:1 to receive nivolumab (3 mg/kg IV day 1, cycles 1–6), Cy (200 mg/m^2 IV day 1, cycles 1–2), GVAX (5×10^8 cells day 2, cycles 1–2), and CRS-207 (1×10^9 day 2, cycles 3–6) or the same regimen without nivolumab. Key inclusion criteria are Eastern Cooperative Oncology Group (ECOG) performance status (PS) of 0–1, measurable disease, and adequate bone marrow and organ function. Patients are excluded if they have penicillin or sulfa allergies, ascites, significant effusions, autoimmune disease, recent thrombosis within 2 months, or prior treatment with GVAX, CRS-207, or checkpoint inhibitors. The primary endpoint is OS, and secondary endpoints include safety, response by tumor measurement and CA19-9 levels, and correlation of survival and clinical responses with specific CTL responses.

Pancreatic Tumor Cell Vaccine (GVAX), Low-Dose Cyclophosphamide, Fractionated Stereotactic Body Radiation Therapy (SBRT), and FOLFIRINOX Chemotherapy in Patients with Resected Adenocarcinoma of the Pancreas (NCT01595321)

This pilot adjuvant study has enrolled 19 patients with resected PDA. The first 6 patients will receive 6.6 gray (Gy) of SBRT over 5 days within 6–10 weeks of surgery followed by 6 cycles of FOLFIRINOX at least 14 days after SBRT. The other patients will receive 1 dose of GVAX with Cy (200 mg/m^2) after surgery followed by SBRT and FOLFIRINOX and then up to 4 additional doses of GVAX with Cy. The primary objective is safety and tolerability of this regimen, and the secondary objectives are to determine survival (OS, DFS, and distant metastases-free survival) and to correlate progression with mesothelin-specific CTL responses. Patients must have an ECOG PS of 0–1, age 18–76, be within 10 weeks of surgical resection, and have adequate organ function. Patients are excluded if they have metastatic disease or have received other anticancer treatment other than surgery within 28 days.

Study with CY, Pembrolizumab, GVAX, and SBRT in Patients with Locally Advanced Pancreatic Cancer (NCT02648282)

This second-line phase II study plans to enroll 54 patients with locally advanced PDA who have already received at least 4 cycles of mFOLFIRINOX or gemcitabine plus nab-paclitaxel (last dose 2–5 weeks prior to study enrollment). All patients receive GVAX with Cy, pembrolizumab (anti-PD-1 antibody, 200 mg IV over 30 min), and SBRT (6.6 Gy over 5 days). Patients must have an ECOG PS of 0–1, no metastatic disease, no autoimmune disease, and no prior treatment with checkpoint inhibitors. The primary objective is to determine the distant metastasis-free survival, and secondary objectives are to determine OS, local progression-free survival (PFS), and immune-related toxicities. This study exploits the abscopal effect, in which radiation stimulates the release of TAAs that activate APCs, and potential synergism with checkpoint inhibitors by further enhancing of the T cell response [149].

A Phase II, Multicenter Study of FOLFIRINOX Followed by Ipilimumab with Allogenic GM-CSF Transfected Pancreatic Tumor Vaccine in the Treatment of Metastatic Pancreatic Cancer (NCT01896869)

This phase II study aims to enroll 92 patients with mPDA with SD after 8–12 doses of FOLFIRINOX and randomize them 1:1 to receive ipilimumab (3 mg/kg) and GVAX or to continue FOLFIRINOX (which can be modified according to the patient's tolerability to 5-FU, capecitabine, FOLFOX, FOLFIRI, or FOLFIRINOX every 21 days). Patients must have an ECOG PS of 0–1 and adequate organ function, and they cannot have been off FOLFIRINOX for more than 70 days or have received prior immunotherapy or chemotherapy (other than FOLFIRINOX or adjuvant therapy). The primary objective is to determine OS; secondary endpoints include adverse events, PFS, immune-related PFS (irPFS), objective response rate, duration of response, and CA19-9 kinetics. This trial will help establish GVAX/anti-CTLA-4 as an effective maintenance regimen relative to conventional cytotoxic chemotherapy.

Dendritic Cell Vaccine and Chemotherapy for Patients with Pancreatic Cancer (PancVax, NCT02548169)

This phase I study with an estimated enrollment of 20 PDA patients (resectable, borderline, locally advanced, or metastatic) aims to establish safety of combining an antigen-loaded DC vaccine with standard of care chemotherapy (FOLFIRINOX or gemcitabine plus nab-paclitaxel). PancVax is an autologous DC vaccine in which the patient's monocytes are cultured with GM-CSF and IFNα and loaded with mesothelin peptides. Patients receive 4 doses of the DC vaccine every 2 weeks with concurrent chemotherapy. Secondary endpoints include response rates, OS, PFS, surgical conversion rate at 6 months (if applicable), measurement of T cell responses, and quality of life assessment. Patients must have an ECOG PS of 0–2, adequate organ function, and cannot be on immunosuppressive medications or have autoimmune disease. This pilot trial will be helpful in establishing tolerability of concurrent DC vaccination and chemotherapy.

Inovio TRT-001: Telomerase DNA Immunotherapy in Breast, Lung, and Pancreatic Cancers (NCT02327468)

As described above, hTERT is frequently expressed on PDA cells and can be recognized by CTLs via MHCs (see description of telomerase in vaccine targets section). Vonderheide and colleagues are enrolling 54 patients with resected cancers in a dose-escalation 3 + 3 design of an hTERT DNA plasmid vaccine (INO-1400) administered via electroporation with or without an IL-12 plasmid (INO-9012) [150]. Electroporation allows the incorporation of exogenous DNA in vivo through creation of a temporary electric field that allows transmission of large molecules into the cell [151, 152]. Adding IL-12 to hTERT increased immune responses in preclinical mouse models [153]. In this study, patients receive 4 monthly treatments. Allowed tumor types include breast, lung, pancreatic, head and neck, ovarian, colorectal, gastroesophageal, or hepatocellular carcinoma.

A Phase I/II Trial of the PD-L1 Inhibitor, Durvalumab (MEDI4736) plus PANVAC in Combination with Maintenance Chemotherapy for Patients with Metastatic Colorectal or Pancreatic Adenocarcinoma

Finally, this study aims to determine the safety of combining a PD-L1 inhibitor (durvalumab) with PANVAC (see section on MUC-1 in vaccine targets above) and the recommended phase II dose of durvalumab in patients with mPDA or mCRC who have SD on first-line therapy. The addition of a different anti-PD-L1 antibody (atezolizumab) in combination with FOLFOX and bevacizumab in mCRC patients has previously been shown to be well tolerated [154]. The phase II portion seeks to determine the PFS rate at 8.5 months in mCRC (50% in the CAIRO3 study) and PFS rate at 4 months in mPDA (second-line PFS typically around 50%) [155, 156]. Patients with mPDA will receive capecitabine 1000 mg PO BID Monday–Friday, and patients with mCRC will also receive bevacizumab 5 mg/kg IV every 2 weeks. The dose of durvalumab is 750 mg IV every 2 weeks, and if 0–1 of 6 patients or 2 of 12 patients in phase I portion have a DLT, then 750 mg will be the recommend phase II dose. The study plans to enroll 26 mPDA and 26 mCRC patients in the phase II portion. Patients receive PANVAC-V (vaccinia, 2×10^8 plaque-forming units (PFUs) on week 1 then PANVAC-F (fowlpox, 1×10^9 PFUs) every 2 weeks for four doses starting week 3, then every 4 weeks for 4 doses. Durvalumab is also started on week 3 and continues every 2 weeks through week 52. Patients must have SD on first-line therapy for metastatic disease, measurable disease that is amenable to serial biopsies, and adequate organ function. Patients with known central nervous system metastases are excluded. This study will provide meaningful data not only regarding the combination of PD-L1 inhibition and PANVAC but also its tolerability and efficacy when administered with maintenance chemotherapy.

Conclusions

PDA remains a devastating illness with few effective treatment options, and numerous attempts have been made at adding vaccine therapy to the armamentarium. Several excellent vaccine targets exist, notably CEA, MUC-1, and telomerase, but generating an immune response that translates into a clinical response has been fraught with difficulty. These shortfalls have persisted despite the addition of immunomodulating drugs designed to augment the immune response, such as IFA, GM-CSF, IL-2, IL-12, IFNα, Cy, and conventional chemotherapy. The GVAX vaccine has also been extensively studied and has shown activity even in patients with treatment-refractory mPDA. More recent studies that integrate checkpoint inhibition with priming using vaccine therapy hold promise and are still ongoing. The optimal sequence of chemotherapy, radiation therapy, checkpoint inhibition, and vaccine administration remains to be determined.

References

1. Cancer of the Pancreas—SEER Stat Fact Sheets. SEER database. 2016. http://seer.cancer.gov/statfacts/html/pancreas.html. Accessed 8 Jul 2016.
2. Neoptolemos JP, Palmer D, Ghaneh P, Valle JW, Cunningham D, Wadsley J, et al. ESPAC-4: a multicenter, international, open-label randomized controlled phase III trial of adjuvant combination chemotherapy of gemcitabine and capecitabine versus monotherapy gemcitabine in patients with resected pancreatic ductal adenocarcinoma. J Clin Oncol. 2016;34(suppl):abstr LBA4006.
3. Von Hoff DD, Ervin T, Arena FP, et al. Increased survival in pancreatic cancer with nab-paclitaxel plus gemcitabine. N Engl J Med. 2013;369(18):1691–703.
4. Conroy T, Desseigne F, Ychou M, et al. FOLFIRINOX versus gemcitabine for metastatic pancreatic cancer. N Engl J Med. 2011;364(19):1817–25.
5. Brahmer JR, Tykodi SS, Chow LQ, et al. Safety and activity of anti-PD-L1 antibody in patients with advanced cancer. N Engl J Med. 2012;366(26):2455–65.
6. Lutz ER, AA W, Bigelow E, et al. Immunotherapy converts nonimmunogenic pancreatic tumors into immunogenic foci of immune regulation. Cancer Immunol Res. 2014;2(7):616–31.
7. Rosenberg SA, Yannelli JR, Yang JC, et al. Treatment of patients with metastatic melanoma with autologous tumor-infiltrating lymphocytes and interleukin 2. J Natl Cancer Inst. 1994;86(15):1159–66.
8. Atkins MB, Kunkel L, Sznol M, Rosenberg SA. High-dose recombinant interleukin-2 therapy in patients with metastatic melanoma: long-term survival update. Cancer J Sci Am. 2000;6(Suppl 1):S11–4.
9. Fyfe G, Fisher RI, Rosenberg SA, Sznol M, Parkinson DR, Louie AC. Results of treatment of 255 patients with metastatic renal cell carcinoma who received high-dose recombinant interleukin-2 therapy. J Clin Oncol. 1995;13(3):688–96.
10. Dutcher JP, Fisher RI, Weiss G, et al. Outpatient subcutaneous interleukin-2 and interferon-alpha for metastatic renal cell cancer: five-year follow-up of the cytokine working group study. Cancer J Sci Am. 1997;3(3):157–62.
11. Lamm DL, Blumenstein BA, Crissman JD, et al. Maintenance bacillus Calmette-Guerin immunotherapy for recurrent TA, T1 and carcinoma in situ transitional cell carcinoma of the bladder: a randomized southwest oncology group study. J Urol. 2000;163(4):1124–9.
12. Caraux J, Weigle WO. Anti-idiotype antibody-dependent cell-mediated cytotoxicity (ADCC) against idiotype-bearing cells. Cell Immunol. 1983;78(1):23–32.
13. Jerne NK. Towards a network theory of the immune system. Ann Immunol (Paris). 1974;125C(1-2):373–89.
14. Laheru DA, Jaffee EM. Potential role of tumor vaccines in GI malignancies. Oncology (Williston Park). 2000;14(2):245–56. discussion 259-260, 265
15. Levy B, Deeken JF, Holt G, Marshall JL. Immunologic therapies for gastrointestinal cancers. Clin Colorectal Cancer. 2005;5(1):37–49.
16. McDonnell WM, Askari FK. DNA vaccines. N Engl J Med. 1996;334(1):42–5.
17. Kaufman H, Schlom J, Kantor J. A recombinant vaccinia virus expressing human carcinoembryonic antigen (CEA). Int J Cancer. 1991;48(6):900–7.
18. Kajihara M, Takakura K, Kanai T, et al. Advances in inducing adaptive immunity using cell-based cancer vaccines: clinical applications in pancreatic cancer. World J Gastroenterol. 2016;22(18):4446–58.
19. Kanodia S, Kast WM. Peptide-based vaccines for cancer: realizing their potential. Expert Rev Vaccines. 2008;7(10):1533–45.
20. Waldmann TA. Immunotherapy: past, present and future. Nat Med. 2003;9(3):269–77.
21. Koido S, Hara E, Homma S, et al. Dendritic/pancreatic carcinoma fusions for clinical use: comparative functional analysis of healthy- versus patient-derived fusions. Clin Immunol. 2010;135(3):384–400.
22. Steinman RM, Banchereau J. Taking dendritic cells into medicine. Nature. 2007;449(7161):419–26.

23. Palena C, Zhu M, Schlom J, Tsang KY. Human B cells that hyperexpress a triad of costimulatory molecules via avipox-vector infection: an alternative source of efficient antigen-presenting cells. Blood. 2004;104(1):192–9.
24. Gabrilovich D. Mechanisms and functional significance of tumour-induced dendritic-cell defects. Nat Rev Immunol. 2004;4(12):941–52.
25. Kortylewski M, Kujawski M, Wang T, et al. Inhibiting Stat3 signaling in the hematopoietic system elicits multicomponent antitumor immunity. Nat Med. 2005;11(12):1314–21.
26. Ghiringhelli F, Puig PE, Roux S, et al. Tumor cells convert immature myeloid dendritic cells into TGF-beta-secreting cells inducing CD4+CD25+ regulatory T cell proliferation. J Exp Med. 2005;202(7):919–29.
27. Aspord C, Pedroza-Gonzalez A, Gallegos M, et al. Breast cancer instructs dendritic cells to prime interleukin 13-secreting CD4+ T cells that facilitate tumor development. J Exp Med. 2007;204(5):1037–47.
28. Heyderman E, Larkin SE, O'Donnell PJ, et al. Epithelial markers in pancreatic carcinoma: immunoperoxidase localisation of DD9, CEA, EMA and CAM 5.2. J Clin Pathol. 1990;43(6):448–52.
29. Berinstein NL. Carcinoembryonic antigen as a target for therapeutic anticancer vaccines: a review. J Clin Oncol. 2002;20(8):2197–207.
30. Thompson J, Zimmermann W. The carcinoembryonic antigen gene family: structure, expression and evolution. Tumour Biol. 1988;9(2-3):63–83.
31. Gold P, Goldenberg N. The carcinoembryonic antigen (CEA): past, present, and future. McGill J Med. 1997;3:46–66.
32. Benchimol S, Fuks A, Jothy S, Beauchemin N, Shirota K, Stanners CP. Carcinoembryonic antigen, a human tumor marker, functions as an intercellular adhesion molecule. Cell. 1989;57(2):327–34.
33. Zaremba S, Barzaga E, Zhu M, Soares N, Tsang KY, Schlom J. Identification of an enhancer agonist cytotoxic T lymphocyte peptide from human carcinoembryonic antigen. Cancer Res. 1997;57(20):4570–7.
34. Geynisman DM, Zha Y, Kunnavakkam R, et al. A randomized phase I study of modified carcinoembryonic antigen (CEA) peptide (CAP1-6D)/montanide/GM-CSF vaccine (CEA-vac) in patients (pts) with pancreatic adenocarcinoma (PC). J Clin Oncol. 2012;30(suppl):abstr 2561.
35. Tsang KY, Zaremba S, Nieroda CA, Zhu MZ, Hamilton JM, Schlom J. Generation of human cytotoxic T cells specific for human carcinoembryonic antigen epitopes from patients immunized with recombinant vaccinia-CEA vaccine. J Natl Cancer Inst. 1995;87(13):982–90.
36. Zhu MZ, Marshall J, Cole D, Schlom J, Tsang KY. Specific cytolytic T-cell responses to human CEA from patients immunized with recombinant avipox-CEA vaccine. Clin Cancer Res. 2000;6(1):24–33.
37. Horig H, Lee DS, Conkright W, et al. Phase I clinical trial of a recombinant canarypox virus (ALVAC) vaccine expressing human carcinoembryonic antigen and the B7.1 co-stimulatory molecule. Cancer Immunol Immunother. 2000;49(9):504–14.
38. Marshall JL, Hawkins MJ, Tsang KY, et al. Phase I study in cancer patients of a replication-defective avipox recombinant vaccine that expresses human carcinoembryonic antigen. J Clin Oncol. 1999;17(1):332–7.
39. von Mehren M, Arlen P, Tsang KY, et al. Pilot study of a dual gene recombinant avipox vaccine containing both carcinoembryonic antigen (CEA) and B7.1 transgenes in patients with recurrent CEA-expressing adenocarcinomas. Clin Cancer Res. 2000;6(6):2219–28.
40. Chen L, Ashe S, Brady WA, et al. Costimulation of antitumor immunity by the B7 counter-receptor for the T lymphocyte molecules CD28 and CTLA-4. Cell. 1992;71(7):1093–102.
41. von Mehren M, Arlen P, Gulley J, et al. The influence of granulocyte macrophage colony-stimulating factor and prior chemotherapy on the immunological response to a vaccine (ALVAC-CEA B7.1) in patients with metastatic carcinoma. Clin Cancer Res. 2001;7(5):1181–91.
42. Finn OJ, Jerome KR, Henderson RA, et al. MUC-1 epithelial tumor mucin-based immunity and cancer vaccines. Immunol Rev. 1995;145:61–89.

43. Dotan E, Alpaugh RK, Ruth K, et al. Prognostic significance of MUC-1 in circulating tumor cells in patients with metastatic pancreatic adenocarcinoma. Pancreas. 2016;45(8):1131–5.
44. Goydos JS, Elder E, Whiteside TL, Finn OJ, Lotze MT. A phase I trial of a synthetic mucin peptide vaccine. Induction of specific immune reactivity in patients with adenocarcinoma. J Surg Res. 1996;63(1):298–304.
45. Lepisto AJ, Moser AJ, Zeh H, et al. A phase I/II study of a MUC1 peptide pulsed autologous dendritic cell vaccine as adjuvant therapy in patients with resected pancreatic and biliary tumors. Cancer Ther. 2008;6(B):955–64.
46. Kaufman HL, Kim-Schulze S, Manson K, et al. Poxvirus-based vaccine therapy for patients with advanced pancreatic cancer. J Transl Med. 2007;5:60.
47. Hodge JW, Sabzevari H, Yafal AG, Gritz L, Lorenz MG, Schlom J. A triad of costimulatory molecules synergize to amplify T-cell activation. Cancer Res. 1999;59(22):5800–7.
48. Sedegah M, Jones TR, Kaur M, et al. Boosting with recombinant vaccinia increases immunogenicity and protective efficacy of malaria DNA vaccine. Proc Natl Acad Sci U S A. 1998;95(13):7648–53.
49. Kaufman HL, Wang W, Manola J, et al. Phase II randomized study of vaccine treatment of advanced prostate cancer (E7897): a trial of the eastern cooperative oncology group. J Clin Oncol. 2004;22(11):2122–32.
50. Goitre L, Trapani E, Trabalzini L, Retta SF. The Ras superfamily of small GTPases: the unlocked secrets. Methods Mol Biol. 2014;1120:1–18.
51. Bryant KL, Mancias JD, Kimmelman AC, Der CJKRAS. Feeding pancreatic cancer proliferation. Trends Biochem Sci. 2014;39(2):91–100.
52. Van Cutsem E, Lenz HJ, Kohne CH, et al. Fluorouracil, leucovorin, and irinotecan plus cetuximab treatment and RAS mutations in colorectal cancer. J Clin Oncol. 2015;33(7):692–700.
53. Douillard JY, Siena S, Cassidy J, et al. Final results from PRIME: randomized phase III study of panitumumab with FOLFOX4 for first-line treatment of metastatic colorectal cancer. Ann Oncol. 2014;25(7):1346–55.
54. Cremolini C, Loupakis F, Antoniotti C, et al. FOLFOXIRI plus bevacizumab versus FOLFIRI plus bevacizumab as first-line treatment of patients with metastatic colorectal cancer: updated overall survival and molecular subgroup analyses of the open-label, phase 3 TRIBE study. Lancet Oncol. 2015;16(13):1306–15.
55. Witkiewicz AK, McMillan EA, Balaji U, et al. Whole-exome sequencing of pancreatic cancer defines genetic diversity and therapeutic targets. Nat Commun. 2015;6:6744.
56. Cerny WL, Mangold KA, Scarpelli DG. K-ras mutation is an early event in pancreatic duct carcinogenesis in the Syrian golden hamster. Cancer Res. 1992;52(16):4507–13.
57. Furukawa T, Sunamura M, Horii A. Molecular mechanisms of pancreatic carcinogenesis. Cancer Sci. 2006;97(1):1–7.
58. Eser S, Schnieke A, Schneider G, Saur D. Oncogenic KRAS signalling in pancreatic cancer. Br J Cancer. 2014;111(5):817–22.
59. Cox AD, Fesik SW, Kimmelman AC, Luo J, Der CJ. Drugging the undruggable RAS: mission possible? Nat Rev Drug Discov. 2014;13(11):828–51.
60. Lu S, Jang H, Gu S, Zhang J, Nussinov R. Drugging Ras GTPase: a comprehensive mechanistic and signaling structural view. Chem Soc Rev. 2016;45:4929–52.
61. Gjertsen MK, Bakka A, Breivik J, et al. Vaccination with mutant RAS peptides and induction of T-cell responsiveness in pancreatic carcinoma patients carrying the corresponding RAS mutation. Lancet. 1995;346(8987):1399–400.
62. Gjertsen MK, Bakka A, Breivik J, et al. Ex vivo ras peptide vaccination in patients with advanced pancreatic cancer: results of a phase I/II study. Int J Cancer. 1996;65(4):450–3.
63. Gjertsen MK, Bjorheim J, Saeterdal I, Myklebust J, Gaudernack G. Cytotoxic CD4+ and CD8+ T lymphocytes, generated by mutant p21-ras (12Val) peptide vaccination of a patient, recognize 12Val-dependent nested epitopes present within the vaccine peptide and kill autologous tumour cells carrying this mutation. Int J Cancer. 1997;72(5):784–90.

64. Gjertsen MK, Buanes T, Rosseland AR, et al. Intradermal ras peptide vaccination with granulocyte-macrophage colony-stimulating factor as adjuvant: clinical and immunological responses in patients with pancreatic adenocarcinoma. Int J Cancer. 2001;92(3):441–50.
65. Weden S, Klemp M, Gladhaug IP, et al. Long-term follow-up of patients with resected pancreatic cancer following vaccination against mutant K-ras. Int J Cancer. 2011;128(5):1120–8.
66. Toubaji A, Achtar M, Provenzano M, et al. Pilot study of mutant ras peptide-based vaccine as an adjuvant treatment in pancreatic and colorectal cancers. Cancer Immunol Immunother. 2008;57(9):1413–20.
67. Rahma OE, Hamilton JM, Wojtowicz M, et al. The immunological and clinical effects of mutated ras peptide vaccine in combination with IL-2, GM-CSF, or both in patients with solid tumors. J Transl Med. 2014;12:55.
68. Lotem M, Shiloni E, Pappo I, et al. Interleukin-2 improves tumour response to DNP-modified autologous vaccine for the treatment of metastatic malignant melanoma. Br J Cancer. 2004;90(4):773–80.
69. Rosenberg SA, Yang JC, Schwartzentruber DJ, et al. Immunologic and therapeutic evaluation of a synthetic peptide vaccine for the treatment of patients with metastatic melanoma. Nat Med. 1998;4(3):321–7.
70. Dudley ME, Wunderlich JR, Robbins PF, et al. Cancer regression and autoimmunity in patients after clonal repopulation with antitumor lymphocytes. Science. 2002;298(5594):850–4.
71. Abou-Alfa GK, Chapman PB, Feilchenfeldt J, et al. Targeting mutated K-ras in pancreatic adenocarcinoma using an adjuvant vaccine. Am J Clin Oncol. 2011;34(3):321–5.
72. Carbone DP, Ciernik IF, Kelley MJ, et al. Immunization with mutant p53- and K-ras-derived peptides in cancer patients: immune response and clinical outcome. J Clin Oncol. 2005;23(22):5099–107.
73. Palmer DH, Dueland S, Valle JW, Otterhaug T, Eriksen JA, Muller H, et al. A prospective, single-arm, phase I/II trial of ras peptide vaccine G01/GM-CSF and gemcitabine as adjuvant therapy for patients with resected pancreatic adenocarcinoma. J Clin Oncol. 2015;33(Suppl):Abstr 4121.
74. Hartley ML, Bade NA, Prins PA, Ampie L, Marshall JL. Pancreatic cancer, treatment options, and GI-4000. Hum Vaccin Immunother. 2014;10(11):3347–53.
75. Cohn A, Morse MA, O'Neil B, Bellgrau D, Duke RC, Franzusoff AJ, et al. Treatment of Ras mutation-bearing solid tumors using whole recombinant S. cerevisiae yeast expressing mutated Ras: preliminary safety and immunogenicity results from a phase 1 trial. J Clin Oncol. 2005;16S(Suppl):2571.
76. Muscarella P, Wilfong LS, Ross SB, Richards DA, Raynov J, Fisher WE, et al. A randomized, placebo-controlled, double blind, multicenter phase II adjuvant trial of the efficacy, immunogenicity, and safety of GI-4000 plus gem versus gem alone in patients with resected pancreas cancer with activating RAS mutations/survival and immunology analysis of the R1 subgroup. J Clin Oncol. 2012;30(Suppl):Abstr e14501.
77. Soussi T, Beroud C. Assessing TP53 status in human tumours to evaluate clinical outcome. Nat Rev Cancer. 2001;1(3):233–40.
78. Yachida S, Iacobuzio-Donahue CA. Evolution and dynamics of pancreatic cancer progression. Oncogene. 2013;32(45):5253–60.
79. Vogelstein B, Lane D, Levine AJ. Surfing the p53 network. Nature. 2000;408(6810):307–10.
80. Chai K, Ai YQ, Jiang LW. Phase II study of dendritic cell vaccination combinated with recombinant adenovirus-p53 in treatment of patients with advanced pancreatic carcinoma. J Clin Oncol. 2013;31(Suppl):Abstr 3049.
81. Braunstein GD, Vaitukaitis JL, Carbone PP, Ross GT. Ectopic production of human chorionic gonadotrophin by neoplasms. Ann Intern Med. 1973;78(1):39–45.
82. Louhimo J, Nordling S, Alfthan H, von Boguslawski K, Stenman UH, Haglund C. Specific staining of human chorionic gonadotropin beta in benign and malignant gastrointestinal tissues with monoclonal antibodies. Histopathology. 2001;38(5):418–24.

83. Iversen P, Yoshihara P, Moulton H, et al. Active beta-hCG specific immunotherapy in patients with advanced pancreatic cancer. Proc Am Soc Clin Oncol. 2002;23(25a):Abstract #96.
84. Shin S, Sung BJ, Cho YS, et al. An anti-apoptotic protein human survivin is a direct inhibitor of caspase-3 and -7. Biochemistry. 2001;40(4):1117–23.
85. Satoh K, Kaneko K, Hirota M, Masamune A, Satoh A, Shimosegawa T. Expression of survivin is correlated with cancer cell apoptosis and is involved in the development of human pancreatic duct cell tumors. Cancer. 2001;92(2):271–8.
86. Ambrosini G, Adida C, Altieri DC. A novel anti-apoptosis gene, survivin, expressed in cancer and lymphoma. Nat Med. 1997;3(8):917–21.
87. Kameshima H, Tsuruma T, Torigoe T, et al. Immunogenic enhancement and clinical effect by type-I interferon of anti-apoptotic protein, survivin-derived peptide vaccine, in advanced colorectal cancer patients. Cancer Sci. 2011;102(6):1181–7.
88. Kameshima H, Tsuruma T, Kutomi G, et al. Immunotherapeutic benefit of alpha-interferon (IFNalpha) in survivin2B-derived peptide vaccination for advanced pancreatic cancer patients. Cancer Sci. 2013;104(1):124–9.
89. Gigante M, Mandic M, Wesa AK, et al. Interferon-alpha (IFN-alpha)-conditioned DC preferentially stimulate type-1 and limit Treg-type in vitro T-cell responses from RCC patients. J Immunother. 2008;31(3):254–62.
90. Monstein HJ, Ohlsson B, Axelson J. Differential expression of gastrin, cholecystokinin-a and cholecystokinin-B receptor mRNA in human pancreatic cancer cell lines. Scand J Gastroenterol. 2001;36(7):738–43.
91. Brett BTKK, Savage K, et al. The effect of antibodies raised against Gastrimmune on the proliferation of human pancreatic carcinoma cell lines. Gut. 1999;44(Suppl 1):W190.
92. Brett BT, Smith SC, Bouvier CV, et al. Phase II study of anti-gastrin-17 antibodies, raised to G17DT, in advanced pancreatic cancer. J Clin Oncol. 2002;20(20):4225–31.
93. Gilliam AD, Broome P, Topuzov EG, et al. An international multicenter randomized controlled trial of G17DT in patients with pancreatic cancer. Pancreas. 2012;41(3):374–9.
94. Vasef MA, Ross JS, Cohen MB. Telomerase activity in human solid tumors. Diagnostic utility and clinical applications. Am J Clin Pathol. 1999;112(1 Suppl 1):S68–75.
95. Hiyama E, Kodama T, Shinbara K, et al. Telomerase activity is detected in pancreatic cancer but not in benign tumors. Cancer Res. 1997;57(2):326–31.
96. Bernhardt SL, Gjertsen MK, Trachsel S, et al. Telomerase peptide vaccination of patients with non-resectable pancreatic cancer: a dose escalating phase I/II study. Br J Cancer. 2006;95(11):1474–82.
97. Middleton G, Silcocks P, Cox T, et al. Gemcitabine and capecitabine with or without telomerase peptide vaccine GV1001 in patients with locally advanced or metastatic pancreatic cancer (TeloVac): an open-label, randomised, phase 3 trial. Lancet Oncol. 2014;15(8):829–40.
98. Gunturu KS, Rossi GR, Saif MW. Immunotherapy updates in pancreatic cancer: are we there yet? Ther Adv Med Oncol. 2013;5(1):81–9.
99. Huff V. Wilms' tumours: about tumour suppressor genes, an oncogene and a chameleon gene. Nat Rev Cancer. 2011;11(2):111–21.
100. Oji Y, Nakamori S, Fujikawa M, et al. Overexpression of the Wilms' tumor gene WT1 in pancreatic ductal adenocarcinoma. Cancer Sci. 2004;95(7):583–7.
101. Oka Y, Elisseeva OA, Tsuboi A, et al. Human cytotoxic T-lymphocyte responses specific for peptides of the wild-type Wilms' tumor gene (WT1) product. Immunogenetics. 2000;51(2):99–107.
102. Oka Y, Tsuboi A, Taguchi T, et al. Induction of WT1 (Wilms' tumor gene)-specific cytotoxic T lymphocytes by WT1 peptide vaccine and the resultant cancer regression. Proc Natl Acad Sci U S A. 2004;101(38):13885–90.
103. Kaida M, Morita-Hoshi Y, Soeda A, et al. Phase 1 trial of Wilms tumor 1 (WT1) peptide vaccine and gemcitabine combination therapy in patients with advanced pancreatic or biliary tract cancer. J Immunother. 2011;34(1):92–9.
104. Takahara A, Koido S, Ito M, et al. Gemcitabine enhances Wilms' tumor gene WT1 expression and sensitizes human pancreatic cancer cells with WT1-specific T-cell-mediated antitumor immune response. Cancer Immunol Immunother. 2011;60(9):1289–97.

105. Nishida S, Koido S, Takeda Y, et al. Wilms tumor gene (WT1) peptide-based cancer vaccine combined with gemcitabine for patients with advanced pancreatic cancer. J Immunother. 2014;37(2):105–14.
106. Koido S, Homma S, Okamoto M, et al. Treatment with chemotherapy and dendritic cells pulsed with multiple Wilms' tumor 1 (WT1)-specific MHC class I/II-restricted epitopes for pancreatic cancer. Clin Cancer Res. 2014;20(16):4228–39.
107. Takakura K, Koido S, Kan S, et al. Prognostic markers for patient outcome following vaccination with multiple MHC class I/II-restricted WT1 peptide-pulsed dendritic cells plus chemotherapy for pancreatic cancer. Anticancer Res. 2015;35(1):555–62.
108. Mayanagi S, Kitago M, Sakurai T, et al. Phase I pilot study of Wilms tumor gene 1 peptide-pulsed dendritic cell vaccination combined with gemcitabine in pancreatic cancer. Cancer Sci. 2015;106(4):397–406.
109. Itakura J, Ishiwata T, Friess H, et al. Enhanced expression of vascular endothelial growth factor in human pancreatic cancer correlates with local disease progression. Clin Cancer Res. 1997;3(8):1309–16.
110. Itakura J, Ishiwata T, Shen B, Kornmann M, Korc M. Concomitant over-expression of vascular endothelial growth factor and its receptors in pancreatic cancer. Int J Cancer. 2000;85(1):27–34.
111. Seo Y, Baba H, Fukuda T, Takashima M, Sugimachi K. High expression of vascular endothelial growth factor is associated with liver metastasis and a poor prognosis for patients with ductal pancreatic adenocarcinoma. Cancer. 2000;88(10):2239–45.
112. Miyazawa M, Ohsawa R, Tsunoda T, et al. Phase I clinical trial using peptide vaccine for human vascular endothelial growth factor receptor 2 in combination with gemcitabine for patients with advanced pancreatic cancer. Cancer Sci. 2010;101(2):433–9.
113. Yamaue H, Tsunoda T, Tani M, et al. Randomized phase II/III clinical trial of elpamotide for patients with advanced pancreatic cancer: PEGASUS-PC study. Cancer Sci. 2015;106(7):883–90.
114. Niethammer AG, Lubenau H, Mikus G, et al. Double-blind, placebo-controlled first in human study to investigate an oral vaccine aimed to elicit an immune reaction against the VEGF-receptor 2 in patients with stage IV and locally advanced pancreatic cancer. BMC Cancer. 2012;12:361.
115. Schmitz-Winnenthal FH, Hohmann N, Niethammer AG, et al. Anti-angiogenic activity of VXM01, an oral T-cell vaccine against VEGF receptor 2, in patients with advanced pancreatic cancer: a randomized, placebo-controlled, phase 1 trial. Oncoimmunology. 2015;4(4):e1001217.
116. Jain RK, Duda DG, Willett CG, et al. Biomarkers of response and resistance to antiangiogenic therapy. Nat Rev Clin Oncol. 2009;6(6):327–38.
117. Verheul HM, Pinedo HM. Possible molecular mechanisms involved in the toxicity of angiogenesis inhibition. Nat Rev Cancer. 2007;7(6):475–85.
118. Schmitz-Winnenthal FH, Podola L, Hohmann N, Friedrich T, Lubenau H, Springer M, et al. A phase 1 trial extension to assess immunologic efficacy and safety or prime-boost vaccination with VXM01, an oral T cell vaccine against VEGF-receptor 2 in patients with advanced pancreatic cancer. J Clin Oncol. 2016;34(Suppl):Abstr 3091.
119. Taniuchi K, Nakagawa H, Nakamura T, et al. Down-regulation of RAB6KIFL/KIF20A, a kinesin involved with membrane trafficking of discs large homologue 5, can attenuate growth of pancreatic cancer cell. Cancer Res. 2005;65(1):105–12.
120. Stangel D, Erkan M, Buchholz M, et al. Kif20a inhibition reduces migration and invasion of pancreatic cancer cells. J Surg Res. 2015;197(1):91–100.
121. Imai K, Hirata S, Irie A, et al. Identification of HLA-A2-restricted CTL epitopes of a novel tumour-associated antigen, KIF20A, overexpressed in pancreatic cancer. Br J Cancer. 2011;104(2):300–7.
122. Asahara S, Takeda K, Yamao K, Maguchi H, Yamaue H. Phase I/II clinical trial using HLA-A24-restricted peptide vaccine derived from KIF20A for patients with advanced pancreatic cancer. J Transl Med. 2013;11:291.

123. Suzuki N, Hazama S, Ueno T, et al. A phase I clinical trial of vaccination with KIF20A-derived peptide in combination with gemcitabine for patients with advanced pancreatic cancer. J Immunother. 2014;37(1):36–42.
124. Yamaue H, Miyazawa M, Katsuda M, Maguchi H, Ishii H, Yamo K, et al. Phase II clinical trial using novel peptide vaccine cocktail as a postoperative adjuvant treatment for surgically resected pancreatic cancer patients. J Clin Oncol. 2016;34(Suppl):Abstr e14587.
125. Tanaka H, Suzuki N, Iguchi H, Uesugi K, Hirakawa K, Amano R, et al. A phase II study of novel three peptides combination with gemcitabine as first-line therapy for advanced pancreatic cancer (VENUS-PC). J Clin Oncol. 2015;33(Suppl):Abstr 3045.
126. Xia Y, Rocchi P, Iovanna JL, Peng L. Targeting heat shock response pathways to treat pancreatic cancer. Drug Discov Today. 2012;17(1-2):35–43.
127. Maki RG, Livingston PO, Lewis JJ, et al. A phase I pilot study of autologous heat shock protein vaccine HSPPC-96 in patients with resected pancreatic adenocarcinoma. Dig Dis Sci. 2007;52(8):1964–72.
128. Hardacre JM, Mulcahy M, Small W, et al. Addition of algenpantucel-L immunotherapy to standard adjuvant therapy for pancreatic cancer: a phase 2 study. J Gastrointest Surg. 2013;17(1):94–100. discussion p 100-101
129. Watier H, Guillaumin JM, Piller F, et al. Removal of terminal alpha-galactosyl residues from xenogeneic porcine endothelial cells. Decrease in complement-mediated cytotoxicity but persistence of IgG1-mediated antibody-dependent cell-mediated cytotoxicity. Transplantation. 1996;62(1):105–13.
130. Watier H, Guillaumin JM, Vallee I, et al. Human NK cell-mediated direct and IgG-dependent cytotoxicity against xenogeneic porcine endothelial cells. Transpl Immunol. 1996;4(4):293–9.
131. Jaffee EM, Abrams R, Cameron J, et al. A phase I clinical trial of lethally irradiated allogeneic pancreatic tumor cells transfected with the GM-CSF gene for the treatment of pancreatic adenocarcinoma. Hum Gene Ther. 1998;9(13):1951–71.
132. Jaffee EM, Schutte M, Gossett J, et al. Development and characterization of a cytokine-secreting pancreatic adenocarcinoma vaccine from primary tumors for use in clinical trials. Cancer J Sci Am. 1998;4(3):194–203.
133. Dranoff G, Jaffee E, Lazenby A, et al. Vaccination with irradiated tumor cells engineered to secrete murine granulocyte-macrophage colony-stimulating factor stimulates potent, specific, and long-lasting anti-tumor immunity. Proc Natl Acad Sci U S A. 1993;90(8):3539–43.
134. Huang AY, Golumbek P, Ahmadzadeh M, Jaffee E, Pardoll D, Levitsky H. Role of bone marrow-derived cells in presenting MHC class I-restricted tumor antigens. Science. 1994;264(5161):961–5.
135. Jaffee EM, Hruban RH, Biedrzycki B, et al. Novel allogeneic granulocyte-macrophage colony-stimulating factor-secreting tumor vaccine for pancreatic cancer: a phase I trial of safety and immune activation. J Clin Oncol. 2001;19(1):145–56.
136. Lutz E, Yeo CJ, Lillemoe KD, et al. A lethally irradiated allogeneic granulocyte-macrophage colony stimulating factor-secreting tumor vaccine for pancreatic adenocarcinoma. A phase II trial of safety, efficacy, and immune activation. Ann Surg. 2011;253(2):328–35.
137. Laheru D, Lutz E, Burke J, et al. Allogeneic granulocyte macrophage colony-stimulating factor-secreting tumor immunotherapy alone or in sequence with cyclophosphamide for metastatic pancreatic cancer: a pilot study of safety, feasibility, and immune activation. Clin Cancer Res. 2008;14(5):1455–63.
138. Royal RE, Levy C, Turner K, et al. Phase 2 trial of single agent Ipilimumab (anti-CTLA-4) for locally advanced or metastatic pancreatic adenocarcinoma. J Immunother. 2010;33(8):828–33.
139. Hurwitz AA, Yu TF, Leach DR, Allison JP. CTLA-4 blockade synergizes with tumor-derived granulocyte-macrophage colony-stimulating factor for treatment of an experimental mammary carcinoma. Proc Natl Acad Sci U S A. 1998;95(17):10067–71.
140. O'Day SJ, Maio M, Chiarion-Sileni V, et al. Efficacy and safety of ipilimumab monotherapy in patients with pretreated advanced melanoma: a multicenter single-arm phase II study. Ann Oncol. 2010;21(8):1712–7.

141. Robert C, Thomas L, Bondarenko I, et al. Ipilimumab plus dacarbazine for previously untreated metastatic melanoma. N Engl J Med. 2011;364(26):2517–26.
142. Le DT, Lutz E, Uram JN, et al. Evaluation of ipilimumab in combination with allogeneic pancreatic tumor cells transfected with a GM-CSF gene in previously treated pancreatic cancer. J Immunother. 2013;36(7):382–9.
143. Le DT, Wang-Gillam A, Picozzi V, et al. Safety and survival with GVAX pancreas prime and Listeria Monocytogenes-expressing mesothelin (CRS-207) boost vaccines for metastatic pancreatic cancer. J Clin Oncol. 2015;33(12):1325–33.
144. Brockstedt DG, Giedlin MA, Leong ML, et al. Listeria-based cancer vaccines that segregate immunogenicity from toxicity. Proc Natl Acad Sci U S A. 2004;101(38):13832–7.
145. Le DT, Brockstedt DG, Nir-Paz R, et al. A live-attenuated Listeria vaccine (ANZ-100) and a live-attenuated Listeria vaccine expressing mesothelin (CRS-207) for advanced cancers: phase I studies of safety and immune induction. Clin Cancer Res. 2012;18(3):858–68.
146. Nomi T, Sho M, Akahori T, et al. Clinical significance and therapeutic potential of the programmed death-1 ligand/programmed death-1 pathway in human pancreatic cancer. Clin Cancer Res. 2007;13(7):2151–7.
147. Soares KC, Rucki AA, AA W, et al. PD-1/PD-L1 blockade together with vaccine therapy facilitates effector T-cell infiltration into pancreatic tumors. J Immunother. 2015;38(1):1–11.
148. Le DT, Crocenzi TS, Uram JN, et al. Randomized phase 2 study of the safety, efficacy, and immune response of GVAX pancreas (with cyclophosphamide) and CRS-207 with or without nivolumab in patients with previously treated metastatic pancreatic adenocarcinoma (STELLAR). J Clin Oncol. 2016;34(suppl):abstr TPS4153.
149. Levy A, Chargari C, Marabelle A, Perfettini JL, Magne N, Deutsch E. Can immunostimulatory agents enhance the abscopal effect of radiotherapy? Eur J Cancer. 2016;62:36–45.
150. Vonderheide RH, Aggarwal C, Bajor DL, Goldenberg J, Loch C, Lee JC, et al. Study of hTERT and IL-12 DNA immunotherapy using electroporation in patients with solid tumors after definitive surgery and adjuvant therapy. J Clin Oncol. 2015;33(Suppl):Abstr TPS3014.
151. Low L, Mander A, McCann K, et al. DNA vaccination with electroporation induces increased antibody responses in patients with prostate cancer. Hum Gene Ther. 2009;20(11):1269–78.
152. Trimble CL, Morrow MP, Kraynyak KA, et al. Safety, efficacy, and immunogenicity of VGX-3100, a therapeutic synthetic DNA vaccine targeting human papillomavirus 16 and 18 E6 and E7 proteins for cervical intraepithelial neoplasia 2/3: a randomised, double-blind, placebo-controlled phase 2b trial. Lancet. 2015;386(10008):2078–88.
153. Yan J, Chu JS, Obeng-Adjei N, Morrow MP, Kraynyak K, Slager AM, et al. Induction of potent cytotoxic and antitumor activity by a highly optimized hTERT DNA vaccine. *American Society of Gene and Cell Therapy Annual Meeting.* 2015:Abstr 417.
154. Bendell JC, Powderly JD, Lieu CH, Eckhardt SG, Hurwitz H, Hochster HS, et al. Safety and efficacy of MPDL3280A (anti-PDL1) in combination with bevacizumab (bev) and/or FOLFOX in patients (pts) with metastatic colorectal cancer (mCRC). J Clin Oncol. 2015;33(Suppl 3):Abstr 704.
155. Koopman M, Simkens L, May AM, Mol L, van Tinteren H, Punt CJA. Final results and subgroup analyses of the phase 3 CAIRO3 study: maintenance treatment with capecitabine + bevacizumab versus observation after induction treatment with chemotherapy + bevacizumab in metastatic colorectal cancer (mCRC). J Clin Oncol. 2014;32(5s(Suppl)):Abstr 3504.
156. Altwegg R, Ychou M, Guillaumon V, et al. Second-line therapy for gemcitabine-pretreated advanced or metastatic pancreatic cancer. World J Gastroenterol. 2012;18(12):1357–64.

Chapter 17
Virotherapies in Pancreatic Cancer

Daniel H. Ahn and Ramesh Ramanathan

Pancreatic cancer remains the fourth leading cause of cancer deaths in the United States with a poor prognosis and a five-year survival of <5% across all stages [1]. In 2014, there were approximately 53,070 new cases of pancreatic cancer with only 9% of patients having localized, resectable disease [2]. Given that the vast majority of patients have advanced disease at presentation, much of the focus for drug development has been in the metastatic setting, which is evident with the advent of two combination chemotherapy regimens for advanced disease [3, 4]. While conventional cytotoxic chemotherapy remains the standard of care, an ongoing search for novel therapeutic approaches continues. One approach that has garnered much interest over the past several decades has been investigating the therapeutic potential of biologic therapy, specifically viral therapy. Herein, we will highlight and review viral therapy, with an emphasis on oncolytic viruses.

Viral Therapy

Oncolytic Virotherapy

Viral therapies represent one of many immunotherapeutic strategies in the treatment of pancreatic cancer. Historical evidence has shown tumor regression and remission of several advanced malignancies after the inoculation with naturally

D.H. Ahn, D.O. • R. Ramanathan, M.D. (✉)
Mayo Clinic, Department of Hematology/Medical Oncology, 5777 E. Mayo Blvd, Phoenix, AZ 85054, USA
e-mail: Ramanathan.Ramesh@mayo.edu

T. Bekaii-Saab, B. El-Rayes (eds.), *Current and Emerging Therapies in Pancreatic Cancer*, DOI 10.1007/978-3-319-58256-6_17

occurring viruses [5]. These observations have led to the investigation of viral therapies as a treatment for cancer. Oncolytic viral therapies have the potential to preferentially infect and replicate in malignant cells while sparing the surrounding normal healthy cells [6]. Oncolytic viral replication can be undertaken by selecting a virus that is either non-virulent to humans or by the genetic modification of the viral genome. The anticancer activities from oncolytic viruses result from the direct lysis of cancer cells by the virus and by cytotoxicity to cancer and the surrounding stromal cells by activated innate and tumor-specific immune cells (Fig. 17.1).

Death of cancer and stromal cells result in the release of tumor-specific epitopes in conjunction with the damage-associated molecular pattern (DAMP), oncolytic virus pathogen-derived pathogen-associated molecular pattern (PAMP) molecules, and inflammatory cytokines that can elicit antitumor immunity [7, 8]. The ability of oncolytic viral therapy to induce tumor cell apoptosis and stimulate an antitumor immune response has resulted in its interest as a potential treatment in several malignancies, including pancreatic cancer [7]. Several OV have been and are under current investigation in the treatment of pancreatic cancer and will be reviewed in detail below (Table 17.1).

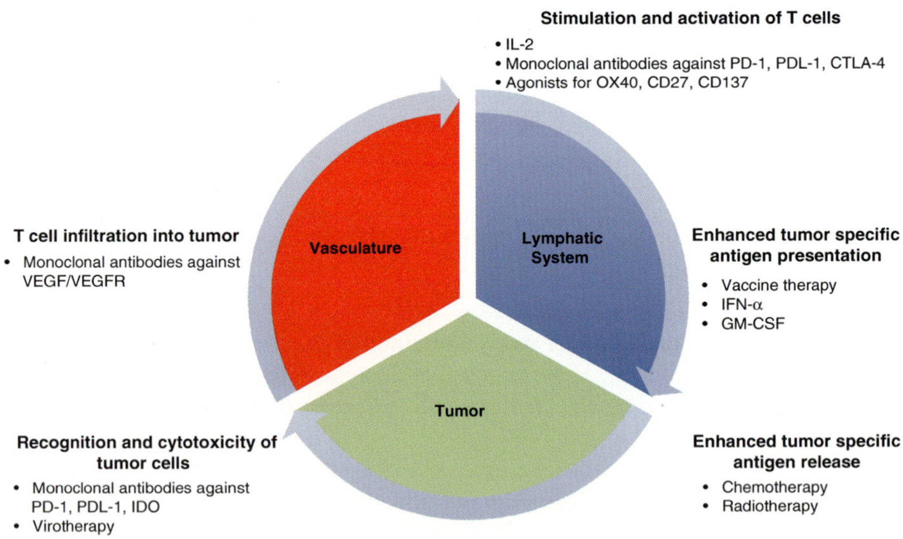

The figure above provides an overview of varying immunotherapeutic approaches, including viral therapies, in the treatment of pancreas cancer.

VEGF-vascular endothelial growth factor; VEGFR-vascular endothelial growth factor receptor; PD-1-program death one; PDL-1 program death ligand-1; IFN-interferon, GM-CSF –granulocyte macrophage colony stimulating factor; IDO-indoleamine-2,3 dioxygenase

Fig. 17.1 Immunotherapeutic treatment strategies in pancreatic cancer

Table 17.1 Summary of ongoing or completed phase I/II clinical trials investigating oncolytic viruses in pancreatic cancer

Study	Virus	Phase	Primary endpoint	Median PFS[a]	Median OS[a]	Comments	Ref/NCT
Mulvihill et al.	*Adenovirus*	I	Safety, tolerance	N/A	N/A	11 of 23 patients experienced prolonged SD	Mulvihill et al. [9]
Hetcht et al.	*Adenovirus*	I/II	Safety, tolerance	N/A	N/A	Administered intratumorally with IV gemcitabine. Out of 21 patients, 2 patients with PR, 4 with SD	Hecht et al. [10]
Noonan et al.	*Reovirus*	II	PFS	4.9	7.31	In combination with carboplatin and paclitaxel for treatment of naive patients	Noonan et al. [11]
De Bono et al.	*Reovirus*	II	CBR	Pending	Pending	In combination with IV gemcitabine for treatment of refractory patients	NCT00998322
Nakao et al.	*Herpes*	I	Safety, tolerance	N/A	N/A	Out of 6 patients, 3 patients with SD, 1 patient with PR	Nakao et al. [12]
Mahalingam	*Reovirus*	I	Safety, tolerance	Pending	Pending	In combination with pembrolizumab	NCT02620423

PFS progression-free survival, *OS* overall survival, *SD* stable disease, *PR* partial response, *IV* intravenous
[a]In months

Reovirus

Respiratory enteric orphan virus or *Reovirus* is a family of non-enveloped double-stranded *RNA virus* that occurs naturally in humans and can affect the gastrointestinal system and respiratory tract. It has innate oncolytic properties, where its replication is dependent upon cellular activity of *RAS*; specifically, it is cytopathic in transformed cells possessing an activated *RAS* signaling pathway [13–16].

Early preclinical studies with *Reovirus* demonstrated its ability to infect, replicate, and induce oncolysis with no activity in normal tissue across several solid tumor malignancies [17–19]. Reolysin (pelareorep) is a propriety formulation of the naturally occurring *Reovirus* Serotype3-Dearing strain, a live replication-competent *Reovirus* [20]. While acquired *Reovirus* infections in humans are mild and are limited to the respiratory and gastrointestinal tract, pelareorep demonstrated cytotoxic effects on cancer cells that harbored mutations in the *RAS* signaling pathway with a good safety profile [16, 21–23]. Additionally, when given concomitantly with chemotherapy or radiotherapy, synergistic antitumor activity has been noted, suggesting a potential benefit from a combined modality approach with Reolysin [24, 25].

Given the ubiquitous nature of *RAS* mutations in pancreatic cancer [26, 27], Reolysin has been of interest as a novel therapeutic agent for the treatment of this disease. In preclinical studies, an increase in reovirus-induced oncolytic activity was seen in *RAS*-mutated pancreatic cancer cell lines [28]. Consistent findings were seen with the injection of Reolysin, where tumor regression was seen in injected pancreatic cancer tumors, as well as in those not subjected to injection. In addition to tumor growth suppression, immunohistochemical studies confirmed the presence of *Reovirus* in each of responding tumors. Noonan et al. reported the results of a phase II randomized trial, in which 73 patients with metastatic pancreatic adenocarcinoma were randomized to receive carboplatin/paclitaxel alone or in combination with Reolysin [11]. While this agent was well tolerated overall with minimal treatment-related adverse effects, it failed to show an improvement in outcomes, including in those patients with *K-ras* mutations. Interestingly, patients that received Reolysin compared to the chemotherapy alone group had increased levels of several markers (including IL-6, VEGF, regulatory T cells) associated with immunosuppression. Consistent with preclinical mice models, Reolysin exposure may promote and enhance immunosuppression in a pre-existing immunosuppressive environment [29]. Another single-arm phase II study evaluated the combination of Reolysin with gemcitabine in treatment naïve patients with advanced pancreatic cancer. Thirty-three patients were enrolled, a median PFS was 4 months, and OS of 10.2 months was observed. Of the 29 patients with evaluable disease, 1 patient had a partial response, 23 had stable disease, and 5 patients experienced disease progression. Thus, across two clinical trials, no significant activity was observed with Reolysin compared to historical chemotherapy regimens, suggesting limited utility in the treatment of pancreatic cancer.

Adenovirus

Adenoviruses are non-enveloped, linear double-stranded DNA viruses that have shown oncolytic activity across several tumor types and were the first OV evaluated in a clinical trial for the treatment of pancreatic cancer. ONYX-015 is an E1B 55-kDA region-deleted virus that preferentially replicates in pancreatic cancer cells with *p53* alterations. Based on early preclinical studies that confirmed viral replication in abnormal cells, a phase I study evaluating intratumoral administration of ONXY-015 was conducted in patients with advanced pancreatic cancer. While no objective responses were seen in the 23 patients enrolled in the study, 11 patients experienced prolong stable disease of at least 12 weeks [9]. The treatment was well tolerated with minimal adverse effects. A subsequent phase I/II study was conducted in patients with unresectable pancreatic cancer, where ONYX-015 was administered intratumorally under endoscopic ultrasound guidance in combination with gemcitabine [10]. Of the 21 patients enrolled in the study, 2 patients experienced a partial response. Side effects related to the virus were mild, but several injection-related complications (e.g., infection, duodenal perforation) were observed. While no significant activity was observed from the two studies, the administration of adenovirus was safe and well tolerated.

Herpes Simplex Virus (HSV)

Oncolytic HSV vectors have been under investigation as a therapeutic approach for the treatment of pancreatic cancer. In a Japanese phase I study, HF-10, an unadulterated, naturally occurring oncolytic HSV, showed no treatment-related adverse effects and 16% response rate [12]. Oncovex GM-CSF (talimogene) is a genetically modified live attenuated oncolytic herpes virus that has demonstrated durable responses and was recently FDA approved in the treatment of unresectable metastatic melanoma. Patients who received Oncovex GM-CSF experienced a durable response rate of 16.3% (response >6 months), of which 29.1% had a complete response [30]. While the potential of HSV as therapeutic agent in pancreatic cancer is unknown, a recently completed phase I study assessing the safety of intratumoral Oncovex GM-CSF injection in unresectable pancreatic cancer (clinicaltrials.gov, NCT00402025) should provide further insight.

Vesicular Stomatitis Virus (VSV)

VSV is an *RNA virus* that is non-cell cycle-dependent, resulting in the rapid uptake by cells. In pancreatic cancer cell lines, VSV showed superior oncolytic activity in comparison to RSV and *Sendai virus*. Resistant cell lines demonstrated that viral replication was dependent on type 1 interferon (IFN) activity, where highly viral replication and infectivity were seen in pancreatic cancer cell lines that lacked an intact IFN response [7]. Additionally, in the same resistant cell lines, high-level expression of antiviral IFN-stimulated genes, *MxA* and *OAS*, and the aberrant activation of the *JAK/STAT* signaling pathway were seen and potentially limited the ability for the virus to adequately infect cancer cells [31].

Vaccinia Virus

Vaccinia virus is a replication-competent virus and is a member of the poxvirus family that has demonstrated promising antitumor activity across several gastrointestinal malignancies including in pancreatic cancer. It is highly immunogenic and produces a strong cytotoxic T cell and innate immune response [32]. As a single agent or in combination with gemcitabine chemotherapy, *Vaccinia* (GLV-1h68) has shown the ability to infect, replicate, and induce oncolysis in pancreatic cancer cell lines [33]. A similar genetically modified *Vaccinia virus*, GLV-1h51, was tested across several different malignancies, where pancreatic cancer cell lines were most sensitive to viral infection, resulting in increased tumor size regression [34]. An ongoing phase I study (ClinicalTrials.gov, NCT02432963) is investigating the combination of a modified vaccinia virus Ankara vaccine that expresses p53 with pembrolizumab, an anti-PD1 inhibitor in treatment-refractory patients.

Obstacles with Oncolytic Virotherapy

While the rationale of oncolytic virotherapy (OV) as a therapeutic modality for pancreatic cancer is intriguing and represents a novel approach in the treatment of this disease, OV remains experimental and is still in its infancy stage. A better understanding of the regulation of the antitumor immune response is needed to allow for the development of rational treatment strategies in order to improve on its efficacy.

A significant immunologic barrier in the treatment of pancreatic cancer is the tolerance toward cancer-specific antigens. Most tumor-associated antigens are self-antigens and, thus, weakly immunogenic. Additionally, the pancreatic tumor microenvironment suppresses the activity of tumor-infiltrating lymphocytes that contributes to blunting an antitumor immunogenic response [35]. In order to obtain an effective antitumor response, a lessening in an immunologic tolerance while increasing tumor-specific antigen load is needed. This can potentially be achieved by increasing the tumor-specific antigen load through effective oncolysis. In addition to antigen exposure, an alteration or disruption of the immunosuppressive environment is needed. Pancreatic cancer is mostly considered to be an immunosuppressive cancer, where pancreatic cancer cells produce inflammatory cytokines that mediate an immunosuppressive environment (*to be discussed in detail in the immunotherapy chapter*). Immunotherapeutic approaches—notably agents that target negative immunologic regulatory molecules on activated T cells (e.g., anti-CTLA4, anti-PD1, or anti-PDL-1)—have shown promise as a therapeutic agent in various solid tumor malignancies [36, 37]. The combination of an oncolytic virus with these agents can potentially enhance and produce a synergistic antitumor immune response. Specifically, increased exposure of tumor-specific antigens from oncolysis with checkpoint inhibition can potentiate an immunogenic response [38].

Another limitation that hinders the systemic delivery of oncolytic viruses is the mode of delivery of treatment. While intravenous administration is an efficient and practical methodology, especially in the case for difficult to reach tumor locations, hepatic and splenic sequestration and pre-existing serum antiviral antibodies may result in insufficient viral particle delivery. Studies evaluating techniques to improve OV efficacy include the chemical modification of the viral coat proteins to evade antibody recognition and the utilization of mesenchymal stem cell carriers to increase target virotherapy delivery.

Physical barriers, notably the tumor vasculature and its microenvironment, serve as obstacles in effective virotherapy in treating pancreatic cancer. The large size of virus particles limits efficient extravasation from blood vessels, resulting in an inadequate delivery to tumor cells. Biologic therapies (interleukin-2, vascular endothelial growth factor (VEGF)) can modulate vascular permeability while depleting immunosuppressive regulatory T cells which can increase sufficient delivery to tumor cells and potentiate the efficacy of OV [39, 40]. In addition to the vasculature, the stroma creates a complex microenvironment that not only serves as a physical barrier to prevent effective penetration of oncolytic viruses but also provides an immunosuppressive environment that blunts any innate antitumor immune response [41–48].

Vector-Mediated Virotherapy

In addition to serving as an oncolytic agent, viruses have utilized as vectors to transport therapeutic agents into patients to target tumor cells, contributing toward inhibiting tumor growth and promoting tumor lysis [49]. Viruses are an effective method for transferring genes to specific targeted areas and are extensively used in oncology. In addition to serving as an efficient mode of transportation, viruses have the ability to bypass potential systemic toxicities related to the transported gene (Table 17.2).

Table 17.2 Summary of completed phase I/II clinical trials with viral vector therapy in pancreatic cancer

Study	Treatment	Phase	Results	Comments	Ref
Gordon et al.	Rexin-G	I	PFS up to 9 months; OS > 5.5 months		Gordon et al. [50]
Galanis et al.	Rexin-G	I/II	TTP 32 days; OS 3.5 months		Galanis et al. [51]
Chawla et al.	Rexin-G	I/II	SD- 5 pts.; PR-1 pt.; PFS > 7.6 month; OS 9.2 months		Chawla et al. [52]
Senzer et al.	TNFerade	I	PR in 2 pts	With RT	Senzer et al. [53]
Hecht et al.	TNFerade	I/II	Clinical response in 4 pts.; OS 332 days	With CRT	Hecht et al. [54]
Herman et al.	TNFerade	III	No significant benefit	With CRT	Herman et al. [55]

PFS progression-free survival, *OS* overall survival, *SD* stable disease, *PR* partial response, *CRT* chemoradiation, *RT* radiotherapy

Rexin-G

Rexin-G is a tumor-targeted retroviral vector that is derived from the Moloney murine leukemia virus family [56]. Its modified von Willebrand factor-derived matrix-binding site allows Rexin-G to identify and target abnormal collagen-exposed areas in the tumor stroma. Additionally, Rexin-G bears a cytocidal cyclin G1 construct that inhibits tumor cell proliferation and induces apoptosis by inhibiting cyclin G1, a key regulator of cell cycle functioning. In preclinical studies, intraportal administration of Rexin-G inhibited pancreatic cancer cell growth and regression of liver metastases [57]. These findings translated in early clinical studies where pancreatic cancer patients experienced tumor growth inhibition with durable results [58]. In a phase I study with Rexin-G, five of six patients with treatment refractory pancreatic cancer experienced partial responses with a median overall survival of 6 months [50]. In subsequent phase I/II study, patients with gemcitabine-refractory pancreatic cancer received higher doses of Rexin-G (2×10^{11} CFU 3× weekly for 4 weeks). At the higher dose, one patient experienced a partial response, while five patients had stable disease. Patients experienced a median progression-free survival greater than 7.6 months and a median overall survival of 9.2 months [52]. Based on these findings, Rexin-G has obtained orphan drug status in the United States, and further work is ongoing to validate its efficacy in pancreatic cancer.

TNFerade

Tumor necrosis factor alpha, TNF-α, is an inflammatory cytokine that has well-documented antitumor properties. It alters tumor vasculature permeability in addition to have direct cytotoxic effects on tumor cells [59, 60]. While TNF-α has been recognized as a potential therapeutic agent, its associated systemic toxicities have been a major limiting factor to its development and application in treatment of solid tumor malignancies. Through gene modification, minimization of its side effect profile while maintaining its antitumor properties has rekindled the interest of TNF-α as a treatment in many diseases, including pancreatic cancer. TNFerade is a genetically modified second-generation replication-deficient adenovirus vector that contains the gene for TNF-α. Through the injection of TNFerade, the gene that encodes for TNF-α is transmitted to the cells in the tumor microenvironment. This allows for TNF-α to be secreted locally and provide its antitumor effects while minimizing systemic toxicities [61]. To optimize the local antitumor effects of TNF-α, the radiation-inducible EGR-1 has been incorporated into TNFerade. This alteration promotes gene expression and activation of TNF-α in addition to potentiating the known effect between TNF-α and radiotherapy [62, 63].

Preclinical studies have shown adenovectors that carry TNF-α to be safe while demonstrating local antitumor effects [64, 65]. This included a phase I study where two of four patients with pancreatic cancer experienced a partial response after receiving TNFerade concomitantly with radiation therapy [53]. A subsequent dose escalation phase I/II trial was conducted where 50 patients with local, unresectable pancreatic cancer were injected with TNFerade and received concomitant chemoradiation therapy (CRT) with 5-fluorouracil (5-FU). Four patients experienced a clinical response including 1 complete response, while 12 patients had stable disease. The median overall survival was 297 days, but in patients who received the maximum tolerated dose, the median overall survival was 332 days. Of note, seven patients were able to achieve a response to undergo surgical resection [54]. Based on these promising results, Herman et al. conducted a large, multicenter randomized phase III trial in patients with locally advanced pancreatic cancer [55]. Three hundred four patients were randomized in a 2:1 fashion to receive TNFerade with 5-FU-based CRT followed by gemcitabine (with or without erlotinib). No differences across all patient outcomes (overall survival, progression-free survival, or time to progression) were seen between the two treatment arms [55]. Thus, the promising findings seen from early phase studies did not translate to a significant clinical benefit in a larger patient population. While there appears to be no role for TNFerade for all patients with localized pancreatic cancer, further investigation, including identification of a subgroup of patients likely to benefit from localized therapy, may warrant further studies in the role of TNFerade and other viral vector-mediated therapies in pancreatic cancer.

Conclusion and Future Directions

Despite advances in cancer care and research, pancreatic cancer remains very challenging, with standard treatment regimens providing modest gains at a significant cost. Novel therapeutic approaches, including viral therapy, are needed to improved outcomes in this dismal disease. An increased understanding has provided a strong rationale that has spurred further investigation in both early- and later-phase studies. While the results so far have been disappointing, in order to benefit our patients and their well-being, it is important to continue to aim for significant improvements rather than incremental gains for a disease with such poor outcomes.

References

1. Weir HK, Thun MJ, Hankey BF, Ries LA, Howe HL, Wingo PA, Jemal A, Ward E, Anderson RN, Edwards BK. Annual report to the nation on the status of cancer, 1975–2000, featuring the uses of surveillance data for cancer prevention and control. J Natl Cancer Inst. 2003;95(17):1276–99.
2. Siegel RL, Miller KD, Jemal A. Cancer statistics, 2016. CA Cancer J Clin. 2016;66(1):7–30. doi:10.3322/caac.21332.
3. Conroy T, Desseigne F, Ychou M, Bouche O, Guimbaud R, Becouarn Y, Adenis A, Raoul JL, Gourgou-Bourgade S, de la Fouchardiere C, Bennouna J, Bachet JB, Khemissa-Akouz F, Pere-Verge D, Delbaldo C, Assenat E, Chauffert B, Michel P, Montoto-Grillot C, Ducreux M, Groupe Tumeurs Digestives of Unicancer, PRODIGE Intergroup. FOLFIRINOX versus gemcitabine for metastatic pancreatic cancer. N Engl J Med. 2011;364(19):1817–25. doi:10.1056/NEJMoa1011923.
4. Von Hoff DD, Ervin T, Arena FP, Chiorean EG, Infante J, Moore M, Seay T, Tjulandin SA, Ma WW, Saleh MN, Harris M, Reni M, Dowden S, Laheru D, Bahary N, Ramanathan RK, Tabernero J, Hidalgo M, Goldstein D, Van Cutsem E, Wei X, Iglesias J, Renschler MF. Increased survival in pancreatic cancer with nab-paclitaxel plus gemcitabine. N Engl J Med. 2013;369(18):1691–703. doi:10.1056/NEJMoa1304369.
5. Kelly E, Russell SJ. History of oncolytic viruses: genesis to genetic engineering. Mol Ther. 2007;15(4):651–9. doi:10.1038/sj.mt.6300108.
6. Russell SJ, Peng KW, Bell JC. Oncolytic virotherapy. Nat Biotechnol. 2012;30(7):658–70. doi:10.1038/nbt.2287.
7. Murphy AM, Besmer DM, Moerdyk-Schauwecker M, Moestl N, Ornelles DA, Mukherjee P, Grdzelishvili VZ. Vesicular stomatitis virus as an oncolytic agent against pancreatic ductal adenocarcinoma. J Virol. 2012;86(6):3073–87. doi:10.1128/JVI.05640-11.
8. Tang D, Kang R, Coyne CB, Zeh HJ, Lotze MT. PAMPs and DAMPs: signal 0s that spur autophagy and immunity. Immunol Rev. 2012;249(1):158–75. doi:10.1111/j.1600-065X.2012.01146.x.
9. Mulvihill S, Warren R, Venook A, Adler A, Randlev B, Heise C, Kirn D. Safety and feasibility of injection with an E1B-55 kDa gene-deleted, replication-selective adenovirus (ONYX-015) into primary carcinomas of the pancreas: a phase I trial. Gene Ther. 2001;8(4):308–15. doi:10.1038/sj.gt.3301398.
10. Hecht JR, Bedford R, Abbruzzese JL, Lahoti S, Reid TR, Soetikno RM, Kirn DH, Freeman SM. A phase I/II trial of intratumoral endoscopic ultrasound injection of ONYX-015 with intravenous gemcitabine in unresectable pancreatic carcinoma. Clin Cancer Res. 2003;9(2):555–61.
11. Noonan AM, Farren MR, Geyer SM, Huang Y, Tahiri S, Ahn D, Mikhail S, Ciombor KK, Pant S, Aparo S, Sexton J, Marshall JL, Mace TA, CS W, El-Rayes B, Timmers CD, Zwiebel J, Lesinski GB, Villalona-Calero MA, Bekaii-Saab TS. Randomized phase 2 trial of the oncolytic virus pelareorep (reolysin) in upfront treatment of metastatic pancreatic adenocarcinoma. Mol Ther. 2016;24(6):1150–8. doi:10.1038/mt.2016.66.
12. Nakao A, Kasuya H, Sahin TT, Nomura N, Kanzaki A, Misawa M, Shirota T, Yamada S, Fujii T, Sugimoto H, Shikano T, Nomoto S, Takeda S, Kodera Y, Nishiyama Y. A phase I dose-escalation clinical trial of intraoperative direct intratumoral injection of HF10 oncolytic virus in non-resectable patients with advanced pancreatic cancer. Cancer Gene Ther. 2011;18(3):167–75. doi:10.1038/cgt.2010.65.

13. Battcock SM, Collier TW, Zu D, Hirasawa K. Negative regulation of the alpha interferon-induced antiviral response by the Ras/Raf/MEK pathway. J Virol. 2006;80(9):4422–30. doi:10.1128/JVI.80.9.4422-4430.2006.
14. Bodkin DK, Nibert ML, Fields BN. Proteolytic digestion of reovirus in the intestinal lumens of neonatal mice. J Virol. 1989;63(11):4676–81.
15. Rosen L, Evans HE, Spickard A. Reovirus infections in human volunteers. Am J Hyg. 1963;77:29–37.
16. Strong JE, Coffey MC, Tang D, Sabinin P, Lee PW. The molecular basis of viral oncolysis: usurpation of the Ras signaling pathway by reovirus. EMBO J. 1998;17(12):3351–62. doi:10.1093/emboj/17.12.3351.
17. Min HJ, Koh SS, Cho IR, Srisuttee R, Park EH, Jhun BH, Kim YG, Oh S, Kwak JE, Johnston RN, Chung YH. Inhibition of GSK-3beta enhances reovirus-induced apoptosis in colon cancer cells. Int J Oncol. 2009;35(3):617–24.
18. Norman KL, Coffey MC, Hirasawa K, Demetrick DJ, Nishikawa SG, DiFrancesco LM, Strong JE, Lee PW. Reovirus oncolysis of human breast cancer. Hum Gene Ther. 2002;13(5):641–52. doi:10.1089/10430340252837233.
19. Wilcox ME, Yang W, Senger D, Rewcastle NB, Morris DG, Brasher PM, Shi ZQ, Johnston RN, Nishikawa S, Lee PW, Forsyth PA. Reovirus as an oncolytic agent against experimental human malignant gliomas. J Natl Cancer Inst. 2001;93(12):903–12.
20. Chakrabarty R, Tran H, Selvaggi G, Hagerman A, Thompson B, Coffey M. The oncolytic virus, pelareorep, as a novel anticancer agent: a review. Investig New Drugs. 2015;33(3):761–74. doi:10.1007/s10637-015-0216-8.
21. Bos JL. Ras oncogenes in human cancer: a review. Cancer Res. 1989;49(17):4682–9.
22. Harrington KJ, Karapanagiotou EM, Roulstone V, Twigger KR, White CL, Vidal L, Beirne D, Prestwich R, Newbold K, Ahmed M, Thway K, Nutting CM, Coffey M, Harris D, Vile RG, Pandha HS, Debono JS, Melcher AA. Two-stage phase I dose-escalation study of intratumoral reovirus type 3 dearing and palliative radiotherapy in patients with advanced cancers. Clin Cancer Res. 2010;16(11):3067–77. doi:10.1158/1078-0432.CCR-10-0054.
23. Morris DG, Feng X, DiFrancesco LM, Fonseca K, Forsyth PA, Paterson AH, Coffey MC, Thompson B. REO-001: a phase I trial of percutaneous intralesional administration of reovirus type 3 dearing (Reolysin(R)) in patients with advanced solid tumors. Investig New Drugs. 2013;31(3):696–706. doi:10.1007/s10637-012-9865-z.
24. Comins C, Spicer J, Protheroe A, Roulstone V, Twigger K, White CM, Vile R, Melcher A, Coffey MC, Mettinger KL, Nuovo G, Cohn DE, Phelps M, Harrington KJ, Pandha HS. REO-10: a phase I study of intravenous reovirus and docetaxel in patients with advanced cancer. Clin Cancer Res. 2010;16(22):5564–72. doi:10.1158/1078-0432.CCR-10-1233.
25. Twigger K, Vidal L, White CL, De Bono JS, Bhide S, Coffey M, Thompson B, Vile RG, Heinemann L, Pandha HS, Errington F, Melcher AA, Harrington KJ. Enhanced in vitro and in vivo cytotoxicity of combined reovirus and radiotherapy. Clin Cancer Res. 2008;14(3):912–23. doi:10.1158/1078-0432.CCR-07-1400.
26. Almoguera C, Shibata D, Forrester K, Martin J, Arnheim N, Perucho M. Most human carcinomas of the exocrine pancreas contain mutant c-K-ras genes. Cell. 1988;53(4):549–54.
27. Jones S, Zhang X, Parsons DW, Lin JC, Leary RJ, Angenendt P, Mankoo P, Carter H, Kamiyama H, Jimeno A, Hong SM, Fu B, Lin MT, Calhoun ES, Kamiyama M, Walter K, Nikolskaya T, Nikolsky Y, Hartigan J, Smith DR, Hidalgo M, Leach SD, Klein AP, Jaffee EM, Goggins M, Maitra A, Iacobuzio-Donahue C, Eshleman JR, Kern SE, Hruban RH, Karchin R, Papadopoulos N, Parmigiani G, Vogelstein B, Velculescu VE, Kinzler KW. Core signaling pathways in human pancreatic cancers revealed by global genomic analyses. Science. 2008;321(5897):1801–6. doi:10.1126/science.1164368.
28. Etoh T, Himeno Y, Matsumoto T, Aramaki M, Kawano K, Nishizono A, Kitano S. Oncolytic viral therapy for human pancreatic cancer cells by reovirus. Clin Cancer Res. 2003;9(3):1218–23.
29. Clements DR, Sterea AM, Kim Y, Helson E, Dean CA, Nunokawa A, Coyle KM, Sharif T, Marcato P, Gujar SA, Lee PW. Newly recruited CD11b+, GR-1+, Ly6C(high) myeloid cells augment tumor-associated immunosuppression immediately following the therapeutic

administration of oncolytic reovirus. J Immunol. 2015;194(9):4397–412. doi:10.4049/jimmunol.1402132.
30. Andtbacka RH, Kaufman HL, Collichio F, Amatruda T, Senzer N, Chesney J, Delman KA, Spitler LE, Puzanov I, Agarwala SS, Milhem M, Cranmer L, Curti B, Lewis K, Ross M, Guthrie T, Linette GP, Daniels GA, Harrington K, Middleton MR, Miller WH Jr, Zager JS, Ye Y, Yao B, Li A, Doleman S, VanderWalde A, Gansert J, Coffin RS. Talimogene Laherparepvec improves durable response rate in patients with advanced melanoma. J Clin Oncol Off J Am Soc Clin Oncol. 2015;33(25):2780–8. doi:10.1200/JCO.2014.58.3377.
31. Moerdyk-Schauwecker M, Shah NR, Murphy AM, Hastie E, Mukherjee P, Grdzelishvili VZ. Resistance of pancreatic cancer cells to oncolytic vesicular stomatitis virus: role of type I interferon signaling. Virology. 2013;436(1):221–34. doi:10.1016/j.virol.2012.11.014.
32. Miller JD, van der Most RG, Akondy RS, Glidewell JT, Albott S, Masopust D, Murali-Krishna K, Mahar PL, Edupuganti S, Lalor S, Germon S, Del Rio C, Mulligan MJ, Staprans SI, Altman JD, Feinberg MB, Ahmed R. Human effector and memory CD8+ T cell responses to smallpox and yellow fever vaccines. Immunity. 2008;28(5):710–22. doi:10.1016/j.immuni.2008.02.020.
33. Yu YA, Galanis C, Woo Y, Chen N, Zhang Q, Fong Y, Szalay AA. Regression of human pancreatic tumor xenografts in mice after a single systemic injection of recombinant vaccinia virus GLV-1h68. Mol Cancer Ther. 2009;8(1):141–51. doi:10.1158/1535-7163.MCT-08-0533.
34. Haddad D, Chen N, Zhang Q, Chen CH, YA Y, Gonzalez L, Aguilar J, Li P, Wong J, Szalay AA, Fong Y. A novel genetically modified oncolytic vaccinia virus in experimental models is effective against a wide range of human cancers. Ann Surg Oncol. 2012;19(Suppl 3):S665–74. doi:10.1245/s10434-011-2198-x.
35. Zou W. Immunosuppressive networks in the tumour environment and their therapeutic relevance. Nat Rev Cancer. 2005;5(4):263–74. doi:10.1038/nrc1586.
36. Topalian SL, Hodi FS, Brahmer JR, Gettinger SN, Smith DC, McDermott DF, Powderly JD, Carvajal RD, Sosman JA, Atkins MB, Leming PD, Spigel DR, Antonia SJ, Horn L, Drake CG, Pardoll DM, Chen L, Sharfman WH, Anders RA, Taube JM, McMiller TL, Xu H, Korman AJ, Jure-Kunkel M, Agrawal S, McDonald D, Kollia GD, Gupta A, Wigginton JM, Sznol M. Safety, activity, and immune correlates of anti-PD-1 antibody in cancer. N Engl J Med. 2012b;366(26):2443–54. doi:10.1056/NEJMoa1200690.
37. Topalian SL, Drake CG, Pardoll DM. Targeting the PD-1/B7-H1(PD-L1) pathway to activate anti-tumor immunity. Curr Opin Immunol. 2012a;24(2):207–12. doi:10.1016/j.coi.2011.12.009.
38. Bartlett DL, Liu Z, Sathaiah M, Ravindranathan R, Guo Z, He Y, Guo ZS. Oncolytic viruses as therapeutic cancer vaccines. Mol Cancer. 2013;12(1):103. doi:10.1186/1476-4598-12-103.
39. Kottke T, Galivo F, Wongthida P, Diaz RM, Thompson J, Jevremovic D, Barber GN, Hall G, Chester J, Selby P, Harrington K, Melcher A, Vile RG. Treg depletion-enhanced IL-2 treatment facilitates therapy of established tumors using systemically delivered oncolytic virus. Mol Ther. 2008;16(7):1217–26. doi:10.1038/mt.2008.83.
40. Tseng JC, Granot T, DiGiacomo V, Levin B, Meruelo D. Enhanced specific delivery and targeting of oncolytic Sindbis viral vectors by modulating vascular leakiness in tumor. Cancer Gene Ther. 2010;17(4):244–55. doi:10.1038/cgt.2009.70.
41. Feig C, Gopinathan A, Neesse A, Chan DS, Cook N, Tuveson DA. The pancreas cancer microenvironment. Clin Cancer Res. 2012;18(16):4266–76. doi:10.1158/1078-0432.ccr-11-3114.
42. Hanahan D, Weinberg RA. Hallmarks of cancer: the next generation. Cell. 2011;144(5):646–74. doi:10.1016/j.cell.2011.02.013.
43. Hwang RF, Moore T, Arumugam T, Ramachandran V, Amos KD, Rivera A, Ji B, Evans DB, Logsdon CD. Cancer-associated stromal fibroblasts promote pancreatic tumor progression. Cancer Res. 2008;68(3):918–26. doi:10.1158/0008-5472.can-07-5714.
44. Ikenaga N, Ohuchida K, Mizumoto K, Cui L, Kayashima T, Morimatsu K, Moriyama T, Nakata K, Fujita H, Tanaka M. CD10+ pancreatic stellate cells enhance the progression of pancreatic cancer. Gastroenterology. 2010;139(3):1041–51e1041–8. doi:10.1053/j.gastro.2010.05.084.

45. Lunardi S, Muschel RJ, Brunner TB. The stromal compartments in pancreatic cancer: are there any therapeutic targets? Cancer Lett. 2014;343(2):147–55. doi:10.1016/j.canlet.2013.09.039.
46. Minchinton AI, Tannock IF. Drug penetration in solid tumours. Nat Rev Cancer. 2006;6(8):583–92. doi:10.1038/nrc1893.
47. Tredan O, Galmarini CM, Patel K, Tannock IF. Drug resistance and the solid tumor microenvironment. J Natl Cancer Inst. 2007;99(19):1441–54. doi:10.1093/jnci/djm135.
48. Vonlaufen A, Phillips PA, Xu Z, Goldstein D, Pirola RC, Wilson JS, Apte MV. Pancreatic stellate cells and pancreatic cancer cells: an unholy alliance. Cancer Res. 2008;68(19):7707–10. doi:10.1158/0008-5472.can-08-1132.
49. Seth P. Vector-mediated cancer gene therapy: an overview. Cancer Biol Ther. 2005;4(5):512–7.
50. Gordon EM, Lopez FF, Cornelio GH, Lorenzo CC 3rd, Levy JP, Reed RA, Liu L, Bruckner HW, Hall FL. Pathotropic nanoparticles for cancer gene therapy Rexin-G IV: three-year clinical experience. Int J Oncol. 2006;29(5):1053–64.
51. Galanis E, Carlson SK, Foster NR, Lowe V, Quevedo F, McWilliams RR, Grothey A, Jatoi A, Alberts SR, Rubin J. Phase I trial of a pathotropic retroviral vector expressing a cytocidal cyclin G1 construct (Rexin-G) in patients with advanced pancreatic cancer. Mol Ther. 2008;16(5):979–84. doi:10.1038/mt.2008.29.
52. Chawla SP, Chua VS, Fernandez L, Quon D, Blackwelder WC, Gordon EM, Hall FL. Advanced phase I/II studies of targeted gene delivery in vivo: intravenous Rexin-G for gemcitabine-resistant metastatic pancreatic cancer. Mol Ther. 2010;18(2):435–41. doi:10.1038/mt.2009.228.
53. Senzer N, Mani S, Rosemurgy A, Nemunaitis J, Cunningham C, Guha C, Bayol N, Gillen M, Chu K, Rasmussen C, Rasmussen H, Kufe D, Weichselbaum R, Hanna N. TNFerade biologic, an adenovector with a radiation-inducible promoter, carrying the human tumor necrosis factor alpha gene: a phase I study in patients with solid tumors. J Clin Oncol Off J Am Soc Clin Oncol. 2004;22(4):592–601. doi:10.1200/JCO.2004.01.227.
54. Hecht JR, Farrell JJ, Senzer N, Nemunaitis J, Rosemurgy A, Chung T, Hanna N, Chang KJ, Javle M, Posner M, Waxman I, Reid A, Erickson R, Canto M, Chak A, Blatner G, Kovacevic M, Thornton M. EUS or percutaneously guided intratumoral TNFerade biologic with 5-fluorouracil and radiotherapy for first-line treatment of locally advanced pancreatic cancer: a phase I/II study. Gastrointest Endosc. 2012;75(2):332–8. doi:10.1016/j.gie.2011.10.007.
55. Herman JM, Wild AT, Wang H, Tran PT, Chang KJ, Taylor GE, Donehower RC, Pawlik TM, Ziegler MA, Cai H, Savage DT, Canto MI, Klapman J, Reid T, Shah RJ, Hoffe SE, Rosemurgy A, Wolfgang CL, Laheru DA. Randomized phase III multi-institutional study of TNFerade biologic with fluorouracil and radiotherapy for locally advanced pancreatic cancer: final results. J Clin Oncol Off J Am Soc Clin Oncol. 2013;31(7):886–94. doi:10.1200/JCO.2012.44.7516.
56. Hall FL, Liu L, Zhu NL, Stapfer M, Anderson WF, Beart RW, Gordon EM. Molecular engineering of matrix-targeted retroviral vectors incorporating a surveillance function inherent in von Willebrand factor. Hum Gene Ther. 2000;11(7):983–93. doi:10.1089/10430340050015293.
57. Gordon EM, Liu PX, Chen ZH, Liu L, Whitley MD, Gee C, Groshen S, Hinton DR, Beart RW, Hall FL. Inhibition of metastatic tumor growth in nude mice by portal vein infusions of matrix-targeted retroviral vectors bearing a cytocidal cyclin G1 construct. Cancer Res. 2000;60(13):3343–7.
58. Gordon EM, Cornelio GH, Lorenzo CC 3rd, Levy JP, Reed RA, Liu L, Hall FL. First clinical experience using a 'pathotropic' injectable retroviral vector (Rexin-G) as intervention for stage IV pancreatic cancer. Int J Oncol. 2004;24(1):177–85.
59. Asher A, Mule JJ, Reichert CM, Shiloni E, Rosenberg SA. Studies on the anti-tumor efficacy of systemically administered recombinant tumor necrosis factor against several murine tumors in vivo. J Immunol. 1987;138(3):963–74.
60. Feinberg B, Kurzrock R, Talpaz M, Blick M, Saks S, Gutterman JU. A phase I trial of intravenously-administered recombinant tumor necrosis factor-alpha in cancer patients. J Clin Oncol Off J Am Soc Clin Oncol. 1988;6(8):1328–34.
61. Rasmussen H, Rasmussen C, Lempicki M, Durham R, Brough D, King CR, Weichselbaum R. TNFerade biologic: preclinical toxicology of a novel adenovector with a radiation-inducible promoter, carrying the human tumor necrosis factor alpha gene. Cancer Gene Ther. 2002;9(11):951–7. doi:10.1038/sj.cgt.7700518.

62. Hallahan DE, Beckett MA, Kufe D, Weichselbaum RR. The interaction between recombinant human tumor necrosis factor and radiation in 13 human tumor cell lines. Int J Radiat Oncol Biol Phys. 1990;19(1):69–74.
63. Hallahan DE, Vokes EE, Rubin SJ, O'Brien S, Samuels B, Vijaykumar S, Kufe DW, Phillips R, Weichselbaum RR. Phase I dose-escalation study of tumor necrosis factor-alpha and concomitant radiation therapy. Cancer J Sci Am. 1995;1(3):204–9.
64. Marr RA, Addison CL, Snider D, Muller WJ, Gauldie J, Graham FL. Tumour immunotherapy using an adenoviral vector expressing a membrane-bound mutant of murine TNF alpha. Gene Ther. 1997;4(11):1181–8. doi:10.1038/sj.gt.3300528.
65. Marr RA, Hitt M, Muller WJ, Gauldie J, Graham FL. Tumour therapy in mice using adenovirus vectors expressing human TNFa. Int J Oncol. 1998;12(3):509–15.

Chapter 18
Novel Radiotherapy Modalities

Lauren M. Rosati, Shalini Moningi, Lauren Colbert, Sweet Ping Ng, and Joseph M. Herman

Abbreviations

3DCRT	Three-dimensional conformal radiation therapy
4D-DWI	Four-dimensional diffusion-weighted MRI
BED	Biological equivalent dose
BRPC	Borderline resectable pancreatic cancer
DS	Double scattering
EBRT	External beam radiation therapy
GI	Gastrointestinal
GTV	Gross tumor volume
HIGRT	Hypofractionated image-guided radiation therapy
IMRT	Intensity-modulated radiation therapy

L.M. Rosati, B.S. (✉)
Department of Radiation Oncology and Molecular Radiation Sciences, The Johns Hopkins University School of Medicine, Baltimore, MD 21287, USA
e-mail: lrosati2@jhmi.edu

S. Moningi, M.D. • L. Colbert, M.D., M.S. • S.P. Ng, M.B.B.S., B.Med.Sci.
Department of Radiation Oncology, MD Anderson Cancer Center, University of Texas, 1515 Holcombe Blvd. Unit 1422, Houston, TX 77030, USA
e-mail: smoningi@mdanderson.org; lcolbert@mdanderson.org; spng@mdanderson.org

J.M. Herman, M.D., M.Sc.
Department of Radiation Oncology and Molecular Radiation Sciences, The Johns Hopkins University School of Medicine, Baltimore, MD 21287, USA

Department of Radiation Oncology, MD Anderson Cancer Center, University of Texas, 1515 Holcombe Blvd. Unit 1422, Houston, TX 77030, USA
e-mail: JMHerman@mdanderson.org

T. Bekaii-Saab, B. El-Rayes (eds.), *Current and Emerging Therapies in Pancreatic Cancer*, DOI 10.1007/978-3-319-58256-6_18

IOERT	Intraoperative electron beam radiation therapy
IPMN	Intraductal papillary mucinous neoplasm
IRE	Irreversible electroporation
LAPC	Locally advanced pancreatic cancer
LET	Linear energy transfer
MRI	Magnetic resonance imaging
OARs	Organs at risk
OS	Overall survival
PBS	Pencil beam scanning
PET	Positron emission tomography
QOL	Quality of life
RECIST	Response Evaluation Criteria in Solid Tumors
RFA	Radiofrequency ablation
SBRT	Stereotactic body radiation therapy

Introduction

Shorter courses, otherwise known as hypofractionated courses (>2.2 Gy per fraction, typically in 1–15 fractions), of radiation therapy have been proposed with the goal of decreasing time away from systemic therapy and potentially decreasing time to surgical resection. These regimens are thought to increase the biological equivalent dose (BED) that is delivered to the tumor, which should, in theory, improve tumor control and response. This is important because the pancreatic tumor is rarely surgically resectable at presentation due to either local invasion of adjacent vessels or evidence of metastatic disease at presentation.

Highly conformal radiation therapy is achieved by using multiple beams of photon radiation that can converge on the tumor. Each beam is modulated with multileaf collimators in order to specifically treat the pancreatic tumor with a high dose of radiation while avoiding adjacent normal tissues including the stomach and small bowel. This approach is termed intensity-modulated radiation therapy (IMRT). When IMRT is delivered in 1–5 treatments and small beam apertures are utilized, this is considered stereotactic body radiation therapy (SBRT). Since the pancreas can move with respiration, SBRT often requires motion management techniques including gating and/or breath hold techniques. SBRT has been shown to improve tumor-related pain without a decrease in quality of life (QOL) [1, 2]. Therefore, SBRT can be more easily integrated with systemic and targeted therapies than traditional chemoradiation. Since hypofractionated IMRT can be delivered in only 15 fractions, it can be given concurrently with chemotherapy, including multi-agent regimens. Heavy ion radiation includes proton and carbon radiotherapy. Both of these forms of radiation can deliver high doses of radiation at the target with very little to no scatter radiation to adjacent normal structures. While promising, incorporating proton and carbon radiation therapy for pancreatic cancer has several challenges before being considered a standard of care option. In this chapter, we will outline these novel radiation technologies, review the clinical outcomes, and discuss ways to improve patient selection for these radiation modalities moving forward.

Stereotactic Body Radiation Therapy

SBRT (≥5 Gy per fraction for 1–5 fractions) is increasingly recognized as an important local treatment modality in pancreatic cancer, both in the neoadjuvant setting for resectable and borderline resectable disease (BRPC) and in the definitive setting for locally advanced disease (LAPC). The role of conventional chemoradiation (1.8–2.2 Gy per fraction for 25–28 fractions) is controversial in the neoadjuvant setting. However, in patients with resectable, borderline resectable, and select patients with locally advanced disease who receive neoadjuvant chemotherapy and SBRT/IMRT may have similar or even improved rates of pathologic complete response, node-negative and margin-negative resections, and overall survival when compared to conventional chemoradiation [3–9]. Although the role of chemoradiotherapy is not fully established, chemotherapy alone does improve overall survival in these patients, whether given in the metastatic, neoadjuvant, or adjuvant setting [10, 11], and interest has therefore developed with SBRT.

Fractionation and Timing

Shorter courses of radiation therapy have been proposed with hopes to decrease time away from systemic therapy and time to surgical resection. Patients with pancreatic cancer who underwent shorter treatment course were found to have significantly better QOL outcomes compared to those who had longer radiation therapy courses [12]. A significant amount of literature has looked into toxicity associated with different number of fractions (i.e., 3–5) of SBRT and has shown that SBRT is well tolerated in terms of short- and long-term toxicity (Table 18.1).

By using SBRT, we have the ability to deliver higher doses of radiation therapy to the pancreas while limiting dose to surrounding normal tissue. Initially, the Stanford group investigated a single fraction of 25 Gy regimen for patients with LAPC. They found excellent local control rates but high rates (~20%) of late grade 2–4 gastrointestinal (GI) toxicities [13, 14]. Schellenberg et al. reported on 16 LAPC patients who also received a single fraction of 25 Gy along with concurrent gemcitabine and showed 100% local control at 1 year and a lower rate of acute GI toxicity compared to previous reports [15]. A follow-up study reported an excellent rate of local control at 1 year (94%) and low late grade ≥ 3 toxicity rates (5%) [16]. Mahadevan et al. evaluated 36 LAPC patients receiving 8–12 Gy in 3 fractions followed by gemcitabine chemotherapy [17]. The 1-year local control rate was 78%, and the median OS was 14.3 months with similar low rates of toxicities. Only 33%

Table 18.1 Pancreas SBRT in LAPC

	N	Regimen	1-year FFLP	Median OS (mos)	Acute grade ≥ 3 toxicity	Late grade ≥ 2 toxicity	Resection	R0 resection
Historically definitive setting (LAPC)								
Koong et al. 2004 (Stanford)	6	25 Gy SBRT, 1 fraction	100%	8.0	33%	–	–	–
Hoyer et al. 2005 (Denmark)	22	45 Gy SBRT, 3 fractions	57% (6 months)	5.4	79%	94%	–	–
Schellenberg et al. 2008 (Stanford)	16	Gem → 25 Gy SBRT, 1 fraction → Gem	100%	11.4	19%	47%	–	–
Chang et al. 2009 (Stanford)	77[a]	25 Gy SBRT, 1 fraction	95%	11.9	5%	13%	–	–
Mahadevan et al. 2010 (Beth Israel)	36	Median 30 Gy SBRT, 3 fractions → Gem	78%	14.3	41%	6%		
Polistina et al. 2010 (Italy)	23	Gem → 30 Gy SBRT, 3 fractions	50%	10.6	0	0	9%	100%
Schellenberg et al. 2011 (Stanford)	20	Gem → 25 Gy SBRT, 1 fraction → Gem	94%	11.8	15%	20%	–	–
Mahadevan et al. 2011 (Beth Israel)	39	Gem → median 24 Gy SBRT, 3 fractions → Gem	85%	20	0%	9%	–	–
Rwigema et al. 2011 (UPMC)	40	Median 24 Gy SBRT	38%	8.0!	4%	0%	–	–
Goyal et al. 2012 (Case Western)	20	Median 25 Gy SBRT, 1 fraction	65%	14.4	0%	16%	–	–
Tozzi et al. 2013 (Italy)	30	Gem → 45 Gy SBRT, 6 fractions	86%	11.0	20%	0%	–	–

	N	Regimen	1-year FFLP	Median OS (mos)	Acute grade ≥ 3 toxicity	Late grade ≥ 2 toxicity	Resection	R0 resection
Gurka et al. 2013 (Georgetown)	10	Gem → 25 Gy, 5 fractions	40%	12.2	0%	0%	–	–
Pollom et al. 2014 (Stanford)	76[b]	25 Gy SBRT, 1 fraction	90%	13.6	8%	4%		3%
	91	33 Gy SBRT, 5 fractions	88%		5%	1%		1%
Herman et al. 2015 (Johns Hopkins, Stanford, MSKCC)	49	Gem → Median 33 Gy, 5 fractions → Gem	78%	13.9	12%	11%	8%	100%
Comito et al. 2016 (Italy)	45	Chemo (71%) → median 45 Gy, 6 fractions	93%	13.0	0%	4%	–	–
Neoadjuvant setting (BRPC/ LAPC)								
Boone et al. 2013 (Pittsburgh)	25 (12 BR, 13 LA)	FOLFIRINOX +/– median 36 Gy SBRT (57%), 3 fractions	–	–	–	8%[c]	43% (58% BR, 15% LA)	33% (55% BR, 10% LA)
Chuong et al. 2013 (Moffitt)	73 (57 BR, 16 LA)	Gem-based chemo → median 25 Gy SBRT, 5 fractions	81%[d]	16.4 BR, 15.0 LA	0%	5%[e]	44% (56% BR, 0% LA)	97% (97% BR, N/A LA)
Rajagopalan et al. 2013 (Pittsburgh)	12 (7 BR, 5 LA)	Chemo → median 36 Gy SBRT, 3 fractions	–	47.2	0%	–	11%[f]	92% (86% BR, 100% LA)

(continued)

Table 18.1 (continued)

	N	Regimen	1-year FFLP	Median OS (mos)	Acute grade ≥ 3 toxicity	Late grade ≥ 2 toxicity	Resection	R0 resection
Mellon et al. 2015 (Moffitt)	159 (110 BR, 49 LA)	Chemo → median 30 Gy SBRT, 5 fractions	78%[d]	18.1 (19.2 BR, 15.0 LA)	2%	6%[e]	38% (51% BR, 10% LA)	97% (96% BR, 100% LA)
Moningi et al. 2015 (Johns Hopkins)	88 (14 BR, 74 LA)	Chemo → median 33 Gy SBRT, 6 fractions	61%	18.4 (14.4 BR, 18.4 LA)	3%	6%	22% (29% BR, 20% LA)	84% (84% BR, 80% LA)
Chuong et al. 2016 (Moffitt)	36 BR	GTX → median 35 Gy SBRT, 5 fractions	–	22.5	–	–	100%[g]	97%

FFLP freedom from local progression, *BR* borderline resectable, *LA* locally advanced, *Gem* gemcitabine, *IMRT* intensity-modulated radiation therapy

! Estimated from survival curve

[a]Includes 62% of patients who were treated for medically inoperable, metastatic, and locally recurrent disease

[b]Patients had unresectable (80%), borderline resectable (7%), medically inoperable (12%), or resectable (1%) disease

[c]Unknown time from SBRT

[d]Includes unresected patients only

[e]Late grade 2 toxicity not reported

[f]Percentage calculated based on the total number of patients who were treated with definitive SBRT ($n = 105$)

[g]Surgical resection was a criterion for inclusion in the study

of patients experienced any grade 1–2 toxicities, and as low as 8% of patients experienced any grade 3 toxicity.

A phase II multi-institutional trial further investigated SBRT in the neoadjuvant setting for LAPC patients, utilizing a 6.6 Gy × 5 fractionation regimen with gold fiducial marker placement, image guidance, and respiratory gating. In this study, the median OS was 13.9 months with 11% of patients experiencing grade 2 or higher acute and late toxicities. Overall, the regimen was well tolerated with minimal high-grade toxicities (Table 18.1) [1]. Interestingly, patients who had positron emission tomography (PET) avid tumors at baseline in this study were found to have significantly worse survival after controlling for known risk factors in a multivariate model. Moningi et al. retrospectively evaluated 74 LAPC or BRPC patients at Johns Hopkins Hospital who received SBRT to 25–33 Gy in 5 fractions following gemcitabine or FOLFIRINOX chemotherapy [5]. They found that these patients had a median OS of 18.4 months with 20% of patients undergoing successful surgical resection following neoadjuvant SBRT with an 84% margin-negative (R0) resection rate. Colleagues at Stanford University investigated single (25 Gy × 1) vs. 5 (6.6 Gy × 5)-fraction SBRT [18] and demonstrated that 5-fraction SBRT resulted in significantly less GI toxicity (25% vs. 9%, $p = 0.005$) with no difference in rates of local progression or survival. Furthermore, grade ≥ 2 toxicity was an independent predictor for worse overall survival, therefore suggesting the superiority of 5-fraction over single-fraction SBRT.

As seen in Table 18.1, there is limited literature evaluating the role of neoadjuvant SBRT in BRPC. Moffitt Cancer Center recently investigated 30 BRPC patients who received neoadjuvant SBRT with concurrent gemcitabine, docetaxel, and capecitabine [19]. The investigators found that 70% of their cohort underwent surgical resection following neoadjuvant therapy, with a 95% margin-negative (R0) and a 76% node-negative (N0) resection rate. One of the 30 patients had a complete response, and 2 patients had a partial response on surgical pathology. Chuong et al. retrospectively analyzed LAPC in addition to BRPC patients who received neoadjuvant chemotherapy along with SBRT [20]. The majority (78%) of their cohort had BRPC; 44% of the cohort underwent surgical resection following neoadjuvant therapy with a 97% margin-negative and 66% node-negative resection rate. Moffitt Cancer Center recently published a report on perioperative morbidity and mortality in patients who underwent up-front resection ($n = 241$) vs. patients with BRPC or LAPC who underwent neoadjuvant therapy ($n = 61$) [21]. Patients who received neoadjuvant therapy had similar or improved perioperative and long-term survival outcomes in comparison with patients who underwent up-front resection.

Currently, the optimal dose and fractionation of stereotactic body radiation therapy have not been established. Brunner et al. reviewed the existing literature on SBRT and found no clear benefit above a biological equivalent dose of 100 Gy [22]. It suggested that SBRT above 100 Gy likely resulted in toxicity that led to decreased survival. However, it is important to note that several of the studies included in the review were outdated and did not include image-guided radiation therapy or fiducial markers. In addition, most of the studies did not specifically designate dose constraints for normal tissues or rules for dose heterogeneity (dose range delivered to the tumor). A phase I dose escalation study for BRPC determined that a dose of 36 Gy with a 9 Gy simultaneous infield boost to the positive posterior resection margin (total of 45 Gy) delivered over 3 fractions was achievable while meeting normal tissue constraints [23]. While encouraging, longer follow-up for potential late bowel- or stomach-related toxicity of this regimen is needed.

It is unclear what number of SBRT fractions is optimal (1, 3, or 5 fraction) or whether it is the dose per fraction that ultimately determines tumor control or toxicity. Alternatively, the total BED may be what determines tumor control, and, therefore, dose and dose per fraction are irrelevant. Table 18.2 includes the BED for various dose and fractionation regimens for chemoradiation, SBRT, and hypofractionation regimens.

In some cases, it may be difficult to safely deliver full-dose radiation therapy with a 5-fraction SBRT regimen. Therefore, rather than focus on one fractionation approach, it is ideal to determine the treatment approach based on the spatial relationship of the tumor with the bowel and stomach. For example, if the tumor is located away (at least 1 cm) from dose-limiting structures (e.g., small bowel), delivering a single large fraction(s) of radiation may be effective and safe assuming the patient's radiation delivery is consistent and reliable (small setup error). However, when the tumor is located in close proximity to dose-limiting structures—which is

Table 18.2 Proposed dose constraints for dose escalation with IMRT, SBRT, and HIGRT

Structure	Standard dose constraints for 15-fraction IMRT [24]	Dose constraints for 5-fraction SBRT[a]	Dose constraints for 5-fraction HIGRT[a]
Spinal cord	DMax <30 Gy	V20 < 1 cm^3	V20 < 1 cm^3
Liver	700 cc < 24 Gy, mean dose <24 Gy	V12 < 50%	Mean < 15Gy
Kidneys	V12 < 25% (combined)	V12 < 25% (combined)	70% <15Gy for each kidney
Stomach	V20 < 20 cc		
	V35 < 1 cc	V20 < 20 cm^3	V27.5 < 1 cm^3
		V35 < 1 cm^3	V20 < 30 cm^3
Duodenum	V20 < 20 cc		
	V35 < 1 cc	V20 < 20 cm^3	V27.5 < 1 cm^3
		V35 < 1 cm^3	V20 < 30 cm^3
Small bowel	V20 < 20 cc		
	V35 < 1 cc	V20 < 20 cm^3	V27.5 < 1 cm^3
		V35 < 1 cm^3	V20 < 30 cm^3
Colon	DMax <50 Gy	–	–
Heart	V40 < 10%	–	–
Bile duct (common)	DMax <70 Gy	–	–

[a]Per the Alliance A021501 protocol for borderline resectable pancreatic cancer. Stereotactic body radiation therapy (SBRT) and hypofractionated image-guided radiation therapy (HIGRT) deliver RT over 5 days to a total dose of 40 Gy and 25 Gy, respectively

Table 18.3 Estimated biological equivalent dose (BED) of fractionation schedules

Dose (Gy)	No. fractions	Dose per fraction	Technique	Concurrent chemotherapy	BED early	BED late
					$\alpha/\beta = 10$	$\alpha/\beta = -3$
36.0	18	2.0	IMRT	Yes	43.2	60.0
50.4	28	1.8	IMRT	Yes	59.5	80.6
67.5	15	4.5	IMRT	Yes	97.9	168.8
25.0	5	5.0	SBRT	No	37.5	66.7
33.0	5	6.6	SBRT	No	54.8	105.6
40.0	5	8.0	SBRT	No	72	146.7

often the case—increasing the number of fractions will likely decrease the risk of late toxicity but may not be ablative. It is also unknown whether it is necessary to deliver 100% of the prescribed dose to the tumor or if the tumor can be sterilized with a heterogeneous dose of radiation. In the neoadjuvant setting, it may be reasonable to deliver a very high dose to the tumor that abuts or invades the adjacent artery or vein while giving a slightly lower dose to the rest of the tumor with the anticipation of resection. Yang et al. has been able to demonstrate that doses in excess of 60 Gy can be delivered to the tumor-vessel interface while still limiting the dose to organs at risk [25]. This approach is also being evaluated in the upcoming Alliance A021501 trial that randomizes BRPC patients to either modified FOLFIRINOX chemotherapy alone or FOLFIRINOX followed by SBRT prior to surgical resection. If the full dose of SBRT cannot be delivered because of anatomy or challenges with image guidance, the protocol allows hypofractionated image-guided radiation therapy (HIGRT), in which patients will receive 5 Gy × 5 to the tumor plus a 3 mm margin. The dose constraints used for each approach and for a 15-fraction regimen are highlighted in Table 18.3.

Sequencing of SBRT with Chemotherapy and Surgery

There have been no formal studies evaluating how SBRT should be sequenced with other therapies. Given the high risk of systemic progression and improved efficacy of multi-agent chemotherapy, most centers deliver at least 2–6 months of chemotherapy prior to considering SBRT. If the patient is a surgical candidate, then surgical exploration is typically recommended 4–8 weeks after SBRT. While surgery can be performed greater than 12 weeks after SBRT, there may be extensive treatment-related fibrosis that may make surgical resection difficult. Although there are limited data for using SBRT in the adjuvant setting, it may be reasonable to deliver SBRT after surgery and prior to systemic therapy if the patient was found to have positive margins (R1 or R2 resection) as SBRT should not induce toxicity that would preclude subsequent treatment [26].

Dose-Escalated Hypofractionation

As an alternative to SBRT, hypofractionated IMRT may allow for a slower and safer technique to reach the higher BED that is needed to provide ablative doses to pancreatic tumors. Although the only definitive treatment for LAPC was resection previously, it is possible that long-term local control may be achieved with radiation or chemoradiation with ablative doses as shown in this treatment plan (Fig. 18.1). Willet et al. demonstrated long-term survival (>5 years) for 8 patients in a series of 150 patients with small, unresectable tumors treated with external beam radiation therapy (EBRT) and intraoperative electron beam radiation therapy (IOERT) boost [27]. This cohort also demonstrated a 3-year survival of nearly 20%. The limitation to this treatment regimen is the dose tolerance of surrounding organs at risk (OARs), including the stomach, duodenum, and other small bowel. The BED of 70–100 Gy required to ablate the majority of the pancreatic tumor can cause severe and potentially fatal toxicity to these structures, including bleeding, stricture, fistula, and perforation. As radiation delivery techniques including improved respiratory motion control and image guidance advance, the ability to deliver ablative doses in a more conformal fashion may allow for delivery of dose-escalated radiation. This technique also allows for a shorter treatment course than a standard dose 28-fraction course, improving patient convenience while also improving patient outcomes.

A dosimetric study from MD Anderson Cancer Center of dose-escalated hypofractionation treatment courses compared three-dimensional conformal radiation therapy (3DCRT), IMRT, and proton radiation techniques using tumor GTV (gross tumor volume) with a 3 mm margin radially and a 7 mm margin superiorly-inferiorly, expanded into an ITV (internal target volume) based on respiratory motion and a 5 mm PTV (planning target volume) [28]. This volume was then translated to 11 potential tumor positions from the pancreatic head to pancreatic tail, and the dose volume histograms for surrounding OARs were produced. In this study, 3DCRT could not produce dose-escalated plans which met OAR constraints in any position; however, in patients with a distance between duodenum and GTV of between 13 and 22 mm, depending on tumor location, dose-escalated radiation to 72 Gy could safely be delivered with IMRT. The distance required between duodenum and tumor was approximately 17–26 mm for a passive scattered proton plan. Overall, the tumor dose coverage was better with IMRT plans than passive scattered proton plans in most tumor locations

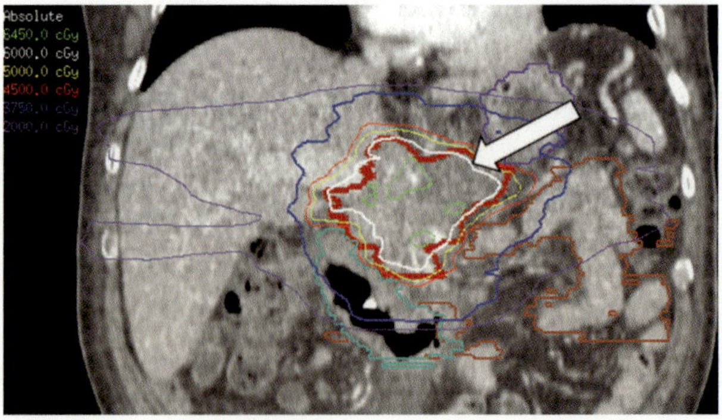

Fig. 18.1 Coronal view of a hypofractionated intensity-modulated radiation (IMRT) plan of a patient with LAPC. This plan delivers a total dose of 60 Gy (*arrow*) delivered over 15 fractions. The plan delivers a simulated integrative boost to the tumor (higher dose gradient) while giving a lower dose to the tumor bowel interface (inferior to the tumor)

due to more conformality in higher doses circumferentially. The one dosimetric advantage noted for proton therapy was the low dose to bowel, with a lower V15 Gy to GI structures than even standard dose 3DCRT plans (Table 18.3). This study has not been repeated using scanning beam proton planning, which may offer more similar conformality to IMRT or volumetric modulated arc therapy (VMAT) planning, which may also be superior due to better radial conformality.

Based on these results, MD Anderson Cancer Center also reported the largest series of patients treated using dose-escalated hypofractionated regimens in which doses in the range of 60–75 Gy were delivered over 15–25 fractions, and volumes treated to this dose were adjusted for proximity to OARs including the duodenum, stomach, liver, and small bowel [24]. Volumes with less than 1 cm distance to OARs were treated to conventional dose/fractionation of 50.4 Gy in 28 fractions, while GTVs with a 3–5 mm margin with a larger distance from tumor to OARs were escalated using a simultaneous integrated boost technique where possible.

In this retrospective series of 200 patients with LAPC, 24% were eligible for dose-escalated radiation therapy due to tumor location and clinical characteristics, and these patients demonstrated improved overall survival (17.8 months vs. 15 months) when they received a BED >70 Gy. No prospective analysis of dose-escalated radiation has been performed due to limitations in patient eligibility, among other limitations. A comparison of toxicity in these patients demonstrated decreased grade ≥ 3 toxicity in this cohort of patients over those treated with standard dose 4-field RT, indicating no excess toxicity in carefully selected patients (*paper under review*). This study also demonstrated the importance of respiratory management and tumor motion evaluation when treating with dose-escalated radiation, including simulation with deep inspiration, breath hold, and/or 4D-CT technique. Simulation with pancreatic protocol contrast administration and with additional imaging including magnetic resonance imaging (MRI) simulation can also improve visualization. Future directions include exploration of scanning beam proton therapy over passive scatter proton therapy.

Heavy Particle Therapy

Heavy particle therapy is the use of charged or inert large particles that are accelerated to the speed of light to deposit energy within tissue. In this chapter, we will focus on only proton and carbon therapy. Both have multiple theoretical advantages, some of which have been realized clinically. While photon irradiation with IMRT focuses the radiation dose to the tumor, there is scatter dose as the photon beam enters and exits tissue. Heavy particle therapy delivers lower entrance doses, higher depth doses, and very little exit dose. This is known as the Bragg peak. Consequently, it presents a theoretical advantage in delivering radiation to the target and minimal damage to surrounding tissues (Fig. 18.2). Given the proximity of small bowel to the pancreas, less scatter dose could be beneficial. The most common type of heavy particle therapy used in pancreatic cancer is proton therapy, which theoretically has a slightly higher radiobiological effect on the tumor than photon radiation therapy.

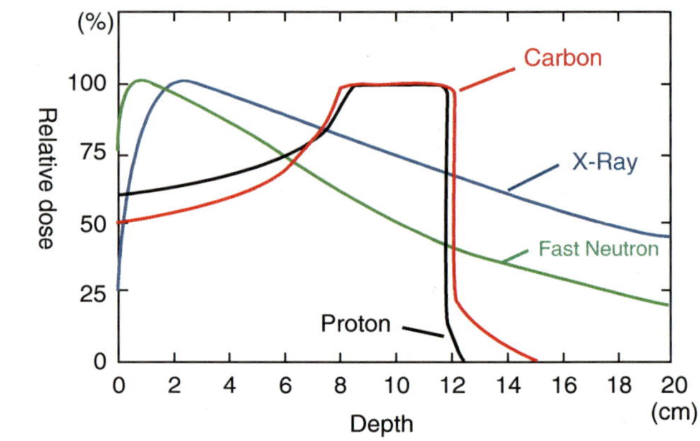

Fig. 18.2 Comparison of radiation therapy modalities. *Permission to republish granted by Ebner, D. K., & Kamada, T. (2016). The emerging role of carbon ion radiotherapy. Frontiers in Oncology, 6, 140. doi:10.3389/fonc.2016.00140 [doi]*

The largest barriers to the universal implementation of heavy particle therapy include the size of the machine, cost, and challenges with insurance reimbursement [29]. Another major challenge with heavy ion therapy includes the inability to utilize daily image guidance in the same manner as IMRT and SBRT [30].

Proton Therapy in Resectable Pancreatic Cancer

Massachusetts General Hospital (MGH) reported results of a phase I/II trial of neoadjuvant proton therapy to 25 Gy in five fractions with concurrent capecitabine followed by surgical resection (1–6 weeks after RT) and adjuvant gemcitabine chemotherapy [31]. Of the 35 patients, only 4% were observed to have grade ≥ 3 GI toxicity. Interestingly, 22% of patients did not undergo surgery due to the change in diagnosis (2%), metastatic progression (4%), or unresectable disease at the time of exploration (16%). The node-negative resection rate was reported to be very low at 19%, whereas 84% had a margin-negative resection. Median OS was 17.3 months, with 42% of patients surviving 2 years, and median progression-free survival was 10.4 months. Of the 37 resected patients, median OS and PFS were 27.0 months and 14.5 months, respectively. At median follow-up of 38 months, 16% of the resected patients had recurred locoregionally. The approach used in this study is in contrast to SBRT where concurrent chemotherapy is typically not included and nodal basins are not treated (tumor plus 1–5 mm only).

The University of Pennsylvania conducted studies comparing dosimetric data between proton and photon therapy treatment plans in patients with pancreatic cancer. The study compared 3DCRT with IMRT and different approaches with proton therapy in patients receiving adjuvant radiation therapy to 50.4 Gy [32]. The study reported that all proton plans had significantly lower doses to the left kidney, stomach, and spinal cord (maximum dose) compared with all the photon plans, except in the case of 3-field 3DCRT with lower spinal cord maximum dose. The dosimetric advantage of proton therapy may allow for more tolerable dose-escalated RT to the tumor bed or be used in cases where there is recurrence after standard adjuvant chemoradiation.

Proton Therapy in Locally Advanced Pancreatic Cancer

In unresectable, LAPC tumors, proton therapy may be able to deliver higher doses that may, in theory, sterilize tumors. However, given the proximity of the duodenum, small shifts during therapy may deliver even higher doses to the duodenum than with photon therapy and place the patient at risk of duodenal toxicity. One study evaluated 55 Gy delivered to patients with LAPC via double scattering (DS) and pencil beam scanning (PBS) proton therapy vs. IMRT [33]. DS and PBS proton therapy were shown to decrease stomach, duodenum, and small bowel dose in low-dose regions compared to IMRT ($p < 0.01$). However, protons yielded increased doses in the mid- to high-dose regions and increased generalized equivalent uniform dose to the duodenum and stomach although these differences were minimal (<5% and 10%, respectively, $p < 0.01$). This study suggests that proton therapy results in decreased low-to-intermediate dose to the treatment volume although high dose of radiation to OARs was not significantly reduced. One Japanese study reported on the use of proton radiation in patients with LAPC and found it to be extremely tolerable (0–10% grade ≥ 3 toxicity) [34, 35]. Interestingly, however, a follow-up report of this study reported that 49% of patients had radiation-induced gastric and duodenal ulcers (grade 1) found on endoscopy though the rate of grade ≥ 3 toxicity was only 3% [36]. In Fig. 18.3, we have provided an example patient who was planned

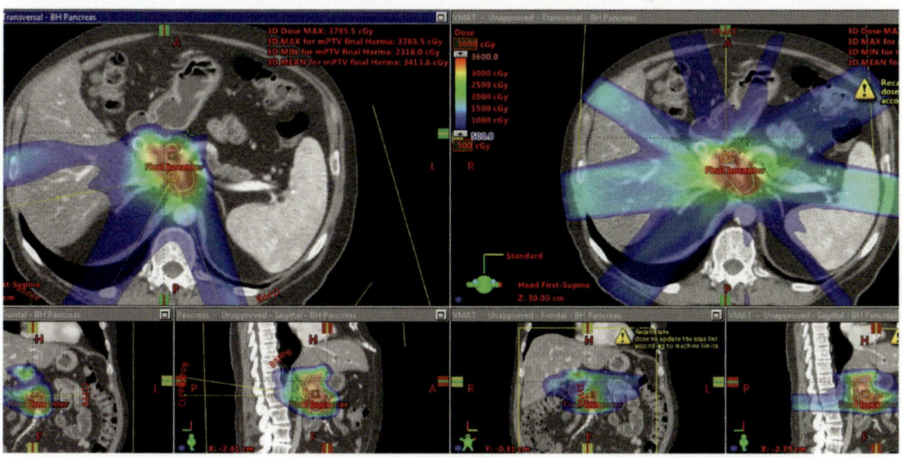

Fig. 18.3 Proton (*left*) and photon (*right*) stereotactic body radiation therapy plan performed on the same patient with locally advanced pancreatic cancer (LAPC). Notice that the proton plan uses only three fields, while the photon field requires eight fields. The proton plan contributes significantly less radiation dose (*color wash*) to adjacent normal structures than the photon plan including the liver, bowel, kidneys, and spinal cord

for both photon and proton SBRT. Note the lower scatter dose in the proton plan. Both plans were able to achieve the dose objectives for tumor coverage and sparing of organs at risk. One challenge with proton SBRT is controlling/monitoring tumor motion due to breathing.

Carbon Ion Therapy

Some experts argue that the biological impact of protons mirrors that of photon therapy, and, therefore, attention has turned to heavier ions due to a higher biological impact owing to higher linear energy transfer (LET) [37]. Progress has been limited as there are currently only eight carbon facilities worldwide and none in the United States. Shinoto et al. set out to determine the maximum tolerated dose of carbon ion radiation therapy and gemcitabine delivered concurrently [38]. Gemcitabine was administered on days 1, 8, and 15, and the dose levels were escalated from 400 to 1000 mg/m^2 with the starting carbon ion radiation therapy dose at 43.2 GyE. The dose levels of RT were escalated from 43.2 to 55.2 GyE at 12 fractions under the fixed recommended gemcitabine dose determined. Among the 72 patients treated, dose-limiting toxicity was observed in 3 (4%) patients: grade 3 infection in 1 patient and grade 4 neutropenia in 2 patients. Only one patient experienced a late grade 3 gastric ulcer and bleeding 10 months after radiation therapy. The recommended dose of gemcitabine with carbon ion RT was found to be 1000 mg/m^2. The dose of carbon ion radiation therapy with the full dose of gemcitabine (1000 mg/m^2) was safely increased to 55.2 GyE. The freedom from local progression rate was 83% at 2 years using the Response Evaluation Criteria in Solid Tumors (RECIST) criteria. The 2-year OS rates in all patients and in the high-dose group (≥45.6 GyE) were 35% and 48%, respectively. Longer-term follow-up is needed to determine the true efficacy of this approach, but the results are encouraging.

At this time, it is unclear what radiation approach is ideal in terms of obtaining long-term control with limited toxicity. Ultimately, an adaptive approach that takes into account each individual patient's anatomy (location of tumor and proximity of the duodenum, small bowel, and/or stomach) will be the most efficacious. For example, if there is a large tumor in the head of the pancreas, adjacent to the duodenum, a hypofractionated approach (10–15 fractions) can still achieve a BED with limited toxicity. In contrast, a body tumor that is at least 1 cm away from any dose-limiting structures could be treated with 3- or 5-fraction SBRT. Taking this same approach with protons and carbon ion therapy (assuming motion management is optimized) will likely result in even better tumor control rates based on some modeling reported by a comprehensive review by Durante et al. [39]. Future studies will likely evaluate the interplay of dose, fractionation, and targeted/immunotherapy to optimize multimodality therapy for this disease.

Image-Guided Therapy and Motion Management in Pancreatic Cancer

With IMRT and SBRT, the smaller field sizes can be potentially undertreat tumor if respiratory tumor motion is not accounted for. Pancreatic tumors can have respiratory motion at times greater than 2 cm craniocaudally [40]. If patients have ≥3 mm breathing motion on fluoroscopy or 4D-CT scan, tumor immobilization techniques should be utilized [41]. Two approaches to motion management are commonly employed: immobilization of the target (abdominal compression or breath hold techniques) or physiologically monitoring of tumor motion (tracking or gating) [42]. Generally, if breathing motion is <3 mm, patients can be treated free breathing with an internal target volume (ITV) based on extreme phases (superior and inferior) of the breathing cycle or using gating. In these patients, a PET or MRI simulation may improve the ability to delineate the tumor and adjacent structures as well as provide a baseline to determine treatment response.

For SBRT, specifically, gold fiducials are placed by endoscopy in or near the tumor under ultrasound guidance and are used to assist in targeting the tumor during radiation delivery. Respiratory gating is used to track the tumor during respiration and/or during breath hold. Both of these methods decrease the margin needed to cover the tumor, decrease dose to the bowel and stomach, and result in less acute and chronic toxicity. These approaches are also essential in order to achieve radiation dose levels that may be potentially ablative.

Locally Ablative Techniques

Other locally ablative techniques, such as radiofrequency ablation (RFA), irreversible electroporation (IRE), and intraluminal brachytherapy, have also been explored with little success. RFA generates high temperatures within tumor by the use of needle electrodes, while IRE involves high-voltage electric fields that produce cell death. Thus, both require direct contact with tumor through open, laparoscopic, or percutaneous approaches, all of which increase the risk of complications and morbidity. RFA can also produce very high temperatures and tissue necrosis, particularly in the vasculature, under endoscopic ultrasound (EUS) guidance. IRE has been evaluated as a method to accentuate positive margins in BRPC or LAPC patients who undergo surgical resection after neoadjuvant therapy as well as an exclusive treatment modality in unresectable tumors. Both RFA and IRE appear to be safe and feasible in patients with localized disease, and survival outcomes are promising [43–47]. Although IRE may have more value in areas close to vital blood vessels, further exploration of endoscopic and laparoscopic techniques continues.

Exploration into endoscopic or interstitial brachytherapy for pancreatic cancer continues, both in the early-stage setting and in the setting of obstruction causing jaundice. The Ohio State University designed a 3D high-resolution optical coherence tomography (OCT) imaging technique to detect early-stage pancreatic tumors and deliver treatment through the pancreatic duct using an HDR source [48]. This technique has not yet been tested in humans. A recent study in China used interstitial brachytherapy with iodine-125 stranded seeds to treat patients with local tumor causing obstructive jaundice and reported successful bile drainage in all patients with low rates of stent dysfunction or morbidity [49]. Small retrospective studies have shown the EUS-guided interstitial brachytherapy improved pain in patients with advanced pancreatic cancer; however, the impact on clinical outcomes such as survival and tumor response remains unclear [50–53].

Planning and Quality Assurance

Radiation therapy quality assurance is essential to ensure pancreatic cancer patients receive safe and efficacious local therapy, especially when utilizing high doses of radiation such as IMRT and SBRT. An analysis on the locally advanced SCALOP trial elucidates the importance of quality assurance and central review of imaging and treatment plans prior to and during the delivery of RT in pancreatic cancer [54]. After retrospective central review of radiation treatment plans, it was made clear that a tumor was completely missed in one patient, and >50% of a tumor was missed in three patients. Moreover, major deviations in planning were observed in 5% of cases, and a Jaccard conformity index (JCI) value for GTV ≥ 0.7 had a 7.12 (95% CIs: 1.83–27.67, $p = 0.005$) higher odds of progressing within 9 months on multivariate analysis.

In order to improve the accuracy and standardization of pancreatic tumor delineation for radiation therapy treatment planning, collaborators at multiple institutions recently published guidelines for MRI-based contouring [55]. Specific recommendations with respect to contouring the GTV, OARs, and blood vessels using MRI are outlined. Four-dimensional diffusion-weighted MRI (4D-DWI) in particular and respiratory-gated PET (4D-PET) may also be helpful in delineating respiratory motion during treatment planning and delivery [56, 57].

Immunotherapy, Vaccines, and Targeted Therapy

Radiotherapy coupled with immunotherapy has become more popular over the past decade with the hypothesis that a synergy between radiotherapy and immune response exists. With hypofractionated radiotherapy, specifically, it is believed that antitumor abscopal effects may occur with high-dose radiation [58]. Although the current data are limited, investigators at Johns Hopkins reported that 12 Gy × 1 SBRT primes an endogenous antigen-specific immune response in breast cancer and melanoma [59]. The immune-stimulating effects were amplified when the SBRT was combined with anti-PD-1 or regulatory T-cell depletion therapy. Similar results were also reported by investigators at the University of Pennsylvania after analyzing the outcomes of 20 Gy × 1 SBRT combined with checkpoint inhibitors in melanoma, breast cancer, and pancreatic cancer in mice [60].

To our knowledge, the first study to evaluate immunotherapy and SBRT in the adjuvant setting of pancreatic cancer explored the feasibility and efficacy of GM-CSF-secreting allogeneic pancreatic cancer (GVAX) vaccine combined with low-dose cyclophosphamide integrated with 5-fraction SBRT and FOLFIRINOX (NCT01595321). Although the final results of the study have not yet been published, the preliminary data demonstrated limited toxicity [26]. A current study open at Johns Hopkins (NCT02648282) is evaluating the role of the GVAX vaccine combined with PD-1 blockade antibody and SBRT in patients with LAPC. Future clinical trials are necessary to prospectively evaluate the role of high-dose radiotherapy with immunotherapy. There are several studies combining SBRT with various targeted therapies including SBRT and nelfinavir. A list of current SBRT studies can be found in Table 18.4.

Table 18.4 Current and future clinical trials evaluating novel radiation therapy techniques for the definitive management of patients with localized pancreatic cancer

Identifier	Phase	Institution	RT technique	Patient population	Date opened	Primary outcome
Stereotactic body radiation therapy						
NCT02035072	II	Istituto Scientifico Romagnolo per lo Studio e la cura dei Tumori	Gemox → hypofractionated RT (35 Gy in 7 fx) → Gemox	LAPC	November 2010	Toxicity
NCT01342354	I	University of Chicago	Dose-escalated SBRT	Unresected	April 2011	MTD
NCT01357525	II	University of Pittsburgh	SBRT	Resected	May 2011	LPFS
NCT01781728	II	Johns Hopkins University	Chemo → SBRT	BRPC, LAPC, recurrent	August 2012	Toxicity
NCT01872377	I	Ottawa Hospital Research Institute	SBRT Boost	LAPC	October 2012	Toxicity
NCT02707315	I	Cooper Health System	Gem → SBRT	Resectable, BRPC	January 2013	Resection
NCT01918644	I	University of Wisconsin, Madison	Cap with SBRT → surgery	Resectable	August 2013	Toxicity
NCT01926197	III	Stanford University	FFX +/– SBRT	LAPC	August 2013	PFS
NCT01959672	II	University of Nebraska	Gem, LV, 5-FU +/– oregovomab → SBRT + nelfinavir	Resectable, BRPC	September 2013	PFS
NCT01992705	I	University of Maryland	FFX → SBRT	BRPC	March 2014	Resection
NCT02128100	II	James Graham Brown	FFX + SBRT	LAPC	April 2014	Toxicity
NCT02454140	I	University of California, San Diego	Dose-escalated SBRT	LAPC or medically inoperable	June 2014	MTD
NCT02208024	I	University of Cincinnati	SBRT	Resectable	July 2014	Toxicity

NCT02292745	II	Erasmus Medical Center	FFX + SBRT	LAPC	July 2014	OS
NCT02416609	II	Universitaria di Modena	Low-Dose RT → Gemox → SBRT	LAPC	January 2014	PFS
NCT02311361	I	NCI	Tremelimumab +/− MEDI4736 + SBRT	LAPC	December 2014	Feasibility, toxicity
NCT02308722	I	University of Oxford	Dose-escalated SBRT	BRPC	December 2014	MTD
NCT02347618	II	University of Rochester	SBRT → Surgery	Resectable	December 2014	Toxicity
NCT02241551	II	University of Pittsburgh	GNP vs. FFX → SBRT → Surgery	BRPC	December 2014	Toxicity, pathologic complete response
NCT02707328	I	Cooper Health System	Gem → Dose-escalated SBRT (up to 55 Gy, 5 fx) → Gem	LAPC	January 2015	MTD
NCT02153450		Case Comprehensive Cancer Center	Metformin → SRS with metformin	BRPC, LAPC	May 2015	Toxicity
NCT02461836	II	Zhejiang University	Gem +/− SBRT	Resected	August 2015	DFS
NCT02643498	I	Memorial Sloan Kettering Cancer Center	Dose-escalated SBRT	LAPC	December 2015	MTD
NCT02704156	II	Changhai Hospital	SBRT	LAPC	March 2016	OS
NCT02716207	I	Changhai Hospital	Dose-escalated SBRT	LAPC, medically inoperable	March 2016	MTD
NCT02745847	II	Changhai Hospital	Re-irradiation with SBRT	Recurrent	April 2016	OS
NCT02734680	II	Cancer Institute and Hospital, Chinese Academy of Medical Sciences	IORT → Gem-based CRT vs. SBRT → S-1	LAPCC	April 2016	OS

(continued)

Table 18.4 (continued)

Identifier	Phase	Institution	RT technique	Patient population	Date opened	Primary outcome
NCT02780648	I	Indiana University	SBRT	BRPC, LAPC, recurrent	May 2016	Toxicity
NCT02723331	II	University of Colorado, Denver	GNP → SBRT → surgery	Resectable, BRPC	May 2016	R0 resection
NCT02791503	II/III	Vanderbilt University	FFX + SABR vs. IRE	LAPC	May 2016	OS
NCT02648282	II	Johns Hopkins University	Cyclophosphamide + GVAX vaccine + pembrolizumab + SBRT	LAPC	July 2016	DMFS
NCT02873598	I	University of Colorado, Denver	GNP or FFX → dose-escalated SBRT	LAPC	August 2016	MTD
NCT02868632	Ib	New York University	SBRT + MEDI4736, tremelimumab, or both	LAPC	August 2016	OS
NCT02704143	II	Changhai Hospital	SBRT + S-1	LAPC	October 2016	OS
NCT02839343 A021501	II	Alliance for Clinical Trials in Oncology	mFFX +/− HIGRT or SBRT → surgery → FOLFOX	BRPC	December 2016	OS
NCT02950025	II	Washington University	SBRT +/− adaptive planning	LAPC	January 2017	Toxicity
Proton beam therapy						
NCT02207465	I	University of Pennsylvania	Dose-escalated GNP + PBT and IMRT	BRPC, LAPC	July 2014	Toxicity
NCT01683422	II	Loma Linda University	Gem + erlotinib → PBT + CapOx	LAPC	December 2011	OS
NCT01821729	II	Massachusetts General Hospital	FFX + losartan → PBT	LAPC	July 2013	DFS
NCT02598349	II	University of Florida	PBT	BRPC, LAPC, medically inoperable	November 2015	OS

Other						
NCT01027221	I/II	German Cancer Research Center	Low-dose IMRT	Resectable	December 2009	T-Cell activity
NCT01372735	I/II	German Cancer Research Center	IMRT → surgery + IORT	Resectable	June 2011	Local recurrence
NCT01972919	II	Medical College of Wisconsin	Dose-escalated MR-guided IMRT	LAPC	August 2013	Efficacy, toxicity
NCT02283372	I	Washington University	GNP + dose-escalated IMRT	BRPC, LAPC	January 2015	MTD
NCT02303990	I	University of Pennsylvania	Pembrolizumab + hypofractionated RT	LAPC, metastatic	February 2015	Toxicity
NCT02394535	I	MD Anderson	Cap + NP + dose-escalated IMRT	LAPC	March 2015	MTD
NCT02481635	I/II	University Health Network, Toronto	GNP + IMRT → surgery	BRPC	June 2015	Toxicity
NCT02439593	II	University of Zurich	Gem-based CRT +/− thermoCRT	LAPC	October 2015	OS
NCT02599662	I	Loyola University	IORT	Resectable	November 2015	MTD
NCT02981641	II	Chinese Academy of Medical Sciences	IORT vs. Gem-based 3DCRT	LAPC	December 2015	OS
NCT02024009 SCALOP-2	I/II	University of Oxford	Conventional or dose-escalated CRT +/− nelfinavir	LAPC	March 2016	OS, PFS
NCT02843945	II	CivaTech Oncology	LDR brachytherapy	Resected	July 2016	Toxicity
NCT02318095	I	Duke University	GNP + HIGRT → surgery	Resectable, BRPC	December 2014	Feasibility

Imaging as a Prognostic Factor

Although major strides have been made in the management of pancreatic cancer in the past few decades, there is a large need for prediction of outcomes and response to therapies. A large contributing factor to early detection and evaluation of prognostic factors relies on imaging studies. Investigators at MD Anderson Cancer Center have studied imaging biomarkers in pancreatic cancer. Evaluating mass transport properties of tumors measured on CT scans may provide insight into patterns of disease progression and/or response to therapies [61, 62]. Another report investigated the malignant potential of intraductal papillary mucinous neoplasms (IPMNs) [63]. Using distinct imaging features as a prognostic factor, oncologists can determine optimal management for patients with IPMNs (i.e., seek a more aggressive therapy regimen such as resection for high-grade IPMNs that are likely to progress to pancreatic ductal adenocarcinoma).

Furthermore, PET avidity has been shown to be a prognostic factor in patients who received SBRT [1, 64]. The prognostic signature developed by colleagues at Stanford University may be utilized to predict overall survival and guide treatment recommendations for select patients. As science and technologies advance, we move toward personalized medicine, and larger prospective trials are needed to deliver state-of-the-art care specific to each patient.

References

1. Herman JM, Chang DT, Goodman KA, Dholakia AS, Raman SP, Hacker-Prietz A, Iacobuzio-Donahue CA, Griffith ME, Pawlik TM, Pai JS, O'Reilly E, Fisher GA, Wild AT, Rosati LM, Zheng L, Wolfgang CL, Laheru DA, Columbo LA, Sugar EA, Koong AC. Phase 2 multi-institutional trial evaluating gemcitabine and stereotactic body radiotherapy for patients with locally advanced unresectable pancreatic adenocarcinoma. Cancer. 2015a;121(7):1128–37.
2. Rao AD, Sugar EA, Chang DT, Goodman KA, Hacker-Prietz A, Rosati LM, Columbo L, O'Reilly E, Fisher GA, Zheng L, Pai JS, Griffith ME, Laheru DA, Iacobuzio-Donahue CA, Wolfgang CL, Koong A, Herman JM. Patient-reported outcomes of a multicenter phase 2 study investigating gemcitabine and stereotactic body radiation therapy in locally advanced pancreatic cancer. Pract Radiat Oncol. 2016;6(6):417–24.
3. Colbert LE, Hall WA, Nickleach D, Switchenko J, Kooby DA, Liu Y, Gillespie T, Lipscomb J, Kauh J, Landry JC. Chemoradiation therapy sequencing for resected pancreatic adenocarcinoma in the national cancer data base. Cancer. 2014;120(4):499–506.
4. Katz MH, Shi Q, Ahmad SA, Herman JM, Marsh Rde W, Collisson E, Schwartz L, Frankel W, Martin R, Conway W, Truty M, Kindler H, Lowy AM, Bekaii-Saab T, Philip P, Talamonti M, Cardin D, LoConte N, Shen P, Hoffman JP, Venook AP. Preoperative modified FOLFIRINOX treatment followed by capecitabine-based chemoradiation for borderline resectable pancreatic cancer: alliance for clinical trials in oncology trial A021101. JAMA Surg. 2016;151(8):e161137.
5. Moningi S, Dholakia AS, Raman SP, Blackford A, Cameron JL, Le DT, De Jesus-Acosta AM, Hacker-Prietz A, Rosati LM, Assadi RK, Dipasquale S, Pawlik TM, Zheng L, Weiss MJ, Laheru DA, Wolfgang CL, Herman JM. The role of stereotactic body radiation therapy for pancreatic cancer: a single-institution experience. Ann Surg Oncol. 2015;22(7):2352–8.

6. Roland CL, Yang AD, Katz MH, Chatterjee D, Wang H, Lin H, Vauthey JN, Pisters PW, Varadhachary GR, Wolff RA, Crane CH, Lee JE, Fleming JB. Neoadjuvant therapy is associated with a reduced lymph node ratio in patients with potentially resectable pancreatic cancer. Ann Surg Oncol. 2015;22(4):1168–75.
7. Stessin AM, Meyer JE, Sherr DL. Neoadjuvant radiation is associated with improved survival in patients with resectable pancreatic cancer: an analysis of data from the surveillance, epidemiology, and end results (SEER) registry. Int J Radiat Oncol Biol Phys. 2008;72(4):1128–33.
8. Talamonti MS, Small W Jr, Mulcahy MF, Wayne JD, Attaluri V, Colletti LM, Zalupski MM, Hoffman JP, Freedman GM, Kinsella TJ, Philip PA, McGinn CJ. A multi-institutional phase II trial of preoperative full-dose gemcitabine and concurrent radiation for patients with potentially resectable pancreatic carcinoma. Ann Surg Oncol. 2006;13(2):150–8.
9. Turrini O, Ychou M, Moureau-Zabotto L, Rouanet P, Giovannini M, Moutardier V, Azria D, Delpero JR, Viret F. Neoadjuvant docetaxel-based chemoradiation for resectable adenocarcinoma of the pancreas: new neoadjuvant regimen was safe and provided an interesting pathologic response. Euro J Surg Oncol. 2010;36(10):987–92.
10. Neoptolemos JP, Dunn JA, Stocken DD, Almond J, Link K, Beger H, Bassi C, Falconi M, Pederzoli P, Dervenis C, Fernandez-Cruz L, Lacaine F, Pap A, Spooner D, Kerr DJ, Friess H, Buchler MW, European Study Group for Pancreatic Cancer. Adjuvant chemoradiotherapy and chemotherapy in resectable pancreatic cancer: a randomised controlled trial. Lancet, 2001;358(9293):1576–85.
11. Regine WF, Winter KA, Abrams RA, Safran H, Hoffman JP, Konski A, Benson AB, Macdonald JS, Kudrimoti MR, Fromm ML, Haddock MG, Schaefer P, Willett CG, Rich TA. Fluorouracil vs gemcitabine chemotherapy before and after fluorouracil-based chemoradiation following resection of pancreatic adenocarcinoma: a randomized controlled trial. JAMA. 2008;299(9):1019–26.
12. Herman JM, Wild AT, Wang H, Tran PT, Chang KJ, Taylor GE, Donehower RC, Pawlik TM, Ziegler MA, Cai H, Savage DT, Canto MI, Klapman J, Reid T, Shah RJ, Hoffe SE, Rosemurgy A, Wolfgang CL, Laheru DA. Randomized phase III multi-institutional study of TNFerade biologic with fluorouracil and radiotherapy for locally advanced pancreatic cancer: final results. J Clin Oncol Off J Am Soc Clin Oncol. 2013;31(7):886–94.
13. Hoyer M, Roed H, Sengelov L, Traberg A, Ohlhuis L, Pedersen J, Nellemann H, Kiil Berthelsen A, Eberholst F, Engelholm SA, von der Maase H. Phase-II study on stereotactic radiotherapy of locally advanced pancreatic carcinoma. Radiother Oncol. 2005;76(1):48–53.
14. Koong AC, Le QT, Ho A, Fong B, Fisher G, Cho C, Ford J, Poen J, Gibbs IC, Mehta VK, Kee S, Trueblood W, Yang G, Bastidas JA. Phase I study of stereotactic radiosurgery in patients with locally advanced pancreatic cancer. Int J Radiat Oncol Biol Phys. 2004;58(4):1017–21.
15. Schellenberg D, Goodman KA, Lee F, Chang S, Kuo T, Ford JM, Fisher GA, Quon A, Desser TS, Norton J, Greco R, Yang GP, Koong AC. Gemcitabine chemotherapy and single-fraction stereotactic body radiotherapy for locally advanced pancreatic cancer. Int J Radiat Oncol Biol Phys. 2008;72(3):678–86.
16. Schellenberg D, Kim J, Christman-Skieller C, Chun CL, Columbo LA, Ford JM, Fisher GA, Kunz PL, Van Dam J, Quon A, Desser TS, Norton J, Hsu A, Maxim PG, Xing L, Goodman KA, Chang DT, Koong AC. Single-fraction stereotactic body radiation therapy and sequential gemcitabine for the treatment of locally advanced pancreatic cancer. Int J Radiat Oncol Biol Phys. 2011;81(1):181–8.
17. Mahadevan A, Jain S, Goldstein M, Miksad R, Pleskow D, Sawhney M, Brennan D, Callery M, Vollmer C. Stereotactic body radiotherapy and gemcitabine for locally advanced pancreatic cancer. Int J Radiat Oncol Biol Phys. 2010;78(3):735–42.
18. Pollom EL, Alagappan M, von Eyben R, Kunz PL, Fisher GA, Ford JA, Poultsides GA, Visser BC, Norton JA, Kamaya A, Cox VL, Columbo LA, Koong AC, Chang DT. Single- versus multifraction stereotactic body radiation therapy for pancreatic adenocarcinoma: outcomes and toxicity. Int J Radiat Oncol Biol Phys. 2014;90(4):918–25.

19. Chuong MD, Springett GM, Weber J, et al. Induction gemcitabine-based chemotherapy and neoadjuvant stereotactic body radiation therapy achieve high margin-negative resection rates for borderline resectable pancreatic cancer. J Radiat Oncol. 2012;1:273–81.
20. Chuong MD, Frakes JM, Figura N, Hoffe SE, Shridhar R, Mellon EA, Hodul PJ, Malafa MP, Springett GM, Centeno BA. Histopathologic tumor response after induction chemotherapy and stereotactic body radiation therapy for borderline resectable pancreatic cancer. J Gastrointest Oncol. 2016;7(2):221–7.
21. Mellon EA, Strom TJ, Hoffe SE, Frakes JM, Springett GM, Hodul PJ, Malafa MP, Chuong MD, Shridhar R. Favorable perioperative outcomes after resection of borderline resectable pancreatic cancer treated with neoadjuvant stereotactic radiation and chemotherapy compared with upfront pancreatectomy for resectable cancer. J Gastrointest Oncol. 2016;7(4):547–55.
22. Brunner TB, Nestle U, Grosu AL, Partridge M. SBRT in pancreatic cancer: what is the therapeutic window? Radiol Oncol. 2015;114(1):109–16.
23. Shaib WL, Hawk N, Cassidy RJ, Chen Z, Zhang C, Brutcher E, Kooby D, Maithel SK, Sarmiento JM, Landry J, El-Rayes BF. A phase 1 study of stereotactic body radiation therapy dose escalation for borderline resectable pancreatic cancer after modified FOLFIRINOX (NCT01446458). Int J Radiat Oncol Biol Phys. 2016;96(2):296–303.
24. Krishnan S, Chadha AS, Suh Y, Chen HC, Rao A, Das P, Minsky BD, Mahmood U, Delclos ME, Sawakuchi GO, Beddar S, Katz MH, Fleming JB, Javle MM, Varadhachary GR, Wolff RA, Crane CH. Focal radiation therapy dose escalation improves overall survival in locally advanced pancreatic cancer patients receiving induction chemotherapy and consolidative chemoradiation. Int J Radiat Oncol Biol Phys. 2016;94(4):755–65.
25. Yang W, Reznik R, Fraass BA, et al. Dosimetric evaluation of simultaneous integrated boost during stereotactic body radiation therapy for pancreatic cancer. Med Dosim. 2015;40(1):47–52.
26. Herman JM, Parkinson R, Onners B, et al. Preliminary results of a pilot study evaluating an allogeneic GM-CSF pancreatic tumor cell vaccine (GVAX) and Cytoxan (cy) with stereotactic body radiation therapy (SBRT) and Folfirinox (FFX) in patients with resected pancreatic adenocarcinoma. Int J Radiat Oncol Biol Phys. 2015c;93(3):S154.
27. Willett CG, Del Castillo CF, Shih HA, Goldberg S, Biggs P, Clark JW, Lauwers G, Ryan DP, Zhu AX, Warshaw AL. Long-term results of intraoperative electron beam irradiation (IOERT) for patients with unresectable pancreatic cancer. Ann Surg. 2005;241(2):295–9.
28. Bouchard M, Amos RA, Briere TM, Beddar S, Crane CH. Dose escalation with proton or photon radiation treatment for pancreatic cancer. Radiother Oncol. 2009;92(2):238–43.
29. Herman JM, Koong AC. Stereotactic body radiation therapy: a new standard option for pancreatic cancer? J Natl Compr Canc Netw. 2014;12(10):1489–93.
30. Hong TS, DeLaney TF, Mamon HJ, Willett CG, Yeap BY, Niemierko A, Wolfgang JA, Lu HM, Adams J, Weyman EA, Arellano RS, Blaszkowsky LS, Allen JN, Tanabe KK, Ryan DP, Zhu AX. A prospective feasibility study of respiratory-gated proton beam therapy for liver tumors. Pract Radiat Oncol. 2014a;4(5):316–22.
31. Hong TS, Ryan DP, Borger DR, Blaszkowsky LS, Yeap BY, Ancukiewicz M, Deshpande V, Shinagare S, Wo JY, Boucher Y, Wadlow RC, Kwak EL, Allen JN, Clark JW, Zhu AX, Ferrone CR, Mamon HJ, Adams J, Winrich B, Grillo T, Jain RK, DeLaney TF, Fernandez-del Castillo C, Duda DG. A phase 1/2 and biomarker study of preoperative short course chemoradiation with proton beam therapy and capecitabine followed by early surgery for resectable pancreatic ductal adenocarcinoma. Int J Radiat Oncol Biol Phys. 2014b;89(4):830–8.
32. Ding X, Dionisi F, Tang S, Ingram M, Hung CY, Prionas E, Lichtenwalner P, Butterwick I, Zhai H, Yin L, Lin H, Kassaee A, Avery S. A comprehensive dosimetric study of pancreatic cancer treatment using three-dimensional conformal radiation therapy (3DCRT), intensity-modulated radiation therapy (IMRT), volumetric-modulated radiation therapy (VMAT), and passive-scattering and modulated-scanning proton therapy (PT). Med Dosim. 2014;39(2):139–45.
33. Thompson RF, Mayekar SU, Zhai H, Both S, Apisarnthanarax S, Metz JM, Plastaras JP, Ben-Josef E. A dosimetric comparison of proton and photon therapy in unresectable cancers of the head of pancreas. Med Phys. 2014;41(8):081711.

34. Nichols RC, Huh S, Li Z, Rutenberg M. Proton therapy for pancreatic cancer. World J Gastrointest Oncol. 2015;7(9):141–7.
35. Terashima K, Demizu Y, Hashimoto N, Jin D, Mima M, Fujii O, Niwa Y, Takatori K, Kitajima N, Sirakawa S, Yonson K, Hishikawa Y, Abe M, Sasaki R, Sugimura K, Murakami M. A phase I/II study of gemcitabine-concurrent proton radiotherapy for locally advanced pancreatic cancer without distant metastasis. Radiol Oncol. 2012;103(1):25–31.
36. Takatori K, Terashima K, Yoshida R, Horai A, Satake S, Ose T, Kitajima N, Kinoshita Y, Demizu Y, Fuwa N. Upper gastrointestinal complications associated with gemcitabine-concurrent proton radiotherapy for inoperable pancreatic cancer. J Gastroenterol. 2014;49(6):1074–80.
37. Ebner DK, Kamada T. The emerging role of carbon-ion radiotherapy. Front Oncol. 2016;6:140.
38. Shinoto M, Yamada S, Terashima K, Yasuda S, Shioyama Y, Honda H, Kamada T, Tsujii H, Saisho H, Working Group for Pancreas Cancer. Carbon ion radiation therapy with concurrent gemcitabine for patients with locally advanced pancreatic cancer. Int J Radiat Oncol Biol Phys, 2016;95(1):498–504.
39. Durante M, Tommasino F, Yamada S. Modeling combined chemotherapy and particle therapy for locally advanced pancreatic cancer. Front Oncol. 2015;5:145.
40. Santoro JP, Yorke E, Goodman KA, Mageras GS. From phase-based to displacement-based gating: a software tool to facilitate respiration-gated radiation treatment. J Appl Clin Med Phys. 2009;10(4):2982.
41. Herman JM, Crane CH, Iacobuzio-Donahue C, Abrams RA. Pancreatic cancer. In: Gunderson LL, Tepper JE, editors. Clinical radiation oncology: expert consult. 4e ed. Amsterdam: Elsevier; 2015b. p. 934–59.
42. Moningi S, Marciscano AE, Rosati LM, Ng SK, Teboh Forbang R, Jackson J, Chang DT, Koong AC, Herman JM. Stereotactic body radiation therapy in pancreatic cancer: the new frontier. Expert Rev Anticancer Ther. 2014;14(12):1461–75.
43. Marsanic P, Mellano A, Sottile A, De Simone M. Irreversible electroporation as treatment of locally advanced and as margin accentuation in borderline resectable pancreatic adenocarcinoma. Med Biol Eng Comput. 2017. doi:10.1007/s11517-016-1603-9.
44. Martin RC 2nd, Durham AN, Besselink MG, Iannitti D, Weiss MJ, Wolfgang CL, Huang KW. Irreversible electroporation in locally advanced pancreatic cancer: a call for standardization of energy delivery. J Surg Oncol. 2016;114(7):865–71.
45. Martin RC 2nd, Kwon D, Chalikonda S, Sellers M, Kotz E, Scoggins C, McMasters KM, Watkins K. Treatment of 200 locally advanced (stage III) pancreatic adenocarcinoma patients with irreversible electroporation: safety and efficacy. Ann Surg. 2015;262(3):486–94; discussion 492–4.
46. Paiella S, Salvia R, Girelli R, Frigerio I, Giardino A, D'Onofrio M, De Marchi G, Bassi C. Role of local ablative techniques (radiofrequency ablation and irreversible electroporation) in the treatment of pancreatic cancer. Updat Surg. 2016;68(3):307–11.
47. Tasu JP, Vesselle G, Herpe G, Richer JP, Boucecbi S, Velasco S, Carretier M, Debeane B, Tougeron D. Irreversible electroporation for locally advanced pancreatic cancer. Diagn Interv Imaging. 2016;97(12):1297–304.
48. Lu L, Hu Z, Frankel W, et al. Endoscopic 3-dimensional OCT-guided brachytherapy for early-stage pancreatic cancers. Int J Radiat Oncol Biol Phys. 2016;96(2 Suppl):S167–8.
49. Yang M, Yan Z, Luo J, Liu Q, Zhang W, Ma J, Zhang Z, Yu T, Zhao Q, Liu L. A pilot study of intraluminal brachytherapy using 125I seed strand for locally advanced pancreatic ductal adenocarcinoma with obstructive jaundice. Brachytherapy. 2016;15(6):859–64.
50. Fuccio L, Guido A, Larghi A, Antonini F, Lami G, Fabbri C. The role of endoscopic ultrasound in the radiation treatment of pancreatic tumor. Expert Rev Gastroenterol Hepatol. 2014;8(7):793–802.
51. Jin Z, Du Y, Li Z, Jiang Y, Chen J, Liu Y. Endoscopic ultrasonography-guided interstitial implantation of iodine 125-seeds combined with chemotherapy in the treatment of unresectable pancreatic carcinoma: a prospective pilot study. Endoscopy. 2008;40(4):314–20.

52. Sun S, Xu H, Xin J, Liu J, Guo Q, Li S. Endoscopic ultrasound-guided interstitial brachytherapy of unresectable pancreatic cancer: results of a pilot trial. Endoscopy. 2006;38(4):399–403.
53. Xu W, Liu Y, Lu Z, Jin ZD, Hu YH, Yu JG, Li ZS. A new endoscopic ultrasonography image processing method to evaluate the prognosis for pancreatic cancer treated with interstitial brachytherapy. World J Gastroenterol. 2013;19(38):6479–84.
54. Fokas E, Spezi E, Patel N, Hurt C, Nixon L, Chu KY, Staffurth J, Abrams R, Mukherjee S. Comparison of investigator-delineated gross tumour volumes and quality assurance in pancreatic cancer: analysis of the on-trial cases for the SCALOP trial. Radiol Oncol. 2016;120(2):212–6.
55. Heerkens HD, Hall WA, Li XA, Knechtges P, Dalah E, Paulson ES, van den Berg CA, Meijer GJ, Koay EJ, Crane CH, Aitken K, van Vulpen M, Erickson BA. Recommendations for MRI-based contouring of gross tumor volume and organs at risk for radiation therapy of pancreatic cancer. Pract Radiat Oncol. 2016;7(2):126–36.
56. Kishi T, Matsuo Y, Nakamura A, Nakamoto Y, Itasaka S, Mizowaki T, Togashi K, Hiraoka M. Comparative evaluation of respiratory-gated and ungated FDG-PET for target volume definition in radiotherapy treatment planning for pancreatic cancer. Radiol Oncol. 2016;120(2):217–21.
57. Liu Y, Zhong X, Czito BG, Palta M, Bashir MR, Dale BM, Yin FF, Cai J. Four-dimensional diffusion-weighted MR imaging (4D–DWI): a feasibility study. Med Phys. 2017;44(2):397–406.
58. Popp I, Grosu AL, Niedermann G, Duda DG. Immune modulation by hypofractionated stereotactic radiation therapy: therapeutic implications. Radiol Oncol. 2016;120(2):185–94.
59. Sharabi AB, Nirschl CJ, Kochel CM, Nirschl TR, Francica BJ, Velarde E, Deweese TL, Drake CG. Stereotactic radiation therapy augments antigen-specific PD-1-mediated antitumor immune responses via cross-presentation of tumor antigen. Cancer Immunol Res. 2015;3(4):345–55.
60. Twyman-Saint Victor C, Rech AJ, Maity A, Rengan R, Pauken KE, Stelekati E, Benci JL, Xu B, Dada H, Odorizzi PM, Herati RS, Mansfield KD, Patsch D, Amaravadi RK, Schuchter LM, Ishwaran H, Mick R, Pryma DA, Xu X, Feldman MD, Gangadhar TC, Hahn SM, Wherry EJ, Vonderheide RH, Minn AJ. Radiation and dual checkpoint blockade activate non-redundant immune mechanisms in cancer. Nature. 2015;520(7547):373–7.
61. Koay EJ, Amer AM, Baio FE, Ondari AO, Fleming JB. Toward stratification of patients with pancreatic cancer: past lessons from traditional approaches and future applications with physical biomarkers. Cancer Lett. 2016;381(1):237–43.
62. Koay EJ, Baio FE, Ondari A, Truty MJ, Cristini V, Thomas RM, Chen R, Chatterjee D, Kang Y, Zhang J, Court L, Bhosale PR, Tamm EP, Qayyum A, Crane CH, Javle M, Katz MH, Gottumukkala VN, Rozner MA, Shen H, Lee JE, Wang H, Chen Y, Plunkett W, Abbruzzese JL, Wolff RA, Maitra A, Ferrari M, Varadhachary GR, Fleming JB. Intra-tumoral heterogeneity of gemcitabine delivery and mass transport in human pancreatic cancer. Phys Biol. 2014;11(6):065002.
63. Hanania AN, Bantis LE, Feng Z, Wang H, Tamm EP, Katz MH, Maitra A, Koay EJ. Quantitative imaging to evaluate malignant potential of IPMNs. Oncotarget. 2016;7(52):85776–84.
64. Cui Y, Song J, Pollom E, Alagappan M, Shirato H, Chang DT, Koong AC, Li R. Quantitative analysis of (18)F-fluorodeoxyglucose positron emission tomography identifies novel prognostic imaging biomarkers in locally advanced pancreatic cancer patients treated with stereotactic body radiation therapy. Int J Radiat Oncol Biol Phys. 2016;96(1):102–9.

Chapter 19
The Role for Palliative Surgical Interventions in Pancreatic Cancer

Alexandra G. Lopez-Aguiar and Shishir K. Maithel

The Challenge of Treating Locally Advanced and Metastatic Pancreatic Cancer

Despite increasing research and constant innovations in medical treatment, pancreatic cancer continues to be a devastating and lethal disease worldwide. It is one of the most aggressive malignancies, such that 50% present with metastatic disease and 35% with locally advanced disease [1]. As the fourth leading cause of cancer death in Western societies, it has an abysmal 5-year survival rate of approximately 5% [2] and an overall median survival of 4.4 months [1]. Its poor prognosis is often attributed to the fact that the symptoms of pancreatic cancer are usually late and non-specific, thus leading to delays in early diagnosis [1]. Likewise, while multiple risk factors have been identified—for example, older age, African American race, female gender, and smoking—there is no specific high-risk group to directly target for screening protocols.

Operative resection remains the primary treatment modality and the only curative option for pancreatic cancer, but only 10–20% of patients initially present with localized, nonmetastatic disease that is amenable for complete surgical extirpation. [2]. Even with curative resection, however, there is only a modest increase in long-term survival to a median of 20 months, with a 5-year survival increase to 15–26% overall [1]. Even if adjuvant chemotherapy is added, the median survival after complete resection still only ranges between 14 and 24 months [3]. In the face of such a poor prognosis, and with the knowledge that the vast majority of patients present with unresectable disease due to metastasis or local advancement, the role for surgical intervention in the palliative setting becomes controversial and debatable. Other less invasive options that are available for patients with biliary obstruction, gastric

A.G. Lopez-Aguiar, M.D. • S.K. Maithel, M.D. (✉)
Winship Cancer Institute, Division of Surgical Oncology, Department of Surgery, Emory University Hospital, 1365C Clifton Road NE, Atlanta, GA 30322, USA
e-mail: smaithe@emory.edu

T. Bekaii-Saab, B. El-Rayes (eds.), *Current and Emerging Therapies in Pancreatic Cancer*, DOI 10.1007/978-3-319-58256-6_19

outlet obstruction, or malignant bowel obstruction must be considered. The feasibility and efficacy of systemic therapy in the context of the patient's performance status, which is often poor, must weigh heavily into the clinical decision-making. Although surgery continues to be a valid option to address many of these concerns, current evidence suggests that the least invasive intervention is often associated with the best outcomes, specifically in terms of quality of life.

Management of Biliary Obstruction

Biliary obstruction—often caused by either tumor invasion within the biliary tree or extrinsic mass effect—is a frequent symptom noted upon initial presentation of patients with unresectable pancreatic cancer. In fact, as many as 70% of patients have some degree of biliary obstruction at the time of their diagnosis [4]. Malignant bile duct obstruction has been associated with worse patient outcomes, as it may lead to cholangitis, delay in disease treatment, decreased quality of life, and increased mortality [4]. Jaundice in itself can impair cellular immunity and thus allow tumor growth and metastatic progression if left untreated [5]. By preventing the usual flow of bile through the enteric tract, the absorption of lipid-soluble vitamins such as vitamin K is compromised and may even lead to increased bleeding due to a resulting coagulopathy [5]. More concerning still is the possibility of bacterial and endotoxin translocation through intestinal mucosa causing a systemic inflammatory response or sepsis that is sometimes seen in jaundiced patients [5]. From a palliation perspective, relieving a biliary obstruction can significantly improve patient comfort by eliminating pruritus, and the resulting normalized bilirubin level also can prevent toxicity that could otherwise be caused by some chemotherapy regimens [4]. It is therefore imperative that, in most cases, an intervention be performed for patients who present with biliary obstruction to relieve their jaundice.

While there are many options for the timely treatment of biliary obstruction, studies to date support endoscopic biliary stenting as the standard of care for biliary decompression [4]. Endoscopic stent placement into the common bile duct is a reasonably well-tolerated procedure and is technically successful in over 90% of cases [5]. For patients with borderline resectable disease that may eventually come to surgical resection, biliary decompression via stenting can quickly decrease bilirubin levels and thus decrease chemotoxicity from a cholestatic liver during the use of gemcitabine- or 5-FU-based chemotherapy regimens for neoadjuvant treatment [4]. Self-expanding metal stents (SEMS) have been found to be the most effective stents in these cases, as they are more likely to remain patent until surgery and are associated with fewer complications as compared with plastic stents [4]. There are two types of widely used SEMS: uncovered SEMS (USEMS) and covered SEMS (CSEMS), each with their advantages and limitations. On the one hand, USEMS use a mesh design that favors easy incorporation into the biliary duct wall, but they also are more susceptible to tissue ingrowth that may lead to increased incidence of occlusion [4]. Furthermore, should the patient come to resection, these stents can be difficult to remove during surgery. CSEMS, on the other hand, are designed specifically to prevent tissue ingrowth and thus increase duration of patency, but because of this they are known to have higher rates of migration [4]. The rate of stent-induced cholecystitis is reportedly higher with CSEMS compared to USEMS due to cystic duct occlusion; however, this is a rarely encountered clinical problem.

Stenting also plays a major role in the palliative setting. The purpose of stenting in inoperable patients is similar to that of those with borderline resectable disease: largely to relieve jaundice and pruritus, to normalize bilirubin levels to allow for administration of chemotherapy, and to improve the patient's quality of life. While it is generally agreed that SEMS have better outcomes and long-term patency, in situations where the patient's life expectancy is only a few weeks to months, plastic stents may sometimes be preferred. SEMS cost 15–40 times more than plastic stents and are only cost effective when the patient lives longer than 4 months after insertion [4]. Unfortunately, for patients with liver or distant metastases, median survival in pancreatic cancer can be as low as 2.7 months [6]. It is in these cases that plastic stents prove most useful, as they can provide inexpensive yet quick relief that usually lasts about 3 months [5]. Double-layer stents (DLSs) are also an option getting growing attention within the medical community. These economical stents are designed with a stiff outer layer to allow cannulation, along with a smooth inner layer that is less likely to occlude [4]. In this way, patients with inoperable disease may receive the intervention necessary to ensure the most comfort for the longest time possible. Figure 19.1 demonstrates a suggested algorithm for treatment of biliary obstruction based on disease stage.

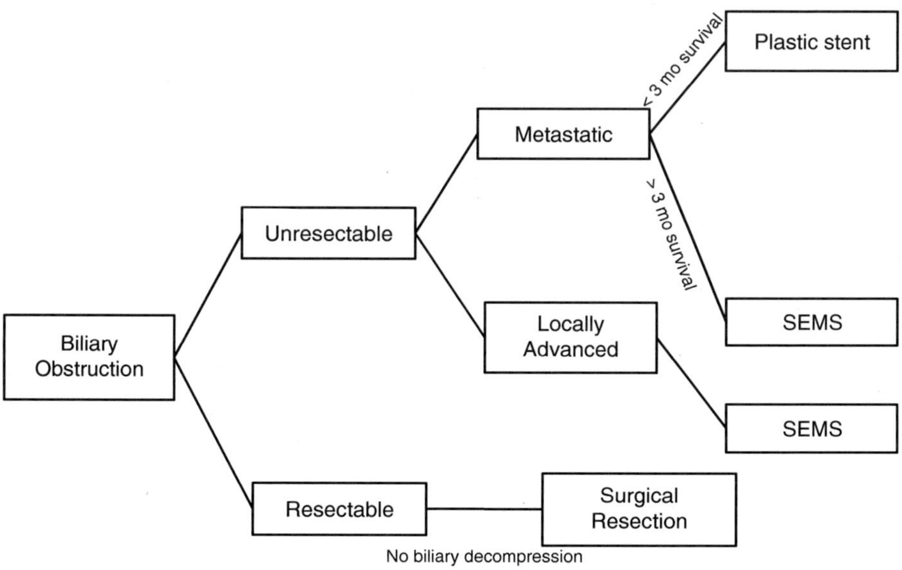

Fig. 19.1 Algorithm for treatment of biliary obstruction. SEMS, self-expanding metallic stent

Although stenting is the least invasive and preferred treatment for biliary obstruction, patients who are not candidates for or have previously failed ERCP still have options for non-operative biliary decompression. Percutaneous transhepatic biliary drainage (PTBD) has been used particularly for this population of individuals. In most cases, internal bile drainage is reestablished via an internal-external biliary drain that is passed through the site of malignant obstruction into the duodenum [4]. Once enterohepatic circulation is restored, the drain is often internalized to facilitate management and decrease likelihood of infection [4]. If the biliary drain is unable to successfully traverse the site of obstruction during the procedure, exclusively external drainage remains an option for decompression [4]. PTBD is associated with more complications than endoscopically placed stents; however, as they can more frequently predispose to cholangitis, bacteremia, and hemobilia after puncture of the liver [4]. They also have a proclivity for leakage, dislodgement, and recurrent obstruction [4].

Surgical biliary bypass in the form of hepaticojejunostomy may also be used to relieve biliary obstruction in patients with unresectable pancreatic cancer [7]. In fact, a meta-analysis by Glazer et al. showed that surgically treated patients are significantly less likely to have recurrent biliary obstruction (3.1 vs. 28.7%) compared to endoscopic stenting [8]. Unsurprisingly, studies have also shown that surgical bypass is associated with a higher rate of complications and longer hospital stays (21.8 days on average), as it is the most invasive treatment for biliary decompression [4, 9]. While it may provide more permanent resolution, most would argue that the recovery time and complication rate can drastically decrease the quality of the little remaining time patients with such a poor prognostic disease may have. Moreover, surgical biliary bypass also delays the initiation of potentially life-extending palliative chemotherapy, as the patient's recovery time from surgery is significantly prolonged compared to the endoscopic or percutaneous approach [9]. It is thus recommended that, if possible, endoscopic stenting be the chosen path of intervention for biliary decompression in the palliative setting. If that is not possible, a percutaneous approach should be utilized. Surgical biliary bypass should be reserved for select cases and only after a thorough discussion with the patient and family regarding goals of care and realistic expectations of recovery.

Gastric Outlet Obstruction and Possible Interventions

Biliary obstruction is not the only challenging symptom from which patients with pancreatic cancer may suffer. Gastric outlet obstruction may affect 15–20% of patients in the course of their disease [10], and those who suffer with it have their clinical conditions deteriorate rapidly due to vomiting, dehydration, and malnutrition [11]. The resultant weakness both hastens their decline and causes extreme discomfort for the patient who is no longer able to eat. Usually, patients who present with this symptom have disease that has progressed to unresectability, with a median survival of 3–6 months [10]. Therefore, intervention is primarily aimed toward palliation to resume oral intake, along with quality-of-life improvement.

Much like biliary obstruction, there are both an endoscopic route for intervention and a more invasive surgical option. Endoscopic placement of a SEMS in the duodenum is increasingly being used to treat patients with gastric outlet obstruction [11]. Endoscopic stenting has been shown to relieve symptoms faster than surgery, has shorter hospital stays, and improves pain scores sooner after intervention [11]. Of note, stent placement is also significantly less expensive than surgical intervention—a benefit for patients and their families who already may suffer under the burden of high healthcare costs [11]. This technique does have its limitations though, with increased recurrence of obstructive symptoms, often which require re-intervention and repeat stent placement [11]. While both uncovered and covered stents are used, covered stents are usually the stent of choice due to longer patency [11]. Consideration for biliary decompression must be done prior to placing a duodenal stent, as endoscopic access to the ampulla, particularly in the setting of covered stents, is severely compromised once the duodenal stent is in place. If the goals of care are only to provide optimal comfort as the patient transitions to hospice care, a simple percutaneous endoscopic gastrostomy (PEG) tube can be placed to relieve the obstruction and prevent vomiting. This also facilitates oral liquid intake that can be vented out the tube, which can greatly improve the patient's quality of life.

Gastrojejunostomy is the surgical intervention of choice to treat gastric outlet obstruction. The procedure may be done laparoscopically or with an open technique, and it is used to bypass the area of obstruction at the duodenum by anastomosing the distal stomach directly to the jejunum. Doing so allows the patient to continue to eat with the aim of preventing dehydration and malnutrition. Bile from the biliary tree still joins enteric content downstream at the jejunum and thus is able to also preserve hepato-enteric circulation. Given the invasive nature of this procedure, it is associated with longer hospital stays, as it often takes patients more time than stents to have return of bowel function [11]. Furthermore, the recovery from a surgical procedure is longer compared to an endoscopic intervention. There is evidence, however, to suggest better outcomes in patients undergoing a laparoscopic approach instead of an open gastric bypass—with shorter hospital stays, lower morbidity and mortality, and decreased hospital costs [12]—which may increase the appeal of intervening surgically. Nonetheless, the time to functional recovery of bowel motility to enable proper oral nutrition intake, regardless of the approach, can be substantially delayed and frustratingly long. Another option for palliation to relieve vomiting and promote enteric nutrition is to combine an endoscopic and surgical approach with placement of a PEG tube and a surgically placed jejunostomy feeding tube. The feeding tube can be placed utilizing a laparoscopic or open approach as well. This treatment strategy has the advantage of allowing the patient to drink liquids for comfort that can be vented through the PEG tube while initiating enteric feeds via the jejunostomy tube almost immediately.

Although gastrojejunostomy initially has slower relief of symptoms, studies have shown that, over time, patients experience fewer episodes of recurrent obstruction and thus require fewer re-interventions [11]. Quality of life is reportedly similar for both gastrojejunostomy and stenting, and there is no survival advantage for either procedure [11]. Thus, due to the initially slower resolution of symptoms and longer hospital stays, many physicians agree that gastrojejunostomy should be reserved only for patients with a survival expectancy of greater than 2 months. It is this population alone that would benefit from the lower rates of re-intervention seen with surgical intervention [11]. Otherwise, the endoscopic approach is usually more in line with the minimally invasive goals of palliation that prioritize comfort, fewer hospital days, and less physiologic stress to the patient [10].

The Late-Stage Presentation of Malignant Bowel Obstruction

Another possible presentation of patients with advanced pancreatic cancer is malignant bowel obstruction, either partial or complete. In the setting of high tumor burden with metastatic peritoneal disease, the bowels may become functionally affected, or they may suffer from mechanical blockage due to tumor invasion or mass effect. Such a presentation is almost invariably associated with poor survival [13]. The resulting dilemma is the desire to relieve the symptoms—bilious emesis, nausea, poor oral tolerance, pain, and distention that could ultimately culminate with bowel perforation—without causing further morbidity from operating on an already significantly deconditioned patient [13]. Studies have shown that operative intervention by either bowel resection with anastomosis, bypass, or creation of a stoma is often associated with high morbidity and mortality, with limited success in symptom relief [13]. In fact, operating on malnourished patients can have a death rate of over 70%, and the presence of shock, ascites, or abdominal masses serves as particular predictors of poor outcome [13]. Likewise, postoperative complications—which range from pneumonia to renal failure to wound infections—occur in over 60% [13]. Thus, operative intervention is only recommended in a very select group of patients that is usually not inclusive of those suffering from advanced pancreatic cancer.

The alternative to operative intervention is primarily gastric decompression, which is often ineffective or only temporarily successful. Nasogastric (NG) tube decompression has a re-obstruction rate that is 15% higher than with operative intervention, but an initial trial with it is still recommended [13]. Long-term NG tube decompression in poor surgical candidates is not recommended though, as it is associated with psychological distress, as well as complications including wing necrosis, otitis media, and aspiration pneumonia [14]. PEG tube placement is a well-tolerated alternative to long-term NG tube for symptom improvement [14]. The success rate of PEG tube placement is between 86 and 100%, and adequate control of symptoms occurs in 84–100% of patients [14]. PEG tubes are not recommended for patients with life expectancies shorter than 30 days, but they can provide successful palliation by relieving intractable vomiting via gastric venting and by providing an avenue for enteral nutrition in patients with at least partially functioning gastrointestinal tracts [13]. For those unable to tolerate PEG tube feeds, parenteral supplementation has been shown to have some beneficial effects by maintaining nutritional status [14], and, finally, the simultaneous use of antiemetics and analgesics can also be used to maintain maximal comfort, both in- and outside the hospital [13]. In most cases of malignant bowel obstruction from metastatic pancreatic cancer, the most palliative and humane course of action is decompressive PEG tube placement and transition to hospice care.

Irreversible Electroporation: A Promising New Frontier for Locally Advanced Disease

After reviewing the palliative options for the most frequent symptoms in patients with locally advanced or widely metastatic pancreatic cancer, it is important to address the potentially therapeutic surgical options for such patients as well. Although these patients may not be candidates for curative resection, there remain surgical procedures including irreversible electroporation, liver resection in the setting of liver metastases, and cytoreduction with hyperthermic intraperitoneal chemotherapy (HIPEC) as possible interventions. While some of these alternatives may be promising, data to date favor less invasive procedures and palliation for such a poor prognostic disease.

Irreversible electroporation (IRE) is a nonthermal ablation technology in which short, high-voltage pulses are applied to tissues to increase the permeability of cell membranes and thus cause cells to undergo cell death [26]. This modality can be used to treat locally advanced disease while safely navigating around vital vascular and ductal structures, as it uses a nonthermal-based method of action and has minimal effect on blood vessel scaffolding [26]. Furthermore, some early studies have suggested that it may, in fact, improve both local (14 vs. 6 months) and distant (15 vs. 9 months) progression-free survival in locally advanced pancreatic cancer compared with chemoradiation [15]. Even overall survival has been shown to be increased about 6 months compared with chemoradiation in some series [15].

IRE is not without its morbidities, as patients who undergo IRE can suffer bile leaks, ileus, DVTs, and wound infections [26]. Patients also spend a median of 9 days in the hospital, and the expense of the IRE device is around $2000 per probe [26]. Another limiting factor for this intervention is the requirement for the physician to have significant experience with thermal ablation such as radiofrequency, microwave, and cryoablation, as well as a thorough understanding of the mechanism of action for IRE to ensure its appropriate and safe use [26]. Thus, although promising, IRE remains in the early stages of evaluation of its use and efficacy.

Surgical Options for Widely Metastatic Pancreatic Cancer

Liver metastases are a common presentation of patients with pancreatic cancer. Yet due to the diffuse nature of their disease and extremely poor prognosis, these patients are usually not candidates for surgical resection or even for IRE. Metastases to the liver are usually a dismal prognostic indicator, with such patients living an average of only 3–6 months [16]. Of late, select cases of oligometastatic disease in the setting of otherwise resectable pancreatic cancer have been considered as a population that may benefit from aggressive operative intervention [16]. In these cases, patients may successfully undergo simultaneous resection of their primary cancer, as well as the liver metastases [16]. This approach is not universally recommended at this point, but some early studies have suggested a positive impact on overall survival for those patients who undertake this treatment compared with traditional palliative chemotherapy [16]. Indeed, a study by Bahra et al. showed an increase in median overall survival to 10.4 months after cytoreductive pancreatic surgery and consecutive gemcitabine-based chemotherapy versus the 7.2 months of overall survival for patients treated only with chemotherapy [17]. Unfortunately, studies have yet to explore the effect on quality of life, and the numbers of patients examined have been relatively low for reliable conclusions to be made [16]. Some evidence also supports that the extended resection approach may increase length of ICU or hospital stay, and it may increase surgical morbidity [18]. As it stands, it appears that liver resection is only an option for patients with resectable pancreatic disease and only on a very individualized, case-by-case basis. This approach is not recommended as a standard of care.

There is a group of patients who may present with metachronous liver metastases years after initial curative resection of an early pancreatic cancer, but due to the aggressiveness and poor 5-year overall survival of <15% for resectable disease, this group is fairly small [19]. Although treatment with chemotherapy is the standard of care in such cases, there have been some instances where hepatic arterial infusion chemotherapy, as well as additional treatment using radiofrequency ablation, has been used with complete remission [20]. There have also been select cases where hepatectomy has been performed for patients in good overall condition with liver metastases years after successful pancreaticoduodenectomy for pancreatic cancer [21, 22]. Unfortunately, data remains sparse and limited to case reports, thus making it difficult to broadly apply the findings of such studies. Appropriate patient selection is paramount when choosing a liver-directed approach, particularly resection, for patients with metastatic disease. A long disease-free interval after primary resection and a small number of tumors, ideally solitary, are necessary features of selecting patients for this aggressive therapy.

There are some studies that take a more preemptive approach to liver metastases by using prophylactic hepatic irradiation (PHI) following curative resection for pancreatic cancer to decrease the incidence of future liver metastases. With PHI, the whole liver is irradiated 5 days per week starting 2–4 weeks after surgery [23]. Compared to patients treated with chemoradiation, those treated with PHI both had less incidence of future liver metastases and higher 5-year overall survival [23]. Of course, studies have been limited by small numbers, a lack of randomized control trials, and a minimal assessment of quality of life for patients undergoing such an aggressive postoperative treatment regimen.

The final aggressive surgical approach that has been entertained as a possible treatment modality for pancreatic cancer is cytoreduction combined with HIPEC. Much like the evidence for liver resection in pancreatic cancer, the data for cytoreduction/HIPEC is sparse, as it has mostly been studied in the setting of appendiceal and colorectal cancer. Nonetheless, a number of studies have implied a potential survival benefit for patients with resectable pancreatic cancer, as there may be a resulting decrease in locoregional recurrence for these patients [24]. The potential advantage only applies to those who undergo an R0 resection and HIPEC simultaneously, thus limiting its applicability, since patients who present with metastases or locally advanced disease that precludes resection would not be candidates for this treatment modality. Ultimately, while HIPEC has proven its efficacy in managing peritoneal metastases in appendiceal and colorectal cancer [25], further studies evaluating its role in pancreatic cancer are required before it should be considered for disease management.

Conclusions

Pancreatic cancer remains a fatal disease that frequently presents in late stages with a poor overall survival. Although surgical resection serves as the only treatment modality with a chance for cure, the commonly unresectable presentation of this disease limits the management options available. Nonetheless, there do remain some instances where surgical intervention may play a palliative role, particularly when patients present with symptoms including biliary obstruction, gastric outlet obstruction, and malignant bowel obstruction. Of course, when balancing the morbidity of surgery and the effect on quality of life it may have, it may behoove patients with such an aggressive disease to undergo less invasive treatment options. Indeed, this is the precise population that may benefit most from endoscopic stenting, percutaneous procedures, and palliative PEG tubes. While some evidence supports the use of newer techniques such as IRE, data is still scant to support more aggressive approaches like liver resection or HIPEC. Until further studies suggest otherwise, the emphasis and goals of care for most patients should focus on optimizing comfort and quality of life for patients who suffer from advanced and metastatic pancreatic cancer.

References

1. Weledji EP, Enoworock G, Mokake M, Sinju M. How grim is pancreatic cancer? Oncol Rev. 2016;10:294.
2. Chang DK, Johns AL, Merrett ND, Gill AJ, Colvin EK, Scarlett CJ, Nguyen NQ, Leong RW, Cosman PH, Kelly MI, Sutherland RL, Henshall SM, Kench JG, Biankin AV. Margin clearance and outcome in resected pancreatic cancer. J Clin Oncol. 2009;27:2855–62.
3. Gurusamy KS, Kumar S, Davidson BR, Fusai G. Resection versus other treatments for locally advanced pancreatic cancer. Cochrane Database Syst Rev. 2014:CD010244. doi:10.1002/14651858.CD010244.pub2.
4. Boulay BR, Parepally M. Managing malignant biliary obstruction in pancreas cancer: choosing the appropriate strategy. World J Gastroenterol. 2014;20:9345–53.

5. Boulay BR, Birg A. Malignant biliary obstruction: from palliation to treatment. World J Gastrointest Oncol. 2016;8:498–508.
6. Kaassis M, Boyer J, Dumas R, Ponchon T, Coumaros D, Delcenserie R, Canard JM, Fritsch J, Rey JF, Burtin P. Plastic or metal stents for malignant stricture of the common bile duct? Results of a randomized prospective study. Gastrointest Endosc. 2003;57:178–82.
7. Ueda J, Kayashima T, Mori Y, Ohtsuka T, Takahata S, Nakamura M, Tanaka M. Hepaticoch olecystojejunostomy as effective palliative biliary bypass for unresectable pancreatic cancer. Hepato-Gastroenterology. 2014;61:197–202.
8. Glazer ES, Hornbrook MC, Krouse RS. A meta-analysis of randomized trials: immediate stent placement vs. surgical bypass in the palliative management of malignant biliary obstruction. J Pain Symptom Manag. 2014;47:307–14.
9. Maire F, Sauvanet A. Palliation of biliary and duodenal obstruction in patients with unresectable pancreatic cancer: endoscopy or surgery? J Visc Surg. 2013;150:S27–31.
10. Nagaraja V, Eslick GD, Cox MR. Endoscopic stenting versus operative gastrojejunostomy for malignant gastric outlet obstruction-a systematic review and meta-analysis of randomized and non-randomized trials. J Gastrointest Oncol. 2014;5:92–8.
11. Jeurnink SM, Steyerberg EW, Van Hooft JE, Van Eijck CH, Schwartz MP, Vleggaar FP, Kuipers EJ, Siersema PD, Dutch SSG. Surgical gastrojejunostomy or endoscopic stent placement for the palliation of malignant gastric outlet obstruction (SUSTENT study): a multicenter randomized trial. Gastrointest Endosc. 2010;71:490–9.
12. Masoomi H, Nguyen NT, Stamos MJ, Smith BR. Overview of outcomes of laparoscopic and open Roux-en-Y gastric bypass in the United States. Surg Technol Int. 2012;22:72–6.
13. Miller G, Boman J, Shrier I, Gordon PH. Small-bowel obstruction secondary to malignant disease: an 11-year audit. Can J Surg. 2000;43:353–8.
14. Zucchi E, Fornasarig M, Martella L, Maiero S, Lucia E, Borsatti E, Balestreri L, Giorda G, Annunziata MA, Cannizzaro R. Decompressive percutaneous endoscopic gastrostomy in advanced cancer patients with small-bowel obstruction is feasible and effective: a large prospective study. Support Care Cancer. 2016;24:2877–82.
15. He J, Page AJ, Weiss M, Wolfgang CL, Herman JM, Pawlik TM. Management of borderline and locally advanced pancreatic cancer: where do we stand? World J Gastroenterol. 2014;20:2255–66.
16. Tachezy M, Gebauer F, Janot M, Uhl W, Zerbi A, Montorsi M, Perinel J, Adham M, Dervenis C, Agalianos C, Malleo G, Maggino L, Stein A, Izbicki JR, Bockhorn M. Synchronous resections of hepatic oligometastatic pancreatic cancer: disputing a principle in a time of safe pancreatic operations in a retrospective multicenter analysis. Surgery. 2016;160:136–44.
17. Bahra M, Pratschke J, Klein F, Neuhaus P, Boas-Knoop S, Puhl G, Denecke T, Pullankavumkal JR, Sinn M, Riess H, Pelzer U. Cytoreductive surgery for pancreatic cancer improves overall outcome of gemcitabine-based chemotherapy. Pancreas. 2015;44(6):930.
18. Sinn M, Bahra M, Denecke T, Travis S, Pelzer U, Riess H. Perioperative treatment options in resectable pancreatic cancer – how to improve long-term survival. World J Gastrointest Oncol. 2016;8:248–57.
19. Taniguchi H, Mizuma M, Motoi F, Abe T, Okada R, Kawaguchi K, Karasawa H, Masuda K, Yabuuchi S, Fukase K, Sakata N, Okada T, Nakagawa K, Hayashi H, Morikawa T, Yoshida H, Naito T, Katayose Y, Egawa S, Unno M. A case of pancreatic cancer with local recurrence and liver metastases eight years after surgery. Gan To Kagaku Ryoho. 2014;41:2193–5.
20. Nakayama A, Tajima H, Kitagawa H, Shoji M, Nakanuma S, Makino I, Hayashi H, Nakagawara H, Miyashita T, Takamura H, Ohta T. A case report of hepatic arterial infusion chemotherapy and RFA for liver metastasis from pancreatic cancer. Gan To Kagaku Ryoho. 2014;41:2205–7.
21. Iida T, Nakabayashi Y, Okui N, Shiba H, Otsuka M, Yanaga K. Successful management of metachronous liver metastasis after pancreaticoduodectomy for pancreatic ductal carcinoma using hepatectomy and chemotherapy: a case report. Anticancer Res. 2014;34:2417–20.

22. Fujisaki S, Takashina M, Sakurai K, Tomita R, Takayama T. A case of successful management of liver metastases of pancreatic carcinoma by hepatectomy and adjuvant chemotherapy. Gan To Kagaku Ryoho. 2008;35:2109–11.
23. Hishinuma S, Ogata Y, Tomikawa M, Ozawa I, Inoue K, Katano S, Tsukiyama I. Prophylactic hepatic irradiation following curative resection of pancreatic cancer. J Hepato-Biliary-Pancreat Surg. 2005;12:235–42.
24. Tentes A, Stamou K, Pallas N, Karamveri C, Kyziridis D, Hristakis C. The effect of Hyperthermic intraoperative Intraperitoneal chemotherapy (Hipec) as an adjuvant in patients with Resectable pancreatic cancer. Int J Hyperth. 2016;32(8):1–11.
25. Roesch M, Mueller-Huebenthal B. Review: the role of hyperthermia in treating pancreatic tumors. Indian J Surg Oncol. 2015;6:75–81.
26. Robert CG Martin, McFarland K, Ellis S, Velanovich V. Irreversible electroporation therapy in the management of locally advanced pancreatic adenocarcinoma. J Am Coll Surg. 2012;215(3):361–369

Chapter 20
Current and Emerging Therapies in Pancreatic Cancer: Do They Provide Value?

Astrid Belalcazar and Olatunji B. Alese

Introduction

The economic burden of cancer treatment is substantial. In 2010 alone, cancer cost in the USA was estimated at $124 billion. Breast cancer treatment accounted for most expenditure ($16.10 billion), followed by colorectal, lymphoma, lung, and prostate cancers, each with costs above $11 billion [1]. The cost is estimated to reach $173 billion by 2020, a 40% increase over a decade [1]. Pancreatic cancer was close to the bottom of the list in cancer costs ($2.27 billion), exceeding only stomach, cervix, and esophageal cancers. However, costs associated with treatment of metastatic pancreatic cancer are relatively high due to the remarkably short survival of these patients. Information regarding cost-effectiveness of pancreatic cancer treatment derives from a limited number of studies. Their results are variable and reflect the impact of factors such as willingness-to-pay (WTP) threshold used in various analyses, price changes across health systems and over timelines, and the methods used for calculation. This chapter looks at the value of various diagnostic and treatment modalities employed in the care of pancreatic cancer patients.

Resectable Pancreatic Cancer

Surgery remains the mainstay of treatment for pancreatic cancer and offers the only chance for cure [2]. Up-front surgical resection is advocated for early stages of the disease, when the tumor is localized within the pancreas, without vascular or

A. Belalcazar • O.B. Alese (✉)
Winship Cancer Institute, Emory University, Atlanta, GA, USA
e-mail: olatunji.alese@emory.edu

T. Bekaii-Saab, B. El-Rayes (eds.), *Current and Emerging Therapies in Pancreatic Cancer*, DOI 10.1007/978-3-319-58256-6_20

neighboring tissue involvement. Although the morbidity and mortality is significant, the progressive decline in direct surgical costs for pancreatic cancer patients, despite rising overall healthcare costs, is encouraging [3]. In keeping with the trend in better outcomes in high-performing centers, length of hospital stay, postoperative complications, and substantial cost-effective utilization of surgery are associated with volume of resections per center [4, 5]. What is yet to be fully clarified is the cost utilization of minimally invasive surgical treatment of pancreatic cancer. Numerous studies evaluating open versus laparoscopic pancreatectomy give conflicting evidence regarding the cost-effectiveness of laparoscopic surgery. While patients' preference of minimally invasive techniques complements the shorter duration of hospital stay, lower operative morbidity, and better cosmetics, data supporting lower complications and reduced overall costs is more controversial. The postoperative enzyme supplementation, frequent use of proton pump inhibitors for reflux symptoms, and inadequate insulin function with glucose intolerance are significant although these are mainly indirect surgical costs. Emergency room visits and hospitalizations for other side effects such as dumping syndrome, late-onset vitamin, and elemental insufficiencies in cancer survivors are other contributing cost factors that should be taken into account. Nevertheless, the cost implications of potential for cure through resection of early-stage pancreatic cancer are favorable compared to the high recurrence and metastatic disease rate in these patients.

Imaging plays a crucial role in patient selection for surgical resection [6]. Although there is limited data regarding comparative effectiveness, currently available imaging tests that are used to assess resectability of pancreatic cancer appear to be equivalent in effectiveness. A study evaluating a strategy of computed tomography (CT), diagnostic laparoscopy, and laparoscopic ultrasonography (US) showed significantly lower costs than other imaging modalities, with an incremental cost-effectiveness ratio (ICER) of $87,502 per life-year gained [6]. The modeling employed showed that the strategy was more cost-effective than CT followed by magnetic resonance (MR) imaging, while retaining the difference in life-year gains. Arguably, proceeding with up-front surgery without comprehensive imaging would be cheaper but less effective than all imaging strategies.

Preoperative or neoadjuvant chemoradiation allows for the identification of pancreatic cancer patients who are not likely to benefit from definitive surgical resection, due to early metastases or poor performance status. A retrospective analysis using a decision analytic model evaluated 164 patients who completed preoperative therapy, compared to patients who underwent up-front surgical resection [7]. Costs associated with the surgery-first approach were about $46,830, with a survival of 8.7 quality-adjusted life-months (QALMs). The second group had significantly less costs ($36,583) and improved survival of 18.8 QALMs. Significant morbidity and mortality associated with surgical treatment of pancreatic cancer are thus avoided, and this approach improves survival at considerably lower cost than a surgery-first approach. It is a strategy with undeniably more cost-effectiveness in this selected group of patients.

A novel attempt at decreasing post-op complications such as leakage rates after Whipple procedure is prophylactic pasireotide. The somatostatin analog has been shown in a prospective randomized study to significantly decrease complications such as pancreatic fistula, postoperative leak, and infections [8]. A cost-effectiveness analysis to determine the cost-effective analysis of prophylactic pasireotide however showed a paltry net savings of $390 or 1% of total costs per patient [9]. Despite the 56% reduction in postoperative complications, the intervention strategy was not more cost-effective compared to usual care, due to the current pricing regimen for pasireotide.

Even in the absence of nodal disease, the role of adjuvant therapy is widely accepted in pancreatic cancer unlike most other solid tumors. Since the survival advantage of gemcitabine was established by CONKO-001 trial [10], it has widely replaced the more cost-effective infusional 5-fluorouracil as demonstrated in ESPAC-1 trial [11] due to more complex administration of the latter over several days. For high-risk patients who go on to receive chemoradiation, the added expense of oral capecitabine over the older intravenous 5-FU in combination with external beam radiation is significant. Notwithstanding, statistical models evaluating different treatment strategies showed that surgery with adjuvant chemotherapy is the most cost-effective, biologically plausible treatment option [12]. Combined with high-volume treatment settings, the indices of cost-effectiveness analyses were even more striking [13, 14]. The cost-effectiveness analysis of the recently adopted new adjuvant therapy utilizing gemcitabine and capecitabine [15] would help clarify its impact on health expenditure in pancreatic cancer.

Advanced Unresectable Pancreatic Cancer

To improve patient selection and survival outcomes, nonmetastatic pancreatic tumors that have extended beyond the pancreas have been classified as borderline resectable (BRPC) and locally advanced pancreatic cancer (LAPC). They account for about 30% of all pancreatic cancer presentations [16]. Although the classification methodology often differs considerably between various professional societies and treatment groups, the role of preoperative systemic therapy in these two categories is becoming more clarified and acceptable [17, 18]. Vascular involvement as described in preceding chapters is more commonly treated with chemotherapy in attempts at downstaging, or as definitive therapy. Chemotherapy regimens which were previously developed for metastatic disease have become frontline therapy for unresectable nonmetastatic pancreatic cancer [19, 20]. Although it is likely that the use of preoperative therapy would be more significant in terms of cost-effectiveness, there is paucity of data regarding their use in advanced unresectable pancreatic cancer.

Metastatic Pancreatic Cancer

Cytotoxic Chemotherapy

Chemotherapy regimens consisting of oxaliplatin, irinotecan, fluorouracil, and leucovorin (FOLFIRINOX) [21] or gemcitabine and nab-paclitaxel [22] are most frequently used in the frontline treatment of patients with metastatic pancreatic cancer

Table 20.1 Monthly costs of chemotherapy regimens used in pancreatic cancer treatment

Chemotherapy agents	Medication cost	Administration costs	Toxicity cost	Total cost per month
Gemcitabine	$188	$143	$1032	$1363
Gemcitabine/nab-paclitaxel	$9088	$522	$2692	$12,221
FOLFIRINOX	$763	$531	$5940	$7234
Gemcitabine/erlotinib	$6831	$143	$1032	$8007

Adapted with permission from 2015 ASCO educational book. Costs include the use of growth factors

[23]. Table 20.1 shows the monthly cost in 2013 US dollars of these two regimens compared to single-agent gemcitabine, in addition to the costs of more rarely used gemcitabine and erlotinib combination. The cost-effectiveness of using FOLFIRINOX instead of gemcitabine as first-line treatment for metastatic pancreatic cancer was reported in a 2014 Canadian study. Using the overall (OS) and progression-free survival (PFS) data from the landmark multicenter, randomized, phase III ACCORD trial [21], the Markov model for projection showed that FOLFIRINOX chemotherapy derives more life-years and quality-adjusted life-years (QALYs) than gemcitabine. FOLFIRINOX was associated with QALYs of $57,858 compared to single-agent gemcitabine [24].

A study using data from various phase III trials and information from Canada's health system for cost projections reported incremental cost-effectiveness ratio (ICER) of gemcitabine/nab-paclitaxel at 199,011/QALY and FOLFIRINOX at 115,123/QALY [25]. In the US health system, two studies have reported gemcitabine/nab-paclitaxel as a more cost-effective option than FOLFIRINOX. The first reported the cost per course of therapy for gemcitabine/nab-paclitaxel to be $29,361 in 2013 US dollars, FOLFIRINOX had a cost of $39,704, and gemcitabine was associated with $2566 [26]. This study included costs of administration, growth factor use, and adverse events. A more recent study reinforced this observation, reporting treatment costs of $252,474 for FOLFIRINOX and $136, 202 for gemcitabine/nab-paclitaxel [27].

Because no prospective trial to date has compared FOLFIRINOX to gemcitabine/nab-paclitaxel, some studies have used an indirect comparison to evaluate head-to-head cost-effectiveness. A Canadian analysis of FOLFIRINOX compared to gemcitabine/nab-paclitaxel in metastatic pancreatic cancer reported an ICER of $7380/QALY for FOLFIRINOX. This indirect comparison study used data from the ACCORD and MPACT trials. Another analysis using case data from the ACCORD and MPACT trials was calculated at a university hospital in China. They reported costs associated with gemcitabine/nab-paclitaxel at US$32,080.59, compared to US$37,203.75 for FOLFIRINOX. Survival benefits reported as quality-adjusted life-years (QALYs) showed 0.67 QALY for FOLFIRINOX but a superior 0.51 QALY for gemcitabine/nab-paclitaxel [28]. In a US study, comparison of FOLFIRINOX versus gemcitabine/nab-paclitaxel cost-effectiveness showed that at 3 years gemcitabine/nab-paclitaxel was cheaper at $684 per patient. In addition, FOLFIRINOX showed an incremental cost of $16,012 per additional life-year [29].

A network meta-analysis evaluating the cost-effectiveness across several existent regimens for pancreatic cancer reported that FOLFIRINOX would cost more than $182,723 per QALY, while gemcitabine/5-FU would cost between $15,259 and $182,723, making the latter a more cost-effective option. The authors noted that the cost of FOLFIRINOX was higher due to a lack of generic oxaliplatin [30]. There is even less data about the cost-effectiveness of less frequently used combination chemotherapies like gemcitabine/capecitabine and gemcitabine/erlotinib. In 2013, the ICER for gemcitabine/capecitabine was reported as 84,299/QALY when compared to gemcitabine single agent [31]. Erlotinib combination therapy is discussed below under targeted therapies.

Targeted Therapy

The lack of effective targeted therapies for treatment of metastatic pancreatic cancer is probably contributory to the relative low overall treatment costs compared to other solid tumors such as lung cancer. To date, the only targeted agent approved for use in pancreatic cancer has been erlotinib. In Canada, the calculated ICER for gemcitabine/erlotinib was reported to be $153,631/QALY compared to gemcitabine alone [31]. This regimen is not frequently used as survival benefits at lower costs have been demonstrated with other cytotoxic chemotherapy. Nevertheless, in an era where personalized cancer treatment is developing at a fast pace, the role of targeted agents in pancreatic cancer continues to evolve. Agents such as checkpoint inhibitors, vaccines, RAS, and JAK/STAT pathway inhibitors are being explored for efficacy. Considering that new treatment agents in the USA are priced at an average monthly cost of $5000 [32], it is reasonable to assume that costs of pancreatic cancer care may eventually rise when these agents are introduced.

Supportive Care

Hospice care for pancreatic cancer was estimated at $4500 per patient in 2009 US dollars, corresponding to 7% of the total cost per patient from diagnosis to death or end of follow-up [33]. A study of Medicare patients with pancreatic cancer showed that those with metastatic disease were more likely to use hospice care than those initially treated with curative intent [34]. This is significant since many studies have shown that initiation of palliative or hospice care early in the course of a disease increases overall survival in other malignancies [35]. In pancreatic cancer, more patients receive chemotherapy during the last month of their lives, a practice that reflects frequent misconceptions, inadequate hospice/palliative care, and unrealistic expectations [36]. There is an urgent need to expand the role of palliative care as part of the multidisciplinary approach for the care of patients with pancreatic cancer.

References

1. Mariotto AB, Yabroff KR, Shao Y, et al. Projections of the cost of cancer care in the United States: 2010-2020. J Natl Cancer Inst. 2011;103:117–28.
2. Wagner M, Redaelli C, Lietz M, et al. Curative resection is the single most important factor determining outcome in patients with pancreatic adenocarcinoma. Br J Surg. 2004;91:586–94.
3. Vollmer CM Jr, Pratt W, Vanounou T, et al. Quality assessment in high-acuity surgery: volume and mortality are not enough. Arch Surg. 2007;142:371–80.
4. Gajdos C, Schulick R. Cost-effectiveness of treatment strategies for primary operable pancreatic head adenocarcinoma: do we have more scientific evidence to call for further centralization of care? Ann Surg Oncol. 2013;20:5–6.
5. Abbott DE, Merkow RP, Cantor SB, et al. Cost-effectiveness of treatment strategies for pancreatic head adenocarcinoma and potential opportunities for improvement. Ann Surg Oncol. 2012;19:3659–67.
6. McMahon PM, Halpern EF, Fernandez-del Castillo C, et al. Pancreatic cancer: cost-effectiveness of imaging technologies for assessing resectability. Radiology. 2001;221:93–106.
7. Abbott DE, Tzeng CW, Merkow RP, et al. The cost-effectiveness of neoadjuvant chemoradiation is superior to a surgery-first approach in the treatment of pancreatic head adenocarcinoma. Ann Surg Oncol. 2013;20(Suppl 3):S500–8.
8. Allen PJ, Gonen M, Brennan MF, et al. Pasireotide for postoperative pancreatic fistula. N Engl J Med. 2014;370:2014–22.
9. Abbott DE, Sutton JM, Jernigan PL, et al. Prophylactic pasireotide administration following pancreatic resection reduces cost while improving outcomes. J Surg Oncol. 2016;113:784–8.
10. Oettle H, Post S, Neuhaus P, et al. Adjuvant chemotherapy with gemcitabine vs observation in patients undergoing curative-intent resection of pancreatic cancer: a randomized controlled trial. JAMA. 2007;297:267–77.
11. Neoptolemos JP, Stocken DD, Friess H, et al. A randomized trial of chemoradiotherapy and chemotherapy after resection of pancreatic cancer. N Engl J Med. 2004;350:1200–10.
12. Ansari D, Gustafsson A, Andersson R. Update on the management of pancreatic cancer: surgery is not enough. World J Gastroenterol. 2015;21:3157–65.
13. Moesinger RC, Davis JW, Hill B, et al. Treatment of pancreatic and periampullary cancers at a community hospital: successful application of tertiary care treatment standards. Int J Surg Oncol. 2011;2011:936516.
14. Khorana AA, Mangu PB, Berlin J, et al. Potentially curable pancreatic cancer: American Society of Clinical Oncology clinical practice guideline. J Clin Oncol. 2016;34:2541–56.
15. Neoptolemos JP, Palmer DH, Ghaneh P, et al. Comparison of adjuvant gemcitabine and capecitabine with gemcitabine monotherapy in patients with resected pancreatic cancer (ESPAC-4): a multicentre, open-label, randomised, phase 3 trial. Lancet. 2017;389(10073):1011–24.
16. Shaib WL, Ip A, Cardona K, et al. Contemporary Management of Borderline Resectable and Locally Advanced Unresectable Pancreatic Cancer. Oncologist. 2016;21:178–87.
17. Sultana A, Smith CT, Cunningham D, et al. Meta-analyses of chemotherapy for locally advanced and metastatic pancreatic cancer. J Clin Oncol. 2007;25:2607–15.
18. Wolff RA. Pancreatic cancer: is it time for Dr Whipple's orphans to have a Facebook page? Nat Rev Clin Oncol. 2012;9:553–4.
19. Blazer M, Wu C, Goldberg RM, et al. Neoadjuvant modified (m) FOLFIRINOX for locally advanced unresectable (LAPC) and borderline resectable (BRPC) adenocarcinoma of the pancreas. Ann Surg Oncol. 2015;22:1153–9.
20. Faris JE, Blaszkowsky LS, McDermott S, et al. FOLFIRINOX in locally advanced pancreatic cancer: the Massachusetts General Hospital cancer center experience. Oncologist. 2013;18:543–8.
21. Conroy T, Desseigne F, Ychou M, et al. FOLFIRINOX versus gemcitabine for metastatic pancreatic cancer. N Engl J Med. 2011;364:1817–25.

22. Von Hoff DD, Ervin T, Arena FP, et al. Increased survival in pancreatic cancer with nab-paclitaxel plus gemcitabine. N Engl J Med. 2013;369:1691–703.
23. Teague A, Lim KH, Wang-Gillam A. Advanced pancreatic adenocarcinoma: a review of current treatment strategies and developing therapies. Ther Adv Med Oncol. 2015;7:68–84.
24. Attard CL, Brown S, Alloul K, et al. Cost-effectiveness of FOLFIRINOX for first-line treatment of metastatic pancreatic cancer. Curr Oncol. ASCO Meeting Abstracts. 2012;30:199.
25. Ko Y-J, Tam VC, Mittmann N, et al. A cost-utility analysis of gemcitabine plus nab-paclitaxel in metastatic pancreatic cancer. J Clin Oncol. ASCO Meeting Abstracts. 2013;31:e17569.
26. Milentijevic D, Binder G, Whiting S, et al. Population-based economic impact of nab-paclitaxel plus gemcitabine in metastatic pancreatic cancer. J Clin Oncol. ASCO Meeting Abstracts. 2014;32:16.
27. Gharaibeh M, McBride A, Bootman JL, et al. Optimized economic evaluation for the United States (US) of NAB-paclitaxel plus gemcitabine (NAB-P+GEM), FOLFIRINOX (FFX), and gemcitabine (GEM) as first-line treatment for metastatic pancreatic cancer (mPDA). J Clin Oncol. ASCO Meeting Abstracts. 2016;34:4113.
28. Zhou J, Zhao R, Wen F, et al. Cost-effectiveness analysis of treatments for metastatic pancreatic cancer based on PRODIGE and MPACT trials. Tumori. 2016;2016:294–300.
29. Wang Y, Chen L, Camateros P, et al. Comparative effectiveness of FOLFIRINOX or nab-paclitaxel plus gemcitabine in locally advanced or metastatic pancreatic cancer: a population-based analysis. J Clin Oncol. ASCO Meeting Abstracts. 2016;34:6561.
30. Chan KK, Ko Y-J, Shah K, et al. A network meta-analysis-based cost-effectiveness analysis of systematic therapies in advanced pancreatic cancer. J Clin Oncol. ASCO Meeting Abstracts. 2015;33:6611.
31. Tam VC, Ko YJ, Mittmann N, et al. Cost-effectiveness of systemic therapies for metastatic pancreatic cancer. Curr Oncol. 2013;20:e90–e106.
32. Fojo T, Grady C. How much is life worth: cetuximab, non-small cell lung cancer, and the $440 billion question. J Natl Cancer Inst. 2009;101:1044–8.
33. O'Neill CB, Atoria CL, O'Reilly EM, et al. Costs and trends in pancreatic cancer treatment. Cancer. 2012;118:5132–9.
34. Sheffield KM, Boyd CA, Benarroch-Gampel J, et al. End-of-life care in Medicare beneficiaries dying with pancreatic cancer. Cancer. 2011;117:5003–12.
35. Temel JS, Greer JA, Muzikansky A, et al. Early palliative care for patients with metastatic non-small-cell lung cancer. N Engl J Med. 2010;363:733–42.
36. Smith TJ, Hillner BE. Bending the cost curve in cancer care. N Engl J Med. 2011;364:2060–5.

Index

A
ABO blood group, 8
Acinar cell carcinoma, 70, 86
Active-specific immunotherapy, 282
Adenosquamous carcinoma, 61, 83
Adenoviruses, 313
Advanced unresectable pancreatic cancer, 363
AIO-PK0104 study, 222
Algenpantucel-L, 294
Alliance Trial A021501, 196
All-trans-retinoic acid (ATRA), 238
Americas Hepato-Pancreato-Biliary Association (AHPBA), 185
Anaplastic carcinoma. *See* Undifferentiated carcinoma
Angiogenesis, 223–224
Annular pancreas, 27
Anti-idiotype antibodies (AIAs), 282
Ataxia telangiectasia (AT), 5, 6
Ataxia telangiectasia and Rad3-related protein (ATR), 258
Ataxia telangiectasia mutated (ATM), 258
Atrophic gastritis with hypergastrinaemia, 8
Autoimmune pancreatitis (AIP), 153, 175
AViTA, 223
Axitinib, 223

B
BBI608, 227
β-Catenin expression, 227
β-human chorionic gonadotropin (β-hCG), 289
Bile ducts
  anatomic variations, 40
  extrahepatic, 34, 39, 45
  intrahepatic, 36
Biliary decompression, 160–162
Biliary obstruction
  algorithm, 351
  bacterial and endotoxin translocation, 350
  endoscopic biliary stenting, 350
  gemcitabine/5-FU-based chemotherapy regimens, 350
  hepaticojejunostomy, 352
  PTBD, 352
  SEMS, 350
  stenting, 351
Biliary self-expandable metal stents (SEMS), 160
Biliary tree
  anatomy, 34
  arterial inflow, 32
  cystic duct, 42–44
  drainage, liver, 38
  embryologic development, 35–37
  epithelium-lined ductal structures, 34
  extrahepatic bile duct, 39, 41, 45
  gallbladder, 42–44
  innervation, 46
  intrahepatic bile duct, 38, 39
  lymphatic drainage, regional blood supply, 44, 45
  surgical anatomy, 37
  sympathetic afferent fibers, 46

T. Bekaii-Saab, B. El-Rayes (eds.), *Current and Emerging Therapies in Pancreatic Cancer*, DOI 10.1007/978-3-319-58256-6

Borderline resectable pancreatic cancer (BRPC), 187, 188, 192, 325
  clinical work up
    arterial phase, 187
    biliary decompression, 188
    contrast-enhanced MRI, 187
    EUS, 187
    FDG-PET/CT, 187
    hepatic phase, 187
    MDCT, 187
    pancreatic phase, 187
    tissue diagnosis, 188
  definition, 185, 186
  neoadjuvant regimens, 189–191
    FOLFIRINOX, 192
    gemcitabine combination therapy, 188
Breast cancer-associated gene mutations, 4, 5
BRPC. *See* Borderline resectable pancreatics cancer (BRPC)
Bruton's tyrosine kinase (BTK), 276

C
Capecitabine, 122, 221
Carbon ion therapy, 336–337
Carcinoembryonic antigen (CEA), 283, 284
Carcinoma-associated fibroblast (CAF), 239
Celiac artery (CA), 198
Cell-free nucleic acids, 125
Cetuximab, 222
Checkpoint inhibitors
  algenpantucel-L, 276
  BMS-936559, 275
  completed phase I/II clinical trials, 272–274
  GVAX, 276
  IgG4 monoclonal antibody, 275
  PD-L1-specific monoclonal antibody, 275
  single agent therapeutic approach, 275
Chronic pancreatitis, 6, 59
Circulating tumor cells (CTC), 126
Circulating tumor DNA (ctDNA), 125
Clivatuzumab tetraxetan (PAM4), 225
Colloid carcinomas, 60, 61
Colony-stimulating factor-1 (CSF-1) and its receptor (CSF-1R), 242
Contrast-enhanced endoscopic ultrasound, 157
Covered SEMS (CSEMS), 350
Cystic fibrosis (CF), 6, 7
Cytology
  benign biliary ductal cells, 79
  cell block preparation, 78
  contamination, 79
  cyst fluid analysis, 87, 89
  cytocentrifugation, 78
  diagnostic approach, 79, 87
  diagnostic sensitivity, 78
  endoscopic ultrasound-guided FNA biopsy, 77
  fine needle aspiration biopsy, 77
  liquid-based preparation, 78
  pancreatobiliary tract brushing, 78, 79
  primary indications, 77
  sample preparation, 78
  tissue biopsy, 77
Cytotoxic chemotherapy, 363–365

D
Delayed-type hypersensitivity (DTH) reaction, 287
Dendritic cell (DC) vaccines, 282–283
Diabetes
  and glucose metabolism, 7
  management of, 15
  PDAC, risk factor of, 99
  screening, 103
DNA damage repair, 123, 124, 259, 261
DNA mutational analysis, 157
DNA-targeting cytotoxic chemotherapy, 262–263
Dose-escalated hypofractionation, 332, 333
Double duct sign, 159
Double-layer stents (DLSs), 351
Ductal adenocarcinoma. *See* Pancreatic ductal adenocarcinoma (PDAC)

E
ELISpot, 293
Endoscopic enteral stent placement, 151
Endoscopic retrograde cholangiopancreatography (ERCP), 78
  biliary decompression, 160–162
  biliary stents, 160–161
  diagnosis, 159–160
  neoadjuvant treatment, 162
  preoperative biliary drainage, 161–162
Endoscopic ultrasound (EUS), 152–154, 156
  celiac plexus neurolysis, 157–158
  elastography, 157
  EUS-FNI, 158
  EUS-guided biliary drainage, 159
  limitations, 187
  pancreatic malignancy
    high-risk pancreatic cancer screening, 152

pancreatic cyst evaluation, 152
pancreatic masses
diagnosis, 153
differential diagnosis, 153
stages, 154
sensitivity and negative predictive value, 187
tissue diagnosis
EUS-FNA, 154
EUS-FNB, 156
Endoscopic ultrasound elastography, 157
Enhancer of zeste 2 polycomb repressive complex 2 subunit (EZH2), 257
Epidermal growth factor receptor (EGFR), 222–223
ERCP. *See* Endoscopic retrograde cholangiopancreatography (ERCP)
Erlotinib, 222
EUS. *See* Endoscopic ultrasound (EUS)
EUS-celiac plexus neurolysis (EUS-CPN), 157–158
EUS-fine needle aspiration, 154–156
EUS-fine needle biopsy (EUS-FNB), 156–157
EUS-fine needle injection (EUS-FNI), 158
EUS-guided biliary drainage, 159
EUS-guided direct celiac ganglion injection, 158
Extracellular matrix (ECM), 246–248

F
Familial atypical multiple mole melanoma (FAMMM) syndrome, 5
Familial pancreatic cancer (FPC), 3, 4
Farnesyl transferase inhibitors, 221
Farnesylation, 221
First-line therapy
combination therpy, 206–207
gemcitabine and albumin-bound paclitaxel, 206–208
5-fluorouracil, 206
FISH analysis, 157
5-Fluorouracil (5-FU), 206
Focal adhesion kinase (FAK), 277
Focal pancreatitis, 139
FOLFIRINOX, 208–211
BRPC, 192
chemotherapy, 297
duration of therapy, 209
incidence, 209
LAPC, 193
modified dose/schedule, 210
MPACT vs. ACCORD11/PRODIGE studies, 209–211
objective response rates, 208, 209
phase II randomized study, 208
phase III ACCORD 11/PRODIGE study, 209
prophylactic G-CSF, 210
QoL assessment, 209
side effect profile, 210

G
Gastric outlet obstruction, 163
endoscopic stenting, 353
gastrojejunostomy, 353
prevalance, 352
uncovered and covered stents, 353
Gastrojejunostomy (GJJ), 163, 353
Gemcitabine, 221
Genetic predisposition syndromes, 4
Groove pancreatitis, 59

H
Heat shock proteins (HSPs), 293
Heavy particle therapy, 333–334
Hedgehog pathway, 227
Hepatic plate/sheath system, 41
Hepaticojejunostomy, 352
Hepatoid carcinoma, 62
Her2/neu amplification, 224
Hereditary nonpolyposis colorectal cancer (HNPCC), 6
Hereditary pancreatitis, 4
Herpes simplex virus (HSV), 313–314
Histologic core of tissue, 156
Human equilibrative nucleoside transporter (hENT), 127
Hypofractionated image-guided radiation therapy (HIGRT), 331

I
Imatinib, 219
Immune cells
activated cytotoxic (effector) CD8+ T cells/NK cells, 240
CD40 agonists, 242
CSF-1/CSF-1R signaling, 242
experimental agent, 241
inflammatory monocytes, 240
leukocyte infiltrate, 239
MDSCs, 239
reprogramming, 241
TAMs, 240
therapeutic implications, 241
Tregs, 239

Immunotherapy, 272–276
BTK, 276
checkpoint inhibitors
algenpantucel-L, 276
BMS-936559, 275
completed phase I/II clinical trials, 272–274
GVAX, 276
IgG4 monoclonal antibody, 275
PD-L1-specific monoclonal antibody, 275
single agent therapeutic approach, 275
CXCR2, 277
FAK, 277
IL-6/STAT3 pathway, 277
NF-kB, 277
pancreatic cancer microenvironment, 271–272
tumorigenesis process, 277
Intraductal neoplasms, 64
definition, 64
IPMN (*see* Intraductal papillary mucinous neoplasm (IPMN))
ITPN (*see* Intraductal tubulopapillary neoplasm (ITPN))
Intraductal papillary mucinous neoplasm (IPMN), 17, 152, 344
branch duct type, 64
clinical behavior, 64
combined duct type, 64
cystic lesions, 73
cystic neoplasm, 141
dilated ducts, 64
epithelial dysplasia, 88
gastric type, 64
grading system, 66
histological types, 65
histology, 64
imaging characteristics, 141
intestinal type, 64
invasive adenocarcinoma, 66
ionizing radiation, 141
main duct type, 64
morphological subtypes, 66
MRI, 142
oncocytic type, 65
pancreatobiliary type, 65
patient age, 64
resection margin, 67
surgical resection, 88
Intraductal tubulopapillary neoplasm (ITPN)
diagnosis, 67
molecular genetics, 67
mutation profile, 68
neoplastic proliferation, 67
tubulopapillary structures, 67
Intraluminal brachytherapy, 337
Ipilimumab, 199, 275, 276, 295, 297, 298
Irinotecan, 212, 221
Irreversible electroporation (IRE), 337, 355

J

Janus kinase inhibition (JAK 1/2), 224–225

K

Kinesin family member 20A (KIF20A), 293
KRAS mutations, 122, 125, 286

L

LAP-07 phase III randomized trial, 196
LAPC. *See* Locally advanced pancreatic cancer (LAPC)
Locally advanced pancreatic cancer (LAPC), 187, 188, 193, 195–198, 325
checkpoint inhibitors, 199
clinical work up
arterial phase, 187
biliary decompression, 188
EUS, 187
FDG-PET/CT, 187
hepatic phase, 187
MDCT, 187
pancreatic phase, 187
tissue diagnosis, 188
contrast-enhanced MRI, 187
definition, 185, 186
neoadjuvant regimens, 190, 191, 194
FOLFIRINOX, 193
gemcitabine and nab-paclitaxel, 195
gemcitabine and oxaliplatin, 196
radiation therapy, 196–197
surgical resection
Appleby procedure, 198
determination, 197
vascular resection, 197–198
Low hENT1 and Adenocarcinoma of the Pancreas (LEAP) study, 213
Lurbinectedin, 213
Lymphoepithelial cyst, 76, 77, 89, 90
Lynch syndrome, 6, 100

M

Malignant bile duct obstruction, 350
Marimastat, 221
Matrix metalloproteinases (MMPs), 221
Medullary carcinomas, 60, 62

Metastatic pancreatic cancer
  cytotoxic chemotherapy, 363–365
  ipilimumab with allogenic GM-CSF transfected pancreatic tumor vaccine, 297–298
  targeted therapy, 363–365
MicroRNAs (miRs), 124, 125
Microsatellite instability, 124
Mitogen-activated protein kinase (MAPK) pathway, 286
Mixed adenoneuroendocrine carcinomas (MANEC), 71
Mixed ductal-neuroendocrine carcinomas, 62
Molecularly targeted therapy
  advantages, 219
  angiogenesis, 222–224
  clinical trials, 219, 220
  EGFR, 221–223
  farnesylation, 221
  hedgehog pathway, 227
  Her2/neu amplification, 224
  inhibition, 219
  JAK 1/2, 224–225
  matrix metalloproteinases, 221
  MEK/MAPK and PI3K/Akt/mTOR pathways, 225–226
  MUC 1, 225
  signaling pathways, 219
  STAT3, 227
  targeting *RAS*, 226
Mucin 1 (MUC-1), 225, 285
Mucinous cystadenoma, 145
Mucinous cystic neoplasms (MCN), 75, 76, 88, 145, 146, 152
Multi-detector computed tomography (MDCT), 186
Multiple endocrine neoplasia type 1 (MEN1), 147
Myeloid-derived suppressor cells (MDSCs), 238, 239

N
Nasogastric (NG) tube decompression, 354
Neoadjuvant chemoradiation, 362
Neoadjuvant regimens, 188, 192, 193, 195, 196
  BRPC
    FOLFIRINOX, 192–193
    gemcitabine combination therapy, 188
  LAPC
    FOLFIRINOX, 193
    gemcitabine and nab-paclitaxel, 195
    gemcitabine and oxaliplatin, 196
Neurofibromatosis type 1 (NF1), 147

O
Oncolytic virotherapy (OV), 316, 317
  adenoviruses, 313
  biologic therapies, 315
  HSV, 313
  immunologic barrier, 314
  immunotherapeutic approaches, 315
  immunotherapeutic treatment strategies, 310
  intravenous administration, 315
  mode of delivery, 315
  ongoing/completed phase I/II clinical trials investigating, 311
  pancreatic tumor microenvironment, 314
  physical barriers, 315
  reovirus, 312
  tumor-associated antigens, 314
  vaccinia virus, 314
  vector-mediated virotherapy
    completed phase I/II clinical trials, 316
    Rexin-G, 316
    TNFerade, 316–317
  VSV, 313
Ontario Pancreas Cancer Study (OPCS), 3

P
Palliative surgical interventions, 350–353
  biliary obstruction
    algorithm, 351
    bacterial and endotoxin translocation, 350
    DLS, 351
    endoscopic biliary stenting, 350
    gemcitabine/5-FU-based chemotherapy regimens, 350
    hepaticojejunostomy, 352
    PTBD, 352
    SEMS, 350
    stenting, 351
  chemotherapy, 356
  cytoreduction with HIPEC, 356
  extended resection approach, 356
  gastric outlet obstruction
    endoscopic stenting, 353
    gastrojejunostomy, 353
    prevalence, 352
    uncovered and covered stents, 353
  irreversible electroporation, 354–355
  liver metastases, 355
  locally advanced and metastatic pancreatic cancer, 349–350
  malignant bowel obstruction, 354–355
  PHI, 356
  radiofrequency ablation, 356

Pancreas, 23, 27–34, 51
  anatomy
    accessory duct of Santorini, 31
    arterial inflow, 32
    autonomic innervation, 34
    congenital anomalies and variants
      categorization, 27
    descriptive, 30
    endocrine component, 23
    exocrine component, 23
    head, 29
    in situ, 28
    microscopic structure and functions, 23
    pancreatic duct of Wirsung, 29
    posterior surface of the body, 29
    primordia and ductal system, 27
    regional blood supply, 31–34
    sphincter of Oddi, 31
    splenorenal ligament, 29
    surgical, 28–34
    transampullary septum, 31
    uncinate process, 29
  anomalies, 27
  cellular and molecular interactions, 25
  developmental biology, 23
  embryology, 23, 24, 26, 27
  exocrine acini lobules, 50
  histology, 50
  lymphatic drainage, regional blood supply, 31–34
  pancreas-licensing signals, 26
  pancreatobiliary structures, 42
  parenchymal cells, 26
  tumor classification
    primary, 51
    secondary, 51
  WHO 2010 classification, 51, 52
Pancreas divisum, 26, 27
Pancreatic adenocarcinoma, 262–267, (*see also* Pancreatic ductal adenocarcinoma (PDAC))
Pancreatic cancer (PC), 3, 4, 7–16, 119–123, 126, 127, 206–211
  biliary stenting, 162
  and diabetes (*see* Diabetes)
  and hereditary syndromes, 63
  arterial phase sequence, 136
  biomarkers
    CA19-9, 120, 127
    C-reactive protein, 120, 121
    features, 119
    hENT1, 127
    KRAS, 121, 122
    p21-activated kinases, 123
    Rigosertib, 122
    SMAD4, 123
    SPARC, 126, 127
  clinical presentation, 49
  diagnostic modalities, 49
  dietary habits, 14
  endoscopic retrograde cholangiopancreatography, 137
  environmental risk factors
    alcohol consumption, 13
    smoking, 8–12
  epidemiology, 49
  first-line therapy
    combination therpy, 206
    5-fluorouracil, 206
    gemcitabine and albumin-bound paclitaxel, 207
  FOLFIRINOX
    duration of therapy, 209
    incidence, 209
    modified dose/schedule, 210
    MPACT vs. ACCORD11/PRODIGE studies, 209–211
    objective response rates, 208, 209
    phase II randomized study, 208
    phase III ACCORD 11/PRODIGE study, 209
    primary and secondary end point, 209
    prophylactic G-CSF, 210
    QoL assessment, 209
    side effect profile, 210
  gemcitabine-based chemotherapy, 123
  genetic predisposition (*see* Genetic predisposition syndromes)
  Helicobacter pylori infections, 17
  hepatitis viral infection, 17
  idiopathic, 1
  incidence, 2, 49, 205
  inherited risk factors
    familial, 3, 4
    hereditary pancreatitis, 4
  magnetic resonance cholangiopancreatography, 135, 136
  medications
    angiotensin converting enzyme inhibitors, 15
    angiotensin receptor blockers, 15
    anti-angiogenic effects, 15
    anti-inflammatory effects, 15
    dipeptidyl peptidase-4, 15
    eicosapentaenoic acid, 16
    hyperinsulinemia, 15
    incretin-based drugs, 15
    pro-apoptotic effects, 15
    renin-angiotensin system, 14
    signalling pathways, 15
    Veteran Affairs, 15
  metastatics, 205

MRI, 137
NSAIDs, 16
obesity, 16
occupational exposure, 13, (*see also* Pancreatic ductal adenocarcinoma (PDAC))
prognostic scoring systems, 121
screening, 17, 18
second- line therapy, 211–213
SEER database, 2
selenium, 16
soft tissue imaging, 136
steady-state free precession sequences, 136
survival rates, 1, 205
T1weighted 3D GRE imaging, 136
tumour markers, 17
Pancreatic ductal adenocarcinoma (PDAC), 56, 58–61, 99–106, 281
adenosquamous cell carcinoma, 82
anaplastic/undifferentiated carcinoma, 82
arterial resection, 114, 115
borderline resectability, 112
cellular aspirate, 81
cellularity, 81, 82
chemotherapeutic regimens, 109
clinical classification, 111–113, 115
clinical significance, 84
clinical-radiological correlation, 82–84
conventional ductal carcinoma
differential diagnosis, 59
epidemiology, 56
histology, 56, 58
incidence, 56
risk factors, 56
staging and grading, 60
cross-sectional imaging, 98
with cystic changes, 138
cytomorphology, 82
diagnostic accuracy, 98
diagnostic features, 58
distant metastatic disease, 141
dyshesion and hyperchromasia, 81
epidemiology, 104
exocrine pancreatic tumor, 137
foamy gland pattern, 82
focal pancreatitis, 140
focal steatosis, 139
gastric foveolar epithelium, 82
gene mutations, 63
histologic features, 59
imaging modalities, 115
indications, 140
metastatic disease, 116
molecular genetics, 62, 63
morphologies, 57
poorly differentiated, 81
prognostic implications, 115
radical resection, 109
resectability criteria, 111, 112
screening
APC, 100
benefits and risks, 105, 106
beta cell dysfunction, 103
BRCA1, 100
CDK2NA, 100
clinical factors, 103
diabetes, 99
family history, 100, 102, 106
fine needle aspiration, 103
genetic evaluation, 101, 102, 105
germline mutations, 100–102
imaging modalities, 103
immune therapy, 101
PALB2, 100
patient counseling, 105
platinum-based chemotherapy, 101
poly(ADP-ribose) polymerase inhibitors, 101
PRSS1, 101
risk assessment, 104
STK11, 100
test frequency, 104
TP53, 100
treatment approaches, 101
staging systems, 115–117
superior mesenteric artery, 138
surgical techniques, 109
synthetic lethality
BRCA1/2-mutation, 262
PARP inhibition, 263–267
T1-weighed fat-suppressed imaging, 137
TNM staging, 110, 111
tumor marker, 115
variants
histologic, 61
prognostic value, 60
vascular involvement, 141
vascular resection, 113
venous resection, 113, 114
Pancreatic intraepithelial neoplasia (PanIN), 17
Baltimore consensus, 54
with dysplasia, 55
grading system, 53, 54
histology, 54
intraductal epithelial proliferation, 53
management, 53
molecular genetics, 56
at resection margin, 54
Pancreatic malignancy
high-risk pancreatic cancer screening, 152
pancreatic cyst evaluation, 152–153

Pancreatic masses
diagnosis, 153
differential diagnosis, 153
stages, 154
Pancreatic neuroendocrine tumors (PanNETs), 146, 147
acinar cell carcinoma, 86
arterial phase, 148
aspirate smear, 84
benign acinar cells, 80, 84
cell cytomorphology, 84
clinical symptoms, 147
cystic degeneration, 147
cytoplasmic processes (cercariform), 86
diagnosis, 84
florid islet cell aggregation, 84
grading system, 72
histology, 68
hormonal hypersecretion, 147
imaging method, 147
immunohistochemical stains, 84, 86
incidence, 68, 146
interpretation errors, 84
molecular alterations, 73
non-tumor cell contamination, 84
occurrence, 147
oncocytic variant, 85
poorly differentiated neoplasms, 60, 70, 85
sampling insufficiency, 84
serotonin-producing tumors, 68
solid pseudopapillary tumor, 86
staging, 72
tumor detection and staging, 147
vacuolated and oncocytic, 84
well-differentiated neoplasms, 68, 69, 85
WHO classification, 63, 72
Pancreatic stellate cells (PSCs)
activated stromal index, 237
agonistic, 237
anti-CTLA-4 antibody, 239
ATRA, 238
CAF, 239
CD31+ (endothelial) cells, 238
co-culture assays, 238
co-injection, 237
components, 236
effective antitumor immune response, 238
fibroblasts, 236, 239
in vivo experiments, 238
metastatic, 237
myeloid-derived suppressor cells, 238
oncogenic Kras and mutant p53, 238
pancreatic tumor biology and signaling, 237
sex mismatch study, 237
tumor angiogenesis, 238
VDR, 238
Pancreatic tumor cell vaccine, 297
Pancreatoblastoma, 72
PancVax, 298
PanIN lesions, 152
Paraneoplastic syndrome, 103
Partner and localizer of BRCA2 (PALB2), 261
Pembrolizumab, 275, 297
Peptide vaccines, 282
Percutaneous transhepatic biliary drainage (PTBD), 352
Pernicious anaemia, 8
Peutz-Jeghers (PJ) syndrome, 5, 100
phosphatidylinositol-3-kinase (PI3K)/AKT pathway, 286
Plasmodium falciparum circumsporozoite antigen (PfCSF), 285
Plastic biliary stents, 160
Preoperative Prognostic Score (PPS), 121
ProCore needle, 157
Program death (PD-1) and its ligand (PD-L1), 272
Prophylactic hepatic irradiation (PHI), 356
Proton therapy
in locally advanced pancreatic cancer, 335, 336
in resectable pancreatic cancer, 334–335
Pseudocyst, 73, 89

Q
Quality-adjusted life-months (QALMs), 362

R
RAB6KIFL. *See* Kinesin family member 20A (KIF20A)
Radiation therapy, 325–331, 333–336, 340–343
carbon ion therapy, 336–337
dose-escalated hypofractionation, 332, 333
heavy particle therapy, 334
Bragg peak, 333
in locally advanced pancreatic cancer, 335, 336
in resectable pancreatic cancer, 334–335
HIGRT, 330, 331
image-guided therapy, 337
immunotherapy, 339
IMRT, 330
intraluminal brachytherapy, 337

irreversible electroporation, 337
motion management, 337
prognostic factor, 344
quality assurance, 338
radiofrequency ablation, 337
SBRT
BRPC, 325
with chemotherapy and surgery, 331
clinical trials, 340–343
conventional chemoradiation, 325
dose constraints, 330
estimated biological equivalent dose, 331
fractionation, 325, 329
in LAPC, 325–328
minimal high-grade toxicities, 329
neoadjuvant therapy, 329
optimal dose, 329
resectable disease, 325
targeted therapy, 339
treatment planning, 338
vaccine, 339
Radiofrequency ablation (RFA), 337
Ramucirumab, 223
Rapid on-site cytology evaluation, 155
Reactive ductal epithelia atypia, 83
Recombinant viral DNA vaccines, 282
Regulatory T cells (Tregs), 239
Reovirus, 312
Resectable pancreatic cancer
anastomotic techniques, 177
cost-effectiveness analysis, 362, 363
cross-sectional imaging, 172
decision analytic model, 362
endoscopic retrograde cholangiopancreatography, 174
fine needle aspiration, 174
imaging, 362
infusional 5-fluorouracil, 363
laparoscopy, 176
lymph node involvement, 177
neoadjuvant chemoradiation, 362
neoadjuvant therapy, 171
open vs. laparoscopic pancreatectomy, 362
operative drains, 178
painless jaundice, 171
pancreaticojejunostomy, 177
positron emission tomography scanning, 174
postoperative pancreatic fistula, 177
preoperative biliary drainage, 172
pylorus-preserving pancreaticoduodenectomy, 176
QALMs, 362
serum CA 19-9, 174
somatostatin analog, 362
staging, 175
standard pancreaticoduodenectomy, 176
statistical models, 363
stent complications, 172
superior mesenteric artery, 173
superior mesenteric vein, 173
surgical technique, 176
up-front surgical resection, 361
vascular resections, 178
Whipple procedure, 176
Respiratory enteric orphan virus. *See* Reovirus
Response Evaluation Criteria in Solid Tumors (RECIST), 197, 336
Rexin-G, 316

S
Saxagliptin Assessment of Vascular Outcomes Recorded (SAVOR study), 15
SBRT. *See* Stereotactic body radiation therapy (SBRT)
Secreted protein acidic and rich in cysteine (SPARC), 126
Self-expanding metal stents (SEMS), 188, 350
Serous cystadenoma, 74, 75, 89, 144, 145
Serous microcystic adenoma, 74
SET domain-containing 2 (SETD2) deficiency, 257
Signet ring cell carcinoma, 62
Slow pull/capillary technique, 157
Society for Surgery of the Alimentary Tract (SSAT), 185
Society of Surgical Oncology (SSO), 185
Solid pseudopapillary neoplasms (SPN), 146
Solid pseudopapillary tumor, 71, 86
Solid tumors, cystic degeneration, 77
STAT3, 227–228
Stereotactic body radiation therapy (SBRT), 158, 297
BRPC, 325
clinical trials, 340–343
with chemotherapy and surgery, 331
conventional chemoradiation, 325
dose constraints, 330
estimated biological equivalent dose, 331
fractionation, 325, 329
LAPC, 325–328
minimal high-grade toxicities, 329
neoadjuvant therapy, 329
optimal dose, 329
resectable, 325
Supportive care, 365

Synthetic lethality
  ATM, 258
  ATR, 258
  BRCA1/2 mutations and alterations, 257–262
  BRCA-mutant xenografts, 262
  clinical application, 258–259
  definition, 257
  double-strand breakage repair, 258
  EZH2, 257
  FOLFIRINOX, 262
  PAR-1, 258
  PARP inhibition, 258, 263–267
  SETD2, 257

T
T cell response, 287
Tanomastat, 221
Telomerase, 290, 291
Telomerase DNA immunotherapy, 298
Tipifarnib, 221
Tissue diagnosis
  EUS-FNA, 154
  EUS-FNB, 156
Tuberous sclerosis, 147
Tumor angiogenesis, 238
Tumor microenvironment (TME), 236–242
  blood vessels, 242–243
  chemotherapy agents, 246–249
  extracellular matrix, 243–248
  Hedgehog signaling, 242–245
  immune cells
    activated cytotoxic (effector) CD8+ T cells/NK cells, 240
    CD40 agonists, 241, 242
    CSF-1/CSF-1R signaling, 242
    experimental agent, 241
    inflammatory monocytes, 240
    leukocyte infiltrate, 239
    MDSCs, 239
    reprogramming, 241
    TAMs, 240
    therapeutic implications, 241
    Tregs, 239
  pancreatic stellate cells
    activated stromal index, 237
    agonistic, 237
    anti-CTLA-4 antibody, 239
    ATRA, 238
    CAF, 239
    CD31+ (endothelial) cells, 238
    co-culture assays, 238
    co-injection, 237
    components, 236
    effective antitumor immune response, 238
    fibroblast compartment, 236, 239
    in vivo experiments, 238
    metastatic, 237
    myeloid-derived suppressor cells, 238
    oncogenic Kras and mutant p53, 238
    pancreatic tumor biology and signaling, 237
    sex mismatch study, 237
    tumor angiogenesis, 238
    VDR, 238
Tumor-associated antigens (TAAs), 282
Tumor-associated macrophages (TAMs), 239
Tumor-vessel interface (TVI), 185

U
Uncovered SEMS (USEMS), 350
Undifferentiated carcinoma, 62, 83

V
Vaccine, 283–299
  DC vaccines, 282
  memory B and T cell populations, 282
  multiple oncology settings, 283
  ongoing vaccine clinical trials
    antigen-loaded DC vaccine with chemotherapy, 298
    CRS-207 with/without nivolumab, 296
    CY, 297
    FOLFIRINOX chemotherapy, 297
    GVAX pancreas (with cyclophosphamide), 296, 297
    Inovio TRT-001, 298
    ipilimumab with allogenic GM-CSF transfected pancreatic tumor vaccine, 297–298
    low-dose cyclophosphamide, 297
    PD-L1 inhibitor (durvalumab), 299
    pembrolizumab, 297
    SBRT, 297
  peptide vaccines, 282
  recombinant viral DNA vaccines, 282
  targets
    β-hCG, 289
    CEA, 283, 284
    gastrin, 289, 290
    HSP, 293

KIF20A, 293
MUC-1, 285
RAS, 286–288
survivin, 289
telomerase, 290, 291
TP53, 288–289
VEGFR2, 292, 293
WT1, 291, 292
whole tumor cell vaccines, 282
algenpantucel-L, 294
GM-CSF (GVAX), 294–296
Vaccinia virus, 314
Vascular endothelial growth factor 2 (VEGFR2), 292, 293
Vascular endothelial growth factors (VEGFs), 223
Vesicular stomatitis virus (VSV), 313–314
Viral therapy. *See* Oncolytic virotherapy (OV)
Vitamin D receptor (VDR), 238
von Hippel-Lindau syndrome (vHL), 147
VXM01, 292

W
Whole tumor cell vaccines, 282
algenpantucel-L, 294
GM-CSF (GVAX), 294–296
Wilms tumor gene (*WT1*), 291

Printed by Printforce, the Netherlands